**BY THE EDITORS OF**

# CONSUMER GUIDE®

with Ira J. Chasnoff, M.D., Jeffrey W. Ellis, M.D.,
and Zachary S. Fainman, M.D.

## FUNK & WAGNALLS

# FAMILY
# MEDICAL
# GUIDE

The material in this book has been
previously published under the title
"FAMILY MEDICAL GUIDE"

## Funk & Wagnalls Corporation

Publishers since 1876

**1996 Printing**

Copyright © 1994 Publications International, Ltd.

All rights reserved. This book may not be reproduced or quoted in whole or in part by mimeograph or any other printed or electronic means, or for presentation on radio, television, videotape, or film without written permission from:

Louis Weber, C.E.O.
Publications International, Ltd.
7373 N. Cicero Avenue
Lincolnwood, Illinois 60646

Permission is never granted for commercial purposes.

Manufactured in U.S.A.

10  9  8  7  6  5  4  3  2  1

ISBN: 0-8343-0100-8

Medical Consultants:
  Ira J. Chasnoff, M.D., Pediatrics
  Jeffrey W. Ellis, M.D., Obstetrics and Gynecology
  Zachary S. Fainman, M.D., Internal Medicine
  Earl Schwartz, M.D., Emergency Medicine
Consultant for Prescription Drugs:
  Nicola Giacona, Pharm.D.

Illustrations: Teri J. McDermott, M.A., Medical Illustrator

**Notice:**
In this book, the authors and editors have done their best to outline the indicated general treatment for various conditions, injuries, diseases, ailments, and their symptoms. Also, recommendations are made regarding certain drugs, medications, and preparations; and descriptions of certain medical tests and procedures are offered.

Different people react to the same treatment, medication, preparation, test, or procedure in different ways. This book does not attempt to answer all questions about all situations that you may encounter. Always consult your doctor if you suspect you may be allergic to a specific drug.

Neither the Editors of CONSUMER GUIDE® and Publications International, Ltd., nor the authors or publisher take responsibility for any possible consequences from any treatment, procedure, test, action, or application of medication or preparation by any person reading or following the information in this book. The publication of this book does not constitute the practice of medicine, and this book does not attempt to replace your physician. The authors and publisher advise the reader to check with a physician before administering any medication or undertaking any course of treatment.

# CONTENTS

# INTRODUCTION

The *Family Medical Guide* is designed to help the one person who is responsible for your health—and perhaps for the health of your entire family—you. You are the only one who can observe your health and regulate your personal health habits on a daily basis. You are the only one who decides what you eat, how you exercise, when you sleep, and where you go when a medical problem occurs. You are the one who wants to protect your good health and prevent illness. You are the one who wishes to avoid unnecessary trips to the doctor while at the same time becoming informed about when you should see a physician and what the field of medicine can do. How can you intelligently fulfill these goals?

This *Family Medical Guide* provides the answers. Its wide coverage of health and medical topics shows you how to design and plan health care for yourself and for your family. As medical costs continue to rise and medical testing becomes both more sophisticated and more expensive, average people in need of medical care often find it impossible to keep up with what needs to be known in order to assure good health for themselves and their families. This book provides a guide to medical care and health practices that will help you make the right decisions about what you and your family need.

The *Family Medical Guide* is not a substitute for your doctor. Rather, it gives you the information you need to make the best use of modern medical care—whether you are trying to select the right doctor for your family, decide on which specialist you need to see, or simply make sure that you and your family stay healthy.

You will find advice on how to find a doctor and how to make certain that he or she is the best doctor for you. You will also find an explanation of all the specialties in medicine—from anesthesiology (the study of painkilling substances used in surgery) to urology (the study of disorders of the urinary tract).

You will learn the difference between clinical and laboratory tests and be able to familiarize yourself with commonly administered tests. If you have to have tests done, you will know what to expect, how to prepare yourself for as little discomfort as possible, and what the results may indicate.

If your doctor prescribes a medication, you will learn how to read the prescription and interpret the directions. You can read about buying drugs—and saving money on your prescriptions—as well as about storing and administering your medications. You will learn how your medication works and how to anticipate and, if necessary, cope with any possible side effects of your medicine. Most important, you'll find out how to work with your doctor in developing the best medication program for you.

The heart of the *Family Medical Guide* is a comprehensive medical encyclopedia arranged in alphabetical order for easy and fast reference. This A-to-Z section covers diseases, disorders, conditions, syndromes, symptoms, diagnostic procedures, treatments, and medical terms. Each entry is presented in clear, easy-to-understand language with practical advice about when to treat a problem at home, when to consult a doctor, and when to administer emergency first aid or seek immediate emergency care. Since this section is a reference manual, each entry is designed to be self-contained; for example, terms that may not be part of everyday vocabulary are defined where they occur, even if they have been defined elsewhere. On the other hand, if another entry or section of the book naturally expands or complements a topic, there is a cross reference for you to find the additional information. Furthermore, to make the medical guide as useful as possible, numerous detailed illustrations have been included. These illustrations are designed to clarify the information and expand your knowledge about the topics.

In those entries that discuss a disease or disorder, the description of the problem, the cause (if known), the symptoms, the treatment, the prognosis, and the risk factors are discussed. In addition, preventive action is outlined, if appropriate or possible. In short, each entry attempts to be as inclusive as possible without being too technical or hard to understand.

In addition to diseases and other abnormal problems, the A-to-Z medical guide includes descriptions of body systems (for example, the nervous system) and organs (the heart) as they function normally in a healthy body. These entries give you a reference point for becoming familiar with

the way your body should work; to understand disease as a departure from the normal healthy state of an organ or system, you should understand what is considered normal and healthy.

Finally, the A-to-Z medical guide is followed by an Emergency first aid action guide. These illustrated, step-by-step instructions cover life-threatening emergency situations when minutes or even seconds count. You will be able to see at a glance the emergency procedures for choking, heatstroke, bleeding, shock, and other circumstances that require immediate action. Read this section before an emergency arises.

The aim of the *Family Medical Guide* is to help you take charge of your health care and that of your family. This book will help you develop a personal health plan that fits your lifestyle and meets your health and medical needs. If you need medical care, see your doctor. This book will tell you when and why. Equally important, this guide will help you communicate effectively with your doctor as he or she diagnoses your ailments and prescribes treatment for them. It will help you describe your problem more accurately, thus enabling the doctor to help you with greater understanding.

Maintaining good health is a team effort between you, your doctor, and the other members of your family. Remember, however, that the final responsibility for your health is yours—you are the one in charge of your health on a day-to-day basis. The best way to help yourself and your family is to be informed about your medical needs. You can gain that knowledge by reading the *Family Medical Guide*.

# How to choose a doctor

Most people never think about how to choose a doctor until they need one in a hurry. When a person is injured or suddenly becomes ill, finding a good doctor is a necessity, and there is often no time to spare in the search.

If a person does not have a family doctor, injury or sudden illness often means a quick visit to the emergency room or outpatient section of the nearest hospital, where staff physicians who may know little about the patient's personal medical history must treat them symptomatically and, more often than not, on an urgent basis. This is usually not a good way to establish a lasting physician-patient relationship.

A better way to assure yourself of medical care is to have a personal physician who is familiar with you and your family's medical history and who is available (or has associates who are available) when you need care. In this way, your health needs will be met by someone who knows you and whom you know.

The best time, then, to choose a doctor is when you don't need one. You should never wait until you have no choice about the doctor you see. How do you choose a doctor? Here are some guidelines for making an informed choice.

## Choosing a family doctor

Many families want a doctor who is familiar both with family members as individuals and with the family as a group. Doctors who specialize in family medicine are called family practitioners. Their education and training enable them not only to provide medical care but also to recognize and handle the social, emotional, and psychological factors that affect the health and well-being of patients and their families. Whereas a physician may need to have only one year of internship (postgraduate hospital training, usually divided among several branches of medicine) before being licensed, today's family practitioner completes a one-year internship and a two-year residency in family practice. During that time, they receive more intensive training in general surgery, internal medicine, obstetrics/gynecology, and pediatrics, among other fields.

Family practitioners care for all members of a family, so there is usually no need for a different specialist for each individual. A family practitioner is well equipped to handle most aspects of medical care, such as uncomplicated pregnancies, immunizations, and routine physicals. A family practitioner can generally diagnose and treat all of the common ailments, as well as many of the uncommon ones, and can guide you to the right specialist when you need one.

In addition to providing comprehensive medical care for all family members, today's family practitioner is as interested in *maintaining* your good health as in curing or treating illness. The family practitioner's overall goal is to treat each family member as an individual with physical, emotional, and social needs, as well as medical requirements.

How can you find a family practitioner who is right for your family? You can call the county medical society or your state medical society.

These organizations have uniform requirements for physicians to qualify for membership (for example, completion of appropriate training and board certification). They also can tell you where you can find a specialist. However, these societies do not offer an opinion on the overall quality of a physician. This is something you must judge for yourself. The questions listed below will help you make this assessment.

Another valuable source is the physician referral service of your local hospital. This service will give you the names of family physicians who are on staff and are accepting new patients.

You should also ask people in your neighborhood about their doctors. They may be able to offer suggestions based on personal experience with local physicians. In addition, if you live in a city, you may find that there is a local organization that evaluates the medical profession on behalf of the consumer. Neighborhood consumer groups often will make medical referral information available to you at no charge and will steer you toward physicians who have a record of treating their patients with respect and concern.

In the process of selecting a family physician, you should draw up a list of basic questions to ask the doctor, including:

- Will the doctor treat all family members?
- Does the doctor provide care during pregnancy and perform deliveries?
- Does the doctor have staff privileges at an accredited hospital in a convenient location?
- Does the doctor perform surgery? If so, what kind?
- Does the doctor encourage preventive medicine, such as routine checkups, immunizations, and follow-up tests?

- Does the doctor make emergency house calls for bedridden family members?
- Does the doctor have office hours that are convenient for your family, especially for those who work or attend school?
- What arrangement does the doctor have for a substitute when he or she is unavailable?
- What are the fees for the various services?
- Is the doctor certified by the American Board of Family Practice (or a specialty board of another area)?

The answers to these questions, along with the recommendations of friends and neighbors, will help you select the right doctor for you and your family.

# How to choose a specialist

In approaching the problem of finding a specialist, you should remember that most specialists receive their patients through referrals from family doctors or from other specialists. Many have a policy of not accepting a patient who has not first been examined and referred by a family doctor. This is a method of making sure that those who really need specialists see them and that those who do not need them do not incur the expense of seeing a specialist. Your family doctor will usually decide whether your medical complaint warrants the attention of a specialist. For example, if you have a mild inflammation of the ear canal, your family doctor is quite capable of treating it. If there is chronic inflammation of the ear canal, however, or if you have suffered a partial loss of hearing, your doctor will probably refer you to an otorhinolaryngologist (ear, nose, and throat specialist).

You must also remember that difficulties in one area of the body affect other areas, so a specialist is not always needed to diagnose and treat a problem. For example, visual problems may be limited to abnormalities in the eye itself, but they may also be the result of a wide variety of causes, including diabetes, hardening of the arteries, a stroke, or a tumor in the part of the brain that controls vision. The human body is an organic system. Changes in one part of the system affect other parts, and no part of the system functions in isolation. Consequently, the first task in treating an illness is to discover the underlying primary cause of the ailment. When the culprit is found, you may then be referred to a specialist who deals with the specific area of the body most affected by that problem.

The first line of action in selecting a specialist is to follow your family doctor's advice. He or she will know whether you need a specialist. However, you can always ask for a second opinion or seek out a specialist on your own. You should always try to get as much information as possible about your own or a family member's illness. You may even find something that one of the doctors missed.

If your family doctor refers you to a specialist, or if you seek one on your own, you should know what each specialty consists of and what to expect when you see each specialist. The following section gives you a brief description of more than 30 medical and surgical specialties. As you read about each one, remember that an internship is the period immediately after graduation from medical school, during which a doctor receives supervised practical experience in a hospital setting. A residency, also supervised in a hospital setting, follows an internship; it is a period of advanced training in a doctor's chosen medical specialty. As noted in the following section, the length of residency varies depending on the specialty. Even within a specialty, however, the length of residency may vary from one medical center to another and may change with time. Board certification means that a doctor has been certified as meeting the professional standards of a medical specialty organization called a board, which requires completion of a residency at an accredited institution, acceptable performance on a rigorous set of examinations, and, in some fields, a year or two of clinical experience.

## Allergy and immunology

This branch of medicine is concerned with the study, diagnosis, and treatment of disorders related to immunity (the body's ability to resist disease or threatening substances). The body's immune system fights against the intrusion of outside forces, whether they are irritating substances that cause allergic reactions or microorganisms that cause infection. This is the system that helps us fight off illness every day of our lives. Modern immunological research indicates that many infections can be as much a result of defects in a person's immune system as they are a result of exposure to viruses or bacteria.

Immunologists are also studying the role of the immune system in cancer growth. It may someday be possible to prevent cancer by modifying the immune system to reject cancerous growths in the body. Immunologists are also interested in the opposite effect of the immune system—the rejection of foreign substances that are actually beneficial (the most obvious example is an organ transplant). Immunologists are seeking ways to make the immune system work selectively, so that the body would reject cancer cells but accept a new heart, kidney, or liver.

The best-known branch of immunology deals with allergies, which are responses of the body's immune system to irritating substances in the environment. Doctors who practice as allergists are involved in identifying environmental irritants that cause symptoms and formulating a plan of treatment. Allergists may treat allergies by suggesting environmental modifications to eliminate the offending substance or by using drugs to relieve the symptoms. Another option is a program of desensitization, which involves injecting minute amounts of the offending agent to make the immune system less sensitive to it. Once such a program has been set up, your family doctor can often give the injections. Allergists also consult in the management of certain diseases, such as asthma.

An allergist must complete a residency in internal medicine or pediatrics after graduating from medical school. After this residency, he or she completes a two-year fellowship program in allergy and immunology. Specialty board examinations are also required.

## Anesthesiology

With the use of anesthetics, surgery may be done without pain during the procedure. Many minor procedures may be done with a local anesthetic (a painkiller that is usually injected into or rubbed onto the affected area), but more complex procedures require that the patient be unconscious.

An anesthesiologist is a specialist in the use of those drugs that cause a cessation of the experience of pain. Anesthesiologists must complete medical school, an internship, and a residency in their specialty before starting their practice. They may also receive some training in a field other

than anesthesiology, such as internal medicine, pediatrics, or obstetrics. Some of them also do tours of surgical residency to broaden and deepen their knowledge of surgical techniques and needs.

In the past few years, anesthesiologists have become more concerned with pain management in general. For example, an anesthesiologist may be called in to deal with pain after surgery or to manage chronic pain syndromes on an outpatient basis.

## Bariatrics

Bariatrics is a relatively new field in medicine, brought into popularity by the public's keen interest in the problems of being overweight.

Bariatricians have been making advances in what is known about being overweight or underweight by dispelling myths and substituting hard scientific evidence. Their training usually includes an internship in internal medicine, with a special residency in bariatrics. Bariatricians are certified by their specialty group, the American Society of Bariatric Physicians.

## Cardiology

Cardiology is a branch of internal medicine that deals with the diagnosis and treatment of disorders of the heart and circulatory system, including those that stem from birth abnormalities, childhood diseases, or advancing age. Cardiologists take care of a variety of heart conditions, such as rheumatic heart disease in children and congestive heart failure and heart attacks in adults.

Cardiology and cardiovascular surgery complement each other. Over the years, doctors in these fields have worked together closely in the treatment of heart diseases. For example, the cardiologist may determine that a child has been born with a hole between the chambers of the heart; the cardiovascular surgeon is the one who will repair this hole through open-heart surgery.

In the past few years, many advances in the medical and surgical treatment of heart disease have been made. A cardiologist must be acquainted not only with anatomy and physiology, but also with modern computerized diagnostic equipment. One special diagnostic procedure performed by cardiologists is cardiac catheterization, in which a catheter (a long, thin, flexible tube) is inserted into the heart and adjacent blood vessels, allowing the injection of a special dye that affords visualization of those structures. Angioplasty (the opening of a blocked artery by insertion of a balloon-tipped catheter) is a treatment procedure that is commonly performed by cardiologists. New procedures utilizing lasers and special catheters to diminish blockages within arteries are also performed by cardiologists.

Training in cardiology includes completion of a residency in internal medicine, followed by at least two years of specialized training in cardiology.

# Cardiovascular surgery

The cardiovascular surgeon performs many different types of surgery on the heart and blood vessels, including replacement of heart valves and bypasses of blocked coronary arteries. Open-heart surgery came into its own during the 1950s and underwent further refinement in the 1960s and 1970s. Three decades have passed since the first heart transplant. In 1982, the first implantation of an artificial heart took place.

Training in cardiovascular surgery includes the completion of a general surgery residency (usually five years),

followed by two or three years of specialized training.

# Dentistry

Dentistry is concerned with the prevention, diagnosis, and treatment of diseases, disorders, and malformations of the teeth, mouth, and jaws. Most people select a dentist with a general practice who can provide routine dental care and, if necessary, recommend a dental specialist for those conditions requiring specialized treatment. Some of the dental specialties include:
• Orthodontia (straightening of teeth)
• Periodontia (treatment of gums and underlying bone)
• Endodontia (root canal treatment)
• Exodontia (extraction of teeth)

A dentist planning to establish a general practice will complete four years of dental school and perhaps an optional one-year general residency. Dental specialists have additional specific training in their specialty.

Finding a family dentist is much like finding a family doctor. You should ask friends and neighbors for recommendations or contact your local dental society. Your family doctor may also be able to recommend a dentist.

# Dermatology

Dermatology is the study of diseases and disorders of the skin, ranging from acne to psoriasis to skin cancer.

The dermatologist must also be knowledgeable about diseases that primarily affect other parts of the body but that may have some bearing on the condition of the skin. In addition, dermatologists have training in allergy, since over the years many skin conditions have been recognized as allergic reactions instead of skin diseases.

Dermatologists are required to do an internship, usually in internal medicine, followed by a three-year residency in dermatology.

# Endocrinology

When we think of "messages" being sent throughout the body, we usually think of the nervous system. But there is another communication system in the body, called the endocrine system. It is made up of the ductless glands, including the pituitary gland, the adrenal glands, the thyroid gland, the parathyroid glands, the islet cells in the pancreas, the ovaries (in women), and the testes (in men). These glands secrete hormones that travel as messengers throughout the body to direct and integrate a vast number of bodily functions. Disorders of the endocrine system include diabetes, Cushing's syndrome, and growth abnormalities.

An endocrinologist is a specialist in the diagnosis and treatment of disorders of the endocrine system. He or she must complete an internship and a residency in internal medicine, followed by two years of training in endocrinology.

# Epidemiology

Specialists in this medical field study the outbreak, frequency, distribution, and control of communicable diseases. The unofficial headquarters of this activity is the Centers for Disease Control (once the Communicable Disease Center) in Atlanta, Georgia.

Epidemiology deals not only with communication of disease in general, but also with the specific conditions under which certain diseases seem to flourish. For example, the relatively new field of urban epidemiology specifically addresses itself to those diseases and conditions peculiar to city settings. In addition, epidemiologists work to devise ways of preventing disease, such as developing vaccines.

Epidemiology is also concerned with causes of illness other than infectious diseases. For example, lead poisoning as a result of eating lead-based paint was a major cause of brain damage among children before epidemiologists discovered the connection. Epidemiologists have led the medical field in seeking environmental causes for a host of disorders once attributed to bacteria or other sources. Air and water pollution, toxic substances in foods, toxic substances used in the manufacture of a variety of products—all have come under the scrutiny of the epidemiologist.

Epidemiology attracts physicians not only from internal medicine but also from other fields, such as immunology, occupational medicine, and pediatrics. An epidemiologist will usually have completed three years of specialized training and a year of independent research or teaching.

# Gastroenterology

A gastroenterologist specializes in the diagnosis and treatment of diseases and disorders of the stomach and the intestines, as well as related organs that help in the digestive process, such as the esophagus, liver, and pancreas. Gastritis (inflammation of the stomach), enteritis (inflammation of the intestinal tract), ulcers, inability to digest certain foods, constipation, diarrhea, hyperacidity, and heartburn are among the disorders treated by the gastroenterologist.

Gastroenterologists often use a procedure called endoscopy, in which a flexible tubelike instrument is used to directly view hollow organs, such as the esophagus, stomach, and colon. Diagnosis and treatment of many conditions, such as ulcers and polyps, may be done with this procedure.

Biopsies (in which tissue samples are gathered for testing) are also carried out with endoscopy. Gastroenterologists have recently introduced endoscopic lasers for the treatment of bleeding ulcers, large.tumors, and other conditions.

These specialists are trained as internists or pediatricians with at least an additional two-year fellowship in gastroenterology.

## Hematology

Hematology is the study of diseases and disorders of the blood and the blood-forming tissues, such as the bone marrow and the spleen. A hematologist is proficient in a wide range of diagnostic techniques in which blood and bone marrow samples are used to shed light on disease processes. Blood analyses can aid in developing treatment for a patient. The hematologist's primary concern, however, is the host of diseases and disorders relative to the blood itself, including inability of the red blood cells to carry sufficient oxygen, inability of the white blood cells to fight against invading microorganisms, and inability of the bone marrow to manufacture enough blood cells. The hematologist is also an expert on cancer of the blood (leukemia) and on blood clotting problems, such as hemophilia.

The hematologist must be firmly grounded not only in internal medicine, anatomy, and physiology, but also in biochemistry. Knowledge of computerized diagnostic equipment and sophisticated biochemical analyses is also necessary.

A hematologist completes an internship and a residency in internal medicine plus two years of training in hematology. Hematologists are simultaneously trained as oncologists (cancer specialists).

## Internal medicine

Internal medicine is the branch of medicine that deals with the diagnosis and treatment of diseases of adults, except for those conditions that require management by a surgeon or an obstetrician. Like the family practitioner, the internist is trained to handle a wide range of illnesses; in fact, many people select an internist as their family doctor. The internist is specifically trained to deal with chronic (long-term) illnesses, such as diabetes and high blood pressure, and acute (short-term) diseases, such as infections. In addition, an internist has both the range and the depth to diagnose illnesses that might escape detection by a specialist if they lie outside his or her special field. For this reason, internists are often called diagnosticians.

After graduating from medical school, an internist completes one year of internship, followed by two years of residency in internal medicine. Internal medicine is also the basis for many other specialties, such as cardiology, endocrinology, gastroenterology, hematology, and nephrology. That is why these branches are often referred to as subspecialties, and the doctors who practice them as subspecialists. In order to become a subspecialist, an internist must complete at least two years of additional training, referred to as a fellowship, in his or her chosen subspecialty before becoming eligible for subspecialty board certification.

## Nephrology

Nephrologists treat kidney disorders. Their patients are usually referred to them by internists when kidney problems are diagnosed as requiring special care. In treating kidney disorders, the nephrologist may make use of medications or dialysis (removal of waste and other undesirable substances from the blood by means of a special machine). Referral for surgery (for example, if a transplant is indicated) is also initiated by a nephrologist. Nephrologists also perform kidney biopsies, which are used to diagnose and follow up on a number of kidney diseases.

Nephrologists are thoroughly grounded in internal medicine, with special attention paid to the physiologic processes performed by the kidneys. Because of the complex nature of kidney function, nephrologists must be equally well grounded in biochemistry and the tools of modern biochemical analysis. They must also be familiar with all of the latest computerized diagnostic equipment, as well as the latest in dialysis machines and techniques.

Training includes an internship and a residency in internal medicine, followed by a two-year fellowship in nephrology, after which the specialty board examinations may be taken.

## Neurology

Neurology is the field of medical science that is concerned with the nervous system—the brain, the spinal cord, and the complex network of nerves. Clinical neurology concerns itself specifically with the diagnosis and treatment of diseases of the nervous system, but the neurologist must be familiar with the total functioning of the body because disorders of other systems can affect the nervous system and vice versa.

Training in neurology includes a one-year internal medicine internship, followed by a three-year residency in neurology.

## Obstetrics/gynecology

The fields of obstetrics and gynecology are closely related, and physi-cians generally practice these specialties together. While gynecology encompasses the diagnosis and treatment of disorders of the female reproductive system, obstetrics deals specifically with pregnancy, childbirth, and related conditions.

Many obstetricians are members of a group practice. Most obstetric groups make sure that every doctor in the group either has seen or is familiar with each patient during her pregnancy. Thus, when it comes time for delivery, the mother will generally be taken care of by a doctor whom she knows.

After medical school, an obstetrician/gynecologist completes a four- or five-year residency. During this time, he or she will also receive some training in internal medicine, general surgery, and care of newborn infants.

The obstetrician/gynecologist often acts as the primary care-giver for women. He or she will also cooperate closely with other medical specialists if specific problems occur that do not directly involve the reproductive system itself.

## Occupational medicine

Occupational medicine began with industrial and business clinics, which were usually staffed by a physician and an industrial nurse (one who has specialized in the care of patients within a working environment). Occupational medicine has grown to include the study, diagnosis, and treatment of a vast range of illnesses caused by the industrial environment itself. Asbestos-induced cancer, "black lung" (in which coal dust literally turns the inside of the lungs black, with accompanying damage to the lungs), allergic reactions to industrial fibers, eye damage from welding arcs, and injury to the feet from jobs that require standing are but a few of the hundreds of disorders treated by occupational medicine physicians.

Specialists in occupational medicine generally have a strong background in internal medicine, with special training in the causes of industry-related illnesses. Often these doctors complete a public health program before going on to their specialty residency.

## Oncology

Oncology is the study of tumors, particularly cancer. This field is often associated with hematology (the study of the blood). Strictly speaking, oncology deals only with solid tumors—not with cancers of the blood. Today, however, hematologist-oncologists are certified to deal with both types of cancer.

Oncology requires expertise in a large number of medical and technical disciplines, from surgery to nutrition, from immunology to biochemistry, from diagnosis of symptoms to treatment of tumors with nuclear radiation.

There are subspecialties within the field of oncology. The medical oncologist is primarily responsible for prescribing and implementing chemotherapy, along with diagnosing and treating complications unique to cancer and coordinating the total treatment plan for cancer patients. Surgical oncologists perform cancer surgery. Pediatric oncologists diagnose and treat cancer in children. Gynecologic oncologists deal with cancer that occurs in the female reproductive system. They are also usually surgeons.

After graduating from medical school, a medical oncologist completes an internship and residency in internal medicine, followed by an additional training program in oncology, which includes training in hematology and chemotherapy. Surgical oncologists are usually general surgeons who have completed a fellowship in cancer surgery. Pediatric and gynecologic oncologists are first certified in their respective fields and then go on to oncology fellowships.

## Ophthalmology

An ophthalmologist is a medical doctor who diagnoses and treats diseases and injuries of the eyes. Most ophthalmologists are also eye surgeons. They perform a variety of operations, such as reattaching retinas, removing cataracts, relieving pressure caused by glaucoma, and repairing blood vessel ruptures and other injuries. Ophthalmologists also prescribe corrective lenses.

Ophthalmologists have a background in both internal medicine and surgery. This specialty requires an additional three- or four-year residency in ophthalmology after a one-year general internship before specialty board examinations may be taken.

Optometrists provide eye examinations; diagnose diseases of the eye; prescribe eyeglasses, contact lenses, and other vision aids; and in many states are able to prescribe drugs to treat eye disease.

There are allied health-care workers who are not permitted to treat diseases of the eyes or to prescribe drugs. An optician makes and fits glasses according to the ophthalmologist's or the optometrist's specifications. An ocularist fits artificial eyes.

## Orthopedics

Orthopedics is the branch of surgery that is concerned with the diagnosis and treatment of disorders of the bones and joints. The orthopedist treats broken bones, disorders of the bones and joints that can be corrected surgically, and bone tumors, as well as other problems of the skeletal system. Because of his or her knowledge of the functioning of the musculoskeletal system, the orthopedist often treats sports injuries and may serve as the physician for amateur and professional athletic teams.

The orthopedist is required to complete a one-year internship in general surgery, four years of training in orthopedic surgery, and a year of medical practice before taking specialty board examinations.

# Otorhinolaryngology

This specialty combines the study of the ear, nose, and throat into a single discipline commonly referred to as ENT. The more formal term "otorhinolaryngology" is derived from the Greek roots *ot-* ("ear"), *rhin-* ("nose"), *laryng-* ("voice box"), and *logos* ("study").

The ears and throat are connected by the eustachian tubes, which lead from the middle ear to the throat. The nose leads directly into the part of the throat referred to as the nasopharynx. Inflammations of the nose may spread to the throat, and vice versa. Inflammations of the throat often spread through the eustachian tubes to the ears. Consequently, infection in any of these areas could result in infection in all of them.

Ear, nose, and throat specialists are primarily surgeons. They perform such varied procedures as rhinoplasty (reconstructive nose surgery); removal of tumors from the oral, nasal, and neck areas; reconstructive ear surgery; and sinus surgery. They also function as diagnosticians of diseases of the head and neck, excluding the brain and eyes.

This specialty requires a one-year residency in general surgery and a four-year residency in otorhinolaryn-

gology. Special fellowships such as pediatric otolaryngology (ear, nose, and throat) require extra time.

# Pathology

Pathology is the study of the changes in body tissues brought about by disease and the ways in which these changes provide clues not only to the causes of disease and death, but also to ways in which the spread of disease may be checked.

There are a variety of subspecialties within pathology, including the following:

- Cellular pathology, in which cells are the focus of study
- Clinical pathology, in which laboratory methods are used to aid clinical diagnosis
- Comparative pathology, in which diseases in humans are compared with those in other animals
- General pathology, which is the study of the processes that may occur in various diseases
- Forensic pathology, in which the results of pathologic examinations (such as autopsies and analyses samples) are used as evidence in legal proceedings

Much of the pathologist's work is done with the microscope, preparing and examining biopsy specimens (tissue samples). Pathologists are charged with deciding whether a tissue specimen indicates the presence of a disease. They also perform autopsies to determine the cause or causes of death. The pathologist must be knowledgeable about both the cause and the course of disease processes.

Pathologists ordinarily work in both internal medicine and surgery during their training. A strong laboratory background is a necessity, with extensive training in modern instrumentation. Three- to four-year residencies in pathology are required, depending on the subspecialty.

## Pediatrics

Pediatricians specialize in the diagnosis and treatment of diseases of children from birth through adolescence. They administer the appropriate immunizations to prevent disease and watch for any abnormalities that may appear during the growth of the child. They also advise parents about the child's social and psychological needs.

After completion of medical school, pediatricians must have at least three years of training in general pediatrics. This is followed by an examination by the specialty board.

## Peripheral vascular diseases

While cardiovascular surgeons treat disorders that affect the heart and its blood vessels specifically, surgeons who specialize in peripheral vascular diseases treat conditions that affect the rest of the circulatory system. Among these conditions are the following:

- Atherosclerosis, in which the artery walls become abnormally thickened or hardened (in advanced cases, the arteries may become partially or completely blocked)
- Arterial occlusion and embolism, in which undissolved material in the bloodstream (such as clumps of clotted blood, bacteria, or tissue fragments) blocks the flow of blood in the artery, causing a loss of blood to tissue beyond the blockage and sometimes necrosis (death of tissue)
- Carotid occlusive disease, in which the carotid arteries (the arteries in the neck that supply the brain with blood) become blocked
- Aortic or femoral artery occlusive disease, in which the aorta (the main artery from the heart going through the chest and abdomen) or one of the femoral arteries (the main arteries that carry blood to the legs) becomes blocked
- Venous thrombosis, in which the veins become clogged, usually with blood clots, with the result that pain and swelling occur in the affected extremity
- Pulmonary embolism, in which blood clots travel to the lungs

Allied specialists in this area can be internists with extensive cardiovascular training. They do not perform surgery.

## Physical medicine and rehabilitation

The field of physical medicine and rehabilitation is concerned with the diseases and disorders of the neuromuscular system (the nerves and muscles). Specialists in this field are skilled in using heat, cold, water, electricity, massage, and exercise to help patients regain use and function of parts of the body that have been damaged by stroke, severe arthritis, or spinal or other injury.

After completion of medical school, the physical medicine and rehabilitation specialist is required to complete at least three additional years of training, followed by two years of specialty practice. Specialty board examinations are required.

## Podiatry

Podiatrists treat diseases and injuries of the feet. Only recently have all the states recognized podiatry as a legitimate healing field. Doctors in this area have degrees in podiatric medicine (DPM), but not M.D. degrees; they have not attended medical school. Many podiatrists have joined the ranks of sports medicine practitioners, since many foot injuries result from sports activities.

Many podiatrists are qualified to perform surgery on the feet when it is indicated. They also fit a variety of orthotic devices (inserted into shoes) to correct foot problems. The boom in jogging and running has increased the demand for podiatric services.

## Preventive medicine

Specialists in this relatively new field seek to prevent illnesses from happening. Physicians from every field have made contributions to preventive medicine. Practitioners range from immunologists (who seek to prevent illness with inoculations) to urban epidemiologists (who search out the causes of widespread illnesses, such as childhood lead poisoning, and try to alter the environment so that illnesses can be prevented).

Preventive medicine advocates often recommend regular or periodic physical examinations, prescribe certain regimens, and warn against toxic environments. Critics of the field claim that there are no safeguards against some types of illnesses. Advocates of the field point out that the same was said of infections before antibiotics.

Occupational medicine and public health specialists are important members of this field of medicine. In addition, preventive medicine is concerned with reviewing present health services and anticipating and planning to meet future medical needs.

Preventive medicine specialists complete at least three years of specialized training, one year of research or teaching, and examinations by their specialty board.

## Proctology

The proctologist specializes in diseases and disorders of the anus and rectum. The rectum is the last portion of the large intestine; the anus is the opening to the outside from the rectum. Some of the conditions a proctologist treats include hemorrhoids (enlarged blood vessels around the anus) and rectal cancer.

Proctologists complete a residency in general surgery plus one or two years of training in colon and rectal surgery.

## Psychiatry

A psychiatrist is a medical doctor—with the authority to prescribe medications and make medical decisions—who deals with mental disorders. (Psychologists do not have a medical degree and therefore cannot prescribe drugs.) Many psychiatrists use psychoanalysis as part of their therapeutic or diagnostic method, and all psychiatrists have intensive training in psychology.

There are four chief branches of psychiatry: (1) descriptive psychiatry, which is based on the observation of external factors that may be the cause of mental illness; (2) dynamic psychiatry, which is the study of the processes, origins, and mechanisms of emotional states; (3) forensic psychiatry, which deals with the legal aspects of mental illness; and (4) orthomolecular psychiatry, which is the study of the molecular bases of mental illnesses. Areas such as psychopharmacology (the study of the effects of drugs on a person's emotional and mental state) and psychophysiology (the study of the physiology of mental illness) are offshoots of orthomolecular psychiatry.

Psychiatrists go through the usual medical sequence: medical school, internship, and residency. The psychiatrist may spend five years or more in specialized training in psychiatry and neurology.

## Pulmonary medicine

This field deals with the study, diagnosis, and treatment of diseases and disorders of the lungs and related passageways. Among the diseases included are:

- Lung cancer
- Tuberculosis
- Pneumonia (inflammation of the lungs)
- Bronchitis (inflammation of the passageways from the windpipe into the lungs)
- Tracheitis (inflammation of the windpipe)
- Black lung (in which the lungs become clogged with coal dust)
- Pleurisy (inflammation of the lining of the lungs and the chest cavity)
- Emphysema (in which lung tissue is destroyed, causing air to become trapped within the lungs, often accompanied by severe breathing problems)

These specialists also perform bronchoscopy (examination of the trachea and bronchial passages directly with a flexible, lighted, tubelike instrument) and specialize in managing ventilators (artificial breathing machines).

The pulmonary specialist's training is in internal medicine, followed by two years of specialized training in the diagnosis and treatment of pulmonary diseases and disorders.

## Radiology/radiation oncology/nuclear medicine

A radiologist is a physician who uses X rays to diagnose and treat disorders. Radiologists have training in physics and instrumentation, as well as in biochemistry and the effects of radiation on human tissues.

Diagnostic radiology is primarily concerned with the use of radiation to produce images of the body and the interpretation of the resultant X-ray films. Some procedures involve the injection of special dyes, which are called contrast media. Other procedures performed by radiologists create images through the use of sound waves or magnetic impulses, rather than radiation.

A specialist in diagnostic radiology must complete a four-year residency in that field, which is often preceded by a year of internship in another medical field. Some diagnostic radiologists then subspecialize by completing a fellowship in a branch of radiology, such as neuroradiology (imaging of the nervous system) or uroradiology (imaging of the urinary tract).

Radiation oncology is concerned with the application of radiation in the treatment of cancer. A specialist in radiation oncology must have completed a one-year internship, either rotating among specialties or in internal medicine, followed by a three-year residency in the specialty.

Nuclear medicine is the field in which radioactive substances, called isotopes, are used to diagnose and treat diseases, such as an overactive thyroid gland. A nuclear medicine specialist must have completed a three-year residency in diagnostic radiology, plus a one-year residency in nuclear radiology.

## Rheumatology

Rheumatology is the field of medicine concerned with the study, diagnosis, and medical treatment of diseases and disorders of bones, joints, and muscles. These disorders are often characterized by inflammation or degeneration and include such conditions as arthritis, gout, lupus erythematosus, and other diseases of the connective tissues.

A rheumatologist has completed an internship and residency in internal medicine, followed by two or more years of training.

## Sports medicine

This is one of the newest fields in medicine and has come into its own largely as a result of two factors: the training and rehabilitation needs of both amateur and professional athletes and the tremendous growth in fitness and sports-related activities among members of the public. Doctors from a variety of fields now list themselves as sports medicine practitioners. Many of them have trained as orthopedists, since that specialty field is concerned with the mechanics of muscular and skeletal function. Orthopedists are surgeons and thus are qualified to diagnose and surgically treat many sports injuries. They also apply casts, splints, and many other aids. Since most sprains, fractures, and muscle strains do not require surgery, many nonsurgical physicians also practice sports medicine. Exercise physiology has become an integral part of medical and sports training programs, and what was once a collection of lore on how to get the most out of your body in a game has become a field of medical research and practice.

Sports medicine has made great contributions to the general public welfare by producing hard evidence of the benefits of healthful exercise. As a consequence, information about subjects such as nutrition, kinesiology (the study of body movement), and biomechanics (the study of lever systems and their effect on performance) has become available to the average weekend athlete. Training need no longer be haphazard or hazardous; by using information available from sports medicine practitioners, you can train for strength, power, endurance, or speed, and minimize your chances of becoming injured. Each goal calls for a different kind of training method. Sports medicine and exercise physiology have made a science out of athletic training.

In a sense, with the advent of sports medicine as a medical field, athletics serves the same function for ordinary people that auto racing serves for the development of new ways to make the family car better: The desire for high performance calls for research and ingenuity in converting research findings into practical applications. Sports medicine converts the lessons learned on the playing field and in the laboratory to insights into the medical problems of ordinary people who want to play a little golf, tone up, or trim down.

## Surgery

Surgery is the branch of medicine that uses surgical operations to treat disease, injury, or deformity. Surgeons go into the human body by way of incisions through the skin and muscles to alter, correct, remove, or replace the offending organ or tissue. There are many surgical specialties, among them the following:

- General surgery (including surgery of the abdomen and breasts)
- Thoracic (chest) surgery
- Cardiac (heart) surgery
- Oral (mouth) surgery (usually performed by dentists with a subspecialty in oral surgery)
- Neurosurgery (surgery of the nervous system, particularly the brain and spinal cord)
- Plastic surgery (to correct damage caused by injury or to improve appearance)

• Orthopedic surgery (to correct disorders of the bones, joints, ligaments, and tendons)

Surgeons work closely with internists, pathologists, radiologists, anesthesiologists, and other specialists. In a very real sense, everything that physicians know about diagnosing and treating illnesses is relevant in an operating room.

After the usual four years of medical school, surgeons complete a general surgery internship and a general surgery residency, followed by additional training in their specific field of surgery.

# Urology

Urology deals with diseases and disorders of the kidneys, the urinary tract, the prostate gland, and the male sex organs. The urologist's skills include knowledge of diagnostic procedures and surgical techniques

After completion of medical school, the urologist usually has two years of training in general surgery, followed by a three-year training period in urology and urologic surgery and an 18-month period of clinical practice before specialty board examinations may be taken.

# What you need to know about medical tests

The basis of medical evaluation is a complete medical history and physical examination. Common health problems are primarily detected and diagnosed by this means. Nevertheless, your doctor will also use a variety of diagnostic aids and tests to rule out a disease, to confirm a diagnosis, or to detect a disorder that is not otherwise apparent. Modern technology now enables medical professionals to inspect the structure of a cell, to see the inside of an organ, and to examine a detailed cross-sectional picture of the body. These tests provide essential information to aid your doctor in the diagnosis of illness and the selection of appropriate treatment.

This section is a guide to some of the more common medical tests and how they are performed.

## Common tests

### Blood tests

Although some blood tests can be done on a sample from a finger prick, most tests require a larger sample. The complete blood cell count (the most common of the blood tests) and blood chemistry screening tests are usually based on blood samples drawn by venipuncture (puncture of a vein by a hypodermic needle). The procedure is quick and relatively painless. The doctor who orders the blood tests will most often submit all the test orders together, so that only one venipuncture is needed for several tests.

Although some patients fear that a great volume of blood is being drawn in venipuncture, the usual laboratory tests do not ordinarily require only 10 to 20 milliliters (two to four teaspoons). The total amount of blood circulating in the body of the average person is at least six quarts at any given time and is constantly being replenished. Therefore, fears about unusual blood loss from such testing are groundless. Also, with the use of disposable, single-use needles, the concern about transmission of disease is unfounded.

### Blood chemistry tests

Besides the complete blood cell count, there are other blood tests that together constitute what is known as a blood chemistry panel. These tests, which analyze many components and chemicals in the blood, can be done from a single sample of blood within minutes, using an automated blood chemistry machine.

Blood chemistry studies are performed routinely as screening tests for the detection of certain disorders, such as diabetes and kidney disease. They are also used as diagnostic tests when specific diseases, such as hepatitis, are suspected. Blood chemistry profiles are frequently used to determine the overall function of an organ, especially the liver (the usual profiles contain three or four indicators of liver function). These tests may not pinpoint a specific disease of the liver, but instead provide a general indication of whether the liver is functioning normally and whether specific diagnostic tests need to be performed. Many illnesses affect more than one organ; furthermore, failure in one organ may cause problems in another. It is here that blood chemistry profiles have great utility; using one sample, they give information about the function of several organs (particularly the liver and kidneys).

The following list provides brief explanations as to the purpose of some of the more common blood chemistry tests:

• Blood glucose—to aid in diagnosing diabetes mellitus (glucose is a form of sugar)
• Blood urea nitrogen (BUN)—to assess kidney function
• Creatinine—to assess kidney function
• Electrolytes—to check body fluid and salt balance (salts include sodium, potassium, and chloride)
• Uric acid—to aid in the diagnosis of gout
• Cholesterol or triglycerides—to measure levels of fat, and often lipoproteins, in the blood
• Bilirubin—to assess liver function, to evaluate jaundice, and to help diagnose anemia
• Albumin—to assess general nutritional status and to get a general idea of liver function (albumin is a type of protein produced by the liver)

## Complete blood cell count

A complete blood cell count (CBC) determines the number and types of blood cells in the blood. The CBC includes:

• Hematocrit—to measure how much of the blood is made up of red blood cells alone
• Hemoglobin test—to measure the amount of hemoglobin (the blood substance that carries oxygen to the body tissues) in a given volume of red blood cells
• White blood cell count—to find out how many white blood cells are in the blood
• Differential count—to learn how many of the various types of white blood cells are present in the blood
• Platelet count—to determine the number of platelets (the blood elements that aid in clotting the blood) that are present

## Chest X ray

The most common standard X-ray examination is the chest X ray, usually used to check for signs of lung diseases and abnormalities. Because the heart, parts of the aorta (the large artery that carries blood from the heart to much of the body), the ribs, the upper spine, the shoulders, the upper arm bones, and the collarbones are also seen, diseases other than those that affect the lungs, such as congestive heart failure (enlargement of the heart accompanied by fluid buildup in the lungs and their blood vessels), may be diagnosed and followed up with chest X rays.

The patient undresses from the waist up. The usual chest X ray is taken in two positions: with the patient standing sideways and with either the chest or back resting against the cassette containing the X-ray film. The patient must be correctly positioned and must remain motionless if good X-ray pictures are to be obtained. The test is painless. The actual time of exposure to radiation is quite short; however, if the test is overused, there may be a minimal risk of long-term effects of radiation exposure. Routine X rays should be avoided by pregnant women; if such an examination is necessary, a lead shield can be used to protect the developing baby.

## Electrocardiogram

An electrocardiogram (ECG) is a visual record of the heart's electrical impulses, which control the rate and rhythm of beating and reflect many alterations in the heart muscle. This test, along with the history and physical examination, is used to diagnose a number of heart disorders, including previous and new myocardial infarctions (heart attacks), some congenital (present at birth) abnormalities of the heart, pericarditis (inflammation of the sac surrounding the heart), and abnormal thickness of the muscle (such as is seen in long-term high blood pressure). There is no risk to this test, and it is totally painless.

Electrodes (small metal disks that are sensitive to the heart's impulses) are taped onto the body at various points on the chest, arms, and legs. The electrode cables are connected to the electrocardiograph, a machine that produces a visual record of the impulses. The ECG tracing for a normal heart consists of regularly occurring wave patterns, whereas that for an abnormal heart will show alterations in the rhythm or appearance of the wave patterns.

## Stool blood test

This test is used to detect tiny quantities of occult (hidden) blood in the stool (feces) that are not visible without a microscope. The presence of occult blood may signal bowel disease or bleeding somewhere along the digestive tract.

The test is usually done by the patient at home and mailed to a laboratory. The patient places a small sample of stool on specially coated paper that will reveal any blood when treated with a special developer. The test may have to be done several times, since the bleeding may be intermittent. The patient will be instructed to eat no red meat for at least three days before taking the stool specimen (the blood from meat, including cooked meat, may cause a falsely positive result on the test) and to take no aspirin-containing medications (aspirin may cause bleeding from the stomach).

This test is painless and has no risk. It is a good but not foolproof method of screening for colon cancer.

## Throat culture

This common procedure is used to determine the type of microorganisms causing infection in the throat. A sample of bacteria is obtained by rolling a cotton-tipped applicator around the swollen area. The test is painless but may cause gagging.

The cell samples are placed in a culture medium (a special mixture of chemicals and nutrients designed to support growth of bacteria), so that growth of microorganisms can be detected and measured. Special procedures are used to identify the specific types of bacteria. It usually takes from 24 to 48 hours to get definitive results.

Recently, "instant" throat cultures have become available specifically for the detection of streptococcal infection. The results are known within 15 minutes and are generally reliable.

## Urinalysis

A routine urinalysis is a microscopic examination and chemical analysis of the urine. If red or white blood cells can be seen under the microscope, bleeding or an infection is present somewhere along the urinary tract. Other microscopic elements, such as casts (formations of protein with or without cellular elements, which usually indicate disease in the kidneys) and crystals (of uric acid or calcium, for example) may also be seen. A chemical analysis can determine the presence of sugar, protein, or other substances that may indicate kidney or bladder diseases, as well as disorders unrelated to the urinary tract, such as diabetes mellitus and starvation. There is no risk to this test.

The patient is given a clean container and told to urinate directly into it. When a urine culture is indicated, a "midstream" specimen is usually requested, that is, a specimen obtained after the urinary tract opening has been properly cleansed and the initial spurt of urine has been passed. If you are to collect the specimen at home, you should also be provided with a clean container with a cap. If not, you should use a clean plastic or glass container. A container that has held food, perfume, chemicals, or cosmetics should not be used. Such containers may be difficult to empty and may still contain traces of the original contents, which would invalidate the test results.

# Special diagnostic tests

## Allergy tests

Tests to determine the existence of various allergies are as numerous and complex as the substances (called allergens) that cause the allergic responses. One of the most common allergy tests is the skin test. This procedure can be either a scratch skin test or an intracutaneous skin test. In the scratch test, suspected allergens are applied in small amounts to individual, tiny scratches on the skin, often several at a time and in a prescribed order. In the intracutaneous skin test, small quantities of the suspected allergens are injected into or under the skin. After a short period of time (about half an hour), the doctor notes which substances have caused a reaction. In both of these tests, a swollen, reddish bump at the site of the application is a positive reaction to that allergen. The skin scratches and injections can be uncomfortable while the procedures are being performed. In addition, there is the risk that an extremely sensitive individual may have an allergic reaction.

There is also a blood test to help identify allergens. The test, called a radioallergosorbent test (RAST), measures specific antibodies in the blood. Antibodies are substances formed by the immune system in response to foreign invaders, such as allergens. The test can be used for those people who should not have skin tests—persons with extremely sensitive skin, very young children, and persons suspected of being extremely sensitive to an injected allergen. However, the RAST may not be as sensitive as skin tests and is more expensive.

In the case of food allergies, diagnosis is often difficult. One method of identifying allergens is to have samples of suspected allergy-causing foods eaten in small quantities at times when there is nothing in the digestive system. Symptoms, if any, are noted. Adequate time is required between food samples so that each sample can clear the system before the next food is given. Someone with a history of severe reactions should not be tested in this fashion. Skin testing may be useful.

# Biopsy

A biopsy is the removal of a small sample of tissue for examination under a microscope. This procedure is done to establish a precise diagnosis of abnormalities, including cancer. The tissue may be obtained by cutting, by aspirating (suctioning) with a needle, or by other methods, depending on the part of the body from which the sample is to be removed. For example, endoscopic biopsy is removal of tissue by instruments attached to or passed through an endoscope (a flexible, lighted tube-like device) into a hollow organ, such as the colon.

The procedure varies with the type of biopsy to be performed. Some biopsies require hospitalization, especially if surgery is necessary to obtain a specimen from an internal organ. Other procedures, such as biopsy of small skin growths and needle aspiration of a breast lump, can be done in a doctor's office or an outpatient clinic. Many biopsies are done with some type of anesthesia, and there may be discomfort if a biopsy involves cutting or an invasive technique (one involving the insertion of an instrument or other device into the body). Also, there is some risk, which varies with the procedure being performed. The risks of outpatient biopsies are usually minimal, but complications, such as excessive bleeding, can occur.

# Cardiac stress test

The cardiac stress test, also often called the treadmill test, is done basically to determine the reaction of the cardiovascular system (the heart and blood vessels) to physical exercise. Devices other than a treadmill, such as a bicycle, can also be used, depending on the situation. A stress test is done for many reasons—among them, to determine whether the cause of chest pain is a heart abnormality, to detect the presence of coronary artery disease, and to follow the progress of a patient in cardiac rehabilitation.

At the lab, the patient will put on exercise clothes and running shoes and will be questioned about his or her recent medical history and exercise habits.

For the test, electrodes for continuous electrocardiographic recording are attached so that the tester (usually a cardiologist) can monitor the heart rate and the response of the heart to graded exercise. A blood pressure cuff is also attached to one arm.

The patient then starts walking on the treadmill at a low work load. The work load (determined by the speed and incline of the treadmill) is gradually increased, usually at three-minute intervals, until the patient: (1) attains about 90 percent of the predicted maximum heart rate for his or her age (obtained from standardized tables); (2) experiences symptoms or electrocardiographic changes consistent with heart disease; or (3) cannot continue the test for some reason (for example, leg cramps or shortness of breath).

The time it takes to reach the target heart rate is related to the degree of cardiovascular fitness, but is not necessarily related to the presence or absence of heart disease. That is, an individual who attains his or her peak heart rate at only six minutes is less fit than someone who can exercise for 12 minutes on the treadmill before attaining peak heart rate. However, either individual may have changes or symptoms indicating heart disease.

At the individual's maximum performance level, the closer he or she comes to the predicted maximum heart rate, the more meaningful the test. For example, a negative ECG (indicating that there is no heart disease) would have greater diagnostic significance if it was obtained at a particular patient's age-predicted maximum heart rate of 180 beats per minute than if the patient had had to stop the test at a rate of 130 beats because of a leg cramp, fatigue, or some other noncardiovascular reason.

The addition of thallium, an injected isotope (radioactive molecule), has enabled specialists to create a picture of the heart and increase the accuracy of the conventional treadmill test by actually visualizing areas of decreased circulation. In the case of individuals who for some reason should not undergo a treadmill test, injected agents can actually "stress" the heart and allow either nuclear or echocardiographic visualization of diseased areas.

## Contrast examinations

Contrast media, known popularly as dyes, are materials that, when introduced into the body, alter radiopacity (the capacity to be "seen" on an X-ray examination of one part of the body in comparison with surrounding parts). The contrast materials are opaque, that is, they stop the passage of X rays and are essential to visualize certain internal body organs, such as the stomach and intestines, which normally are not seen on X-ray examinations. When the contrast medium is introduced into the body, the radiologist performing the test often uses fluoroscopy (the projection of X rays through the body onto a special screen) to observe the working of the internal body organs and then takes still X-ray films of the area being examined. Commonly performed contrast examinations include the upper gastrointestinal tract examination (upper GI series), the lower gastrointestinal series (barium enema), the intravenous pyelogram (IVP, or kidney study), the gallbladder series,

and the coronary angiogram (visualization of the heart and its blood vessels).

Barium is an inert (not active) substance that is either swallowed or introduced via enema. It coats the gastrointestinal tract and allows visualization of its anatomy. Ulcers, tumors, and other abnormalities are found in this manner. True allergic reactions to barium probably do not exist.

The contrast medium (dye) used for IVP, angiography, computed tomography scanning, and some other X-ray studies is usually injected directly into a vein. This substance is not inert and can cause severe reactions, such as hives, swelling, and rash. Less severe reactions include hot flashes, nausea, vomiting, and diarrhea. Kidney failure can also occur with this type of contrast if the individual has preexisting kidney disease or certain other illnesses. Prior to receiving these dyes, the patient should provide the physician with a careful medical history.

### Angiography

Angiography (also called arteriography) is visualization of blood vessels (the heart is often included in this term), usually by introduction of a contrast medium (dye) via a tube, called a catheter, that is inserted directly into a blood vessel.

Coronary angiography is required before heart surgery and for diagnosis of some heart diseases. In this procedure, the cardiologist introduces a catheter into the body, usually through a puncture in an artery in the groin or arm, and threads it through the vascular system until it reaches the heart. Through this catheter, an opaque contrast medium is injected, allowing moving pictures of the heart to be obtained. With this procedure, the cardiologist and the cardiovascular surgeon obtain crucial information, such as the location of defects in the walls and valves of the heart, the location and degree of narrowing of the coronary arteries (the arteries that supply blood to the heart muscle itself), and even the different pressures in the chambers (which reflect the overall functioning of the heart).

Nowadays, this procedure is commonly performed and carries a very low risk in the hands of experienced physicians. Balloon angioplasty and laser surgery are performed with the use of angiography. After the procedure, there is sometimes bleeding at the catheter introduction site, as well as mild discomfort there. During contrast injection, many patients complain of a "hot flash" or nausea. As with any X-ray study, there is a minimal risk of radiation exposure. Also, patients with diabetes, kidney disease, or a history of reaction to contrast media may be at risk from the contrast medium. Precautions can be taken to prevent complications if the physician performing the procedure is informed of these problems before the test. Other possible risks should be discussed with the doctor.

## Gallbladder series

A gallbladder series, or oral cholecystogram, is performed to test gallbladder function and to detect gallstones. The oral cholecystogram allows correct diagnosis of gallbladder disease (including both poor function and gallstones) about 96 percent of the time.

For this examination, it is helpful to clear the intestinal tract of fecal matter and gas to allow for adequate viewing of the gallbladder. This is done by giving a spe-cial diet for the 24 hours before the examination and by administering enemas. Avoidance of cream, butter, and other fatty foods is also necessary.

Contrast medium in tablet form is given to the patient after dinner the day before the X-ray study begins. Usually, nothing is then given by mouth until the examination has been completed. If the gallbladder does not show up on the X-ray film (does not concentrate the contrast material), the dose of contrast is repeated the next day, and another film is taken. If the gallbladder still is not visible, this indicates that the gallbladder is diseased (assuming that the gastrointestinal tract and liver are processing the contrast material normally). In some X-ray departments, after the films of the contrast-filled gallbladder have been made, the patient is given a fatty meal to stimulate the gallbladder to empty, and another film is then obtained to evaluate this function. The time required for the actual examination is about one hour, excluding the time for the fatty meal.

There may be side effects, such as nausea, vomiting, and diarrhea. As with any X-ray study, there is a minimal risk from radiation exposure. There is also a risk (although uncommon) of an allergic reaction to the contrast material. Patients with diabetes and kidney disease should inform the radiologist so that precautions can be taken. With the advent of ultrasound and nuclear isotope visualization, this test is becoming uncommon.

## Intravenous pyelogram (IVP)

This test is used to evaluate the size and functioning of the kidneys and the urinary tract, as well as the presence of obstructions. In men, an enlarged prostate gland may also be noted. The test is done by injecting contrast material into a vein in the arm. The contrast material is then eliminated through the kidneys and urinary tract. X-ray films are made at specified time intervals to observe the rate of excretion, the concentration of the contrast medium inside the kidneys, and the outlines of the ureters (tubes from the kidneys to the bladder) and the bladder. Since fecal matter and gas in the intestinal tract obscure the observation of urinary tract structures, the lower bowel needs to be cleared for this examination. As with any X-ray study, there is a minimal risk from the effects of radiation exposure.

Patients with diabetes mellitus, kidney disease, or a history of previous reactions to X-ray contrast materials may be at risk of kidney damage or serious allergic reactions. These patients should inform the radiologist of such risk factors, because precautions can be taken to minimize the chance of complications.

## Lower GI series

The lower GI series, or barium enema, is a contrast examination of the colon (large intestine), which is useful in detecting tumors, polyps (abnormal outgrowths of tissue from the bowel's inner surface), and other problems. For this examination, the colon must be cleared of all fecal matter. This is usually accomplished by taking a liquid diet for 24 to 48 hours, accompanied by laxatives and enemas. Nothing is then allowed by mouth until the examination has been completed. The time for the examination itself is usually about 30 minutes. The patient is given an enema consisting of a barium solution (which makes the colon opaque) introduced into the large intestine through a tube inserted into the anus; the solution must be retained until all the films have been obtained. When looking for polyps or when a detailed view of the lining of the colon is required, air is put into the colon to form a double contrast with the barium. This procedure is referred to as an "air-contrast barium enema" and is rapidly becoming more common than the plain lower GI series.

At the time of the examination, the radiologist observes the colon fluoroscopically as it fills with barium. X-ray films are made before, during, and after emptying of the barium-coated colon. Afterward, the patient is usually given a cleansing enema or a mild laxative to rid the colon of barium.

Although rare, obstruction of the colon by impacted (hardened) barium or perforation of the colon by the enema tube may occur. As with any X-ray study, there is the usual minimal risk from radiation exposure.

## Upper GI series

The upper GI series is a contrast examination of the esophagus, stomach, and duodenum (first part of the small intestine). This X-ray study is used to detect ulcers, cancer, and other abnormalities. The contrast medium used is barium sulfate, which is introduced by having the patient drink it after fasting overnight. The patient's stomach must be empty to accommodate the barium meal and also to avoid having food particles confuse the results. The radiologist observes the filling of the stomach on the fluoroscope as the patient drinks. The time required for the exam is about 30 minutes. In some instances, the doctor will order what is known as a small bowel follow-through, a series of X rays taken to follow the movement of the barium through the small intestine. In this procedure, many films are taken at specified time intervals. This study may take hours. Patients can expect very light-colored stools after the test because of the presence of the barium sulfate. As with any X-ray examination, there may be a risk of effects from radiation exposure, but modern equipment and techniques have minimized this.

## Electroencephalogram

An electroencephalogram, or EEG, is a visual record of electrical impulses discharged by brain cells. The EEG is used to detect abnormalities in the brain. The test is painless and without risk.

Electrodes (small metal disks) are placed at specified points on the surface of the head (in special circumstances, disks may be inserted through the nose into the throat, which may be uncomfortable) and then attached to the electroencephalograph, which is a machine that produces a visual tracing of the brain's electrical waves. If, for instance, the brain has been damaged or the patient has epilepsy, the waves produced by the electrical discharges form characteristic patterns. Tracings are taken when the patient is awake and calm; when he or she has been asked to hyperventilate (breathe rapidly) and has been stimulated with a flashing light, which may evoke changes characteristic of epileptic grand mal seizures; and when the patient is asleep. An EEG usually takes about one hour to complete.

Careful pretest preparation of the patient is essential for accurate results. On the day of the test, no coffee, tea, cola drinks, or other stimulants are permitted. Alcohol, which as a depressant would affect the accuracy of the EEG, must also be avoided. The physician ordering the test must be informed of any medications the patient is taking, as these can have profound effects on the EEG. After shampooing, no hair preparations should be used until after the tracing has been made. If sleep recording is planned, it is helpful if no naps are taken on the day of the test.

## Endoscopy

Endoscopy is a method of directly viewing the inside of hollow organs by inserting an endoscope (a flexible, lighted tubelike instrument) into the organ. Five common endoscopic examinations are described here (in order, from the most frequently performed to the least frequently performed).

### Proctosigmoidoscopy

This is an examination of the rectum and colon for detection of cancers and other ailments of the lower 12 inches of the large intestine. In addition to cancer, the examination can reveal hemorrhoids (swollen veins), infected areas, anal fistulas (abnormal passageways), rectal polyps (abnormal growths), and abnormal narrowing of the intestine, among other problems.

The examination is frequently recommended as part of a complete checkup. It is a must for anyone with rectal bleeding or a change in bowel habits. The examination usually takes place on a tilting-top table with the patient in the knee-chest position (resting on the knees and chest, with the face turned to the side) or lying in a head-down position. After a manual examination (insertion of the physician's gloved finger into the anus), the doctor inserts a lubricated anoscope (an instrument that enlarges the anus and lower rectum to allow close inspection). Then a proctosigmoidoscope (a lighted, hollow instrument, also known as a proctoscope or sigmoidoscope) is inserted through the anal canal into the large intestine. Formerly, such scopes were rigid, but these have largely been replaced by flexible ones. The advantages of the flexible devices are that they cause less discomfort and generally allow more accurate visualization of a greater length of intestine than was allowed by the traditional proctoscope.

Patients are advised to prepare for this examination by eating a light diet for 24 to 48 hours before the test and by emptying the lower intestinal tract with one or two enemas. If a barium X ray of the colon is to follow the proctosigmoidoscopy, more detailed preparation, involving laxatives and a number of enemas, is undertaken.

There are few risks to a routine screening. Perforation of the colon is possible, but quite rare. There may be some discomfort or cramping during the examination, but there should be no actual pain.

## Gastroscopy (Esophago-gastro-duodenoscopy, or EGD)

Gastroscopy is an examination of the interior of the esophagus, stomach, and duodenum (the first part of the small intestine). The test is performed to detect and examine ulcers or tumors and to determine the cause of gastrointestinal bleeding or any other known or suspected abnormalities. The response of an ulcer to treatment can also be followed up endoscopically

rather than by X-ray studies. During this procedure, biopsy specimens (tissue samples) can be collected, and stomach contents can be suctioned out for examination.

Recently, techniques utilizing lasers, chemical injections, and electrocautery (use of a heated needle to destroy tissue) have been developed for use through an endoscope. With these instruments, treatment as well as diagnosis can be accomplished.

The patient can have no solid food for the evening meal the night before the test is done. Water cannot be taken within eight hours before the test. Smoking is prohibited on the day of the test until the examination has been completed, since smoking stimulates secretion of digestive juices by the stomach. Any other stimulation, such as that triggered by alcohol, caffeine, or colas, should also be avoided.

In the procedure, the throat is first anesthetized with a spray or a gargle (or both). The patient is then given a sedative to induce relaxation. A gastroscope (a flexible, lighted, tubelike instrument) is then passed down the throat, through the esophagus, and into the stomach and duodenum.

There is little risk involved. The patient may gag and experience a temporary sore throat afterward. On very rare occasions, the gastroscope may injure or perforate an organ, or the patient may vomit and inhale the contents of the stomach.

## Colonoscopy

This procedure is similar to proctosigmoidoscopy, but the entire colon (large intestine) is examined. The instrument used is a long, flexible, lighted, tubelike device. Usually, colonoscopy is performed to detect or remove polyps (small abnormal growths), to do a biopsy of tumors or suspicious areas, to look for sites of occult (hidden) or obvious bleeding, and to detect inflammatory bowel disease. The patient is asked to stay on a liquid diet for about 48 hours before the procedure. Laxatives and enemas are also given to cleanse the colon thoroughly. During the test, mild sedatives are given so the patient is usually asleep, experiences little or no discomfort, and recalls little of the procedure.

Some discomfort and cramping are common, but actual pain should not occur. The main risks are perforation and bleeding from the site of biopsy or growth removal; both are uncommon.

## Cystoscopy

Cystoscopy is the direct viewing of the interior of the urinary bladder and the urethra (the passageway from the bladder to the outside of the body). A flexible, lighted, tube-like instrument called a cystoscope is passed through the urethra into the bladder. The bladder and urethra are examined for cancer, polyps, and other abnormalities. If indicated, biopsy specimens can be collected for later examination.

Men generally enter the hospital for the procedure, and are usually given a sedative before the test and a spinal or general anesthetic during the procedure. Women frequently need only local anesthesia and often have the procedure done as outpatients. There is little risk involved in diagnostic cystoscopy, although there may be a slight chance of damage to the lining of the urethra, of perforation of the bladder, and of temporary retention of urine after the test.

Part of the prostate gland is viewed during this procedure in men, and an overgrown prostate gland can be "shaved down" through the cystoscope. This is referred to as a transurethral resection of the prostate and is considered a surgical procedure. Some bladder cancers can be burned off via electrocautery (use of a heated needle to destroy tissue) through a cystoscope, and this process completely does away with the need for a surgical procedure.

## Bronchoscopy

Bronchoscopy is the direct examination of the trachea (windpipe), larynx (voice box), and bronchi (the breathing tubes through which air travels from the trachea into the lungs). This examination can pinpoint the cause of an unexplained persistent cough, wheeze, or pneumonia. It is also used to investigate an unexplained abnormality on a chest X ray or to diagnose a lung tumor. Bronchoscopy may also be used to obtain a tissue sample or to remove a small obstruction.

A lighted tube, either flexible or rigid, is inserted from the mouth or nose through the trachea into the bronchi. Some bronchoscopes are small enough in diameter to offer a view of even the smallest structures in the bronchial tree. A sedative and an anesthetic are used; the anesthetic may be in the form of a spray for the mouth and nose or a lubricating jelly to protect and anesthetize the tissues of the nose and throat. The patient fasts for at least eight hours prior to the test.

Patients with a history of heart disease and those over age 50 are frequently monitored with an electrocardiograph. There is a minor risk of damage to the teeth, throat, and bronchial structures, but damage to the respiratory tract is very rare. Bleeding from biopsy sites and areas of growth removal also occurs, but uncommonly. This procedure is almost always done in a hospital setting on an outpatient basis.

## Lumbar puncture

The lumbar puncture (also called a spinal tap) is a procedure used to withdraw a small amount of cerebrospinal fluid from an area (the subarachnoid space) surrounding the spinal cord. The cerebrospinal fluid is then examined microscopically and analyzed chemically to detect conditions that may exist in the central nervous system. These conditions include bleeding, infections, and other abnormalities of the brain and spinal cord. Often the appearance of the fluid, which is normally crystal clear, will suggest a preliminary diagnosis of a problem; if, for example, the fluid is cloudy, it may indicate the presence of an infection.

The patient usually lies on his or her side with the knees drawn up sufficiently to bow the back. After administration of a local anesthetic, the subarachnoid space (where the cerebrospinal fluid circulates) is entered with a special needle inserted through the skin and soft tissues and between two of the lower lumbar vertebrae (bones of the spinal column). The pressure of the cerebrospinal fluid in the central nervous system is measured with a manometer (an instrument for measuring the pressure of liquids and gases). Some fluid is then collected in a series of small, sterile test tubes for subsequent laboratory analysis.

Although patients are sometimes apprehensive about the lumbar puncture procedure, it is usually not painful. Headache after the tap is common, but lying flat for an hour or so after the procedure appears to decrease the incidence and ease the pain of headache.

There is a slight risk of nerve damage from the needle, but this is extremely rare. The site of the puncture is below the end of the spinal cord, so the cord itself cannot be injured in any way. Special precautions are necessary if the pressure in the central nervous system is elevated due to swelling of the brain or the presence of a tumor. Computed tomography or magnetic resonance imaging may be used to evaluate the brain before a spinal tap is performed. Although any procedure that invades the body carries a risk of infection, the incidence of infections following lumbar punctures is quite low.

## Magnetic resonance imaging

Magnetic resonance imaging (MRI), sometimes referred to as nuclear magnetic resonance (NMR), is one of the newest and most versatile imaging techniques currently available. With it, physicians are able to distinguish the fine details of internal body structures.

The main component of an MRI facility is a massive cylindrical magnet, which weighs as much as one hundred tons. The patient is positioned at the center of the magnet, and a radio signal is transmitted through the patient's body while a powerful magnetic field is simultaneously generated around him or her.

The magnetic field generated by such a huge magnet is extremely powerful—powerful enough to temporarily modify the position of the protons (charged particles in the center of each atom) in the patient's body. Under the influence of the magnet, these protons line up parallel to the magnetic field, in much the same way that a compass needle points toward the North Pole. The radio signal causes the protons to move out of alignment. When the radio signals are stopped, the protons once again align with the magnetic field, releasing energy in the process. This energy can be detected as tiny alterations in the magnetic field. The information can then be transmitted to a computer for analysis. The images generated by the computer are very thin cross-sectional "slices" through the body, which can show details unobtainable by any other means.

Physical effects from undergoing an MRI procedure are rare, but may include headache, nausea, and a warm, tingling sensation. No health risks from either the radio waves or the magnetic field have yet been reported. Any metal object present in the body should be reported to the physician prior to this procedure. Individuals who are claustrophobic may experience anxiety during this test due to the close quarters imposed by the machine. Mild sedation is commonly used and is quite effective in easing or preventing anxiety.

Contrast may also be used with MRI, but generally it does not carry the risk of the intravenous contrast agents used for conventional X rays. MRI of the vascular system is a very promising method of noninvasively imaging blood vessels.

# Nuclear medicine (or radioisotope) scanning

Radioactive isotopes, or radioisotopes, are used primarily as a diagnostic tool to detect tumors, blood clots, and malfunctioning of organs in the body.

A radioisotope is a form of a chemical element in which the nucleus of each atom is unstable because it does not contain the usual number of neutrons. (The nucleus is the central portion of an atom, which is the smallest particle of an element.) Because the nucleus is unstable, it disintegrates and gives off electrically charged particles and energy (ionizing radiation).

Certain elements are concentrated in, or are used by, particular organs. For example, iodine, when given by mouth or injected, will travel to and be concentrated by the thyroid gland. Radioactive iodine, when administered to a patient, will also travel to the thyroid gland, where, because of its special properties, it will show up on X-ray films. A machine called a scanner is placed near the patient. It detects the radiation emitted by the radioactive isotope as it travels to the organ being studied. The scanner converts the radiation into flashes of light that form an image on X-ray film or are projected onto a special screen.

Using this technique, a physician can determine the position, shape, and size of an organ or the presence of a tumor. By looking at the rate at which the radioisotope is absorbed and eliminated, the doctor can also evaluate how the organ is functioning.

Radioisotopes are used mainly to study organs such as the thyroid gland, brain, liver, gallbladder, spleen, and kidneys, which do not show up well on ordinary X-ray images. The most recent advance in radioisotope diagnosis has allowed doctors to observe the heart muscle. Although the procedure is still quite costly, it appears promising for victims of heart attack and other abnormalities. This type of imaging, when coupled with a cardiac stress test, is excellent for detecting and localizing areas of heart muscle that are not getting enough oxygen. Some of the other conditions that can be detected by using radioisotopes are tumors, blood clots, injuries, bone marrow disease, red blood cell irregularities, cirrhosis of the liver (a condition in which the tissues of the liver are scarred and otherwise damaged), hepatitis (inflammation of the liver), nonabsorption of vitamin $B_{12}$, and certain anemias.

There is no danger of radiation poisoning with this study. Because very small amounts of radiation can be detected and measured, only a minute amount of a radioisotope is required.

## Photon absorptiometry

Due to increasing awareness of the risks associated with osteoporosis (a disease in which the bones become thinner and more easily breakable), a reliable means of determining the presence and degree of this disorder has been sought. Photon absorptiometry (also known as densitometry), a technique for measuring bone density, is being used increasingly for this purpose. Although this procedure is probably not harmful, its usefulness as a screening procedure is not yet fully known.

## Pulmonary function testing

Pulmonary function testing (PFT) is a procedure for assessing how well the lungs are working. The results of this group of tests may reveal the existence of various diseases of the lungs, including asthma and emphysema. Diseases that cause restriction of lung movement can be diagnosed and differentiated from those that cause airway obstruction. Pulmonary function tests are also used to obtain baseline values when monitoring the course of a disease and the effects of therapy.

Routine PFT is done with a spirometer—long tubes resembling vacuum-cleaner hoses are connected to a device that measures the volume of air breathed in and out over a period of time and then displays that information on a graph. The patient breathes into the spirometer according to instructions given during the test. The amount of air inhaled and exhaled and the rate of inhalation and exhalation are measured; sometimes, specific exhaled gases are also measured. Some pulmonary function tests also require a blood sample from an artery to determine if the arterial blood (freshly oxygenated in the lungs) has adequate oxygen and a normal concentration of carbon dioxide.

The test is painless and without risk, with the possible exceptions of discomfort during, and complications after, an arterial puncture for the blood sample.

## Tomography

Tomography is a type of X-ray examination in which the shadows in front of and behind the part of the body being studied are blurred out on the X-ray picture. Successive exposures are made at different depths within the structure of the body part under study and from different angles. The effect is the same as that achieved when a microscope is adjusted back and forth and up and down while looking at a piece of tissue—it is possible to get a picture of a structure at different levels, each one pinpointed and sharply focused.

The combination of the tomographic X-ray technique and expanded computer capabilities led to the development of a highly sophisticated form of diagnostic imaging called computed tomography (also known as computerized axial tomography, CAT scanning, and CT scanning). With this special procedure, X rays are not used to create images directly on film. Instead, the X rays are detected by a scanner as they leave the body, and that information is analyzed by a computer to construct a cross-sectional "map" of the body part under study.

The most widely known use of the CT scan has been in the detection of brain disorders. However, in recent years, use of the technique has been extended to other parts of the body, so that, for example, cross-sectional images of organs in the abdomen, such as the liver and pancreas, can now be produced. These scans are quite sensitive and have greatly aided in the early detection of tumors. One of the breakthroughs that has made this possible is the development of equipment that can complete a scan in five seconds or less. Brain scanning does not require such speed, since the head can easily be immobilized. The abdominal area, however, is in constant movement, because of the action of the stomach, the intestines, and the diaphragm. Consequently, the scan must be made fast enough to provide a clear image, in the same way that a fast shutter speed on an ordinary camera can "stop" the motion of the subject.

The test is painless and there is minimal risk from radiation exposure. Also, intravenous X-ray contrast medium is sometimes used to enhance the picture. Persons with kidney disease or diabetes may be at risk of kidney damage when contrast medium is used, and persons with a sensitivity to such dyes may suffer serious allergic reactions. These individuals should tell their radiologist of such risk factors so that adequate precautions can be taken to minimize the chance of complications. Oral contrast agents, similar to barium, are also routinely used. CT scanning is relatively expensive and therefore not done as a screening procedure.

## Ultrasonography

Ultrasonography (often called ultrasound) is a method of visualizing the structures of the body by recording the reflections of high-frequency sound waves off those structures. The procedure is painless and uses no radiation. Ultrasound, the sound range used in this diagnostic procedure, is a vibration beyond the range of human hearing.

The instrument used in ultrasonography is called a transducer. The transducer, placed over the area to be examined, directs ultrasonic waves at the tissue. The sounds returning from the internal structure are processed by machines that produce a multidimensional, detailed image of the structure. Formerly, only still pictures could be obtained; now, however, moving pictures in "real time" are possible—for example, in pregnancy, the fetus' movements and beating heart can actually be visualized.

Sonography does not involve the use of contrast medium or invasive procedures (for example, injections, catheterization, and incisions). There is no known risk involved in sonography, although the long-term effects of sound waves have not been determined.

# Tests for women

## Amniocentesis

Amniocentesis is performed during pregnancy. A hollow needle is inserted through the abdominal and uterine walls into the amniotic sac surrounding the fetus in order to withdraw some amniotic fluid for testing. The analysis of amniotic fluid is useful in determining the condition of the fetus, since the amniotic fluid contains discarded fetal cells. Examination of these cells for chromosomal and chemical makeup can detect a large number of genetic defects and hereditary disorders. Testing certain chemicals in the fluid itself is done to determine fetal lung maturity and to detect certain fetal abnormalities, such as spina bifida. The fetal cells will also indicate the sex of the baby, which is important if a sex-linked hereditary disorder, such as hemophilia (a blood-clotting disease that occurs almost exclusively in males), is suspected. However, amniocentesis is never performed simply to satisfy curiosity about the sex of a baby.

The test is performed most often in women who are over the age of 35 or who have a family history of certain hereditary disorders. The incidence of chromosome abnormalities of the fetus increases rapidly after a woman reaches the age of 35. As each year passes, the chances of chromosome abnormalities increase.

The procedure is relatively painless, since a local anesthetic is used around the injection site. The test is usually done during the sixteenth to eighteenth week of pregnancy (before this time the test results are inconclusive). The final results are not available for three to four weeks; therefore, the waiting period can be the most difficult part of the test. However, approximately 95 percent of amniocentesis results are normal.

There is some risk to this test, which is why it is not routinely used. There is a risk of miscarriage, as well as a chance of striking the placenta or the fetus. However, this risk is minimized by the use of ultrasonography to reveal the position of both the fetus and the placenta before the needle is inserted. In addition, as with any invasive technique (that is, one that involves an incision, an injection, or the insertion of something into the body), there is a chance of infection. A patient experiencing pain, fever, or discharge from the puncture site or from the vagina should notify her doctor immediately.

# Mammography

Mammography is a simple, generally painless examination of the breasts by means of a special X-ray machine that is designed to be used for soft tissues. This procedure is especially valuable for the detection of early breast cancers before they can be felt manually by the woman or her doctor. Mammography can frequently help to differentiate between malignant (cancerous) and nonmalignant (noncancerous) lumps and can provide information about fibrocystic breast disease.

Many medical experts recommend that a mammogram of the normal breasts be made when a woman is around the age of 35. This baseline study can then be used for comparison with subsequent mammograms to detect changes in the breasts. After the first mammogram, it is recommended that the test be repeated every one to two years, depending on individual risk factors, such as a family history of breast cancer. Most doctors suggest a mammogram every year for women past the age of 50, regardless of risk factors. However, a mammogram should not replace monthly breast self-examinations (see page 135) and regular breast examinations by a doctor; rather, the mammogram should be done in conjunction with these manual examinations.

Other related techniques for breast examination are xerography and thermography. Xerography is a form of mammography that records the image using a photoelectric process rather than standard X-ray film. Thermography is a diagnostic technique that uses no X rays and thus can be repeated as often as desired. Thermography records differences in temperature among various parts of the breast. The basic premise of thermography is that rapidly growing cancer cells give off more heat than normal cells do. Thermography, however, is not as accurate as mammography and should be used only to augment information obtained from a physical examination and a mammogram.

There is some question about the risk of radiation exposure in mammography, especially for those women who receive a yearly mammogram. The radiation dosage has been reduced in modern testing, and many physicians feel that the benefits of early detection outweigh any risks. However, because of these risks, most doctors are conservative about the use of mammography. A woman should discuss the benefits and risks of this procedure with a doctor who knows her medical history. As a general rule, mammography should not be performed on a pregnant woman.

## Pap test

The Pap test is a standard part of the gynecological examination for women. (Pap is an abbreviation of Papanicolaou, the name of the physician who developed the test.) Analysis of the specimen obtained is used to detect early cell changes that might indicate cancer or other abnormalities of the cervix.

The Pap test involves scraping some cells from the surface of the area where the cervix opens into the vagina. The scraping is done with a small plastic or wooden spatula. The scrapings are smeared onto a glass slide for microscopic examination. The test is relatively painless, and there is virtually no risk.

The test results are reported according to the degree of dysplasia (extent of characteristics) of the cells. Thus, the pap smear may be reported as normal, mild dysplasia, severe dysplasia, and cancer. The system of reporting that used Classes I through V is no longer used.

A woman should have her first Pap test at about 18 years of age. It should be repeated every one to two years. Women over age 40 should have an annual test. Any woman with a history of cervical or uterine cancer or of abnormal Pap tests should have the test done every six months.

## Pelvic examination

The pelvic examination is a manual and visual inspection of the female reproductive tract. It is done to detect disorders in the reproductive organs, including the vagina, cervix, uterus, and ovaries. A pelvic examination can also reveal pregnancy.

The patient lies on an examination table and places her heels in metal holders resembling the stirrups on a horse's saddle. The doctor inserts into the vagina a speculum, a special instrument that expands the vagina to permit visual examination of the vagina and cervix. A specimen for a Pap test may then be obtained. After removing the speculum, the doctor inserts two gloved fingers into the vagina while simultaneously pressing lightly on the patient's abdomen; this procedure enables the doctor to detect abnormalities in the uterus and ovaries. Sometimes, the doctor also inserts a finger into the rectum while pressing on the abdomen; this, too, enables the doctor to feel the uterus and ovaries.

A pelvic examination takes only a few minutes, is relatively painless, and entails virtually no risk.

# What you need to know about prescription drugs

Because of the variety of drugs now available, both over the pharmacy counter and by prescription from a physician, a wide range of illnesses and disorders can be controlled, relieved, or even cured. We can control hypertension, eliminate the irritating effects of allergies and hay fever, relieve cold discomfort, cure a variety of stomach and intestinal disorders, control stress and insomnia, and end bacterial and fungal infections—all by taking a medication.

Along with the benefits of modern drug therapy, however, comes responsibility. There is a great deal that the informed patient ought to know about the medicine he or she is taking: how to take it, how often to take it, what its possible side effects are, and how it might react with other medications, foods, or alcohol.

The process of buying and taking a prescription drug starts when your doctor writes out a prescription. The choice of drug is determined by many facts you have already told your doctor, including information about drugs that you have taken at various times in your life, any allergic reactions you might have suffered, any chronic conditions for which you are still taking medication, any special side effects that you have experienced with certain drugs or classes of drugs, and any chronic health problems you have. Based on this information, the doctor makes a decision about the right drug for your particular condition. The doctor's part of the process is now complete; your part is just beginning.

You need to know many facts before you take your first pill or swallow your first spoonful of medicine. You need to know how to administer the medicine. You need to understand the dosage schedule—how often to take the drug, how much each time, whether to schedule medication at night as well as in the daytime. You need to know something about common side effects in order to distinguish between those that are truly "minor side effects" and those that are signs of a serious drug reaction. You need to know whether you should continue the medicine after your symptoms have completely disappeared, or whether you should stop the medication when you no longer show symptoms. You need to know if the drug might interact negatively with other drugs you are taking (even nonprescription drugs, such as cold pills, aspirin, or vitamins), with alcohol, with caffeine, with foods, and, if you are a woman, with the form of birth control that you use. You need to know the possible consequences of overdosage or underdosage. In short, you need to assume responsibility for taking your prescription drugs.

As you read on, you will learn how some common types of drugs work to relieve certain conditions or symptoms. You will learn how to read a prescription correctly and how to buy, store, and use drugs. You will learn how to administer the most common forms of medication either to yourself or to someone else. You will learn how to save money, in many cases, by substituting a less expensive generic drug for a more expensive brand-name medication. Finally, you will learn to identify some common side effects of the most widely used prescription drugs and to recognize symptoms that will help you decide when your drug response is not a cause for concern and when it calls for prompt medical attention.

This chapter is not a substitute for informed advice from your doctor and pharmacist. You should keep these two persons informed at all times of your condition and of any reactions you are experiencing, as well as of other medication you take on a regular basis. You should also ask your doctor or pharmacist for the latest information about your medications; although every effort has been made to ensure that the information here is up-to-date, new developments occur rapidly in drug research. What this chapter can do is help you to work better with your pharmacist and your doctor by becoming a well-informed, aware patient who receives the maximum benefits from your medication and treatment.

# How drugs work

Prescription drugs fall into a number of groups, according to the conditions for which they are prescribed. In the following pages we will provide you with a better understanding of the types of medications that are prescribed for different medical conditions. We will describe the intended actions of drugs and the therapeutic effects you can expect from various types of medications. The generic drug names have been used here. If a brand-name product has been prescribed for you, read the label or ask your pharmacist for its generic name.

## *Cardiovascular drugs*

### Antianginals

Since the heart is a muscle that must work continuously, it requires a constant supply of nutrients and oxygen. The chest pain known as angina pectoris occurs when there is an insufficient supply of blood, and consequently of oxygen, to the heart. There are several types of antianginal drugs. These include vasodilators (which act by causing relaxation of blood vessels, thereby allowing more blood to flow through), such as nitroglycerin and isosorbide dinitrate; calcium-channel blockers (which are also vasodilators), such as diltiazem, nifedipine, and verapamil; and beta blockers (which act by decreasing the work load of the heart), such as atenolol, metoprolol, nadolol, pindolol, propranolol, and timolol. All of these drugs act ultimately by increasing the amount of oxygen that reaches the heart muscle.

### Antiarrhythmics

If the heart does not beat rhythmically or smoothly (a condition called arrhythmia), it does not perform efficiently. This state of affairs can be dangerous and usually (but not in all cases) requires correction. Antiarrhythmic drugs, including disopyramide, procainamide, beta blockers, and quinidine, prevent or alleviate some cardiac arrhythmias by altering nerve impulses within the heart. Phenytoin, most frequently used as an anticonvulsant in the treatment of epilepsy, can also act as an antiarrhythmic agent. The digitalis drugs, commonly used to strengthen heart contractions, are also helpful in treating arrhythmias. It is important to know that all of these drugs can actually also cause arrhythmias and must be carefully regulated by a physician.

## Anticoagulants

Drugs that prevent blood from clotting are called anticoagulants. These drugs are commonly referred to as "blood thinners," but they do not actually thin the blood.

There are two categories of anticoagulants. The first category contains only one drug, heparin. Since heparin must be given by injection, its use is generally restricted to hospitalized patients.

The second category includes oral anticoagulants, principally derivatives of the drug warfarin. Warfarin can be used in the treatment of stroke, heart disease, and abnormal blood clotting. It is also used to prevent the enlargement of an existing clot, which could cause serious problems by embolizing (breaking off and moving to another part of the body). It acts by preventing the liver from manufacturing the proteins responsible for blood clot formation.

Persons taking warfarin must avoid using many other drugs (including aspirin) because their interaction with the anticoagulant could cause profuse bleeding. Patients taking warfarin should check with their pharmacist or physician before using any other medications, including over-the-counter products for coughs or colds. In addition, they must have blood samples checked frequently by their physician to ensure that the drug is maintaining the correct degree of anticoagulation.

Drugs such as aspirin and dipyridamole are also, in a very broad sense, anticoagulants in that they inhibit the action of platelets, which aid in clot formation.

## Antihyperlipidemics

Antihyperlipidemic drugs are used to treat elevated serum levels of cholesterol and triglycerides (fats), which form plaques (deposits) on the walls of arteries. Some antihyperlipidemics, such as cholestyramine and colestipol, bind to bile acids in the gastrointestinal tract, thereby decreasing the body's retention of cholesterol. Clofibrate, probucol, and lovastatin appear to decrease the body's production of cholesterol. Use of such drugs is generally recommended only after dietary therapy and changes in lifestyle have failed to lower blood lipids to desirable levels. Even then, dietary therapy should continue.

## Antihypertensives

Hypertension, or high blood pressure, is a condition in which the pressure of the blood against the walls of the blood vessels is higher than what is considered normal. Hypertension is controllable. If a medication for high blood pressure has been prescribed, it is very important that you continue to take it regularly, even if you don't notice any symptoms of hypertension. If hypertension is controlled, other diseases can be prevented. Drugs that counteract or reduce high blood pressure may effectively prolong a hypertensive patient's life and reduce the risk of heart attack, stroke, and kidney failure.

Several different types of drugs have an antihypertensive effect (that is, they reduce blood pressure). Some drugs block nerve impulses that cause arteries to constrict (narrow); others slow the heart rate and decrease its force of contraction; still others reduce the amount of certain hormones in the blood that cause blood pressure to rise. Diuretics (drugs that reduce the volume of body fluids) are frequently prescribed for the treatment of hypertension as well.

## Beta blockers

Beta-blocking drugs block the response of the heart and blood vessels to specific nerve stimulation, resulting in slower heart rate and reduced blood pressure. They are used in the treatment of angina, hypertension, arrhythmias, and migraine headaches. Propranolol and metoprolol are two examples of beta blockers.

## Calcium-channel blockers

Calcium-channel blockers (diltiazem, nifedipine, verapamil) are primarily used for the prevention and treatment of angina pectoris (chest pain). Verapamil in particular is also useful in correcting certain arrhythmias. They all are useful in lowering blood pressure. This group of drugs is thought to prevent angina and arrhythmias by blocking the effects of calcium on nerve transmission and blood vessel tone. This effect results in vasodilation and the delivery of greater quantities of oxygen to the heart muscle.

Calcium-channel blockers have recently been found to be beneficial in the treatment of migraine headache and Raynaud's phenomenon (spasmodic constriction of small blood vessels, usually on exposure to cold, which causes color and temperature changes and pain in the fingers and toes).

## Cardiac glycosides

Cardiac glycosides include drugs that are derived from digitalis (for example, digoxin and digitoxin). They affect the heart rate, but are not strictly antiarrhythmics. This type of drug can slow the rate of the heart but increases its force of contraction. Cardiac glycosides may be used to regulate the heart rhythm or to increase heart output.

## Diuretics

Diuretic drugs, such as chlorothiazide, chlorthalidone, furosemide, hydrochlorothiazide, methyclothiazide, and spironolactone, promote the loss of water and salt from the body (this is why they are sometimes called "water pills"). Because some antihypertensive drugs cause the body to retain sodium and water, they are often used concurrently with diuretics. Most diuretics act directly on the kidneys, but there are various types of diuretics, each with different actions. Thus, therapy for high blood pressure can be individualized for each patient's specific needs.

Thiazide diuretics are the most commonly prescribed water pills available today. They are generally well tolerated. Since patients do not develop a tolerance to their antihypertensive effect, they can be taken for prolonged periods. However, a major drawback to thiazide diuretics is that they often deplete the body of potassium. This depletion can be compensated for with a potassium supplement. Potassium-rich foods and liquids, such as bananas, apricots, and orange juice, can also be used to help correct a potassium deficiency. However, these alone are often not enough, and potassium supplements must be taken. Salt substitutes are another source of potassium. (Too much potassium may also be dangerous, however. Do not make any change in your diet or use a supplement without first consulting your doctor.)

Loop diuretics, such as furosemide, act more vigorously than thiazide diuretics. (The term "loop" refers to the loop-shaped structures in the kidneys on which these medications act.) Loop diuretics promote more water loss.

To remove excess water from the body but retain its store of potassium, manufacturers developed potassium-sparing diuretics, such as amiloride, spironolactone, and triamterene. Potassium-sparing diuretics have been combined with thiazide diuretics (for example, spironolactone and hydrochlorothiazide combination) to enhance the antihypertensive effect and reduce the loss of potassium; they are very commonly used.

## Vasodilators

Vasodilating drugs cause the blood vessels to widen. Some of the antihypertensive agents, such as hydralazine and prazosin, lower blood pressure by dilating the arteries or veins.

# *Gastrointestinal drugs*

## Anticholinergics

Anticholinergic drugs (for example, dicyclomine) slow the action of the bowel and reduce the amount of stomach acid. Because these drugs relax the intestinal muscles and relieve spasms, they are said to have an antispasmodic action. They are frequently used to relieve abdominal cramps.

## Antidiarrheals

Diarrhea may be caused by many conditions, including influenza and ulcerative colitis, and can sometimes occur as a side effect of drug therapy. Narcotics and anticholinergics are used in the treatment of diarrhea because they slow the action of the bowel. A medication such as a diphenoxylate and atropine combination contains both a narcotic and an anticholinergic. These drugs can sometimes prolong certain infections, however; accordingly, they should never be used without the advice of a physician.

## Antinauseants

Antinauseants reduce the urge to vomit. Perhaps the most effective antinauseant is a phenothiazine derivative such as prochlorperazine. This medication acts on the vomiting center in the brain. It is often administered rectally, and usually alleviates nausea and vomiting within a few minutes to an hour.

Antihistamines are also commonly used to prevent nausea and vomiting, especially when those symptoms are due to motion sickness. This type of medication may also work at the vomiting center in the brain.

## Antiulcer medications

Antiulcer medications are prescribed to treat peptic ulcers. The antisecretory ulcer medications, cimetidine, ranitidine, and omeprazole, work by suppressing the secretion of stomach acid. Another antiulcer drug, sucralfate, probably works by forming a chemical barrier (rather like a bandage) over an exposed ulcer, thereby protecting it from stomach acid. These medications provide sustained relief from ulcer pain and promote healing.

# Respiratory drugs

## Antiallergy medications

Histamine is a body chemical that, when released in the body, typically causes swelling and itching. Antihistamines counteract these symptoms of allergy by blocking the effects of histamine. For mild respiratory allergies, such as hay fever, antihistamines can be used. Diphenhydramine and other antihistamines act relatively slowly. Severe allergic reactions sometimes necessitate the use of epinephrine, which is not an antihistamine but which acts on the circulatory system to prevent shock; in its injectable form, it acts very rapidly.

## Antitussives

Antitussives control coughs by acting on the cough center in the brain. There are numerous over-the-counter (nonprescription) antitussives available. Codeine is a narcotic antitussive that is an ingredient in many prescription cough medications.

## Bronchodilators

Bronchodilators (agents that open the airways in the lungs) are used to stop wheezing and improve breathing. Theophylline and similar drugs are commonly used to relieve the symptoms of asthma as well as pulmonary emphysema. Albuterol and metaproterenol are inhalant bronchodilators, which act directly on the bronchi of the lungs.

## Decongestants

Decongestants constrict the blood vessels in the nose and sinuses to open up air passages. Decongestants can be taken orally or as nose drops or spray. Oral decongestants act slowly, but they do not interfere with the production of mucus or the movement of the cilia (hairlike structures) in the respiratory tract. They can, however, increase blood pressure, so they should be used cautiously by patients with high blood pressure. Topical decongestants (nose drops or spray) provide almost immediate relief. At standard dosages, they do not usually increase blood pressure as much as oral decongestants, but they do slow the movement of the cilia.

People who use these products may develop a tolerance for them. (Tolerance can be described as a need for increasing dosages to achieve the same beneficial effect, accompanied by an increasing risk of side effects.) Therefore, these drugs should not be used for more than a few days at a time. "Rebound," or worsening of the original congestion, can occur with abrupt cessation after long-term use.

## Expectorants

Expectorant drugs are used to change a nonproductive cough to a productive one (one that brings up phlegm). Expectorants are supposed to make mucus less viscous (thinner). (Drinking water or using a vaporizer or humidifier is probably as effective as using most expectorants, however.) Many popular cough preparations include an expectorant, such as ammonium chloride or potassium guaiacolsulfonate, in combination with other types of drugs (for example, an antitussive and an antihistamine).

# Central nervous system drugs

## Analgesics

Pain is not a disease, but a symptom. Drugs used to relieve pain are called analgesics. We do not fully understand how most analgesics work. Generally, analgesics fall into two categories: narcotic and nonnarcotic.

Narcotics are derived from the opium poppy. They act on the brain to cause deep analgesia and often drowsiness. Narcotics, particularly codeine, relieve coughing spasms; codeine is used in many cough syrups. Narcotics relieve pain and also give the patient a feeling of euphoria (well-being). They are also addictive.

Of the many nonnarcotic pain relievers, salicylates (such as aspirin) are the most commonly used in the United States today. While aspirin does not require a prescription, many doctors recommend it to treat such diseases as arthritis. The aspirin substitute acetaminophen may be used in place of aspirin to relieve pain. It does not, however, reduce inflammation (such as that caused by arthritis).

A number of analgesic medications combine codeine or another narcotic with a nonnarcotic analgesic (such as aspirin or acetaminophen). These analgesics are not as potent as pure narcotics, but frequently they are as effective. Because these medications contain narcotics, they have the potential for abuse and must be used with caution.

## Anticonvulsants

Drugs such as phenytoin and phenobarbital can effectively control the occurrence of seizures in grand mal epilepsy. They act by selectively reducing electrical nerve discharges in the brain.

## Anti-inflammatory drugs

Inflammation is the body's response to injury. It is characterized by swelling, pain, warmth, and redness. Aspirin is one of the most effective anti-inflammatory drugs, but other nonsteroidal anti-inflammatory drugs (NSAIDs), such as fenoprofen, ibuprofen, indomethacin, naproxen, and tolmetin may be more effective than aspirin in certain individuals. Steroids are also used to treat inflammatory diseases.

The tensing of sore muscles is commonly associated with inflammation. Skeletal muscle relaxants, such as orphenadrine and chlorzoxazone, may relieve the symptoms of muscle spasm. Skeletal muscle relaxants are often given in combination with an anti-inflammatory drug, such as aspirin, to relieve the inflammation that often comes with muscle spasm.

## Antiparkinsonism agents

Parkinson's disease is a progressive disorder that is due to a chemical imbalance in the brain. Victims of Parkinson's disease have uncontrollable tremors, develop a characteristic stoop, and eventually may become unable to walk. Drugs such as benztropine, trihexyphenidyl, levodopa, and bromocriptine are used to alleviate the symptoms of the disease; they provide control, but not cure.

## Sedatives

Medications used in the treatment of anxiety or insomnia selectively reduce activity in the central nervous system (brain and spinal cord). Drugs that have a sedating effect include barbiturates, chlordiazepoxide, clorazepate, diazepam, meprobamate, and oxazepam. Drugs to induce sleep (known as hypnotics) include flurazepam, temazepam, and triazolam.

## Tranquilizers

Tranquilizers calm the activity of certain areas of the brain but allow the rest to function normally; in other words, they act as a screening device to allow the transmission of some nerve impulses and to restrict others. The two types of tranquilizers are antipsychotics (major) and antidepressants (minor).

Antipsychotics are used to treat the symptoms of severe psychiatric disorders. The drugs most frequently used are the phenothiazines, such as chlorpromazine, thioridazine, and trifluoperazine. Haloperidol, a butyrophenone, has effects that are similar to chlorpromazine.

Antidepressants are used to treat mental depression. The most commonly used antidepressants are the tricyclic antidepressants, such as amitriptyline and amoxapine, and the monoamine oxidase (MAO) inhibitors, such as pargyline and phenelzine. Antidepressants must be used with caution, since they often produce dangerous side effects and can interact with other drugs in harmful ways. The MAO inhibitors must be used with particular care because they can interact with certain cheeses and other foods and beverages to greatly increase blood pressure.

# Topical drugs

Topical drugs are applied directly to the skin to treat skin disorders with minimal systemic (throughout the body) side effects. Antibiotic creams or ointments are used to treat skin infections, and adrenocorticosteroids are used to treat inflammatory skin conditions. Another common dermatologic (skin) problem is acne. Acne can be—and often is—treated with over-the-counter drugs, but sometimes prescription medication is necessary. Antibiotics such as tetracycline, erythromycin, and clindamycin are used orally or applied topically to slow the growth of the bacteria responsible for acne pustules. Keratolytics (agents that soften the skin and cause the outer cells to slough off) are also sometimes prescribed.

Some drugs applied to the skin do have prominent effects within the body. For example, nitroglycerin is absorbed into the bloodstream from ointment or patches placed on the skin. The absorbed nitroglycerin dilates blood vessels and prevents anginal pain. Other medications, such as antihypertensives, motion sickness preparations, and nicotine, are also available in patch form.

# Drugs for the ears

For an ear infection, a physician usually prescribes an antibiotic and steroid combination in drop form. The antibiotic attacks the infecting bacteria, and the steroid reduces the inflammation and pain. A local anesthetic, such as benzocaine or lidocaine, may also be prescribed to relieve pain.

# Drugs for the eyes

Glaucoma is one of the major disorders of the eye, especially in people over 40 years of age. It is caused by increased pressure within part of the eyeball. Although glaucoma is sometimes treated surgically, the pressure in the eye can usually be reduced, and blindness prevented, through the use of eye drops. Two frequently used medications are epinephrine and pilocarpine.

Pilocarpine is a cholinergic drug. Cholinergic drugs act by stimulating the parasympathetic nerve endings. These are nerve endings that assist in the control of the heart, lungs, bowels, and eyes. When used in the eyes, pilocarpine causes constriction of the pupils, increasing the outflow of the fluid called aqueous humor and thereby reducing the pressure.

Epinephrine is an adrenergic agent. Drugs with adrenergic properties have actions similar to those of adrenaline. Adrenaline is a chemical that is secreted in the body when one must flee from danger, resist attack, or combat stress. Adrenaline increases the amount of sugar in the blood, accelerates the heartbeat, and dilates the pupils. The mechanism by which epinephrine lowers eye pressure is not completely understood, but it appears to involve both a decrease in production of aqueous humor and an increase in the outflow of this fluid from the anterior (front) chamber of the eye.

Beta blockers in drop form are also very effective antiglaucoma drugs. Antibiotics are used to treat bacterial eye infections. Steroids can also be used to treat noninfectious eye inflammations, as long as these medications are not used for too long a period of time.

Pharmacists carefully monitor requests for eye drop refills, particularly for drops that contain steroids, and may refuse to refill a prescription until you have revisited your doctor, because such products can cause further eye problems with long-term use.

# Hormones

A hormone is a substance produced and secreted by a gland. Hormones stimulate and regulate body functions. Hormone drugs are given to mimic the effects of naturally produced hormones.

Hormone drugs are prescribed to treat various endocrine conditions, such as Addison's disease, Cushing's syndrome, and diabetes. Most often, they are used to replace hormones that are not being produced by the body in amounts sufficient to regulate specific functions. This category of medication also includes oral contraceptives and certain types of drugs that are used to combat inflammatory reactions.

## Antidiabetic drugs

Insulin, which is secreted by the pancreas, regulates the level of sugar in the blood, as well as metabolism of carbohydrates and fats. Glucagon stimulates the liver to produce glucose (a form of sugar). Both insulin and glucagon must be present in the right amounts to maintain proper blood sugar levels.

Treatment of diabetes (the condition in which the body is unable to produce or utilize insulin) may involve dietary adjustments with or without the use of insulin or oral antidiabetic drugs.

Oral antidiabetic drugs induce the pancreas to secrete more insulin by acting on small groups of cells within the pancreas that make and store insulin. They also increase the number of insulin receptor (activator) sites on other cells, thus making the available insulin more effective. Oral antidiabetic medications are prescribed for diabetic patients who are unable to regulate their blood sugar levels by diet and exercise alone. These drugs are also occasionally used in conjunction with insulin.

## Sex hormones

Although the adrenal glands secrete small amounts of sex hormones, these hormones are produced mainly by the sex glands. Testosterone, or androgen, is the male hormone responsible for secondary sex characteristics, such as beard growth and enlargement of muscles. Testosterone reduces elimination of protein from the body, thereby producing an increase in muscle size. People sometimes take drugs called anabolic steroids (chemicals similar to testosterone) for this effect, but such use of these drugs is dangerous. Anabolic steroids can adversely affect the heart, nervous system, and kidneys.

Estrogens are the female hormones responsible for secondary sex characteristics, such as development of the breasts, maintenance of the lining of the uterus, and enlargement of the hips at puberty. Progesterone, another female hormone, prepares the uterus for pregnancy.

Most oral contraceptives (birth control pills) combine estrogen and progesterone, but some contain only progesterone. The estrogen in birth control pills prevents egg production. Progesterone aids in preventing ovulation, alters the lining of the uterus, and thickens cervical mucus—processes that help to prevent conception and implantation of a fertilized egg. Oral contraceptives have many side effects, so their use should be discussed thoroughly with a doctor.

Conjugated estrogens are used as replacement therapy to treat symptoms of menopause in women who are no longer producing sufficient amounts of estrogen. They are also used to prevent osteoporosis in post-menopausal women. Medroxyprogesterone is used to treat uterine bleeding and menstrual problems. It prevents uterine bleeding by inducing and maintaining a lining in the uterus that resembles the lining produced during pregnancy. In addition, it suppresses the release of the pituitary gland hormone that initiates ovulation.

## Steroids

The pituitary gland secretes adrenocorticotropic hormone (ACTH), which directs the adrenal glands to produce adrenocorticosteroids. Oral steroid preparations (for example, methylprednisolone and prednisone) can be used to treat inflammatory diseases, such as arthritis, or to treat poison ivy, hay fever, or insect bites. Steroids can also be applied to the skin to treat certain inflammatory skin conditions.

## Thyroid drugs

Originally, thyroid preparations were made by drying and pulverizing the thyroid glands of animals and then forming them into tablets. Such preparations are still used in the treatment of patients who have reduced levels of thyroid hormone production. A synthetic thyroid hormone (levothyroxine) is also available and is now more commonly used than the animal-based variety.

# Anti-infectives

## Antibiotics

Antibiotics are used to treat a wide variety of bacterial infections. They are usually derived from molds or are produced synthetically. Antibiotics slow the growth of bacteria or actually cause their death by interfering with their production of necessary nutrients or by damaging their cell membranes. The body's natural defenses then have a much easier time in eliminating the infection.

When used properly, antibiotics are usually effective. To adequately treat an infection, antibiotics must be taken regularly for a specific period of time. If you do not take an antibiotic for the prescribed period, microorganisms are given the opportunity to continue growing, and your infection could recur or become resistant. Aminoglycosides, cephalosporins, erythromycins, penicillins (including ampicillin and amoxicillin), and tetracyclines are some examples of antibiotics.

Antibiotics do not counteract viruses, such as those that cause the common cold. Their use in treating the common cold is, therefore, inappropriate.

## Antivirals

Antiviral drugs are used to combat viral infections. Amantadine is used to prevent or treat infections by influenza A virus. A drug called acyclovir is being used in the management of herpes. Although acyclovir does not cure herpes, it does reduce the reproduction of the herpes virus in initial outbreaks, lessen the number of recurring outbreaks, and speed the healing of herpes blisters. It is also effective in treating herpes zoster, or "shingles." Another antiviral drug, zidovudine (also called azidothymidine, or AZT), is used in the treatment of the acquired immune deficiency syndrome (AIDS) to prevent viral replication.

## Vaccines

A vaccine contains weakened or dead disease-causing microorganisms, which activate the body's immune system to produce a natural defense against a particular disease (such as polio or measles). A vaccine is most commonly used to prevent a specific disease.

## Other anti-infectives

Drugs called anthelmintics are used to treat worm infestations. Fungal infections are treated with antifungal agents (such as nystatin), which destroy and prevent the growth of fungi. A pediculicide is a drug used to treat head, body, and pubic lice infestations.

# Prostaglandins

Prostaglandins are fatty acids, similar in chemical structure to hormones, that occur naturally in the human body. The first of the prostaglandins to be isolated came from the human prostate gland, which is how the substances got their name. More than 16 prostaglandins in six groups have now been identified.

Prostaglandins regulate or trigger various activities in every organ system. For example, prostaglandins stimulate smooth muscle, affect heart rate, influence blood pressure, cause the uterus to contract, and initiate release of growth hormone by the pituitary gland.

Medical researchers have been experimenting with various preparations of synthetic prostaglandins for use in both diagnosis and treatment of disease. Because it was found that one prostaglandin stimulates contractions of the uterus in childbirth, a prostaglandin preparation was developed to help speed up some cases of difficult labor. Another prostaglandin has been used to reduce blood pressure in research subjects, but is not yet available as a prescription drug. Use of prostaglandins is being studied in the treatment of asthma, emphysema, shock, the common cold, and prevention of certain types of stomach ulcers. Researchers have also used a prostaglandin to halt the progress of leukemia and melanoma (two types of cancer) in cells in laboratory experiments.

## Antineoplastics

Antineoplastic drugs are used in the treatment of cancer. Most of the drugs in this category prevent the growth of rapidly dividing cells, such as cancer cells. Antineoplastics are usually extremely toxic and can cause serious side effects, but in most cases the benefits received from chemotherapy with antineoplastic drugs far outweigh the risks involved.

## Vitamins and minerals

Vitamins and minerals are chemical substances vital to the maintenance of normal body function. Some people have vitamin deficiencies, but most people obtain enough vitamins and minerals in their diet. People who have an inadequate or restricted diet, those with certain disorders or debilitating illnesses, and pregnant or breast-feeding women are among those who may benefit from taking supplemental vitamins and minerals. However, even these people should consult a doctor to see if a true vitamin deficiency exists.

# How to read and understand your prescription

Part of the process of becoming an informed patient is understanding as much as possible about the medications you are taking. This process starts in the doctor's office. Make sure

that you understand what medication is prescribed for you, how often and how it should be taken, and for how long. Ask specifically if you should continue the medication once the symptoms subside. Some drugs, such as antibiotics, should be taken for a certain minimum period of time, even if all the symptoms have disappeared. Other drugs should be discontinued when the symptoms subside. Make sure, too, that you understand your dosage schedule, any precautions you need to take into account to prevent or reduce possible side effects, and how (if at all) you should alter your normal eating or drinking habits while you are taking the medication. You should also learn what side effects are to be expected, as well as which ones are within the "normal" range and which ones are signals that you need to consult your doctor again. Be sure that you know and fully understand all of these considerations before you leave your doctor's office.

A more detailed, step-by-step review follows.

Step 1: Read your prescription.

You cannot be sure that your prescription has been filled correctly unless you can read it, so your first step is to read the prescription. There is nothing mysterious or secret about a prescription; the "indecipherable" notations are simply abbreviations of Latin or Greek words and phrases (holdovers from a time when doctors wrote in Latin). The following chart will help you understand the abbreviations—for example, "gtt" is an abbreviation for the Latin word *guttae*, meaning drops; "ut dict" is from the Latin *ut dictum*, meaning as directed; and "bid" stands for the Latin *bis in die*, or twice daily.

# COMMON ABBREVIATIONS AND SYMBOLS USED IN WRITING PRESCRIPTIONS

| Abbreviation | Meaning | Derivation and Notes |
|---|---|---|
| $A_2$ or au | both ears | *auris* (Latin) |
| aa | of each | *ana* (Greek) |
| ac | before meals | *ante cibum* (Latin) |
| AD | right ear | *auris dextra* (Latin) |
| AL | left ear | *auris laeva* (Latin) |
| AM | morning | *ante meridiem* (Latin) |
| AS | left ear | *auris sinistra* (Latin) |
| bid | twice a day | *bis in die* (Latin) |
| c | with | *cum* (Latin) |
| cap | capsule | — |
| cc or cm³ | cubic centimeter | 30 cc equals one ounce |
| disp | dispense | — |
| dtd# | give this number | *dentur tales doses* (Latin) |
| ea | each | — |
| ext | for external use | — |
| gt | drop | *gutta* (Latin) |
| gtt | drops | *guttae* (Latin) |
| h | hour | *hora* (Latin) |
| hs | at bedtime | *hora somni* (Latin) |
| M ft | make | *misce fiat* (Latin) |
| mitt# | give this number | *mitte* (Latin) |
| ml | milliliter | 30 ml equals one ounce |
| O | pint | *octarius* (Latin) |
| $O_2$ | both eyes | *oculus* (Latin) |
| OD | right eye | *oculus dexter* (Latin) |
| OL | left eye | *oculus laevus* (Latin) |
| OS | left eye | *oculus sinister* (Latin) |
| OU | each eye | *oculus uterque* (Latin) |
| pc | after meals | *post cibum* (Latin) |
| PM | evening | *post meridiem* (Latin) |
| po | by mouth | *per os* (Latin) |
| prn | as needed | *pro re nata* (Latin) |
| q | every | *quaqua* (Latin) |
| qd | once a day | *quaque die* (Latin) |
| qid | four times a day | *quater in die* (Latin) |
| qod | every other day | — |
| s | without | *sine* (Latin) |
| sig | label as follows | *signa* (Latin) |
| sl | under the tongue | *sub lingua* (Latin) |
| SOB | shortness of breath | — |
| sol | solution | — |
| ss | half unit | *semis* (Latin) |
| stat | at once; first dose | *statim* (Latin) |
| susp | suspension | — |
| tab | tablet | — |
| tid | three times a day | *ter in die* (Latin) |

| Abbreviation | Meaning | Derivation and Notes |
|---|---|---|
| top | apply topically | — |
| ung or ungt | ointment | *unguentum* (Latin) |
| UT | under the tongue | — |
| ut dictas | directed | *ut dictum* (Latin) |

Once you have familiarized yourself with this simple table, you will be able to check your prescription against the label on the drug container to make sure that the two coincide. The chart lists the most commonly used symbols and abbreviations that doctors use in writing prescriptions. Read it; then check your skills in Step 2.

Step 2: Try reading a sample prescription.

The sample prescription is for Darvon Compound-65 (appearing on the prescription as Darvon cpd-65). The prescription tells the pharmacist to give you 24 capsules (#24). It also directs you to take one capsule (cap i) every four hours (q4h) as needed (prn) for pain. In the space for refill information, the prescription indicates that you may receive up to five refills (5x). The prescription says that the label on the drug container should state the name of the drug

(LABEL-yes). The prescription also says that the pharmacist may substitute a less expensive equivalent product (indicated by signing the SUBSTITUTION line). It also gives your name and address, your age, the date of the prescription, and the name of the physician. Many prescription blanks also give the doctor's office address and telephone number in case the pharmacist needs to call for clarification or verification.

Step 3: Talk with your pharmacist.

Once you have read the prescription, you may feel that you understand the instructions. But you may not understand them clearly enough. Using the sample Darvon prescription as an example, the prescription states that you can take one capsule every four hours as needed. What does "as needed" mean? How many capsules is your maximum for the day? You need to know your daily limit on this prescription.

---

Sarah Jones, MD
Anytown, U.S.A.

DEA# 123456789          PHONE# (123)456-7890

NAME YOUR NAME          AGE 25
ADDRESS ANYTOWN, U.S.A. DATE 2/13/94

Rx  Darvon cpd-65
       #24
    sig: cap i q̄4h p̄rn pain

REFILLS 5x                _____

                         MD
LABEL YES                Sarah Jones, M.D.
                         SUBSTITUTION

As another example, suppose your prescription states that you should "take one tablet four times a day." Does that mean one tablet every six hours around the clock (which means getting up at night to take a tablet) or one tablet in the early morning, one at noon, one in the late afternoon or early evening, and one at bedtime? For other medications, it might mean one tablet every hour for the first four hours after arising in the morning. If you are confused about these instructions, be sure to ask the pharmacist while you are there in the pharmacy. He or she can always call the physician for clarification, if necessary.

Step 4: Check with your pharmacist about how to take this medication.

For some medications, it makes a difference whether you take the drug before a meal, after a meal, or along with it. When you take the drug can make an important difference; often, the effectiveness of the drug depends on exactly following the directions for its use. Your pharmacist can help you understand directions such as "take with fluid," "as directed," and "as needed." With some drugs you may take water, whereas with others you should take milk or fruit juice. Some diuretics, for example, should be taken with orange or other citrus juice or with tomato juice to decrease potassium loss, since these foods contain natural potassium. Also, be sure to ask about the maximum number of doses per day if your prescription simply says "as needed."

Step 5: Ask about any foods, beverages, or other drugs that you should avoid.

This is a very important step, because some drugs may interact in negative—even dangerous—ways with tobacco, alcohol, certain foods, or drugs you habitually take (even common nonprescription drugs like aspirin). Ask your pharmacist specif-

ically about all these items, even if you have already discussed them with your doctor. You may have neglected to mention that you will be traveling and taking an antinausea medication, for example, or that you will be going to a dinner party where alcohol will be served, or that you take a certain medication for a chronic condition. Go over the list of items with your pharmacist just to make sure. Ask specifically about alcohol and about avoiding any foods. There are many drugs that interact dangerously with alcohol. If you are taking oral contraceptives, mention the type you take and ask if you should continue to take it along with the new medication. If the pharmacist says no, check with your doctor about an alternative birth control method that can be used safely with the medication.

Step 6: Ask about activities that you should avoid or restrict.

Some drugs now contain warnings on the label that you should not drive or operate equipment or machinery because the drug causes drowsiness and slowed reactions. Even if your medication does not carry such a warning, ask anyway. Drowsiness is a common side effect and, in a driver, can be lethal. Also ask if you need to restrict travel or exposure to the sun. Some drugs, especially in combination with other drugs, cause photosensitivity (sensitivity to light—that is, to the sun), and you may suffer an uncomfortable rash and other side effects.

Step 7: Make sure that you know how long to continue the medication.

The length of time you need to take a medication varies with your condition and also with the drug itself. In some cases, it is advisable to stop the drug as soon as your symptoms disappear in order to minimize side effects or, in some cases, to avoid building up a tolerance to the drug.

In other cases, you should continue taking the drug for a specified length of time regardless of whether you are free from symptoms. In some special cases, such as kidney infection, the treatment is long-term, and you'll need to take the medication for several weeks or months. Some types of chronic conditions, such as high blood pressure, may even require that you take medication indefinitely.

Step 8: Be certain that you are familiar with possible side effects.

This is probably the most important step of all. Your doctor will probably have already mentioned possible side effects to you, but check again with your pharmacist. What are the most common side effects of this drug? Write down the list if you have trouble remembering. Which can you expect and which are rare? Which side effects are not cause for concern and which ones are serious? For example, the drug phenylbutazone may cause a blood disorder, one of the first symptoms of which is a sore throat; thus, your pharmacist will urge you to check with your doctor if your throat becomes sore in the course of taking this medication. (This topic is discussed in more detail in the section on managing side effects.)

Step 9: Learn how to store your medication.

Finally, before you leave the drugstore or pharmacy, ask the pharmacist how to store the medication. This is important because many drugs can lose potency and therefore become ineffective if they are not stored correctly.

# Storing your drugs

All medications should be kept in their original containers to protect them from heat and moisture, which may cause them to lose potency. To prevent confusion, do not mix different medications in one container. Also, some drugs lose their potency when stored with other medications. Never remove the label from the prescription vial. It contains your prescription number (for refills), the name of the medication, and directions for proper use.

You can safely store most prescription drugs at room temperature and out of direct sunlight. Even those drugs dispensed in colored bottles or containers that reflect light should be kept out of direct sunlight.

Some drugs require storage in the refrigerator; other medications should not be refrigerated. For example, some liquid cough suppressants thicken as they become cold, and will not pour from the bottle. Some people keep nitroglycerin tablets in the refrigerator because they mistakenly believe that the drug will be more stable if kept cold; however, nitroglycerin should not be stored in the refrigerator.

Even if the label on your medication states that it should be kept refrigerated, this does not mean that you

## DEFINITIONS OF STORAGE TEMPERATURES

| | |
|---|---|
| Excessive cold | Under 36°F (2°C) |
| Cold (Refrigerated) | Between 36° and 46°F (2°-8°C) |
| Cool | Between 46° and 59°F (8°-15°C) |
| Room temperature | Usually between 59° and 86°F (15°-30°C) |
| Excessive heat | Above 104°F (40°C) |

can keep the drug in the freezer. If frozen and thawed, coated tablets may crack, and some liquid medications may separate into layers that cannot be remixed.

Many people keep prescription drugs and other medications in the bathroom medicine cabinet, but this is one of the worst places to keep drugs. Small children can easily climb onto the sink and reach drugs stored above it. Also, the temperature and humidity changes in the bathroom may adversely affect the stability of both prescription and nonprescription drugs.

It is required by law that all prescription medications for oral use be dispensed in childproof containers. If you find the container difficult to open and if there are no small children in your home, you can request that your pharmacist dispense your medication in a nonchildproof container.

KEEP ALL DRUGS AWAY FROM CHILDREN, and do not keep unused prescription medications. Flush any leftover medication down the toilet or pour it down the sink, and wash and destroy the empty container. Regularly clean out your medicine cabinet and discard all the drugs you are no longer using, as well as those for which the expiration date has passed (the expiration date is often listed on the prescription label). These drugs can be dangerous to your children. Also, you might be tempted to take them in the future if you experience similar symptoms; if those symptoms are not due to the same disease, you may complicate your condition by taking the wrong medication.

If a child accidentally swallows medication or receives too much of a prescribed medication, IMMEDIATELY CALL A POISON CONTROL CENTER OR THE NEAREST EMERGENCY ROOM for instructions and recommendations. These phone numbers should be written down in a readily accessible place. You should also keep a bottle of ipecac syrup (available without a prescription) for each child under five years of age in your home (in case the poison control center or emergency room recommends that you induce vomiting in the child). Do not administer ipecac syrup unless you have been instructed to do so by medical personnel; vomiting should not be induced for certain ingested substances because it may cause further damage.

# Buying drugs

Prescription drugs can be expensive. Therefore, you might want to ask your pharmacist about substituting a generic drug for a trade-name drug when filling your prescription, particularly if your drug therapy is a long-term affair.

A generic drug is one that is not protected by trademark registration. The generic name of a drug is often a shortened form of its chemical name. Any manufacturer can use this generic name (for example, many manufacturers make the drug called tetracycline).

Usually a manufacturer will use both a trade name (or brand name) and a generic name for a drug. A trade name is registered and reserved for the manufacturer who holds that trademark. Thus, to follow the previous example, only Lederle Laboratories can call their tetracycline Achromycin V, and only Upjohn Company can use the name Panmycin for the same drug. (If you're uncertain about what the trade name is, it is usually capitalized in print and is accompanied by the registered symbol ®.)

It is not necessarily true that trade-name drugs are made by large manufacturers and generic drugs by small ones. Often, a manufacturer will market large quantities of a certain drug under a trade name and then sell the base chemical to several other companies, some of which will sell the drug generically, while others will sell it under their own trade name.

The major difference between trade-name drugs and generic drugs is cost. Generic drugs are often priced lower than trademarked equivalents because they are less widely advertised. You should be aware, however, that not all drugs are available generically. Furthermore, not every generic drug is significantly cheaper than, or equivalent to, the trademarked drug. You should seek your pharmacist's advice on these matters, since some trademarked drugs are superior to their generic equivalents, while others are not significantly different either in quality or in price. Remember, however, that although the Food and Drug Administration reports that there is no evidence of "serious differences" between generic and trade-name drugs, private research has demonstrated differences in quality between certain brands.

If you do find an acceptable, safe, generic equivalent for your drug, your cost saving can be significant. One hundred tablets of Inderal (40 mg) may cost more than $40, while one hundred tablets of the generic equivalent (propranolol) can be bought for about $10—a saving of about $30.

All states have some form of substitution law that allows pharmacists to fill prescriptions with the least expensive equivalent product. Your doctor can authorize the use of a specific brand by signing on the appropriate line, checking a box, or otherwise noting this on the prescription form. However, you should be aware that certain patients can sometimes respond in different ways to various equivalent products, and your doctor

may have a good reason for being specific.

Your pharmacist can also help you save money by recommending the use of over-the-counter (OTC) drugs. These are drugs that can be purchased without a prescription and consequently can be sold anywhere. There are no legal limitations on who can buy them.

In general, OTC drugs are safer to use than prescription drugs since they are not as strong as those that require a doctor's signature. Often, a pharmacist or a doctor can recommend an OTC drug that is less costly and less potent than a prescription medication but just as effective for your condition. For example, aspirin, which is inexpensive and widely available, is a highly effective anti-inflammatory drug that is commonly used in the treatment of arthritis and other inflammatory diseases.

Patients with chronic conditions, such as heart disease, high blood pressure, and diabetes, may want to save money by purchasing medications in quantity. Generally, the price per dose decreases with the amount purchased. For example, a drug that costs 6 cents per tablet when bought in amounts of 25 or 30 tablets may cost only 4 to 5 cents per tablet when bought in bottles of 100 or more. Many doctors will prescribe a one- to six-month supply of a drug that you take regularly.

If you have a history of drug reactions or allergies and are concerned about the side effects of a certain drug, you might ask the pharmacist to fill one half or one quarter of the prescription to see if the drug "agrees" with you. You may have to pay more per dose when you buy a small amount, but you will then have a chance to test the drug on yourself. Make sure that the pharmacist realizes that you took only part of the prescription so that you can get the rest if you need it. For many drugs, however, you must get another prescription once any part of the first has been filled.

# Administering medication correctly

You must use medication correctly to obtain its full benefit. If you administer drugs improperly, you may not receive their full therapeutic effects. Furthermore, improper administration can be dangerous. Some drugs become toxic if they are used incorrectly.

## Liquids

Liquid medications are used in several different ways. Some are intended to be used externally on the skin; some are placed into the eye, ear, nose, or throat; still others may be taken internally. Before taking or using any liquid medication, look at the label to see if there are specific directions.

If a liquid product contains particles that settle to the bottom of the container, it must be shaken before you use the medication. If you don't shake it well each time, you may not get the correct amount of the active ingredient; as the amount of liquid remaining in the bottle becomes smaller, the drug becomes more concentrated, and you will get more of the active ingredient with each dose. The concentration may even reach toxic levels.

When opening the bottle, point it away from you. Some liquid medications build up pressure inside the bottle; the liquid could spurt out and stain your clothing. If the medication is intended for application to the skin, pour a small quantity onto a cotton

pad or a piece of gauze. Do not use a large piece of cotton or gauze, as it will absorb the liquid and much will be wasted. Don't pour the medication into your cupped hand; you may spill some of it. If you're using it on only a small area, you can spread the medication with your finger or a cotton-tipped applicator. Never dip applicators or pieces of cotton or gauze into the bottle of liquid, since this might contaminate the rest of the medication.

Liquid medications that are to be swallowed must be measured accurately. When your doctor prescribes one teaspoonful of medication, he or she is thinking of a five-milliliter medical teaspoon. The teaspoons you have at home can hold anywhere from two to ten milliliters of liquid. If you use one of these to measure your medication, you may get too little or too much drug with each dose. Ask your pharmacist for a medical teaspoon or for one of the other plastic devices for accurately measuring liquid medications. Most of these cost only a few cents, and they are well worth their cost in ensuring accurate dosage. Such plastic measuring devices have another advantage. While many children balk at medication taken from a teaspoon, they often seem to enjoy taking it from a "special" spoon.

## Capsules, tablets, and oral powders

Many people find it hard to swallow a tablet or capsule. If tablets or capsules tend to catch in your throat, rinse your mouth with water, or at least wet your mouth, before taking one. Place the tablet or capsule on the back of your tongue, take a drink, and swallow. If it is too large, or still

## EXAMPLES OF DRUGS THAT MUST BE SWALLOWED WHOLE

| | |
|---|---|
| **aminophylline** | (sustained-release or coated tablets and capsules) |
| **cimetidine** | (tablets) |
| **erythromycin** | (delayed-release tablets and capsules) |
| **isosorbide dinitrate** | (sustained-release tablets and capsules) |
| **oxtriphylline** | (sustained-release tablets) |
| **theophylline** | (sustained-release tablets and capsules) |

"sticks" in your throat, empty the capsule or crush the tablet into a spoon and mix it with applesauce, soup, or even chocolate syrup. BE SURE TO CHECK WITH YOUR PHARMACIST FIRST. Some tablets and capsules must be swallowed whole and others should not be taken with certain foods or beverages—your pharmacist can tell you which ones they are.

On the other hand, some capsules that contain beads are made to be opened so that the contents can be sprinkled onto food. These capsules are called sprinkles. They are useful for children and for persons who have difficulty swallowing whole capsules. Once again, however, you should ask your pharmacist if your medication should be taken in this way.

If you have trouble swallowing a tablet or capsule and do not wish to mix the medication with food, ask your doctor to prescribe a liquid drug preparation or a chewable tablet instead, if one is available.

Occasionally, medications come in oral powder form (for example, cholestyramine and colestipol). Such medications should be carefully mixed with a liquid or with applesauce before being swallowed. These medications should NOT be swallowed dry.

## Sublingual tablets

Some drugs, such as nitroglycerin, are prepared as tablets that must be placed under the tongue. Such medications are more rapidly or more completely absorbed into the bloodstream from the lining of the mouth than they are from the stomach and intestines.

To take a sublingual tablet properly, place the tablet under your tongue, close your mouth, and hold the saliva in your mouth and under your tongue for as long as you can before swallowing (until the tablet has completely dissolved). If you have a bitter taste in your mouth after five minutes, the drug has not been completely absorbed. Wait at least five more minutes before drinking water. Drinking too soon may wash the medication into the stomach before it has been absorbed thoroughly. Do not smoke, eat, or chew gum while the medication is dissolving.

## Buccal tablets

Some drugs, such as nitroglycerin, are prepared as tablets that must be placed under the lip or in the cheek. These products are designed to release a dose of the drug over a period of time.

To take a buccal tablet properly, place the tablet between the upper lip and gum (above the front teeth) or between the cheek and gum. If you eat or drink during the three to five hours that it takes for the tablet to dissolve, place the tablet between the upper lip and gum. Do not go to sleep with a tablet in your mouth because it could cause choking. Do not use chewing tobacco when a tablet is in place.

## Eye drops and eye ointments

Before administering eye drops or ointments, wash your hands thoroughly. Then lie down or sit down, tilt your head back and try to relax the muscles in your neck. Using your thumb and forefinger, gently and carefully pull your lower eyelid down to form a pouch. If you're applying eye drops, lay your second finger alongside your nose and apply gentle pressure to your nose. This closes the duct that drains fluid from the surface of the eye into the nose and throat. If you don't close this duct, the drops may drain away too soon. Hold the dropper close to the eyelid but don't allow the dropper to touch the eyelid. Place the prescribed number of drops into the pouch. Do not place the drops directly on the eyeball; doing so might cause you to blink and lose the medication. Close your eye and keep it shut for a few moments. Do not wash or wipe the dropper before replacing it in the bottle—you might contaminate the rest of the medication. Tightly close the bottle to keep out moisture.

To administer an eye ointment, squeeze a line of ointment one-quarter to one-half inch long into the pouch formed as described for administering eye drops, and close your eye. Roll your eye a few times to spread the ointment.

Be sure the drops or ointments you use are intended for use in the eye (all products manufactured for use in the eye must have been sterilized to prevent eye infections). Also, check the expiration date on the label or container of the medication. Do not use a drug product after the specified date, and never use any eye product that has changed color. If you find that the medication contains particles that weren't there when you bought it, do not use it.

## Ear drops

Ear drops must be administered so that they fill the ear canal. To administer ear drops properly, tilt your head to one side, turning the affected ear upward. Grasp the earlobe and gently pull it upward and back to straighten the ear canal. When administering ear drops to a child, GENTLY pull the child's earlobe downward and back. Fill the dropper and place the prescribed number of drops (usually a dropperful) into the ear, but be careful to avoid touching the sides or edge of the ear canal. The dropper can easily become contaminated by contact with the ear canal.

Keep the ear tilted upward for five to ten seconds while continuing to hold the earlobe. Then gently insert a small wad of clean cotton into the ear to ensure that the drops do not escape. Do not wash or wipe the dropper after use; replace it in the bottle and tightly close the bottle to keep out moisture.

Before administering the medication, you may warm the bottle of ear drops by rolling the bottle back and forth between your hands to bring the solution to body temperature. DO NOT place the bottle in boiling water. The ear drops may become so hot that they will cause pain when placed in the ear. Also, boiling water can loosen or peel off the label and might even destroy the medication.

## Nose drops and sprays

Before using nose drops or sprays, gently blow your nose if you can. To administer nose drops, fill the dropper, tilt your head back, and place the prescribed number of drops into your nose. To prevent contamination of the rest of the medicine when the dropper is returned to the container, do not touch the dropper to the nasal membranes. Keep your head tilted for five to ten seconds, and sniff gently two or three times.

Do not tilt your head back when using a nasal spray. Insert the sprayer into the nose, but try to avoid touching the inner nasal membranes. Sniff and squeeze the sprayer at the same time. Do not release your grip on the sprayer until you have withdrawn it from your nose (to prevent nasal mucus and bacteria from entering the plastic bottle and contaminating its contents). After you have sprayed the prescribed number of times in one or both nostrils, gently sniff two or three times.

Unless your doctor has told you otherwise, you should not use nose drops or sprays for more than two or three days at a time. If they have been prescribed for a longer period, do not administer nose drops or sprays from the same container for more than one week. Bacteria from your nose can easily enter the container and contaminate the solution. If you must take medication for more than a week, purchase a new container. NEVER allow anyone else to use your nose drops or spray.

## Inhalers

Aerosol inhalers are used for asthma and other breathing disorders; they assure that a drug gets deep into the lungs where it is most effective. The medication is contained in a pressurized canister that has a mouthpiece attached to it. The drug is actually inhaled into the lungs.

The inhaler must be used properly for maximum benefit. Shake the canister well just before using it. Hold the inhaler about two inches from your open mouth and tilt your head back slightly. Next, exhale fully, but don't force it. Bring the inhaler to your mouth, close your mouth around the mouthpiece, then breath in deeply and slowly for four to five seconds while simultaneously depressing the top of the canister fully. Then hold your breath for five to ten seconds after inhaling the drug to allow the drug to settle in the lungs. If another inhalation is prescribed, wait two to five minutes before repeating the procedure.

Clean the inhaler under warm running water at least once a day. Because the contents of the inhaler are under pressure, do not store it near heat or flame.

## Rectal suppositories

Rectal suppositories are used to deliver various types of medication. They may be used as a laxative, sleeping aid, or tranquilizer, or to relieve the itching, swelling, and pain of hemorrhoids. Regardless of the reason for their use, all rectal suppositories are inserted in the same way.

In extremely hot weather, a suppository may become too soft to handle properly. If this happens, place the wrapped suppository in the refrigerator, in a glass of cool water, or under cold running water until it becomes firm. A few minutes is usually sufficient. Before inserting a suppository, remove any aluminum wrappings. Rubber finger coverings or disposable rubber gloves may be worn when inserting a suppository, but they are not necessary unless your fingernails are extremely long and sharp.

To insert a suppository, lie on your left side with your right knee bent. Push the suppository, pointed end first, into the rectum as far as is comfortable. You may feel like defecating, but lie still for 20 to 30 minutes, until the urge has passed. If you cannot insert a suppository, or if the process is painful, you can coat the suppository with a thin layer of petroleum jelly or mineral oil to make insertion easier.

Manufacturers of many suppositories that are used in the treatment of hemorrhoids suggest that the suppositories be stored in the refrigerator. Be sure to ask your pharmacist if the suppositories you have purchased should be stored in the refrigerator.

## Vaginal ointments and creams

Most vaginal products are packaged with complete instructions for use. If a woman is not sure how to administer vaginal medication, she should ask her pharmacist.

Before using any vaginal ointment or cream, read the directions. They will probably tell you to attach the applicator to the top of the tube and to squeeze the tube from the bottom until the applicator is completely filled. Then lie on your back with your knees drawn up. Hold the applicator horizontally or pointed slightly downward, and insert it into the vagina as far as it will go comfortably. Press the plunger down to empty the cream or ointment into the vagina. Withdraw the applicator and wash it in warm, soapy water. Rinse it thoroughly and allow it to dry completely.

## Vaginal tablets and suppositories

Before using vaginal tablets or suppositories, carefully read the directions.

Remove any foil wrapping. Place the tablet or suppository in the applicator that is provided. Lie on your back with your knees drawn up. Hold the applicator horizontally or tilted slightly downward, and insert it into

the vagina as far as it will go comfortably. Depress the plunger slowly to release the tablet or suppository into the vagina. Withdraw the applicator and wash it in warm, soapy water. Rinse it and let it dry completely.

Unless your doctor has told you otherwise, do not douche for two to three weeks before or after you use vaginal tablets or suppositories. Ask your doctor for specific recommendations on douching.

## Throat lozenges and discs

Lozenges and discs contain medication that is released in the mouth to soothe a sore throat, to reduce coughing, or to treat laryngitis. Neither should be chewed; they should be allowed to dissolve in the mouth. After the lozenge or disc has dissolved, try not to swallow or drink any fluids for a while.

## Throat sprays

To administer a throat spray, open your mouth wide and spray the medication as far back as possible. Try not to swallow—hold the spray in your mouth as long as you can, and do not drink any fluids for several minutes. This gives the medication a greater opportunity to work. Swallowing a throat spray is not harmful, but if you find that your throat spray upsets your stomach, don't swallow it; simply spit it out.

## Topical ointments and creams

Most ointments and creams exert only local effects—that is, they affect only the area on which they are applied.

Most creams and ointments are expensive (especially steroid products, such as betamethasone valerate, fluocinolone, fluocinonide, hydrocortisone, and triamcinolone), and should be applied to the skin as thinly as possible. A thin layer is as effective as (but less costly than) a thick layer; and some steroid-containing creams and ointments can cause toxic side effects if applied too heavily.

Before applying the medication, moisten the skin by immersing it in water or by dabbing the area with a clean, wet cloth. Blot the skin almost dry and apply the medication as directed. Gently massage it into the skin until it disappears. You should feel no greasiness after applying a cream. After an ointment has been applied, the skin will feel slightly greasy.

If your doctor has not indicated whether you should receive a cream or an ointment, ask your pharmacist for the one you prefer. Creams are greaseless and do not stain your clothing. Creams are best to use on the scalp or other hairy areas of the body. However, if your skin is dry, ask for an ointment. Ointments help keep the skin soft for a longer period of time.

If your doctor tells you to place a wrap on top of the skin after the cream or ointment has been applied, you may use a wrap of transparent plastic film like that used for wrapping food. A wrap holds the medication close to the skin and helps to keep the skin moist so that the drug can be absorbed. To use a wrap correctly, apply the cream or ointment as directed, and then wrap the area with a layer of transparent plastic film. Be careful to follow your doctor's directions exactly. If you are told to leave the wrap in place for a certain length of time, do not leave it in place longer. If you keep a wrap on the skin too long, too much of the drug may be absorbed, which may lead to increased side effects. Do not use such a wrap without your doctor's approval.

## Aerosol sprays

Many topical (used on the surface of the skin) items are packaged as pressurized aerosol sprays. These sprays usually cost more than the cream or ointment form of the same medication. On the other hand, they are useful on very tender or hairy areas of the body, where it is difficult to apply a cream or ointment. Aerosols can provide a cooling effect on burns or rashes.

Before using an aerosol, shake the can to evenly disperse the particles of medication. Hold the container upright, four to six inches from the skin. Press the nozzle for a few seconds and then release it.

Never use an aerosol around the face or eyes. If your doctor tells you to use the spray on a part of your face, apply it to your hand and then rub it into the area. If you get it into your eyes or on a mucous membrane, it can be very painful; it may even damage the eyes.

Aerosol sprays may feel cold when they are applied. If this sensation bothers you, ask your pharmacist or doctor whether another form of the same product is available.

## Transdermal patches

Transdermal patches allow controlled, continuous release of medication. They are convenient and easy to use. For best results, apply the patch to a hairless or clean-shaven area of skin, avoiding scars and wounds. Choose a site (such as the chest or upper arm) that is not subject to excessive movement. It is okay to bathe or shower with a patch in place. If the patch becomes displaced, discard it and apply a new one. When replacing a patch, first apply the new unit and then remove the old one. This allows for uninterrupted drug therapy. Also, since you change the site each time, skin irritation is minimized.

If redness or irritation develops at the application site, consult your physician. Some people are sensitive to the materials used to make the patches.

## Medications and children

There are some special considerations when administering medications to children. The fundamental point, however, is that every child needs to understand that taking medicine is an unpleasant but unavoidable fact of life.

A special concern with regard to medications is the danger that they can present to children. Poisoning due to medications—whether they are pills found in a visitor's purse, medications taken from a medicine chest to which the child has access, or overdose of baby aspirin or vitamin or mineral supplements—is a common cause of death in children. It is important to teach children that drugs are not candy and to be vigilant about the risk of poisoning that any medication brought into your home can present to your child. Also, be sure to post the phone number of the local Poison Control Center next to every phone in your home in case of an overdose.

## Coping with side effects

Drugs have certain desirable effects— that's why they are taken. The desirable effects of a drug are known as the drug's activity or therapeutic effects. Drugs may, however, have

undesirable effects as well. These side effects, or adverse reactions, can range from the relatively minor (such as a headache or an upset stomach) to the much more serious (such as heartbeat irregularity or a severe allergic reaction).

Even if you experience minor side effects, it is very important that you take your medication exactly as it was prescribed. You should take the full dose at the appropriate times throughout the day for the length of time prescribed by your doctor. Taking a lesser amount of medication to avoid side effects or because your condition appears to be improving is NOT appropriate. A smaller dose may not provide any benefit whatsoever; that is, half of the dose may not provide half of the therapeutic effects.

Some side effects are expected and unavoidable, but others may surprise the doctor as well as the patient. Unexpected reactions may be due to a person's individual response to the drug.

Side effects generally fall into one of two major groups—those that are obvious and those that cannot be detected without laboratory testing. Discussion between you and your doctor about your medication should not be restricted to easily recognized side effects; other, less obvious side effects may also be harmful.

If you know a particular side effect is expected from a particular drug, you can relax a little. Most expected side effects are temporary and need not cause alarm. You'll merely experience discomfort or inconvenience for a short time. For example, you may become drowsy after taking an antihistamine, or have a stuffy nose after taking reserpine or certain other drugs that lower blood pressure. Of course, if you find minor side effects especially bothersome, you should discuss them with your doctor, who may be able to prescribe another drug or at least reassure you that the benefits of the drug far outweigh its side effects. Sometimes, side effects can be minimized or eliminated by changing your dosage schedule or taking the drug with meals. Consult your doctor or pharmacist before making such a change.

Many side effects, however, signal a serious, perhaps dangerous, problem. If these side effects appear, you should consult your doctor immediately. The following discussion should help you determine whether your side effects require attention from your physician.

## Obvious side effects

Some side effects are obvious to the patient; others can be discerned only through laboratory testing. We have divided our discussion according to the body parts affected by the side effects.

**Ears.** Although a few drugs may cause loss of hearing if taken in large quantities, hearing loss is uncommon. Drugs that are used to treat problems of the ear may cause dizziness, and many drugs produce tinnitus (a sensation of ringing, buzzing, thumping, or hollowness in the ears). Discuss with your doctor any problem with your hearing or your ears if it persists for more than three days.

**Eyes.** Blurred vision is a common side effect of many drugs. For example, digoxin may cause you to see a halo around a lighted object (a television screen or a traffic light), and other drugs may cause night blindness. Chlordiazepoxide and clidinium combination may make it difficult to accurately judge distance while driving and may make the eyes sensitive to sunlight. While the effects caused by digoxin are danger signs of toxicity, the effects caused by chlordiazepoxide and clidinium combination are to be expected. In any case, if you have difficulty seeing while taking a drug, contact your doctor.

### EXAMPLES OF DRUGS THAT MAY BE ASSOCIATED WITH INCREASED INCIDENCE OF ULCERS

aspirin
ibuprofen
indomethacin
methylprednisolone
naproxen
prednisone
sulindac
tolmetin

**Gastrointestinal system.** The gastrointestinal system includes the mouth, esophagus, stomach, small and large intestines, and rectum. A side effect that affects the gastrointestinal system can be expected from almost any drug. Many drugs produce dry mouth, mouth sores, difficulty in swallowing, heartburn, nausea, vomiting, diarrhea, constipation, loss of appetite, or cramping. Other drugs cause bloating and gas, and some cause rectal itching.

### EXAMPLES OF DRUGS THAT MAY CAUSE DIARRHEA

allopurinol
ampicillin
cephalexin
cimetidine
digoxin
erythromycin
haloperidol
imipramine
methyclothiazide
methyldopa
metronidazole
minocycline
oral antidiabetics
oral contraceptives
penicillins
prazosin
procainamide
propranolol
sulfa drugs
tetracycline

Diarrhea can be expected after taking many drugs. Drugs can create localized reactions in intestinal tissue—usually a more rapid rate of contraction, which leads to diarrhea. Diarrhea caused by most drugs is temporary and self-limiting; it should stop within three days. During this time, do not take any diarrhea remedy; drink liquids to replace the fluid you are losing. If the diarrhea lasts more than three days, you should call your doctor.

Diarrhea sometimes signals a problem. For example, some antibiotics can cause severe diarrhea. When diarrhea is severe, the intestine may become ulcerated and begin to bleed. If you have severe diarrhea (diarrhea that lasts for several days or stools that contain blood, pus, or mucus) while taking antibiotics, contact your doctor.

### EXAMPLES OF DRUGS THAT MAY CAUSE CONSTIPATION

clonidine
diazepam
haloperidol
lorazepam
methyldopa
metronidazole
phenytoin
prazosin
prochlorperazine
propranolol
sulindac
thioridazine

As a side effect of drug use, constipation is less serious and more common than diarrhea. It occurs when a drug, such as chlorpromazine, slows the activity of the bowel. Constipation also occurs when drugs cause moisture to be absorbed from the bowel, resulting in a more solid stool. Some drugs, such as methyldopa, act on the nervous system to decrease nerve impulses to the intestine. Constipation produced by a drug can last several days. You may help relieve it by drinking eight to ten glasses of water a day (unless your doctor directs you to do otherwise). Do not take laxatives unless your doctor directs you to do so. If constipation continues for more than three days, call your doctor.

**Circulatory system.** Drugs may speed up or slow down the heartbeat. If a drug slows the heartbeat, you may feel drowsy and tired, or even dizzy. If a drug accelerates the heartbeat, you probably will experience palpitations (a sensation of thumping in the chest). You may feel as though your heart is skipping a beat occasionally. If any of these symptoms occurs, consult your doctor, who may adjust your drug dosage or prescribe other medication.

Some drugs cause edema (fluid retention)—fluid from the blood collects outside the blood vessels. Ordinarily, edema itself is not serious. However, if you are steadily gaining weight or have gained more than two pounds within a week, talk to your doctor.

Drugs may either increase or decrease blood pressure. When blood pressure decreases, you may feel drowsy or tired; you may become dizzy, or even faint, especially when you rise suddenly from a sitting or reclining position. If a medication makes you dizzy or light-headed, sit or lie down for a while. To avoid light-headedness when you stand, contract and relax the muscles of your legs for a few moments before rising. Do this by pushing one foot against the floor while raising the other foot slightly, alternating feet so that you are "pumping" your legs in a pedaling motion. Get up slowly, and be especially careful on stairs. When blood pressure increases, you may feel dizzy, have a headache or blurred vision, hear a ringing or buzzing in your ears, or experience frequent nosebleeds. If you experience any of these symptoms, call your doctor.

### EXAMPLES OF DRUGS THAT MAY CAUSE FLUID RETENTION*

amitriptyline
chlordiazepoxide
conjugated estrogens
disopyramide
fenoprofen
ibuprofen
methylprednisolone
naproxen
oral contraceptives
prochlorperazine
sulfa drugs
sulindac
thioridazine
tolmetin

* Indicated by a weight gain of two or more pounds in a week.

**Nervous system.** Drugs that act on the nervous system may cause drowsiness or stimulation. If a drug causes drowsiness, you may become dizzy or your coordination may become impaired. If a drug causes stimulation, you may become nervous or have insomnia or tremors. Neither drowsiness nor stimulation is cause for concern for most people. When you are drowsy, however, you should be careful around machinery and should avoid driving. Some drugs cause throbbing headaches, and others produce tingling in the fingers or toes. These symptoms should disappear in a few days to a week. If they do not, call your doctor.

**Respiratory system.** Respiratory system side effects include stuffy nose, dry throat, shortness of breath, and slowed breathing. A stuffy nose and dry throat usually disappear several days after starting a medication. If

### EXAMPLES OF DRUGS THAT MAY CAUSE DIZZINESS

cephalexin
cimetidine
disopyramide
flurazepam
imipramine
lorazepam
methyclothiazide
methyldopa
methylprednisolone
metronidazole
nitroglycerin
oral antidiabetics
prazosin
sulindac

these side effects are bothersome, you may use nose drops (consult you doctor first) or throat lozenges or a warm salt-water gargle to relieve them. Shortness of breath is a characteristic side effect of some drugs (for example, propranolol). If shortness of breath continues, check with your doctor. It may be a sign of a serious side effect, or you may simply be overexercising. Barbiturates (drugs that promote sleep) often slow breathing; if your breathing becomes labored, however, contact your doctor immediately.

**Skin.** Skin reactions include rash, swelling, itching, and sweating. Itching, swelling, and rash frequently indicate a drug allergy. You should NOT continue to take a drug if you develop an allergy to it, but consult your doctor before stopping the drug.

Some drugs increase sweating; others decrease it. Drugs that decrease sweating may cause problems during exercise or hot weather, when your body needs to sweat to reduce body temperature.

If you have a minor skin reaction not diagnosed as an allergy, ask your pharmacist for a soothing cream. Your pharmacist may also suggest that you take frequent baths or dust the sensitive area with a suitable powder.

### EXAMPLES OF DRUGS THAT MAY CAUSE A MILD RASH

allopurinol
amitriptyline
ampicillin
chlordiazepoxide
cimetidine
clonidine
diazepam
haloperidol
hydrochlorothiazide
imipramine
indomethacin
lorazepam
methyclothiazide
penicillins
procainamide
prochlorperazine
sulindac

Another type of skin reaction is photosensitivity (also called phototoxicity or sun toxicity)—that is, unusual sensitivity to the sun. If, while taking a drug that can cause photosensitivity, you are exposed to the sun for even a brief period of time (10 or 15 minutes), you may receive a severe sunburn. You do not have to stay indoors while taking these drugs,

### EXAMPLES OF DRUGS THAT MAY CAUSE PHOTOSENSITIVITY

chlorothiazide
chlorpromazine
diphenhydramine
griseofulvin
haloperidol
hydrochlorothiazide
imipramine
methyclothiazide
oral antidiabetics
prochlorperazine
sulfa drugs
tetracycline

but you should be fully clothed while outside, and you should not remain in the sun too long. You should also use a sunscreen while in the sun— ask your pharmacist to help you choose one. Since medications may remain in your bloodstream after you stop taking them, you should continue to follow these precautions for two days after treatment with these drugs has been completed.

# Management of side effects

Consult your physician to determine whether the side effects you are experiencing are minor (relatively common and usually not serious) or major (rare but important signs that something is amiss in your drug therapy). If your side effects are minor, you may be able to compensate for them easily. However, the most prudent course of action is always to consult your doctor if your minor side effects are persistent or particularly bothersome.

If you experience any major side effects, contact your doctor immediately. Your dosage may need adjustment, or you may have developed a sensitivity to the drug. Your doctor may want you to switch to an alternative medication to treat your disorder. Never stop taking a prescribed medication, however, unless you first discuss it with your doctor.

## Subtle side effects

Some side effects are difficult to detect. You may not notice any symptoms at all, or you may notice only slight ones. Therefore, your doctor may want you to have periodic blood tests or eye examinations to ensure that no subtle damage is occurring to any of your organ systems while you are taking certain medications.

# Effects on the blood

A great many drugs affect the blood and the circulatory system but do not produce noticeable symptoms for some time. Some drugs decrease the number of red blood cells—the cells responsible for carrying oxygen throughout the body. If you have too few red blood cells, you become anemic; you appear pale and feel tired, weak, and dizzy. Other drugs decrease the number of white blood cells—the cells responsible for combating bacteria. Having too few white blood cells increases susceptibility to infection and may prolong illness. If a sore throat or a fever begins after you start taking a drug, you may have an infection and too few white blood cells to fight it. Call your doctor.

# Effects on the kidneys

If one of the side effects of a drug is to reduce the ability of the kidneys to remove chemicals and other substances from the blood, these substances begin to accumulate in body tissues. Over a period of time, this accumulation may cause vague symptoms, such as swelling, fluid retention, nausea, headache, and weakness. Obvious symptoms, especially pain, are rare.

# Effects on the liver

Drug-induced liver damage may result in fat accumulation within the liver. Since the liver is responsible for converting many drugs and body chemicals into compounds that can be eliminated by other organs of the body (kidneys, lungs, intestines), drug-induced liver damage can result in a buildup of these substances. Because liver damage may be quite advanced before it produces any symptoms, periodic blood tests of liver function are recommended during therapy with certain drugs.

### EXAMPLES OF DRUGS THAT MAY CAUSE BLOOD DISORDERS*

allopurinol
amitriptyline
chlorthalidone
cimetidine
furosemide
hydrochlorothiazide
imipramine
oral contraceptives
steroids
sulfa drugs
tolbutamide

*Sometimes indicated by a sore throat that doesn't go away in one or two days.

# Drug use during pregnancy and breast-feeding

Because drugs can cross the placenta and can pass into breast milk, it is very important to tell your doctor if you are pregnant, are planning to become pregnant, or are breast-feeding an infant before taking any medications. For most drugs, complete information on safety during pregnancy and while breast-feeding is lacking. This is not due to negligence on the part of regulatory agencies or lack of concern, but rather to the fact that it would be unethical to conduct drug experiments on pregnant and nursing women. Thus, you should discuss with your doctor the risks versus the benefits of taking any medication during pregnancy or while nursing.

# The medical guide to diseases, disorders, syndromes, and medical terms

This section of the medical guide, arranged in alphabetical order for easy and fast reference, covers diseases, disorders, conditions, syndromes, symptoms, diagnostic procedures, treatments, and medical terms. Each entry is presented in clear, easy-to-understand language with practical advice about when to treat a problem at home, when to consult a doctor, and when to administer emergency first aid or to seek immediate emergency care. Since this section can be used as a reference manual, each entry is designed to be self contained; for example, terms that may not be a part of everyday vocabulary are defined where they occur, even if they have been defined elsewhere. On the other hand, if another entry or section of the book naturally expands or complements a topic, there is a cross reference for you to find the additional information.

In those entries that discuss a disease or disorder, the description of the problem, the cause (if known), the symptoms, the treatment, the prognosis, and the risk factors are discussed. In addition, preventive action is outlined, if appropriate or possible. In those entries that define a term or discuss a procedure, the explanation often includes examples to illustrate the concept or idea. In short, each entry attempts to be as inclusive as possible without being technical and hard to understand.

# A

## Acne

Acne is a condition of the skin that ranges in appearance from small raised bumps to pustules (large cysts and pimples). Acne is so common that more than 80 percent of the population will have some form of it at some time in their lives.

Although there are several theories about what causes acne, author-ities generally believe that acne is a by-product of hormonal changes in the body during puberty—that period of life when a child develops the secondary sex characteristics (such as facial and body hair, deepened voice, and increased muscle mass in boys and breast development and menstruation in girls). At this time, production of hormones (particularly the male hormone testosterone) increases and stimulates the sebaceous glands in the skin to produce sebum (an oily secretion). Most excess oil produced by these glands leaves the skin through the hair follicles (the tubelike structures from which hairs develop). Sometimes, oil clogs these tubes and creates comedones (blocked hair follicles). Comedones are what form the initial lumps in acne.

If comedones are open to the surface of the skin, they are called blackheads. They contain sebum from the sebaceous glands, bacteria, and any skin tissue that accumulates near the surface. Comedones that are closed at the surface are called whiteheads. Plugged follicles can rupture internally, resulting in a discharge of their contents into the surrounding tissues. This process begins an inflammatory response that sets the stage for the development of acne.

The role of bacteria in acne is unclear. Bacteria may act by causing chemical reactions in the sebaceous fluid, leading to the release of very irritating compounds called fatty acids. These in turn may cause inflammation that increases susceptibility to infection.

Authorities disagree about the role of diet as a cause of acne. Diet alone does not cure acne, nor does acne stem from an allergic reaction to a specific food. However, some cases of acne appear to improve after eliminating certain foods, particularly chocolates and fats. In addition, emotional stress seems to increase the severity of acne in certain cases.

Acne causes raised swellings, most frequently on the face, neck, back, chest, and shoulders. In severe cases, there may be pus-filled sacs that break open and discharge fluid. Soreness, pain, and itching may accompany the bumps. These symptoms could be acne, or they could indicate other skin reactions to such substances as cosmetics, medications, and grooming or cleaning products.

Since puberty plays a role in the onset of acne, the condition usually appears during the teenage years.

When excess material produced by the sebaceous glands clogs the hair follicle tube, a blackhead results. A blackhead is open on the surface of the skin, but nevertheless blocks the normal release of material from the sebaceous gland to the skin's surface.

When a blocked hair follicle is not open on the surface of the skin, it may eventually rupture internally, discharging its contents into the surrounding tissues. This results in an inflammatory response that sets the stage for the development of acne.

However, it can extend to age 25 and over, particularly in women. Although acne is not life-threatening, it can be problematic. If untreated, acne lesions can leave permanent scars, which can cause embarrassment and emotional stress.

Acne has no prevention or cure, but there are several treatments. The simplest home remedy is to wash the affected areas thoroughly at least twice a day with warm water and mild soap. Washing gently will not dry or irritate sensitive skin. Regular shampooing also helps, especially if the hair is oily. Use of makeup should be limited. In addition, skin may heal with exposure to the sun. However, sunlamps and ultraviolet lamps should be used very cautiously, and only under a doctor's supervision.

One form of treatment not recommended is picking or squeezing pimples, since more inflammation and scarring may result. Also, the risk of infection is increased.

Some over-the-counter acne medications, particularly lotions or creams containing benzoyl peroxide, can help troubled skin. However, most of these preparations tend to dry the skin if the manufacturer's directions are not followed carefully.

For persistent acne, a doctor may prescribe an antibiotic preparation that can be applied to the surface of the skin or an oral antibiotic, such as tetracycline and erythromycin. These antibiotics act to suppress bacterial growth, which may be a factor in worsening acne.

Another drug, tretinoin (vitamin A acid), has reduced acne in more than 50 percent of the persons who have tried it. This drug can be taken independently or in combination with an antibiotic, and must be used under a doctor's supervision. A newer drug, isotretinoin, is related to tretinoin and is used to treat severe cystic acne. It is usually not prescribed, however,

unless all other acne treatments have failed. This drug works by temporarily suppressing the production of secretions by the sebaceous glands. It is important to note that this drug can have very serious side effects and should never be used without the knowledge and supervision of an experienced medical doctor. In addition, isotretinoin should not be used by any woman who is, who thinks she may be, or who intends to become pregnant. Use of this drug in any amount for even short periods during pregnancy is associated with an extremely high risk of fetal abnormalities and spontaneous abortion. Women of childbearing potential should use contraception during therapy with this drug; use of contraception should begin one month prior to starting therapy and should not be discontinued until at least one month after therapy is complete.

See also Boils.

# Addison's disease

Addison's disease is a condition that occurs when the adrenal cortex fails to produce enough of its hormones.

Formerly, the cause of this disease in most cases was tuberculosis or a fungal infection. However, in recent years, the disease is more likely to be idiopathic (of unknown cause). One theory is that most cases are due to autoimmune destruction of the adrenal cortex (that is, the body produces antibodies against its own tissues). Other known causes include partial destruction of the adrenal cortex by cancer, surgery, degeneration of the tissue, or deposition of a substance called amyloid. A similar condition, known as secondary adrenal insufficiency, is caused by failure of the pituitary gland to produce enough adrenocorticotropic hormone (ACTH), which stimulates the adrenal cortex to produce its hormones.

Early symptoms of Addison's disease are weakness, fatigue, and a tendency to become faint when rising suddenly from a bed or chair. Increased pigmentation of the skin, producing a "tan" all over the body, on exposed and unexposed areas alike, with even darker pigmentation on creases and bony pressure points, occurs in most cases. In certain places, the tan may be broken by completely white patches, known as vitiligo. Black freckles appear on the forehead, face, shoulders, and neck. There may be skin discoloration around the nipples, and the mucous membranes of the mouth may have dark-blue patches.

Symptoms that may appear later include weight loss, dehydration (excessive loss of body fluids), low blood pressure, and sometimes loss of appetite, nausea, vomiting, diarrhea, dizziness, and inability to keep warm.

The most alarming symptoms are those of a condition called adrenal crisis, which requires immediate attention and hospitalization. Signs of this are extreme weakness; severe pains in the lower back, abdomen, or legs; shock (collapse of the circulatory system); and renal shutdown (kidney failure). Such a crisis may be brought on by severe stress, such as infection, injury, or surgery, or by a loss of salt through perspiration during hot weather.

One laboratory sign of Addison's disease is a high level of ACTH but a low level of cortisol (one of the adrenal gland hormones) in the blood. This indicates that the pituitary gland is working overtime, stimulating the adrenal cortex with ACTH to produce cortisol, but that the cortex is failing to produce it.

The basic treatment for Addison's disease is to provide steroid hormones, principally cortisone, to replace those not being produced by the adrenal cortex. An additional steroid drug may be prescribed to promote retention of salt, and thereby water, in tissues and blood, so that the low blood pressure of severe Addison's disease can be avoided.

The outlook for patients receiving hormone treatment is excellent. Continued medical supervision is necessary to prevent emergencies caused by a sudden withdrawal of treatment or by an increased need for hormones because of infection, injury, surgery, pregnancy, or other stress on the body. It is important to avoid infection and to treat infection that develops as soon as possible. At all times, patients should carry a card or wear a bracelet describing the condition and the need for cortisone. It is also critical to take the medication exactly as prescribed and to be monitored by a physician who can increase or decrease the dosage as the need arises. With proper care, a person with Addison's disease can lead a nearly normal life.

See also Adrenal glands and Pituitary gland.

# Adenoids

Adenoids are masses of protective lymphoid tissue located in the lining of the nasopharynx. Like the tonsils located below them, the adenoids (technically known as the nasopharyngeal tonsils) are lymph nodes containing the specialized white blood cells that help localize and destroy harmful bacteria and viruses. They thus provide an important defense against diseases that may affect the respiratory system.

It is normal for adenoids to become enlarged during throat infections, just as the tonsils do, and then to diminish in size after the infection has passed. Sometimes, however, as a result of continuing infection or allergies, the adenoids remain enlarged. The resulting obstruction of the nasal passage may cause mouth breathing, the characteristic "nasal" voice, and continuing drainage of pus-filled mucus down the throat. It may also cause a blockage of the eustachian tubes, which connect the throat to the ears, resulting in retention of fluid in the middle ear, impaired hearing, earache, and recurring ear infections.

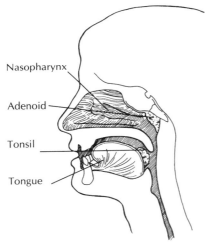

Nasopharynx

Adenoid

Tonsil

Tongue

An adenoid is a mass of lymphoid tissue, located above the throat and behind the nose. Its function is to trap and destroy harmful bacteria and viruses.

Treatment of infection of the adenoids includes antibiotics, taken by mouth. Surgery may be recommended when the infected or enlarged adenoids themselves are the source of the disease (usually the tonsils beneath are infected as well and are removed in the same operation). This would be the case if recurrent or continuing infection of the adenoids could not be eliminated with antibiotics, if the adenoids caused repeated ear infections, or if cancer or an abscess (a mass of pus in a cavity)

was present. If chronically infected adenoids increase susceptibility to a serious condition, such as rheumatic fever or nephritis (a kidney disease), surgical removal of the adenoids may be recommended. However, surgery is generally not performed during an acute attack of tonsillitis, because it may worsen the infection.

Surgery may not be the answer to prevent snoring, mouth breathing, or the nasal voice caused by enlarged adenoids, since the enlargement usually diminishes after childhood.

Adenoid infection and enlargement cannot always be prevented. In fact, enlarging in order to trap and fight infectious organisms is a normal function of the adenoids. Good general health measures can help, however, as can the use of antibiotics prescribed by a physician when the adenoids become infected and enlarged.

See also Tonsillitis.

# Adrenal glands

The adrenal glands are critical to normal body functions, such as maintenance of fluid balance, reaction to stress, and reproduction. There are two adrenal glands, each of which lies above a kidney. The adrenal glands have two distinct parts: the cortex (outer layer), which secretes steroid hormones, and the medulla (inner part), which secretes epinephrine and norepinephrine. The more than 30 steroid hormones regulate a wide array of processes throughout the body. Epinephrine and norepinephrine are responsible for the changes in heart rate, blood pressure, and level of usable glucose (a form of sugar) that are necessary to cope with stress.

See also Addison's disease and Corticosteroids.

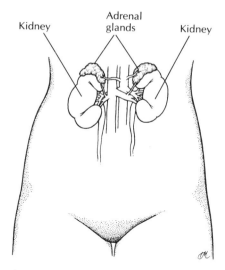

Kidney    Adrenal glands    Kidney

The adrenal glands are two small glands that are located above each kidney and that produce more than 30 different hormones to help regulate body processes.

# AIDS—acquired immune deficiency syndrome

Acquired immune deficiency syndrome (AIDS) is a disease in which the body's natural defense system is disabled, thus allowing organisms that are normally fought off to become deadly.

This disease, discovered in 1979, is caused by a microorganism called the human immunodeficiency virus. This virus is carried and transmitted in bodily fluids (mainly blood, semen, and vaginal secretions). Sexual intercourse (heterosexual or homosexual), use of nonsterile hypodermic needles (a common practice among drug addicts), and infected blood transfusions have all been implicated as means of transmission of the AIDS virus. Transmission from a pregnant woman to her infant or from a mother to her nursing infant may occur. There is currently a great deal of controversy as to whether an infected physician or dentist can infect a patient. There have been isolated reports of transmission by being splashed in the eyes or other mucous membranes with infected blood.

In Western countries, male homosexuals, prostitutes, drug addicts who inject drugs, and hemophiliacs who receive multiple blood transfusions for their disorder are all at high risk for contracting AIDS. In Africa (where the disease seems to have originated), heterosexual transmission is apparently the most common route.

A widespread misconception has been that AIDS can be contracted by *giving* blood—this notion is not true. In addition, since the introduction of a blood screening test for use in blood banks and hospital laboratories, acquisition of the AIDS virus by *receiving* blood transfusions is now extremely unlikely. Furthermore, the evidence to date indicates that casual contacts—such as would occur in school or in the workplace—are not responsible for transmission of the virus.

Clinical illness from AIDS can have its onset as long as ten years after initial infection with the virus. Roughly 75 percent of HIV-positive individuals will develop some signs of disease within seven years of initial infection. Initial symptoms include low-grade fever, swollen lymph nodes, weight loss, fatigue, night sweats, and long-standing diarrhea. (It is important to note that these symptoms can also be present in a large number of less serious illnesses.) Because of impairment of the immune system, people with AIDS easily fall prey to many diseases, including various types of cancer, skin infections, fungal infections, and tuberculosis. About one third of people with AIDS develop a previously rare cancer known as Kaposi's sarcoma, which often appears as purplish bumps on the skin. Many suffer *Pneumocystis carinii* pneumonia. Children with AIDS frequently develop bacterial infections such as sinusitis (sinus infection), otitis media (ear infection), and sepsis (blood infection).

The blood of people with AIDS contains an abnormally small number of specialized white blood cells called lymphocytes. Lymphocytes play an important role in combating infectious diseases and may also be instrumental in destroying malignant growths in their early stages. There are two types of lymphocytes actively engaged in coping with infection: T cells, which directly kill invaders, and B cells, which are involved in the production of infection-fighting antibodies. The finding that people with AIDS have decreased numbers of T cells, particularly a subtype called "helper" T cells, or CD4+T, has proved invaluable in the disease's diagnosis.

A person may be a carrier of the disease without being aware of the fact and without having any of the symptoms. Blood tests for the detection of antibodies to the AIDS virus have recently been developed. The implications of a positive blood test are controversial, however. A confirmed positive blood test definitely indicates exposure to the disease. Newborns whose mothers are infected with the AIDS virus will initially test positive for the antibody to AIDS. However, in only about 30 percent of those infants will this positive test persist after 15 to 18 months of age, and these are the infants who will eventually develop the disease.

No cure for AIDS has been found yet. The drug zidovudine (called azidothymidine or AZT) acts by preventing replication of the AIDS virus in human cells. Although this drug has been shown to prolong survival and improve the quality of life for people with AIDS, it cannot be considered a cure.

Until a cure for AIDS is found, treatment is limited to countering the effects of the disease (for example, nutritional support, surgery to remove skin cancer, chemotherapy, and use of drugs to raise the body's resistance to combat infections).

Since there is no cure for AIDS, prevention is critical. Limiting the number of one's sexual partners and using condoms decrease the risk of sexual exposure to the AIDS virus. Avoiding contact with potentially contaminated hypodermic needles and with blood and blood products is also important. The time between infection with the virus and development of a positive blood test for antibodies can be anywhere from weeks to three or four years. The majority will turn positive within five months of infection. To date, there is no evidence that AIDS can be transmitted by casual contact with an infected individual or by mosquito bite. The most common modes of transmission are sexual contact and intravenous drug use with nonsterile needles. AIDS is a very complex subject, and new discoveries are constantly being made. The information in this section may change from time to time.

Needless to say, the infected person should inform all sex partners and medical and dental personnel with whom he or she comes into contact of his or her immune status and should not donate blood, sperm, organs, or any other body tissues.

See also Immunity.

# Alcoholism

Alcoholism is a disorder in which a person repeatedly drinks excessive amounts of alcoholic beverages, with resulting harm to health, relations with other people, and work performance. The person becomes physically and psychologically dependent on alcohol. There is a genuine craving for alcohol when it is withdrawn for one to three days, and unpleasant responses such as delirium tremens (characterized by a severe stress reaction, hallucinations, and tremors) and convulsions may be seen when alcohol is not available.

Various causes of alcoholism have been suggested. These include depression, self-hatred, and having a shy, lonely, immature, or dependent personality. Some societies and groups within those societies encourage overuse of alcohol as recreation and as an escape from life's problems. There is also evidence that a tendency to alcoholism may be inherited or may be the result of a chemical defect. Whatever the cause, alcoholism is a self-damaging disease and an ineffective way to deal with the hectic pace and challenges of contemporary life.

The fact that a person is an alcoholic is not always obvious. Alcoholics often do not recognize their own alcoholism or try to hide symptoms from spouses, other family members, friends, and employers. Signs of alcoholism include:
- Frequent drunkenness
- Tolerance to alcohol (A great deal of liquor is required before the person shows signs of intoxication; however, this is not true in all cases, especially if alcohol has damaged the liver.)
- Physical dependence, resulting in withdrawal symptoms a day or more after stopping drinking (Symptoms may range from tremors and physical pain to seizures and hallucinations.)
- Poor job performance
- Depression
- Continued drinking even when it is harming the person's health and personal life

Other signs may include an odor of liquor on the breath in the morning, stealthy drinking, suspicious work absences (to sleep off hangovers), and frequent falls, unexplainable accidents, and cigarette burns on hands and body (caused by drunken carelessness).

Alcoholism can cause permanent damage to the liver, brain, heart, and nervous system. Moderate to heavy drinking by a pregnant woman can result in mental retardation in her baby, as well as low birth weight and birth defects.

If an alcoholic has been drinking as much as a gallon of beer or a pint of whiskey a day for several months, sudden withdrawal of alcohol may even result in death because of convulsions or delirium tremens.

Alcoholism is not a cause for shame or embarrassment, nor is it a sign of failure or degeneracy. It is a disease that, like any other, requires professional treatment, not only for the alcoholic's sake but also for the sake of the others—family, friends, and coworkers—whose lives he affects.

Treatment of severe alcoholism involves two stages: immediate and long-term. Both require a physician's attention.

The first step is to stop the drinking while treating the symptoms of withdrawal. The drug disulfiram is sometimes prescribed, to be taken daily by mouth; it causes vomiting if the patient drinks anything alcoholic. It stops the person from drinking, but the patient may refuse to continue taking it because of its unpleasant effects.

In most situations, withdrawal is best done in a hospital alcoholic unit under a doctor's care. Psychological support and reassurance may be enough to comfort the patient during the withdrawal stage. Frequently, however, other measures are necessary. The patient may be undernourished from drinking so much and not eating enough and may need replacement doses of vitamins, particularly thiamin (vitamin B₁). Fluids containing glucose (a form of sugar) and salt water may be added to the blood, which has been robbed of water and glucose by the effects of overuse of alcohol. Tranquilizing drugs are given to help ease withdrawal symptoms, which usually peak at 48 to 72 hours and may continue for days. In severe cases, withdrawal seizures can occur. If the individual is not in a hospital where these can be immediately treated, serious consequences—even death—can result.

Long-term treatment may include psychiatric help to treat the problem that caused the alcoholism in the first place, such as depression or mental illness. For many alcoholics, the solution is to join an organization known as Alcoholics Anonymous (AA). Members help each other overcome their drinking problems and vow to stay away from alcohol completely. In helping each other, they develop confidence and positive feelings about themselves.

Alcoholism is a significant social and medical problem that cannot be easily stopped. However, its threat may be diminished by:

- Learning about the full extent of its dangers
- Finding more healthful ways to deal with life's problems and disappointments—by facing, rather than avoiding, them
- Learning to recognize the symptoms of alcoholism
- Seeking help from a physician or a group such as Alcoholics Anonymous

# Allergy

An allergy is a state of special sensitivity to a particular environmental substance, or allergen. An allergic reaction is the body's response, directed by the immune system, to exposure to an allergen.

Although an allergy can be present almost immediately after exposure to an allergen, it usually develops over time, as the immune system forms antibodies against the foreign substance. Under normal conditions, such antibodies work to protect the body from further attack. In the case of an allergy, however, the antibodies and other specialized cells involved in this protective function trigger an unusual sensitivity, or overreaction, to the foreign substance. The antibodies stimulate specialized cells to produce histamine, a powerful chemical. Histamine causes the small blood vessels to enlarge and the smooth muscles (such as those in the airways and the digestive tract) to constrict. Histamine release can also cause other reactions, such as hives.

No one knows why allergies develop, but it is known that an allergy can appear, disappear, or reappear at any time and at any age. Allergic reactions will rarely occur during the first encounter with the troublesome allergen because the body needs time to accumulate the antibodies. Also, an individual's sensitivity to certain allergens seems to be related to a family history of allergies. People who have a tendency to develop allergies are referred to as atopic. This atopic tendency frequently runs in families.

An allergic reaction can be so mild that it is barely noticeable or so severe that it is life-threatening. Common symptoms of allergy are watery eyes, runny nose, itching or inflamed skin, and a swollen mouth or throat. Some allergic reactions may be accompanied by headaches, sinus stuffiness, a reduced sense of taste or smell, or difficulty in breathing.

An extremely severe allergic reaction, called anaphylactic shock, is characterized by breathing difficulties (caused by swelling of the throat and larynx and narrowing of the bronchial tubes), itching skin, hives, and collapse of the blood vessels, as well as by vomiting, diarrhea, and cramps. This condition can be fatal if not properly treated.

There are four categories of allergens: inhalants, contactants, ingestants, and injectants.

Inhalant allergens are those that are breathed in, including such substances as dust, pollen, feathers, and animal dander (small scales from an animal's skin). Hay fever is an inhalant allergy in which the mucous membranes react to various inhaled substances, usually the pollens associated with the changing seasons. Year-round "hay fever" may actually be a reaction to pet dander, feathers, mold, or dust.

Contactant allergens are those that are touched, including such substances as poison ivy, poison oak, cosmetics, detergents, fabrics, and dyes. Contact dermatitis is an example of an allergic reaction to a contactant allergen.

Ingestant allergens are those that are swallowed. A variety of foods and medications can act as ingestant allergens. Food allergies occur more frequently in children than in adults. Some common ingestant allergens are milk, eggs, shellfish, fish, peanuts, chocolate, strawberries, tomatoes, and citrus fruits.

Injectant allergens are substances that penetrate the skin, such as insect venom and drugs that are injected. An example of this is people who have severe allergic reactions to insect bites or stings; they are suffer-ing from a reaction to an injectant allergen.

Identifying an offending allergen may be uncomfortable, time-consuming, and expensive, but it is sometimes necessary in order to avoid future allergic reactions. A medical history, a record of any recent changes in daily habits, skin-scratch tests (in which small amounts of suspected allergens are applied to tiny scratches in the skin), and intracutaneous skin tests (in which allergens are injected under the skin) are used to help identify the troublesome foreign substance. A special study called radioallergosorbent testing (RAST) is sometimes performed to detect and measure antibodies in the blood that have been manufactured in response to invading substances.

Once the allergen has been identified, half the battle is won. Avoiding the troublesome substance is the first step toward relieving an allergy problem. If the allergen cannot be avoided or removed, medication or immunotherapy may be recommended. Three types of medications are commonly prescribed: antihistamines, which combat the effect of the histamines in the body; corticosteroids, which reduce inflammation and swelling; and bronchodilators, which ease breathing by opening bronchial tubes.

Allergy immunotherapy, or "desensitization," consists of injections of an allergen in gradually increasing quantities. This allows the body to build up a tolerance to the offending substance. Immunotherapy works best in controlling allergies to pollen, insect venom, and house dust.

A little common sense goes a long way toward controlling allergies. Obviously, the offending allergen needs to be avoided. Natural fibers in the home can be replaced with synthetics. Air conditioners or air filters can be installed for hay fever sufferers. Those susceptible to insect bites can wear protective clothes and avoid wearing bright clothing and perfumes, both of which attract insects. Babies born into allergy-prone families should be breast-fed as long as possible to delay exposure to cow's milk, eggs, and citrus fruits.

In most cases, allergies cannot be prevented, but much can be done to help control or diminish the effects of allergies on overly sensitive individuals.

# Alzheimer's disease

Alzheimer's disease is a disorder in which there is a steady deterioration of brain function resulting in progressive loss of memory, recognition, personality, and mental powers. Although Alzheimer's disease may begin as early as age 40, it is most prevalent in the aged. It accounts for at least half of all serious mental impairment in persons over age 65.

In Alzheimer's disease, as in any senile (characteristic of old age) mental disorder, there is atrophy (shrinkage or wasting) of the cerebral cortex (the outer layer of the brain, which is mostly concerned with intellectual and social functioning). There are also more specific abnormalities, such as the presence of tangles of fibers within the nerve cells and of senile plaques, which are probably deposits of amyloid (a semisolid protein complex seen in many degenerative diseases). These abnormal changes are scattered throughout the cortex of a person with Alzheimer's and serve to distinguish the disease from other forms of senility. Because brain biopsy specimens (tissue samples taken from the brain for laboratory examination) are not obtained without very specific reasons and without intention of specific treatment, these changes

are usually seen only after death has occured.

Theories abound as to the possible causes of Alzheimer's disease. So-called slow viruses (viruses acquired early in life that take many years to do their damage) have been considered, as have environmental factors and damage from previous diseases. Recently, a diminished amount of the enzyme choline-acetyltransferase (which is necessary to manufacture the neurotransmitter acetylcholine) has been found in some patients, and theories about replacement of the enzyme or neurotransmitter are being formulated. Deficiencies of other neurotransmitters are constantly being researched. Heredity seems to play some part, since a family member of an Alzheimer's victim is more likely than others to develop the condition. It is generally agreed that hardening of the arteries is not a cause. The disease does not appear to be contagious, nor is it caused by emotional upsets or stress.

Symptoms vary considerably from one person to another and may occur days or months apart. They begin with small memory lapses, almost always first involving loss of recall for recent events. Such lapses can happen to anyone, but in Alzheimer's disease they grow more serious with time. A person may forget a close relative's name, get lost coming home from the office, forget to turn off the oven, recheck to see if a task was done, or repeatedly ask questions that have already been answered.

Eventually, the gaps in memory and the failure to recognize friends and family members interfere with normal work and social life. The individual starts having trouble with figures when working on bills, with understanding what is being read, and with organizing the day's work.

As the disease progresses, the victim of Alzheimer's disease becomes confused, frustrated, and irritable. Although at first the person seems physically unaffected by the disease, as the condition advances the patient becomes restless, always moving about, and must be watched so that he or she does not wander away or into danger. Endless repetition of unnecessary actions, such as the opening and closing of drawers, is another characteristic of the disease. Some victims of Alzheimer's disease may become extremely agitated with little or no provocation.

The course of the disease, which eventually can result in deterioration of the rest of the nervous system and other parts of the body and in loss of control over bladder and bowels, may range from one to 20 years. It may cut life expectancy by contributing to death from another cause, such as pneumonia or heart or kidney failure.

Other conditions can cause many of the symptoms of Alzheimer's disease, and many of these conditions are treatable. Therefore, it is very important for the patient to undergo a thorough medical evaluation, which may include extensive neurological and psychological examinations and other diagnostic studies, such as computed tomography (a special X-ray technique for obtaining cross-sectional images), electroencephalography (a study of brain waves), magnetic resonance imaging (MRI), blood tests, and sampling of cerebrospinal fluid. These procedures can rule out or identify possible causes of nervous system malfunctioning, such as a series of "little strokes," brain tumors or infections, pernicious anemia (curable with vitamin $B_{12}$), overmedication with barbiturates or bromides, alcoholism, drug side effects, abnormal thyroid function, or hydrocephalus (blockage of cerebrospinal fluid in the head).

Psychological depression is also an important—and treatable—cause of senile symptoms, such as apathy, slowness of thought, inattention, and poor concentration. Death of a spouse or a shock, such as moving to a nursing home, could cause such symptoms temporarily.

Medical science does not yet know how to prevent or treat Alzheimer's disease. However, it is important to find a physician who is able to help the patient and his or her family handle the multitude of problems that are bound to arise. At times, tranquilizers can lessen agitation and anxiety and reduce the incidence of undesirable behavior. Medication may also help to improve sleeping patterns and treat depression caused by the disease.

It is important that the patient continue a daily routine, exercise as usual, and keep in touch with friends. Memory aids, such as lists of daily chores, reminders about safety, and a large calendar, can help in day-to-day living. As care of the patient becomes more difficult, it may be best (for the patient and family alike) to move the patient to a health facility where a professional staff can provide around-the-clock care.

# Amblyopia

Amblyopia is the name for diminished vision in one or both eyes, usually without any obvious defect. (Amblyopia is not the same as nearsightedness, farsightedness, or astigmatism, which can be corrected with eyeglasses or contact lenses.)

There are two main types of amblyopia: "lazy-eye" amblyopia and toxic amblyopia.

Lazy-eye amblyopia occurs frequently in young children whose eyes do not line up correctly (a condition known as strabismus). To prevent double vision (in which the patient sees two images of everything), the brain suppresses the sight of one eye; the other eye does all the work. The brain structures dependent on the eye that is not working may atrophy (waste away) or fail to develop.

There are usually no obvious symptoms of this form of amblyopia. By the time the condition is recognized, the eye may be permanently damaged. Usually, the child appears to see as well as the next child. Sometimes, however, the condition that causes the amblyopia is very noticeable: the eyes may turn either inward or outward, or one eye may be looking up while the other is looking down.

"Lazy eye" amblyopia may be corrected by using a patch to hinder the vision in the good eye, thus forcing the lazy eye to work.

To fully restore sight in the lazy eye, treatment must begin before the child is four to six years of age. If the eyes are out of focus because some of the muscles of the eye are weaker than others, the condition may be corrected by wearing special glasses or contact lenses, by doing eye exercises, by using eyedrops or a patch to diminish the ability of the normal eye to focus (and thereby force the lazy eye to work), or by surgery. Periodic reexaminations are needed until the child is at least ten years old.

Prevention of lazy-eye amblyopia can begin soon after birth. If the eyes of a baby are continually out of alignment in the first weeks of life or are still out of alignment from time to time at six months of age, the condition should be investigated. A simple eye test given in the doctor's office should show whether one eye is not working properly. Evaluations of this type should not be delayed. The child will not "grow out" of either strabismus or amblyopia.

Toxic amblyopia, which usually occurs in both eyes, can result from excessive drinking of alcoholic beverages over a long period of time (and may be due mainly to the poor nutrition of heavy drinkers, who get most of their calories from alcohol and so do not eat enough nourishing food). It may also be found in heavy cigarette smokers and in people exposed to various chemicals and drugs, including lead, methanol (wood alcohol), digitalis, chloramphenicol, and arsenic. The toxic substance causes swelling and irritation of the optic nerve around the site where it leaves the eyeball. If the irritation continues long enough, it can cause lasting damage to the nerve and eventually even total blindness.

Symptoms include pain on moving the eyeball and an increasing area of poor eyesight in or near the center of the field of vision.

Treatment is to stop exposure to the poison, if it can be discovered. In the case of lead poisoning, the patient is given medicine that combines with the lead and draws it out of the body tissues (this treatment is known as chelation therapy). If the cause is removed at once, vision may improve—unless there has been permanent damage to the optic nerve.

See also Strabismus.

# Amenorrhea

Amenorrhea is the absence of menstruation. There are two categories of this disorder. Primary amenorrhea is the failure to begin menstruating by the age of 16. Secondary amenorrhea, the more common of the two conditions, is the absence of three or more periods in a row in a woman who has been menstruating for some time. Primary amenorrhea is specifically defined at the age of 16 and can go on indefinitely. Secondary amenorrhea is usually a temporary condition; the periods generally resume when the underlying cause for the interruption has been corrected.

Primary amenorrhea may be caused by an endocrine gland disorder (such as hyperthyroidism or hypothyroidism); genetic abnormalities; damaged or missing ovaries, uterus, or vagina; or an excessively thick hymen (the membrane that usually covers the vaginal opening in virgins), which blocks the outflow of the menstrual discharge.

Secondary amenorrhea is caused most commonly by pregnancy. It can also be triggered by strenuous sports training, poor nutrition, drastic weight gain, jet lag, certain medications (including corticosteroids, tranquilizers, and birth control pills), major surgery or serious disease, emotional shock, or the loss of a large percentage of body fat.

Primary amenorrhea is commonly accompanied by abnormal or inhibited physical development; the young girl may fail to develop breasts or body hair, indicating that a genetic disorder may be preventing her from attaining sexual maturity. These girls are also usually short.

Secondary amenorrhea has no symptoms other than the absence of menstrual periods.

Diagnostic evaluation of both types of amenorrhea will probably include a test to rule out pregnancy, tests to detect genetic or hormonal disorders, and X rays or ultrasound studies to check the reproductive organs.

Primary amenorrhea may be treated with an extensive hormone therapy program to stimulate physical development. If the cause is a thick hymen, a minor surgical procedure may be performed to open the hymen. Some cases of primary amenorrhea, however, are untreatable (for example, those due to structural abnormalities of the reproductive organs).

Secondary amenorrhea may be treated with a hormone that will trigger ovulation and reestablish the menstrual cycle. However, quite often this condition will reverse itself without treatment, especially if the cause is merely an interruption in the patient's normal routine, an emotional upset, or pregnancy.

Maintaining good nutritional habits and a normal weight and avoiding overly strenuous sports can probably be beneficial in preventing secondary amenorrhea. No specific precautions can be taken, however, to prevent primary amenorrhea.

See also Anorexia nervosa.

# Amino acids

Amino acids are the main building blocks of proteins and are found in all living cells. There are 20 or more different kinds of amino acids, each of which contains carbon, hydrogen, oxygen, and nitrogen. Each protein molecule is made up of thousands of amino acid molecules, linked to each other in chains.

In the body, food proteins are broken down to their amino acids in the small intestine. The amino acids are then transported through the bloodstream to form, maintain, and repair body protein. Sometimes they are also used as fuel. In the cells, enzymes (special proteins that cause or speed up chemical processes in the body) break down some amino acids into simpler compounds, use some for structure, and form others into chains of new proteins.

Nutritionists divide amino acids into two groups:

- Nonessential amino acids, which can be manufactured by the body if not enough of them are supplied by the diet
- Essential amino acids, which must be included in our diets if we are to remain healthy

Rich sources of amino acids include meat, fish, fowl, eggs, milk, cheese, grains, nuts, and legumes (beans and peas). The proteins from animal sources are much more complete—that is, they contain more essential amino acids in the right proportions—than those from plant sources. Therefore, the person who avoids meat and dairy products should include substantial amounts of two or more plant proteins in each day's meals.

# Amnesia

Amnesia is the loss of memory and the inability to form new memories. It can be either temporary or permanent. The causes may range from brain damage to a psychological reason.

**Retrograde amnesia** This type of amnesia usually follows any severe head injury that produces unconsciousness. The patient is not able to recall what happened immediately before the accident that caused the injury, the accident itself, or some of the events of the recovery period. In most cases  this type of amnesia is not significant because no other memory is affected, and no treatment is needed.

**Korsakoff's syndrome** An inability to record new memory along with a defect in recent memory, usually accompanied by confabulation (storytelling of fabricated events), is known as Korsakoff's syndrome. It may be caused by head injury, stroke, encephalitis (inflammation of the lining of the brain), deficiency of vitamin $B_{12}$, cancer of the brain, or poor blood supply to memory tissue or pathways in the brain. However, heavy drinking of alcohol, with resultant brain damage, is commonly the cause.

Although there may be little or no loss of memory or skills that were acquired before the disease began, the person with Korsakoff's syndrome cannot effectively learn new skills or remember recent events. To hide this loss, from himself or herself as well as from others, the patient may describe imaginary or confused experiences to take the place of the missing experiences. Sometimes the stories are so convincing that the patient appears normal.

Treatment of Korsakoff's syndrome is limited to treating the condition that caused it. Permanent brain damage may make it incurable. Frequently, however, the condition will disappear with time, especially if it was caused by a concussion (a swelling in the head that puts pressure on the brain).

**Psychological amnesia** Amnesia of psychological origin is less common but more dramatic and newsworthy than other forms of amnesia. A man disappears from home, job, and family; he travels to a new place and assumes a new identity—all without being aware that anything has changed. After days or weeks, he "awakens," becomes his old self, and wonders what happened. There is no memory of the period of amnesia.

Anxiety is the cause of this type of amnesia. The person is faced with an intolerable situation of high emotional stress or pain. To protect itself, the mind forgets the anxieties and everything related, including the person's identity.

Treatment may not be necessary, since most affected persons recover without help. However, if the problem that caused the amnesia still remains, it must be faced and solved. Family therapy and change of work or activities may help. Hypnosis may be used to bring back the memory of the "lost days" and unlock the ideas and feelings that caused the original flight from home and self.

# Anaphylactoid reactions

Similar to anaphylaxis in effect (but not in cause) are anaphylactoid reactions, which can occur on the first injection of certain drugs, such as morphine, and of contrast media (special solutions used when performing certain x-ray studies). These are not allergic reactions in the pure sense, but they may be just as serious nevertheless.

Anaphylaxis is said to be present if a person is extremely sensitive to a substance on first exposure. If the person is exposed to the substance again, the result may be anaphylactic shock, an explosive overreaction of the body's immune system. Anaphylactic shock is a violent allergic reaction characterized by itching skin, hives, breathing trouble, collapse of the circulatory system, and sometimes vomiting, diarrhea, and cramps in the abdomen.

Anaphylaxis may be triggered by an insect sting, such as that of a bee or wasp; by animal serum used in a vaccine; by desensitizing injections; or by one of various drugs. The allergen (the substance that sets off the reaction) is usually a protein, called an antigen. When it first enters the body, certain body cells treat it like an invading microorganism and create antibodies, which are protective substances that fight infection. On subsequent exposures to the same antigen, the antibodies are ready for the "invader" and stimulate the release of certain chemicals. One of these chemicals, histamine, causes contraction of muscles in the digestive and respiratory tracts, resulting in abdominal cramps and wheezing. Histamine also causes the small blood vessels to enlarge and lose plasma (blood fluid) to surrounding tissues. The decrease in the volume of blood in the vessels results in a drop in blood pressure, which may lead to shock (collapse of the circulatory system).

Symptoms of anaphylactic shock develop rapidly. Within 15 minutes, the victim becomes uneasy, upset, and red in the face. Rapid heartbeat, prickling and itching sensations in the skin, throbbing in the ears, sneezing, coughing, and breathing difficulty are also likely. Vomiting, incontinence (involuntary release of urine and bowel contents), and even convulsions may occur. In another one or two minutes, shock may result, in which blood vessels collapse, the pulse becomes weak and rapid, and the person becomes cold, clammy, and faint. Without immediate medical aid, death may result.

In cases of anaphylactic shock, medical aid should be obtained as quickly as possible—call an emergency squad. Keep the patient's airway open. Have the patient lie down, with his legs elevated. Immediate treatment with the drug epinephrine is critical. It counteracts the action of the histamine released in the blood, which is causing the symptoms of anaphylactic shock. If a drug injection has caused the reaction, a tourniquet is applied above the site of the injection, and epinephrine is often injected into the site. Antihistamine drugs are also given. In extreme cases, especially when shock has occurred or there is great breathing difficulty, intravenous solutions are given to restore blood volume and raise blood pressure. Anyone with a severe reaction can usually expect to be hospitalized for at least 24 hours to guard against a recurrence of the condition.

A preventive measure against anaphylactic shock is routine allergy skin testing before the use of substances that may cause sensitivity or that have been known to cause anaphylaxis, such as animal serums in vaccines. In addition, anyone who has had an allergic reaction to an insect sting should carry a kit containing a syringe of epinephrine and an epinephrine-filled nasal sprayer for prompt self-treatment if stung again. Desensitizing injections of the insect venom should also be considered to allow the body to build up a resistance to the venom, if the doctor feels that such injections will not trigger an anaphylactic reaction.

See also Allergy and Insect bite and sting.

---

# Anemia

Anemia is a general term referring to a shortage of red blood cells or a reduction in their hemoglobin content. (Hemoglobin is the pigment in the blood that carries oxygen in the red blood cells.) A shortage of red blood cells or hemoglobin means that the blood is unable to carry adequate amounts of oxygen to all parts of the body.

Anemia can be caused by vitamin or mineral deficiencies or an inability to absorb certain vitamins, the destruction of red blood cells, inherited abnormalities in the blood, or the failure of the bone marrow to manufacture enough red blood cells. Such diverse conditions as bleeding ulcers, drug allergies, cancer, and exposure to radioactivity can also lead to anemia. People with poor diets or histories of alcoholism are likely to suffer from one of the types of anemia caused by vitamin and mineral deficiencies. A tendency toward certain types of anemia (for example, sickle cell anemia) can also be inherited.

Among the many symptoms of anemia are fatigue, shortness of breath, pounding heartbeat, rapid heart rate, headaches, loss of appetite, dizziness, ringing in the ears, weakness, and faintness. Burning of the tongue or a change in its appearance may also be a clue. Another sign of anemia may be paleness in the creases of the palms, under the fingernails, and in the lining of the eye. Very severe cases may be signaled by swollen ankles; rapid, weak pulse; pale, clammy skin; and a feeling of fullness in the neck or abdomen.

Diagnosis is based on the findings from a physical examination and tests of the blood (and sometimes the bone marrow) to detect shortages of red blood cells or hemoglobin. A specific diagnosis is necessary because each type of anemia has a different cause and, therefore, a different treatment.

**Iron deficiency anemia** Iron deficiency anemia is caused by a shortage of the mineral iron, which is necessary to produce hemoglobin. This shortage can be caused by a variety of conditions, among them a drastic blood loss, such as from an accident; a chronic blood loss, such as from a bleeding ulcer or colon tumor; hookworm infestation; and choosing a diet lacking in good sources of iron, such as dark green vegetables, egg yolks, meats (especially liver), fish, seafood, and dried peas and beans. Women are particularly susceptible to iron deficiency anemia because of regular loss of blood during menstruation as well as depletion of iron by the fetus during pregnancy. This type of anemia can be treated with iron supplements (ferrous sulfate or ferrous gluconate tablets) after the cause has been determined.

**Folic acid deficiency anemia** Folic acid deficiency is caused by insufficient dietary folic acid, which is necessary for hemoglobin production. This deficiency may be caused or aggravated by malnourishment or alcoholism. Some disorders of the small intestine, such as inflammatory bowel disease, may also cause it. It is treated with folic acid and sometimes additional supplements.

**Pernicious anemia** Pernicious anemia arises if the body is unable to absorb vitamin $B_{12}$, which is necessary for the production of red blood cells in the bone marrow. A substance called intrinsic factor, which helps to absorb vitamin $B_{12}$, is lacking in the stomach of a person suffering from this condition. Inability to absorb vitamin $B_{12}$ can also be caused by some parasites, inflammatory bowel disease, and diseases of the small intestine. Pernicious anemia is treated with vitamin $B_{12}$ injections directly into the bloodstream, bypassing the stomach completely.

**Aplastic anemia** Aplastic anemia is a serious condition caused by the inability of the bone marrow to produce white and red blood cells and platelets. Bone marrow function can be inhibited by cancer or exposure to radioactivity, hazardous chemicals, or some drugs. This variety of anemia is treated with blood transfusions and bone marrow transplants.

**Hemolytic anemias** Hemolytic anemias are caused by the destruction of red blood cells. These anemias can be either acquired (developed over time) or congenital (present at birth).

Acquired hemolytic anemias can be caused by mismatched blood transfusions, a drug allergy, cancer, or a serious infection. Treatment of the primary condition is necessary to treat the resulting anemia. Blood transfusions can treat the condition temporarily.

Congenital hemolytic anemias are caused by an inherited abnormality in the red blood cells. The most common type is sickle cell anemia, a disorder that predominantly affects black persons. In this form of anemia, the red blood cells, which are sickle-shaped instead of disklike, cannot carry enough oxygen throughout the body. These cells are also very fragile and hemolyze (break down) easily. This disease is characterized by crisis periods of severe joint or abdominal pain and can lead to complications, such as kidney disease, gallstones, and heart failure. Sickle cell anemia is treated with painkillers, oxygen, and transfusions. Avoiding situations in which oxygen may be scarce, such as high altitudes, is advisable.

There are no specific methods to prevent anemias other than selecting a balanced diet to prevent those anemias caused by vitamin and mineral deficiencies and obtaining genetic counseling if a hereditary condition is a possibility.

See also Sickle cell anemia.

# Aneurysm

An aneurysm is a bulge in a blood vessel, usually an artery, due to a weakness in the vessel wall, particularly in the elastic, muscular middle layer of the artery wall. An artery has three layers: the intima, which is the smooth inner layer; the media, or middle layer; and the adventitia, which is the tough outer layer. A true aneurysm involves all three layers, whereas a false aneurysm is a disruption or clot in one or two of the layers, causing a bulge in the vessel. A dissecting aneurysm occurs when blood separates the layers, thereby creating an extra channel, sometimes extending the full length of the artery, through which blood flow is diverted from the organs or tissues served by the blood vessel. This dangerous condition can develop in a matter of hours or days.

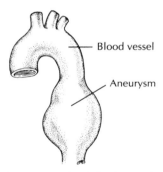

Blood vessel

Aneurysm

An aneurysm is a bulge in an artery due to a weakness in the vessel wall. A true aneurysm involves all three layers of the vessel wall, whereas a false aneurysm is a disruption in one or two of the layers.

The main danger of most untreated aneurysms is that they may rupture, causing death due to loss of blood. Even if death does not occur, blood loss may decrease blood flow to the heart to such an extent that it cannot work properly.

There are various causes of aneurysms. Those occurring in the arteries of the brain are often due to an inherited defect—a weakness or lack of elastic tissue in the media. If an aneurysm in the brain ruptures, a stroke can result. Aneurysms in the small arteries may be caused by blood vessel infections that weaken the vessel wall. Penetrating wounds occasionally can cause aneurysms.

The sexually transmitted disease syphilis may also be a cause of aneurysms. Syphilis can cause vasculitis (inflammation of the smaller arteries that feed a large one). When this occurs, these small arteries are lost, thereby denying nourishment to parts of the large arterial wall and causing scarring and death of tissue. This process leads to weakness of the wall and formation of an aneurysm.

Dissecting aneurysms usually occur in the aorta. Atherosclerosis (hardening of the arteries) is the most common cause, especially in the elderly. If a young person is affected, the condition is usually caused by an inherited defect.

Symptoms of dissecting aneurysms of the aorta, if in the chest, include sudden, severe pain in the area of the aneurysm, often resembling a heart attack. There may be pain under the breastbone or in the back of the neck, difficulty in swallowing, shortness of breath, hoarseness, or a heavy cough. An aneurysm in a neck artery may create a pulsating, swishing sound that the patient can detect.

Evidence of an aneurysm can be a tender, pulsating mass in the abdomen or a painful, tender mass at the back of the knee (the latter can lead to blood clots that can travel downward and may result in death of tissue in the toes). Symptoms of a dissecting aneurysm in the abdomen can include sudden, severe, central or low abdominal pain radiating to the back; a loss of blood flow to the legs; and shock (collapse of circulation, signaled by fainting, pale and clammy skin, and rapid, weak pulse). Death can result quickly.

Computed tomography and ultrasound studies of affected areas are used to locate aneurysms and determine their extent. The most reliable and definitive test is an angiogram (also called an arteriogram). In this procedure, a thin catheter is inserted into an artery in the arm or leg and advanced to the site to be studied; a special dye is then injected through the catheter to outline the area so that X rays may be taken.

Treatment of most aneurysms, especially dissecting aneurysms, should begin as soon as possible. Patients with dissecting aneurysms belong in an intensive care unit. Drugs are given to lower high blood pressure (which worsens a dissecting aneurysm) and thus reduce the chances of rupture. Occasionally, a dissecting aneurysm heals itself if pressure is lessened. Long-term medication that keeps blood pressure low is standard treatment for those who cannot undergo surgery. Surgery, however, is by far the most satisfactory solution when it is possible. The damaged portion of the blood vessel is removed and replaced with a synthetic vessel or a natural vessel taken from elsewhere in the body. Patients with ruptured aortic aneurysms need emergency surgery, as do most patients with dissecting aneurysms. Rapid replacement of blood is necessary, as is intensive monitoring. Surgery for aneurysm repair is usually long and difficult. However, with newer methods of diagnosis, many more people are being spared the risks of surgery by correction of the aneurysm before it becomes a life-threatening problem.

# Angina pectoris

Angina pectoris, usually referred to simply as angina, is a dull constricting pain usually in the center of the chest that indicates that the heart muscle is not getting enough blood and, as a result, is not getting suffi-

cient oxygen. When, during a period of stress or exertion, the oxygen needs of the heart muscle are greater than its blood supply from the coronary arteries can meet, angina occurs. Angina, therefore, is a mechanism for warning the body.

Anginal pain is most often felt in the chest. It can also be felt in the upper part of the abdomen and may extend up the neck and down the arm and hand to the little finger.

An angina attack is not a heart attack. Its pain is usually not as severe or as long-lasting as that experienced during a heart attack, and it does not destroy heart muscle, as does a heart attack. However, those who suffer from this condition are probably more prone to heart attack than are those who do not.

Angina can be caused by any number of factors that prevent the heart muscle from getting enough blood. By far the most common cause of angina is coronary artery narrowing due to atherosclerosis. The coronary arteries supply the heart muscle itself with blood. When an increased demand is placed on the heart by the body, for instance, by exercise, the heart must work harder to supply blood (and thereby oxygen) to keep the muscles and organs nourished. This increased work effort causes the heart muscle itself to require more blood. When narrowing of a coronary artery is present, the areas of heart muscle supplied by that artery cannot get enough blood to keep up with the demand. When this occurs, the muscle reacts by causing the sensation of angina. Exercise, stress, and even cold weather can trigger an attack.

This sensation usually occurs during or after physical exertion or emotional stress, lasts only three to five minutes, and is relieved by resting or relaxing. If the pain does not go away within five minutes or if the pain increases, the condition causing it may not be angina. It may be another disorder unrelated to the heart, or it may be a heart attack.

Overeating and smoking can trigger and aggravate angina—overeating, by drawing much-needed blood to the full stomach to aid in digestion; smoking, by causing the coronary arteries to constrict, thus reducing their diameter and thus their capacity for carrying blood.

Several risk factors are associated with the development of coronary artery disease and angina. A family history of heart disease, smoking, high blood cholesterol levels, and high blood pressure are among the best known. There is much controversy in medicine regarding the degree of impact these factors have. It has not yet been clearly established whether alteration of the last three factors will definitely prevent or delay the onset of heart disease. However, there is much evidence favoring their reduction. Furthermore, common sense dictates that one would make an effort to do so.

The major symptom of angina is the sensation of pressure, squeezing, or burning in the center of the chest behind the breastbone. This discomfort is often compared to that accompanying indigestion. Angina pain may also be felt along the neck, in the jaw or gums, in the upper part of the abdomen, or extending down the arm (most often the left) and hand to the little finger. The location and severity of the pain vary among angina sufferers, but in a given patient the same symptoms usually recur with each episode.

Angina is diagnosed by first eliminating the possibility that the pain is originating from some other disorder, such as gallbladder disease, rib injury, muscle spasm, or pleurisy (an inflammation of the membrane surrounding the lungs and lining the chest cavity). The doctor will take a complete medical history and perform a physical exam and probably a stress test, in which an electrocardiograph (an instrument that records the electrical impulses generated in the heart) is used to evaluate heart function during exercise. This test can indicate abnormalities in the blood supply to the heart.

The most definitive test for the diagnosis of coronary artery disease is coronary angiography (also called coronary arteriography or cardiac catheterization). In this test, radiopaque (which can be seen on X rays) dye is injected through a catheter (tube) placed into the heart through an artery in the leg or arm. Once the dye has been injected, X-ray films are taken, and areas of obstruction to the dye within the coronary arteries can be clearly seen. During this procedure, other important information, such as the overall condition of the heart muscle and its chambers, can also be obtained.

Angina is often treated by recommending changes in the patient's lifestyle to reduce the amount of strain on the heart and by administering medication to modify the relationship of the heart muscle and its blood supply.

A change in lifestyle will be necessary for patients who smoke, overeat, or overexert themselves. Certain types of exercise may be too stressful, but regular exercise is necessary to improve collateral circulation (a system of smaller blood vessels that bypass a blocked artery and increase the blood supply to the area served by that artery). Regular exercise also serves to strengthen the heart muscle and makes it more efficient.

The medication most often used to treat angina attacks is nitroglycerin, which may act by expanding blood vessels to increase blood flow or by altering the volume of blood in the heart. Nitroglycerin is taken as a sublingual tablet that dissolves under the tongue or as an oral spray. Pain should stop within three or four minutes; if it does not, the pain may not be due to simple angina. Nitroglycerin can also be prescribed as a sustained release tablet or capsule, as an ointment, or as a patch applied to the skin. These forms are used for the prevention of attacks, not for the treatment of an acute episode.

Surgery to bypass the obstructions in the coronary arteries is performed only in specific circumstances.

In recent years, the technique of angioplasty has become widely used to treat obstructions that are causing angina pectoris. This procedure consists of inserting a balloon-tipped catheter (tube) into an artery and inflating the balloon at the site of narrowing, thereby decreasing the ob-

struction (the balloon is then deflated and removed). The advantage of this technique is that it saves the patient from having to undergo surgery. Unfortunately, it is not useful in all types of coronary artery disease and can be associated with complications that necessitate emergency surgery. Also, the artery frequently becomes obstructed again, and another angioplasty or surgery must be performed. Laser reduction of plaque and atherectomy (removal of plaque with special catheters) are now also being employed in select circumstances with varying degrees of success.

Incidents of angina can be prevented with several drugs: nitrates (such as nitroglycerin); calcium antagonists (such as diltiazem, nifedipine, and verapamil), which act by blocking the constricting action of calcium on arterial muscle; and beta blockers (such as metoprolol and propranolol), which decrease the work of the heart, thereby lessening its oxygen needs.

See also Atherosclerosis, Coronary bypass surgery, and Heart attack.

# Ankylosing spondylitis

Ankylosing spondylitis is a form of arthritis, mainly affecting the sacroiliac joints, the spine, and nearby structures. Joints become inflamed and eventually stiff and immovable. The elastic cartilage disks between the vertebrae (bones of the spine) become dense, as does adjacent connective tissue. Bony connections form between the vertebrae. The lower vertebrae may become fused together, creating a straight "poker spine," frequently accompanied by a curve in the upper spine.

The cause of ankylosing spondylitis is unknown, but there appears to be an inherited tendency toward the disease. The disease affects men ten times more often than women, and many are born with a certain trait, called HLA-B27, in their blood. Persons carrying this trait are more likely to suffer the disease.

Ankylosing spondylitis is mainly a disease of young men between the ages of 15 and 40. It may progress slowly for 10 to 20 years and then stop or slow down.

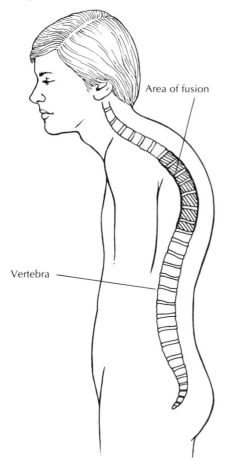

Area of fusion

Vertebra

Ankylosing spondylitis is a form of arthritis in which the vertebrae (bones of the spine) may become fused together, often with a curve in the upper spine.

Chronic low back pain and stiffness in a young man is a chief sign of the disease; hip pain is also quite common, as is an inflammation of the eye known as anterior uveitis. Symptoms begin gradually, usually as low backaches. There may be morning stiffness and pain extending down the leg along the sciatic nerve, commonly alternating from one side to the other. The back pain and stiffness eventually affect the upper spine and sometimes the neck. In up to a third of the cases, large joints (such as those of the hips and shoulders) are affected. Knees and other smaller joints are affected less often, with symptoms matching those of rheumatoid arthritis. The heart is affected in up to three percent of cases (after many years of disease), and inflammation of the lining of the eye occurs in about 25 percent of the cases. As the disease progresses, it is more difficult for the patient to flex the back and expand the chest, and neck movements may be limited. X rays of the back-related joints—especially those between the upper portion of the hip bone and the sacrum (the bony structure at the base of the spine)—reveal changes typical of ankylosing spondylitis. A sign of advanced disease is "bamboo spine," in which bony bands around the disks cement the vertebrae together.

Although there is no cure for ankylosing spondylitis, certain measures can lessen the effects of the disease. These include rest; breathing exercises; and exercises to maintain posture, help with curvature of the upper spine, and keep the back as flexible as possible. To prevent curvature of the upper spine, sleeping on the back on a firm mattress with a small pillow or no pillow is advised. Locking the fingers behind the head and pushing the elbows back as far as possible is a good way to straighten the upper back and stretch the chest muscles. Painkillers and anti-inflammatory drugs may be given. Corticosteroid drugs are generally not prescribed because of their many side effects. Surgery is rarely needed.

# Anorexia nervosa

Anorexia nervosa is an eating disorder that is most common in young women. Anorexics suppress the urge to eat and continue to lose weight to the point of malnutrition and starvation. This disorder can be fatal, because an anorexic can literally starve himself or herself to death.

The reasons for anorexic behavior are still unknown, but theories abound. One theory is that anorexics continue to starve themselves because they mistakenly believe that they are fat and need to diet. The result is not only an unattractively thin appearance but also abnormality of menstrual periods (which very frequently cease when a certain percentage of body fat has been lost) and, most important, the destruction of healthy muscle and organ tissue, which the body uses as sources of energy when faced with starvation.

Ninety-five percent of all anorexics are female; most are teenagers from upper- or upper-middle-class homes. It is estimated that about one in 200 young women of this age and social class has anorexia nervosa.

A person with anorexia nervosa has a distorted body image that makes her think she is fat even when viewing her extremely thin body in a mirror.

Anorexia seems to be mostly a psychiatric disorder, since it often develops in young women with deep-seated problems, although the classic anorexic may not seem to be a "troubled" teenager. The young girl who has always been "perfect" and obedient and who has tried to fulfill all the wishes of her parents, teachers, and friends may become anorexic because of an unconscious need to have total control over at least one area of her life.

Impending adulthood and all that it entails may scare the anorexic into dieting away those characteristics that are symbolic of her developing maturity—larger breasts, fuller hips and thighs, and the monthly cycle of menstrual periods.

Our culture's obsession with thinness as the ideal in beauty can also trigger in an adolescent girl a desire to diet down to her "perfect" weight; often a casual remark that a girl is slightly overweight can lead to a case of anorexia in a susceptible person.

In addition, people with jobs or hobbies that require strict weight control, such as athletes, ballerinas, and fashion models, may begin to find that simply watching their weight has become an obsession with dieting. In fact, the few males who develop this disorder often do so in an attempt to qualify for an athletic team.

The most obvious symptom of anorexia nervosa is drastic weight loss to the point of extreme underweight, which can be accompanied by overly vigorous exercise that burns off the few calories that are consumed. Menstrual periods often stop completely, and a growth of fine, downy hair appears all over the body.

Anorexics cannot be convinced to eat by threats or reasoning. Many have a distorted body image that tells them they are fat even as they view their extremely thin bodies in a mirror. Despite the refusal to eat more than tiny amounts of particular foods, the anorexic may be obsessed with the idea of food and may prepare elaborate meals for others. The anorexic may also suffer from another eating disorder, bulimia, which is characterized by binge-eating, followed by self-induced vomiting and excessive use of laxatives and/or diuretics.

Diagnostic evaluation of anorexia nervosa begins by ruling out the possibility that the extreme weight loss has been caused by a serious physical illness, such as cancer, an infectious disease, a disorder of the digestive organs, or inadequate absorption of vitamins and minerals. Anorexia can usually be diagnosed when the patient displays the classic symptoms before the age of 25 and has lost 25 percent of her body weight.

Anorexia is sometimes treated with hospitalization and forced feeding, but anorexics can usually be treated on an outpatient basis by a medical doctor, psychiatrist, or specialist in eating disorders. The anorexic's distorted body image as well as her eating habits must be changed in order for her to conquer this disorder. Most important, the underlying psychological problems must be resolved. Often, this means psychological therapy for both the anorexic and her family.

See also Bulimia.

# Antibody/antigen

Antibodies are manufactured by the lymph system. Antibodies are specialized proteins that the body produces in response to invasion by a foreign substance. The process of antibody formation begins when an antigen stimulates specialized lymphocytes, called B cells, into action. Antibodies then counteract invading antigens by combining with the antigen to ultimately render it harmless to the body. Some antibodies coat the harmful organisms so that the body's scavenger cells can destroy them more easily. The antibody molecule combines with the antigen molecule by matching combining sites; they fit together like the pieces of a jigsaw puzzle. Other antibodies that neutralize toxins produced by bacteria are called antitoxins.

During periods of active antibody production, lymph nodes often enlarge and become tender to the touch. For example, a vaccination (injection of a natural or artificial antigen to stimulate the body to produce protective antibodies) in the arm can cause swelling of the nodes in the armpit, while mononucleosis causes enlargement of nodes that can be felt under the skin of the armpits, groin, and neck. The spleen (an organ located in the upper left part of the abdomen) is also important in the production of antibodies.

Production of white blood cells and antibodies in reaction to an invading disease organism is called an immune response. This response is one of the body's primary and most efficient lines of defense. In most cases, once antibodies have been produced to fight a certain organism, it no longer poses a great threat to the body. That is why one attack of a disease often prevents that same disease from infecting the body again—the first attack causes production of antibodies that protect the body against subsequent attacks. With measles, for example, antibodies are produced as a result of having the disease or of being immunized with the measles vaccine. These antibodies are able to resist a second attack of the disease, providing protection against recurrence.

Antibodies are not always beneficial. For example, when tissue from another body, such as a transplanted heart, is introduced, antibodies are produced to destroy the "invader." Transplants usually are made possible only by means of drugs that act against the body's natural immune response. Also, when blood is transfused from one person to another, it must be of a matching type; otherwise, the recipient's immune system will manufacture antibodies to destroy the transfused blood.

Sometimes, the immune system causes reactions that make the body unusually sensitive to foreign material. When the immune response is disruptive to the body in this way, it is called an allergic reaction.

An antigen is a substance that can provoke an immune (protective) response by the body. An antigen promotes the manufacture of antibodies that will interact only with that antigen. On the surfaces of all cells are numerous antigens, which cause production of different antibodies. The major blood groups (types A, B, AB, and O) are differentiated on the basis of the presence on the red blood cells of two of those surface antigens: type A blood has antigen A, type B has antigen B, type AB has both antigen A and antigen B, and type O has neither antigen A nor antigen B. A person's blood type must be identified before a blood transfusion can be given because his or her blood may reject transfused blood of the wrong type. Type A blood plasma contains anti-B antibodies but no anti-A antibodies. If type B blood is transfused, the anti-B antibodies in the plasma will destroy the type B red cells, which have type B antigens.

# Apgar score

The Apgar score is a general evaluation of a baby's condition, made soon after birth, to determine immediately whether the newborn needs emergency care. The Apgar scoring system was devised by the late Virginia Apgar, M.D., and the letters of her last name are an acronym for the factors being scored.

At one minute and five minutes after an infant's birth, a delivery room nurse, anesthesiologist, obstetrician, or pediatrician rates five factors, using a scale of 0 to 2:

A (Appearance)—A score of 2 is given if the skin is completely pink; 1 if it is pink except for the hands and feet, which are bluish; and 0 if the entire body is blue (indicating lack of oxygen).

P (Pulse)—A score of 2 is given for a pulse above 100; 1 for a rate of less than 100; 0 for no pulse.

G (Grimace, or reflex irritability)—A score of 2 is given if the baby cries vigorously when slapped lightly on the soles of the feet; 1 if the baby makes only a grimace or slight cry; 0 if there is no response.

A (Activity)—An active infant is given a score of 2; an infant who makes some movement of arms and legs, 1; a limp and motionless infant receives a score of 0.

R (Respiration)—Strong efforts to breathe, together with vigorous crying, score a 2; slow, irregular breathing, 1; no breathing, 0.

Most babies score between 7 and 10 when tested one minute after birth. They are breathing well, crying, pinkish in color, active, and need no emergency measures.

Those babies who score from 4 to 6 usually need help immediately. The throat is suctioned to remove thick mucus, small blood clots, or bits of swallowed membrane (from the amniotic sac that enclosed the baby before birth). Oxygen may be given to assist breathing and restore color.

The baby with an Apgar score of less than 4 is limp, pale or bluish, and perhaps without a heartbeat, and is in grave danger. The throat is suctioned, and the baby is placed on a mechanical respirator, which pumps air in and out of the lungs until the baby can breathe on his or her own once again.

A second Apgar score is determined five minutes after birth and recorded on the baby's chart beside the first score. The second score is a good measure of the baby's adaptation to the world outside the womb.

# Apnea

Apnea is strictly defined as the absence of breathing. The term is also used to refer to an interruption in breathing that occurs in some premature babies and also during the sleep of some children and adults.

The usual cause of apnea in infants is immaturity of the brain centers that regulate breathing. From time to time, the infant suddenly stops breathing completely and turns blue. If the baby is stimulated in some way (for example, by a flick of the finger on the bottom of the foot), he or she will usually start breathing normally at once. Seldom is it necessary to use first-aid measures or a mechanical respirator to restart breathing. However, because a history of apnea is one of the factors that may be associated with sudden infant death syndrome (SIDS), physicians sometimes recommend monitoring high-risk infants with equipment that sounds an alarm if any stoppage of breathing is detected. In some cases, the tendency toward apnea disappears a few weeks after birth, when the breathing control centers have matured.

Apnea in children and adults is generally less immediately life-threatening than apnea in infants, but it can be physically exhausting and, in a severe form, can cause cardiovascular and respiratory problems. In some patients, episodes of sleep apnea can cause the concentration of carbon dioxide in the blood to build up to a dangerously high level.

Recognition of the problem generally cannot be made by the patient. A spouse or parent may be the first to notice an abnormal sleep pattern—for example, loud snoring, followed by silence (when the breathing stops), and then a loud choke or gasp as the sleeper partially awakens, clears the air passage, and resumes breathing. Such a pattern may be repeated many times during the night. As a result, persons with sleep apnea are likely to be drowsy during the day and irritable due to lack of sleep, with decreased memory and attention span. A definitive diagnosis can be made after observation in a hospital sleep laboratory.

In children and adults, apnea may occur because of a disorder in the breathing control centers in the brain, or it may be a result of physical abnormalities of the chest, neck, and back due to obesity; the presence of a disease process; or an inborn structural defect. If apnea is due to an abnormality of the breathing control centers, drugs may be prescribed, or stimulation of the diaphragm (the large muscle separating the chest and abdominal cavities, which is instrumental in breathing) with an electronic pacemaker may be tried. Obesity is a common cause of sleep apnea in adults because the presence of excess tissue may block the airway in certain sleeping positions; the disorder may disappear after weight loss. If a physical abnormality due to disease or a structural defect is the cause, surgical treatment may be necessary; for example, enlarged tonsils and adenoids that are partially obstructing the upper airway may be removed. In extreme cases of airway obstruction, the only solution may be tracheostomy (surgical creation of a hole in the trachea and neck, through which the patient can breathe).

# Appendicitis

Appendicitis is an inflammation of the appendix, frequently caused by some type of hard material getting lodged at its tip.

The appendix is a small, tubular structure located at the end of the right colon (large intestine). Although it may have had a function at some point in evolutionary development, the appendix serves no purpose now.

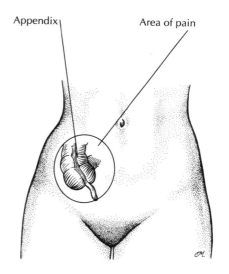

Appendix                    Area of pain

In appendicitis, the lower right side of the abdomen often becomes painful and tender.

Despite its uselessness, the appendix can cause problems when it becomes inflamed. Inflammation occurs when the hollow, tubular structure becomes clogged with masses of waste matter, intestinal worms, or other material that can prevent normal drainage. The blockage provides a fertile environment for bacteria to grow and multiply, thereby causing infection and inflammation.

In the beginning, appendicitis may produce a dull or sharp pain in the navel area of the abdomen. Any movement, coughing, or sneezing can intensify the pain. In early stages, patients may also feel nauseated and may be unable to eat. Constipation can accompany appendicitis; however, about ten percent of patients have diarrhea instead. Adults may run a mild fever (up to 101°F), but children generally experience higher fevers. Occasionally, the pulse rate accelerates to about 100 beats per minute.

Within hours, the pain moves to the lower right side of the abdomen over the appendix and becomes continuous. Because the location of the appendix may vary from one individual to another, pain may emanate from the back, side, or pelvis—or even from the opposite side of the abdomen. The entire area around the appendix becomes extremely tender as abdominal muscles tighten.

As the fever rises and the pain grows more intense, chances of rupture also become greater. Rupture results when the appendix becomes so swollen and filled with pus that it bursts, spreading infection to surrounding organs. One serious complication of rupture is peritonitis (inflammation of the lining of the abdominal cavity).

Any fever with nausea and abdominal pain should be reported to a physician. More severe pain is an immediate medical emergency that must be evaluated and treated to prevent potential complications. Appendicitis can affect anyone, but the disease is more prevalent among persons who are between 10 and 30 years of age.

When confirming appendicitis, the doctor checks for tenderness over the appendix. A blood test determines whether there is an elevated white blood cell count (in response to infection, the body produces extra white blood cells to help fight the disease). The doctor may perform additional tests to rule out disorders sometimes mistaken for appendicitis, such as inflammation of the gallbladder, kidney stones, or a kidney infection. In women, a twisted ovarian cyst (the formation on an ovary of a sac filled with fluid or semisolid material) or a ruptured ectopic pregnancy (a pregnancy that develops outside the uterus) may produce symptoms similar to those of appendicitis.

Although appendicitis cannot be prevented, prompt diagnosis can lead to effective treatment. Patients who suspect appendicitis should not eat, drink, or take drugs to relieve pain until a doctor has been consulted. Eating or drinking any substance, especially taking a laxative, will stimulate activity in the intestine, which may cause the appendix to rupture.

The most common treatment for acute appendicitis is surgery to remove the inflamed organ. To ensure against further infection, antibiotics may also be prescribed after surgery.

# Arrhythmia

See Heartbeat irregularities.

# Arteriosclerosis

See Atherosclerosis.

# Arthritis

Arthritis is an inflammation of the joints (the junctures where the ends of two or more bones meet).

Normal joint

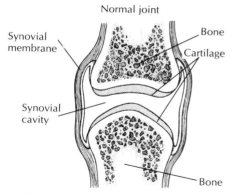

Synovial membrane

Bone

Cartilage

Synovial cavity

Bone

The normal joint is lined by a synovial membrane, which produces the lubricating synovial fluid that fills the synovial cavity. The bone ends are covered by cartilage.

Osteoarthritis

Bone ends may rub together

Eroded cartilage

In osteoarthritis, the cushioning cartilage at the ends of bones wears away or erodes, allowing the bone ends to rub together, which causes swelling and pain.

Rheumatoid arthritis

Inflamed swollen synovium

Rheumatoid arthritis is characterized by swelling and inflammation of the synovial membrane.

Inflammation develops in various ways. With osteoarthritis, there is gradual wearing away of cartilage in the joints. Healthy cartilage is the elastic tissue that lines and cushions the joints and allows bones to move smoothly against one another. When this cartilage deteriorates, the bones rub together, causing pain and swelling. Permanent damage and stiffness of the joints are possible. Although osteoarthritis can result from direct injury to the joint, it commonly occurs in adults over the age of 55 due to long-term wear and tear on the joints.

Rheumatoid arthritis can attack at any age. This form of arthritis affects all the connective tissues, as well as other organs, in the body. The precise cause of rheumatoid arthritis is unknown. Some researchers believe that a virus triggers the disease, causing an autoimmune response whereby the body develops an allergy to its own tissues. However, evidence for this theory is inconclusive as yet. What is confirmed is the progression of the condition. First, the synovium (the thin membrane lining and lubricating the joint) becomes inflamed. The inflammation eventually destroys the cartilage. As scar tissue gradually replaces the damaged cartilage, the joint becomes misshapen and rigid.

Rheumatoid arthritis may damage the heart, lungs, nerves, and eyes. Osteoarthritis can cause permanent damage, stiffness, and deformity of the joints.

Arthritis is not an inherited disease. Nonetheless, people who have a family history of arthritis are more likely to develop the disease. Women are at greater risk than men, although the reason for this is unclear. Excess body weight may promote osteoarthritis because of increased load on the joints. Constant joint abuse may encourage arthritis, but inactivity can also aggravate the problem.

Symptoms of arthritis include swelling, tenderness, pain, stiffness, and redness in one or more joints. For many patients, pain is greatest in the morning and subsides as the day progresses. Damp weather and emotional stress do not actually cause arthritis, but these factors often make symptoms worse.

With rheumatoid arthritis, these symptoms may be accompanied by more generalized feelings of fatigue and fever. This form of arthritis may go into periods of remission, when symptoms disappear. When symptoms return, however, they are often more severe.

To diagnose arthritis, a physician observes the symptoms and administers a standard physical examination. X-ray studies and laboratory tests may be recommended for confirmation of joint swelling and determination of the extent of damage.

The most effective treatment program for arthritis consists of drug therapy, exercise, and rest. Treatment should begin early after diagnosis to prevent permanent damage.

Aspirin is the drug most commonly administered for arthritis. Taking two or three tablets several times a day is often recommended to reduce inflammation and relieve pain. If stomach irritation is a problem, aspirin may be taken after meals or in a coated tablet form. Nonaspirin pain relievers and nonsteroidal anti-inflammatory drugs (such as ibuprofen, naproxen, and sulindac) may also be prescribed. Corticosteroids relieve inflammation, but they can cause adverse side effects. Sometimes, a doctor needs to try several different drugs before finding an effective one that produces few side effects. Oral or injectable gold, when determined to be indicated by a physician, may prove helpful in treating rheumatoid arthritis. Some drugs usually used for cancer chemotherapy, such as methotrexate, may also be helpful.

Moderate daily exercise, such as swimming, walking, or physical therapy, is critical to maintaining mobility in arthritic joints. A supervised exercise program interspersed with rest periods helps to reduce joint inflammation. To lessen pain while increasing movement, moist heat often helps. In addition, maintaining correct posture and body weight reduces the extra burden on sore joints.

Some severe cases of rheumatoid arthritis may require surgery to remove inflamed synovial tissue. With either form of arthritis, artificial joints may be implanted to replace those damaged beyond repair.

# Artificial insemination

Artificial insemination is the introduction of semen (the fluid containing sperm) into a woman's vagina or uterus by means other than sexual intercourse (usually with a special syringe) at or before the time of ovulation in the hope of achieving fertilization. The semen may be from the woman's partner or from a donor.

Artificial insemination using semen from the partner is sometimes done when he has a low sperm count—that is, when there are not enough sperm per unit of fluid to be likely to fertilize an egg. To obtain enough sperm, several collections may be made over a period of days or weeks; the sperm obtained is frozen, pooled, and used in one insertion. Artificial insemination may also be used when one or the other partner cannot perform the sexual act in a normal manner, perhaps because of a physical condition or an emotional problem.

Artificial insemination using semen from a donor can be an alternative to adoption when the partner cannot father a child, whether because of low sperm count, absence of sperm, poor quality of sperm, or lack of motion by sperm or because of inability to perform sexual intercourse. It may also be considered when the partner carries a genetic defect that he does not want to transmit.

# Asthma

Asthma is a respiratory disorder marked by unpredictable periods of acute breathlessness and wheezing. Asthma attacks can last from less than an hour to a week or more and can strike frequently or only every few years. Attacks may be mild or severe and can occur at any time, even during sleep.

The difficult breathing occurs when the small respiratory tubes called bronchioles constrict or become clogged with mucus or when the membranes lining the bronchioles become swollen. When this happens, stale air cannot be fully exhaled but stays trapped in the lungs, so that less fresh air can be inhaled.

Asthma attacks can result from oversensitivity of the bronchial system to a variety of outside substances or conditions. About half of all attacks are triggered by allergies to such substances as dust, smoke, pollen, feathers, pet hair, insects, mold spores, and a variety of foods and drugs. Attacks not related to allergies can be set off by exercise, breathing cold air, stress, and infections, particularly those of the respiratory tract. Heredity may play a part in the tendency to develop asthma; if one or both of a child's parents are asthmatic, he or she has up

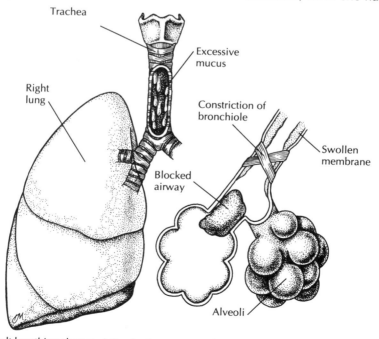

The difficult breathing characteristic of asthma occurs when the small respiratory tubes (bronchioles) constrict or become clogged with mucus, or when the membranes lining the tubes become swollen. Stale air is trapped in the alveoli, and less fresh air can be inhaled.

to a 50 percent chance of developing the condition.

Asthma is rarely fatal, but it can be a very serious condition, especially in young children. Attacks often become less frequent and less severe as a child grows.

Some of the common symptoms of an asthma attack include tightness in the chest, difficulty in breathing, coughing, and wheezing, which is caused by the effort to push air through the narrowed bronchioles. As the attack progresses, muscles surrounding the bronchioles constrict further, breathing becomes even more difficult, and mucus collects in the airways.

Diagnostic procedures may include a complete physical examination and medical history, chest X ray, and allergy testing.

Asthma, for the most part, cannot be cured, but it can be controlled with a variety of drugs. Epinephrine or isoproterenol may be given by injection or inhaled as an aerosol during an acute attack in order to enlarge the bronchioles; however, these drugs may overstimulate the heart and so cannot be used for long periods or by many people with heart conditions. (Individuals on beta-blocking drugs, such as propranolol, are also susceptible to complications from the use of epinephrine and should inform the treating physician that they are taking a beta blocker.) Similar drugs, such as metaproterenol, albuterol, and terbutaline, exert much less of a stimulating effect on the heart and can, therefore, be administered in a larger group of individuals. These drugs can be taken in an oral tablet form but are more commonly used in their aerosol form, which delivers the greatest effect in the bronchial system itself. They act by dilating or relieving the spasm of the bronchial tubes. A new aerosol form of an older drug,

atropine, which blocks certain nerve impulses, probably acts in a similar fashion.

For long-term therapy, the drug theophylline can be used to help keep the bronchioles open. Its dosage, however, must be closely supervised because its rate of absorption into the body varies widely among patients: some persons eliminate the drug so quickly that it is almost ineffective; in others, the drug accumulates in the body, at times to toxic levels. Nausea, vomiting, and agitation are common side effects.

Corticosteroids can control asthma very effectively, but patients may experience such undesirable side effects as weight gain, ulcers, and high blood pressure. Stunting of growth has been reported in children. Consequently, corticosteroids such as prednisone are usually used in large doses in an acute attack and then are tapered as rapidly as possible. Some individuals, however, need relatively low doses chronically. Frequently, aerosol forms of corticosteroids are used to keep the asthmatic as "attack-free" as possible. Since there is less absorption of cortisone into the body with these forms, the likelihood of side effects is lessened.

Cromolyn, a drug that actually prevents attacks, acts to inhibit the release of histamines (the substances produced by the body during an allergic reaction). Cromolyn, however, cannot relieve an attack already in progress.

If an allergy is causing the attacks, the troublesome substance (called an allergen) must be removed from the patient's environment. If this cannot be done or if there are multiple allergies, injections of minute amounts of the allergen may help the body build tolerance to the allergen.

Although there is no way to prevent asthma, several precautions can be taken to reduce the possibility that asthma attacks will occur. Allergy testing to determine sensitivity to common environmental agents such as dust, mold, pet hair, and pollen can be done by a physician. Once allergy is determined, desensitization injections can be tried. Rapid treatment of upper respiratory tract infections can help prevent severe attacks. Chronic preventative medication in known asthmatics will at least lessen the frequency and severity of attacks. With proper medical therapy and supervision, most asthmatics can lead normal lives.

See also Allergy.

# Astigmatism

Astigmatism is a type of distorted vision caused by a defect in the curvature of the cornea or lens of the eye. This prevents the rays of light entering the eye from being properly focused onto the retina at the back of the eyeball. Some rays are misplaced, causing the image to be partially out of focus.

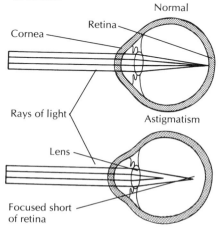

Astigmatism is a form of distorted vision in which rays of light entering the eye are not properly focused on the retina because of a defect in the curvature of the lens or the cornea. This can be corrected by wearing eyeglasses or contact lenses.

Most people with astigmatism can see clearly those objects directly in front of them, but their peripheral vision is defective. They may have vertical astigmatism, in which the areas above and below their direct gaze are imperfectly visualized. They may have horizontal astigmatism, in which the right and left sides of their field of vision are warped (for example, a straight horizontal line may appear curved to the right and to the left). The astigmatism may also be diagonal.

Fortunately, a defect in the curvature of the cornea or lens is usually uniform and can be easily corrected by eyeglasses or contact lenses. The fault is usually in the shape of the cornea (the clear "window" in front of the iris and pupil of the eye), which may be slightly flattened vertically or horizontally. The eyeglass lenses or contact lenses are curved to adjust the angle of rays entering regions of the eye that are defective; they do not bend the rays entering the areas of clear vision.

Although most people with astigmatism were born with a tendency toward the condition, a few cases are caused by eye disease or injury. These may be more difficult to correct. Regardless of the cause, astigmatism—as with any vision problem—should be corrected as early as possible. Children, in particular, are at risk for development of permanently defective vision if astigmatism goes uncorrected.

See also Amblyopia and Myopia.

# Ataxia

Ataxia is a condition characterized by muscular incoordination, producing irregular and inaccurate movements of the body. The result may be a clumsy manner of walking, with feet wide apart; a lack of balance; tremor (shakiness) of the arms; and slurring of speech.

Ataxia may be caused by anything that affects the motor control centers of the brain or the nerve pathways leading from them. Drunkenness can produce a temporary staggering ataxia. Permanent ataxia is caused by damage to the brain, spinal cord, or spinal nerves.

Locomotor ataxia may be a late result of untreated syphilis. Its symptoms include sharp, stabbing pains, usually in the legs; an unsteady walk; and a feeling of walking on foam rubber. There may be an increased sensitivity of the skin, sometimes with burning, prickling, creeping, or crawling sensations.

Ataxia occurs in one case in ten of cerebral palsy, which is a movement disorder caused by damage to the brain or nerve pathways before or around the time of birth. Weakness, unsteadiness, clumsy walking, and difficulty with fine or rapid movements are typical. Physical and occupational therapy help patients handle daily life despite their condition.

Ataxia may also be caused by any one of a group of hereditary diseases that attack the central nervous system. They cause degeneration of the spinal cord and cerebellum (the portion of the brain responsible for fine control of muscle movements) and also frequently damage the brain stem (the portion of the brain that controls the most basic body functions, such as breathing and circulation) and various nerves. Inherited disorders of body chemistry and body chemicals are believed to be involved, but little is known about them. Only one of these disorders—Refsum's syndrome—can be treated, by reducing the excessive level of a body chemical known as phytanic acid.

Symptoms of hereditary ataxias include unsteadiness in walking, tremor of the arms, muscle weakness, and wasting away of muscles. Various other abnormalities may be present, depending on the disease. For example, Friedreich's ataxia, the most common form, causes scoliosis (curvature of the spine) and damages heart tissue.

All of these diseases continue throughout life. With the exception of Refsum's syndrome, none can be treated effectively.

See also Cerebral palsy.

# Atherosclerosis

Atherosclerosis is a slow, progressive disease of the arteries in which fatty deposits partially clog or totally block blood flow. Atherosclerosis is the most common form of arteriosclerosis (hardening of the arteries) and a major cause of coronary artery disease.

Atherosclerosis occurs when the normally smooth, firm linings of the arteries become roughened, thickened, and clogged by deposits of fat, fibrin (a protein involved in blood clotting), calcium, and cellular debris. The condition develops gradually. Lipids (fats), necessary for the production of certain hormones and tissues and as an energy reserve, are constantly present in the bloodstream. When the lipid concentration is greatly increased, however, fatty streaks form along the artery walls. These streaks can cause the development of small nodules of fatty deposits of cholesterol to jut out from the normally smooth linings of the artery walls. Fibrous scar tissue grows under these nodules and attracts calcium deposits. Accumulated calcium develops into a hard, chalky film (called plaque) that cannot be removed. This permanent lining inside the arteries hampers their ability to expand and contract properly and slows the blood flow through the narrowed channels. Clots may then form easily, hindering or preventing the blood from traveling through the artery.

The exact cause of this process has not been pinpointed, but major risk factors have been identified: hyperlipidemia (abnormally elevated concentrations of fats in the blood), hypertension (high blood pressure), a history of smoking, and a family history of atherosclerosis (occurring before the age of 60) or diabetes mellitus. Hyperlipidemia, which promotes the formation of fatty streaks, seems to result from choosing a diet high in saturated fats (fats that are usually solid at room temperature, including all animal fats, such as those found in butter and meats) and cholesterol. Hypertension increases the risk of atherosclerosis because it puts constant strain on the arteries, which speeds

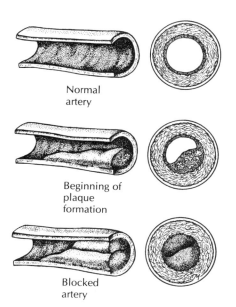

Normal artery

Beginning of plaque formation

Blocked artery

Atherosclerosis occurs when the normally smooth, firm linings of the arteries become roughened, thickened, and clogged with deposits of fat, calcium, and cellular debris, which develop into a hard film called plaque. This deposit eventually may build up and block the artery.

up the clogging and hardening process. Smoking narrows and probably damages the arteries, thus restricting blood flow and setting the stage for atherosclerosis. Diabetes is associated with accelerated atherosclerosis, particularly of small arteries.

Atherosclerosis alone has no visible symptoms. The disease often remains undetected until the arteries leading to a vital organ are blocked. The symptoms that then become apparent are those of the specific condition caused by arterial blockage in that organ. For example, if an artery supplying the heart is partially blocked, angina (chest pain) may be felt; if the artery is totally blocked, heart attack (the death of heart tissue that is supplied by the artery) can result. If atherosclerosis affects an artery in the head, the person may experience dizziness, blurred vision, and faintness, or may suffer a stroke (death of brain tissue supplied by the blocked artery, causing neurologic deficit such as paralysis of the limb[s] controlled by that part of the brain). Kidney failure can develop from obstruction in the arteries leading to the kidneys. Blindness can result from obstruction of vessels leading to the eyes. Diseases of the extremities can result from blockage of their arteries.

Diagnostic evaluation begins with a medical history, physical examination, and analysis of the blood. An exercise tolerance test, or stress test, using an electrocardiograph (an instrument that records the electrical impulses generated in the heart) may indicate whether areas of the heart muscle are damaged or have inadequate blood supply. Nuclear medicine studies and angiography may pinpoint obstructions in blood vessels or areas of the body that are insufficiently supplied with blood. Nuclear medicine studies are X rays taken after the injection of radioisotopes into the bloodstream. Angiography is a procedure in which a thin catheter is inserted into an artery in the arm or leg and advanced to the site to be studied; a special dye is then injected through the catheter to outline the area so that X rays may be taken. Magnetic resonance imaging (MRI) is now in its early stages and may eventually offer a less invasive alternative to conventional angiography with a catheter.

Treatment of this disorder is aimed at reducing the strain on the heart and increasing blood flow to affected organs. Medications, changes in lifestyle and eating habits, and surgery may each be helpful.

Anticoagulants may be prescribed to prevent clotting of the blood. If atherosclerosis has led to angina, nitrates (such as nitroglycerin) and calcium-channel blockers (such as diltiazem, nifedipine, and verapamil) may provide relief by expanding the arteries and increasing blood flow. If high blood pressure contributes to the problem, antihypertensive medication is prescribed. There are not yet any medications that will actually dissolve deposits that are clogging arteries.

Lifestyle changes include quitting smoking, reducing saturated fat and cholesterol intake, losing weight (obesity puts a strain on the heart), and maintaining a moderate (but not strenuous) exercise program (exercise helps develop the collateral circulation, a system of smaller blood vessels that bypass a blocked artery and increase the blood supply to the area served by that artery).

Delicate surgical procedures, called endarterectomies, may be performed to remove deposits that are blocking arteries to vital organs. These procedures can be performed on relatively large vessels entering the brain, heart, kidneys, and legs, but usually cannot remove deposits in small blood vessels of these struc-

tures. If the patient suffers from severe and recurrent chest pain that is not relieved by medication, surgery may be performed to bypass major obstructions in arteries.

Recently, angioplasty (the opening of a vessel via inflation of a tiny balloon at the end of a catheter) has been quite successful in opening arteries to the kidneys and legs. Prior to this procedure, an angiogram must be performed to determine if the individual is an appropriate candidate.

See also Angina, Coronary bypass surgery, Heart attack, Hypertension, and Stroke.

---

# Athlete's foot

Athlete's foot (known medically as *tinea pedis*) is a fungal infection of the foot. It is also known as ringworm of the foot, although it is not caused by a worm.

Athlete's foot causes itching, burning, and stinging sensations. The skin between the toes reddens, cracks open, and crumbles. In extremely longlasting cases, the toenails may become infected, discolored, and overgrown. The fungus may spread to the underside of the foot, beneath the arch, producing groups of itching blisters and peeling of the skin.

It is important to rule out other causes of similar symptoms. For example, hot, tight shoes may make feet sweaty in warm weather; the moisture and friction may cause softening and peeling of the skin on the soles. Dyes, adhesive cements, and other substances inside the shoes may cause irritation, as may powders and nail polishes. Eczema, psoriasis, and scabies are other possible causes of similar symptoms.

Most people can treat athlete's foot at home using one of several good salves, powders, or liquids that may be readily acquired without a prescription from the drugstore in your neighborhood. These include undecylenic acid ointment, tolnaftate, and miconazole. Clotrimazole is another effective medication, but it must be prescribed by a physician. Directions for use normally call for application morning and night, to continue until one week after all symptoms have vanished. As long as loose skin remains, the feet should be soaked before the ointment is applied, and the loose skin removed carefully.

If sweaty feet are the cause, athlete's foot ointments should not be used. Instead, you should ask your doctor for suggestions about controlling the excessive sweating. Changing shoes may eliminate the problem if the feet are sensitive to chemicals inside the shoes.

Severe cases of athlete's foot call for treatment by a physician. To relieve symptoms, the doctor may prescribe soaking the feet three times a day in a solution of aluminum sulfate and calcium acetate (often called Burow's solution), with an antiseptic solution added if a secondary infection is present.

Athlete's foot can recur despite any treatment, especially during hot weather. The organisms that cause athlete's foot thrive in a hot, moist setting. However, there are several things you can do to help prevent the disease. In the first place, you can keep your feet clean, dry between your toes after bathing, and change socks frequently. Use dusting and drying powders to keep the feet dry. In addition, you should separate your toes with small wads of cotton when you are sleeping. Wear wooden or rubber clogs in motel and community showers and wear sandals, opentoed shoes, or no shoes at all (when safe and practical) during hot weather.

# Attention deficit hyperactivity disorder

Attention deficit hyperactivity disorder (ADHD) is a nervous disorder that usually affects children. The condition is characterized by very high levels of physical activity, consistently impulsive and immature behavior, and an extremely short attention span. Because of these behavioral patterns, the condition is also known as minimal brain dysfunction and, in common usage, hyperactivity.

Although ADHD does no physical damage to the body, it can trigger longlasting social, emotional, and educational problems. Because affected children cannot sit still and concentrate for long periods, they may have trouble with schoolwork. They often appear to be immature, uncoordinated, and boisterous and may have trouble getting along with classmates, teachers, and parents; consequently, they often suffer from a poor self-image.

The cause of ADHD is not known, but several theories have been proposed in recent years. None of these theories has been proved or disproved.

The condition may result from a nervous system malfunction or a deficiency of neurotransmitters (chemicals in the brain that transmit impulses between the nerves). According to one theory, based on the supposition that the brain has two systems for responding to situations—one that prompts immediate action and one that encourages hesitation and consideration—the neurotransmitters that control the hesitation response are malfunctioning in the child with ADHD. In some cases, damage to a fetus during pregnancy or a complication of childbirth may have caused a neurologic defect.

Because the condition is four to five times more common in boys than in girls, some researchers believe that the tendency toward ADHD may be inherited as a sex-linked hereditary trait. Support for a genetic basis for ADHD comes from the finding that parents who had ADHD as children tend to have children with ADHD.

ADHD appears to occur more commonly in children of mothers who drank excessive amounts of alcohol or used cocaine during pregnancy. It has also been suggested that the additives, preservatives, and colorings found in processed foods may have a toxic or allergic effect on some children, but no hard evidence is available to support this view.

A variety of symptoms point to ADHD. The child with ADHD is overly active, fidgety, restless, overly talkative or boisterous, impulsive, and seemingly uncoordinated. In school, this child has a very short attention span and seems to forget facts quickly, disrupts the classroom, does schoolwork hastily and incorrectly, skips or adds words when reading, laughs too loud and hard, and prefers to play with younger children.

There are no specific tests to diagnose ADHD. These symptoms seem to be present in all children to some degree, and since ADHD is rather vaguely defined, the symptoms displayed by an individual child should be carefully observed. The quantity, intensity, and duration of these symptoms may single out children with ADHD from others who are merely bored with school or who are having other behavior problems. Care must be taken in diagnosis, since a real danger is that a child will be saddled with the label of hyperactivity not because he or she has an abnormally high energy level, but rather because his or her parents or teachers have a very low level of tolerance.

Although controversial, in some cases drug therapy has proved successful in treating ADHD. Several stimulant drugs appear to have a calming effect on children with ADHD because they seem to affect the hesitation response. However, these drugs have been shown to have unpleasant side effects, such as stomach cramps, susceptibility to colds, nervous mannerisms, and stunted growth. Therefore, many children on this therapy are required by their doctors to take "drug holidays" to give their bodies a break from the side effects of the medication.

Special diets that are designed in an attempt to eliminate all food additives have been prescribed, in keeping with the theory that additives cause ADHD. The findings from studies on this treatment have been contradictory. However, many parents report dramatic changes in behavior after this treatment, although part of the change is most likely to be due to the extra attention paid to the child whose meals have to be specially prepared.

Parents can help to influence the child's actions by praising or rewarding good behavior and ignoring bad behavior.

# Autism

Autism is a form of mental illness in children. The word *autism* comes from *auto*, the Greek word for self, and literally means self-absorption. The autistic child is wrapped up in his or her own inner thoughts, unable to communicate with or relate to other people.

Although the cause of autism remains a mystery, several reasons for the disorder have been suggested. In some cases, an inborn mental defect may play a part, since many affected children do not smile and do not accept or respond to affectionate cuddling. In other instances, severe mental or physical trauma during childhood may have contributed to the disorder. The sex of the child may also be a factor; boys are four times as likely as girls to be autistic.

Autism is a collection of symptoms of unknown cause that appear in the first 30 months of life. The autistic child is very withdrawn, unaffectionate, and uninterested in people, including parents and siblings. The child behaves as if he or she were alone in the world. Accompanying this attitude is a speech and language disorder: The child may learn to speak late or not at all, and, if speech develops, it is odd and limited. One common characteristic is echolalia (repetition of the last phrase or word of everything another person says). Other marks of autism are a total resistance to change (even something so minor as rearrangement of furniture) and the repetition of some meaningless act, such as flapping the arms or banging the head. Mental development is often uneven. Usually the child does best in learning nonverbal skills, and teaching methods that emphasize memorization and drill may be most useful. There are no established signs of nervous system defects, although half of all autistic children experience seizures before reaching their teens.

In diagnosing autism, the doctor must distinguish it from childhood schizophrenia, a mental illness that may also cause a child to be silent and withdrawn. The doctor must also make certain that deafness or severely impaired hearing is not present. The child is given neurologic and intelligence tests to help determine the potential for training and education. A tranquilizer may be prescribed for emergency use.

An autistic child may have to be cared for in an institution or a specialized school. Day-care programs for autistic children are available in some cities, and the trend is to train parents to care for their children at home. The method of treatment most often used by professionals, and taught to parents, is known as behavior therapy. The main goals are to limit self-destructive or meaningless actions, to promote language development, and to make the child more social. In behavior therapy, the professional or parent works to develop a close relationship with the child, so that the child will want to imitate the adult. The adult also uses direct action (such as rewards and praise) to promote speech, play with other children, self-care skills (such as dressing and washing), and helpfulness. With such methods, some autistic children of average or near-average intelligence are able to develop into normal adults.

Unfortunately there are no preventive measures.

# Autoimmune diseases

Autoimmune diseases are disorders in which the body's immune system reacts against some of its own tissue and produces antibodies to it.

Ailments believed to be autoimmune diseases include Hashimoto's thyroiditis and Graves' disease, which are disorders of the thyroid gland; systemic lupus erythematosus, which attacks multiple organ systems; myasthenia gravis, a neuromuscular disease; and autoimmune hemolytic anemia, in which the body's red blood cells are destroyed before the end of their normal 120-day life span. Diseases that are autoimmune disorders, at least in part, include rheumatoid arthritis, a connective tissue disease; pernicious anemia, a serious blood disorder; glomerulonephritis, a disorder that affects the kidneys; and Addison's disease, which attacks the adrenal glands.

Other diseases that have autoimmune features are chronic active hepatitis (a liver disorder), some forms of vasculitis (inflammation of blood vessel walls), and many other diseases that produce inflammation, degeneration, or wasting away of body tissues.

An autoimmune disease can begin in several ways:

- A body substance that ordinarily never enters the bloodstream may do so because of injury. For example, a disease known as sympathetic ophthalmia occurs when tissue from the inside of an injured eye is released into the bloodstream. The tissue is recognized as "out of place" or "foreign" by the body's immune system, and antibodies attack it, causing irritation in both the injured eye and in the noninjured eye. The reaction may be severe enough to cause blindness.
- A body substance may be altered by chemicals, sunlight, or a virus so that it seems foreign to the body's immune system. The substance is then attacked by antibodies. An example of this process occurs when the metal in a bracelet causes chemical changes in the skin on one's wrist. The body reacts against the "different" skin and attacks it, causing the rash of contact dermatitis.
- Infection may cause an immune response so strong that the body reacts against some of its own normal tissues.
- Genetic factors may play a role. Treatment is dependent on the par-

ticular autoimmune disease present. Many treatments involve decreasing the patient's immune response. Other cases require more aggressive therapy to allow repair of damage caused by the body's attack on itself.

See also Antibody/antigen and Immunity.

# B

# Backache

A backache is generally a gripping pain near the inward curve of the back above the base of the spine. It is one of the most common physical ailments, affecting about 80 percent of the population at some time in their lives.

Pain results from a variety of causes. Strains are especially common when overworked or underexercised back muscles perform beyond their normal capacity. The muscles will then contract or go into spasm and become a tight mass of tissue. Meanwhile, the body transmits a sharp pain signal as nearby muscles tighten in an effort to protect strained muscles and prevent further damage. Strain of back muscles can be due to participation in a sport, a sudden jerking motion (such as a car braking), or reflex actions like sneezing.

Overweight is a leading factor in backache because it increases the stress on back muscles. Similarly, pregnancy can produce back pain because of the weight or position of the fetus. For some women, menstruation is also associated with back discomfort.

Many people experience back pain as they age and their joint tissues deteriorate or shift. Psychological tension, stress, or anxiety about everyday problems can also lead to backache. In addition, back pain can result from diseases of the kidneys, heart, lungs, intestinal tract, or reproductive organs.

Backache occasionally stems from a congenital (present from birth) malformation. In such cases, pain generally results from the unusual stresses that the deformity imposes on surrounding muscular structures rather than from the abnormality itself. For example, if one leg is shorter than the other, the muscles in the lower part of the body are forced out of alignment, causing back pain.

Backaches can appear abruptly after physical activity or may develop slowly. The pain may feel like a sharp jab or a dull ache. The pain sometimes becomes so piercing that a person who is bending over may not be able to straighten up. Severe back pain may also be accompanied by pain or numbness radiating down one or both legs. Most muscular back pains disappear within a week or two of their onset, while some will last one to two months. Pain may recur unless preventive measures are taken.

Prolonged back pain (lasting for more than one or two weeks) should be brought to the attention of a physician, who will check for underlying disorders, such as kidney, bone, or lung problems, that may be causing the backache. Once other medical causes have been ruled out, an orthopedic surgeon (a physician who specializes in bone and muscle conditions) may be able to determine the cause of the discomfort.

During the examination, the physician asks questions about the type of pain and its location, general health, previous illnesses, and physical activity routines. The patient walks, sits, stands, and performs exercises while being observed. An X-ray study may reveal the presence of adverse changes in the spine.

If there are no apparent physical causes for the backache, physicians usually recommend an exercise program to strengthen weak muscles. Losing weight can also relieve pressure on the back.

For immediate treatment of symptoms, using a heating pad or, better yet, ice at the site of the pain will usually reduce soreness. Applying nonprescription analgesic creams containing methyl salicylate (oil of wintergreen) or a similar ingredient produce a soothing warm sensation. Muscle relaxants and/or anti-inflammatory drugs may also be prescribed.

When backache is the result of some deformity or damage to a disk (the soft material that lies between the bones of the spine), surgery may be necessary to correct the problem. Braces, corsets, or shoe lifts sometimes improve the condition. Exercises to strengthen affected muscles and counter stress caused by the deformity may be prescribed.

Almost all types of musculoskeletal backaches respond well to rest, which allows muscles to relax and inflammation to subside. Time is often the best healer.

To prevent back pain, stress to the spine should be avoided. Good posture, when awake and asleep, relieves tension on the spinal column. Wearing properly fitted shoes encourages good posture, as does sleeping on a semifirm bed. Contrary to popular belief, a hard mattress distorts alignment of the spine and causes back problems as much as a soft mattress does. A semifirm mattress is recommended in most cases because it conforms to the arch of the back and maintains spinal alignment.

Good posture is also important when performing daily activities. Bending at the knees, rather than from the waist, when lifting large, heavy objects places the stress on the legs and helps prevent back injury. One should avoid looking down for long periods of time while seated at a desk and avoid watching television with the chin on the chest.

---

# Bacteria

Bacteria are one-celled microscopic organisms. Some kinds of bacteria cause disease in humans and animals, but many others are beneficial. Bacteria dispose of organic waste, enrich the soil, and are used to make wine, beer, vinegar, cheese, and yogurt. In human beings, certain beneficial bacteria live in the intestines.

Bacteria are different from viruses in that they are able to multiply outside a living cell, whereas viruses can grow and multiply only in living cells. Bacteria are different from other causes of infection—protozoa (one-celled animals) and fungi (plantlike organisms)—in two ways: they have a primitive nucleus (center where genetic material is located), rather than a well-defined one with an enclosing membrane and chromosomes; and they reproduce simply by splitting in two (binary fission), rather than by means of the more complex process, called mitosis, that is seen in higher organisms.

One way of classifying bacteria is by shape:

Rod-shaped bacteria are known as bacilli. They often have waving projections known as flagella, which they use to propel themselves. Some form thick-walled cells known as spores, which can survive for long periods even after the parent bacteria have been killed by freezing, disinfectants, or other harsh forces. When conditions are favorable, the spores are able to generate new bacteria. Typhoid fever is caused by bacilli.

Round or egg-shaped bacteria are known as cocci. They occur singly (micrococci), in chains (streptococci—the cause of strep throat), in pairs (diplococci—the cause of a common type of pneumonia), or in irregular bunches (staphylococci—a cause of many skin infections). Cocci do not form spores, nor do they usually move about.

Bacteria also exist as comma-shaped organisms called vibrios (the organisms responsible for cholera) and as spiral-shaped organisms, such as the spirochete that causes syphilis.

Another way to classify bacteria is by whether they can live in the presence of air. Those that can are called *aerobic*; those that cannot are called *anaerobic*. Some can live either with or without air and are called *facultative anaerobes*. Tetanus (lockjaw) is an example of a disease caused by anaerobic bacteria that are commonly found in the soil. They pose no danger to humans unless they enter the body through a wound, particularly a puncture wound (such as one made by a nail). The air then cannot get to the organisms to destroy them, and so they multiply within the body, unless the infected person has been vaccinated against tetanus.

Disease-causing bacteria enter the body in many different ways. Those that cause pneumonia and sore throat are carried in droplets that an infected person sneezes or coughs into the air; the bacteria are then inhaled and deposited on the mucous membranes of the throat or lungs of a healthy person, where they multiply and eventually cause disease, unless checked by the body's immune system. The bacteria that cause intestinal diseases like cholera and typhoid can be transmitted in foods that have been handled by an infected person or in water tainted by body wastes from an infected individual. Another important route for infection is any break in the skin, which is why it is important to clean any cut in the skin as soon as possible.

Once inside the body, bacteria do their damage in two main ways: by direct destruction of tissue and by producing toxins (poisons). Certain white blood cells, known as lymphocytes, produce substances called antitoxins, which neutralize the toxins of the bacteria, and substances called antibodies, which destroy the invading bacteria themselves. Once created, the antibodies against a specific disease can persist in the body or be reproduced when needed, providing continuous immunity—sometimes for life. Still other white blood cells, known as phagocytes, entrap and destroy bacteria.

# Baldness

Baldness (or alopecia, as it is known medically) is partial or complete loss of hair on the head. This may be caused by an inherited tendency or by aging, fever, drugs, radiation, or disease.

Male-pattern baldness is the most common form. There seems to be an inherited tendency toward this condition, and androgen (a male hormone) is one of the factors that contributes to it. However, the exact mechanism by which it occurs is not fully understood. Hair loss is gradual, occurring at the forehead, on either side of the front (sometimes leaving a center tuft known as a "widow's peak"), and on top of the head. It can begin as early as age 15 or 16, in which case this early hair loss may indicate that considerable baldness is likely to manifest itself later on in life. Nevertheless, male-pattern baldness does not usually advance at a steady rate of hair loss, nor at a rate that is predictable.

Female-pattern baldness is fairly common in menopausal women and usually involves only the area around the crown of the head. Like male-pattern baldness, it is believed to be due to hormonal causes.

Temporary baldness sometimes occurs up to three or four months following a severe illness, especially one with fever, such as scarlet fever. It can result from decreased activity of the pituitary or thyroid gland, early stages of syphilis, pregnancy, use of birth control pills and certain other med-

Hair loss in male pattern baldness is gradual, beginning at the forehead on either side of the front and continuing to the top of the head.

ications, "crash" dieting or malnutrition, or a diet containing too much vitamin A. When the cause is removed, the missing hair usually returns.

Spotty baldness, or alopecia areata, may affect areas of the head and beard. The cause is unknown. It often clears up after a few months if there are just a few spots and if it first occurs in adulthood; it may recur, however. The outlook is less favorable if it begins in childhood or if hair loss is widespread. Occasionally, all body hair is lost. If there is no apparent cause, such as fever or severe illness, the hair is not likely to return.

Permanent baldness occurs when the scalp is scarred as a result of burns, other injury, or disease. Conditions that can cause scarring baldness include severe bacterial and fungal infections, tuberculosis, ulcers, lupus erythematosus, and certain slow-growing tumors.

There is no totally satisfactory medical treatment at this time to cure or prevent baldness. However, hair transplants can be effective. Scalp plugs containing active hair follicles are taken from the back of the head, which is not affected by male-pattern baldness. The transplanted follicles continue to produce hair just as before, despite the new location.

A topical form of the antihypertensive drug minoxidil has been released for use in treating baldness. This preparation has been shown to stimulate hair growth in some individuals; however, minoxidil must be applied on a continuous basis and is available only by prescription.

# Battered child syndrome

See Child abuse.

# Bell's palsy

Bell's palsy is total or partial paralysis (loss of function or movement) of one side of the face. It is believed to be due to inflammation of the nerve that controls the facial muscles. The inflammation, often of unknown cause but suspected to be the result of viral infection, causes the nerve to swell and to be compressed inside its bony passage in the skull. This compression reduces the blood supply to the nerve and thus its ability to function.

Facial nerve

In Bell's palsy, paralysis of the muscles on one side of the face is probably due to inflammation of the facial nerve and its branches.

This disorder can occur in someone of any age, but is most common from ages 20 to 50. The first sign may be an aching pain behind or below the ear. Paralysis may develop in a few hours or more slowly, causing the entire side of the face to be flat and without expression (this is different from the facial paralysis caused by stroke or brain tumor, in which the weakness is mostly below the forehead). The mouth droops on the weak side, with saliva drooling from the corner. The sense of taste may be impaired. The eyebrow cannot be raised. In most cases, the eye cannot be shut. When the patient tries to close the affected eye, it can be seen to roll upward (which also happens in a healthy person, but is not seen because the eyelid normally closes). Unprovoked tears may come from the affected eye.

In making a diagnosis, the doctor must determine if the paralysis might be caused by other disorders affecting the facial nerve, including ear infections, cancer, or a skull fracture. In such disorders, there is usually involvement of other nerves as well, and distinctive signs and symptoms are frequently present. X-ray studies of the head may be performed.

Primary treatment is aimed at reducing the inflammation of the nerve before any permanent damage is done to it. An oral corticosteroid, such as prednisone, may be given for this purpose. However, in many (if not most) uncomplicated cases, treatment with medication is unnecessary. After two weeks, if there has been no improvement in the ability of the muscles to move, the muscles of the weak side of the face may be stimulated electrically to maintain muscle tone.

The affected eye should be covered with an eye patch, especially when the patient is outdoors, and protected from dirt and wind. Application of moist, moderate heat on the affected side of the face can reduce pain. Brief periods of upward facial massage help maintain muscle tone, as do specific facial exercises.

Fortunately, most Bell's palsy patients recover in one to eight weeks. Elderly patients may take much longer—up to two years. Complete recovery usually follows within several months if the paralysis is partial.

# Beriberi

Beriberi is a disease that is caused by an insufficiency of thiamin (vitamin $B_1$). It has been most common in those parts of the world where people's diets have been limited almost entirely to polished (white) rice. The milling process removes the brown rice husks, which are rich in thiamin.

Other causes of beriberi include the following:

- Increased need for thiamin, such as occurs with fever, pregnancy, breast-feeding, or overactivity of the thyroid gland (which causes the body to increase the rate at which it uses nutrients)
- Failure of the body to absorb enough thiamin, such as may occur with long-lasting diarrhea
- Poor use of the vitamin by the body, as in severe liver disease

A combination of these factors occurs in alcoholism because of lowered food intake, poor vitamin absorption, increased need for thiamin, and poor use of thiamin by the body.

Because thiamin is necessary for the proper use of fats, starches, and sugars and for the normal functioning of nervous tissue and of enzymes (which modulate body processes), symptoms of beriberi usually occur in the digestive and nervous systems. In severe cases, heart muscle is damaged. Early symptoms include fatigue, irritability, poor memory, loss of appetite, constipation, abdominal discomfort, and difficulty in rising from the squatting position. There may be burning of the feet, prickling of the soles, and tenderness and cramps in the calves. Certain muscle reflexes are lost. Mental confusion, paralysis of speech and eye muscles, coma, and death can occur in untreated beriberi affecting the brain. Heart damage from beriberi produces heart failure with buildup of body fluids, seen as swelling in the abdomen and legs, and difficulty in breathing.

Babies who are breast-fed by mothers deficient in thiamin may develop heart failure and loss of speech and certain muscle reflexes.

Treatment for beriberi consists of daily doses of thiamin, at first by injection into a muscle or vein and later by mouth. Improvement usually begins in one or two days.

Eating a well-balanced diet of fruits, vegetables, meat, and whole grains is the best way to prevent such B-vitamin deficiency diseases as beriberi. Beriberi itself is rare in the United States because breads, cereals, and flours are enriched with thiamin.

# Bile

Bile is a fluid produced by the liver, stored in the gallbladder, and discharged into the small intestine, where it helps in the digestion of food, particularly fats. Bile is made up of water, salts, bile acids, cholesterol (a fatlike substance), and lecithin (a fatty acid).

Bile acts like a detergent to break down fat in the intestine into tiny globules that can be dissolved and suspended in water; the tiny globules can then pass through the walls of the small intestine into the bloodstream (to provide fuel for the body). The bile salts are also absorbed through the walls of the intestine but are returned to the liver to form new bile. The yellow-green or golden color of bile is due to the pigments bilirubin and biliverdin. Bilirubin is a yellow pigment derived from decomposed red blood cells. Biliverdin is a green pigment derived from conversion of bilirubin by a chemical reaction.

These pigments are also responsible for some of the coloration of body wastes.

Bile is produced continuously in the liver and passes through ducts to be stored in the gallbladder until mealtime, when it is emptied into the duodenum. Digestive disturbances result if the flow of bile is stopped or reduced, either because of a liver disorder or because a duct has been blocked by inflammation or a gallstone (a solid mass of material—usually composed of calcium, cholesterol, bilirubin, or a combination thereof—formed in the gallbladder). Any of these conditions can also cause jaundice, in which the pigments bilirubin and biliverdin accumulate in the blood. Jaundice is a sign of trouble, not a disease in itself, and shows up as yellow staining of the skin, eyes, and body fluids.

See also Gallstones and Jaundice.

# Birth control

Birth control, also called contraception, is the voluntary prevention of pregnancy. A variety of methods are available for preventing pregnancy. Couples who use no contraceptive method have an 80 to 90 percent chance of achieving pregnancy over a 12-month period, provided that they have no underlying problem that involves infertility.

**Condom** A condom is a thin rubber or synthetic sheath that the man fits over his erect penis just before sexual intercourse. A condom used alone is about 70 percent to 90 percent effective, depending on the care with which it is used. Several problems may occur with the use of the condom. For example, tiny holes or tears may develop in the sheath, causing leakage of sperm. Also, when the penis is withdrawn from the vagina as intercourse is completed, the condom sometimes breaks or partially unrolls inside the vagina, releasing its contents. However, a condom used regularly with a spermicide is approximately 95 percent effective in preventing pregnancy. Condoms have the great advantage of being readily available in any drugstore without a prescription. Condoms also have the advantage of helping to prevent the spread of venereal disease and acquired immune deficiency syndrome (AIDS).

**Diaphragm** The diaphragm is a molded rubber cap that the woman places inside the vagina to cover the cervix. The diaphragm blocks sperm from entering the uterus. It must be inserted for each act of intercourse and left in place for six hours afterward. Diaphragms come in different sizes and must be fitted by a physician. Used alone, diaphragms occasionally fail, either because they were not inserted correctly or because they shifted during sexual intercourse. Used with spermicides, however, diaphragms are quite effective in preventing contraception, with only about a three percent chance of pregnancy.

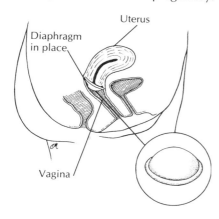

Uterus

Diaphragm in place

Vagina

The diaphragm is a molded rubber cap that a woman places inside the vagina to cover the cervix, the opening of the lower end of the uterus. Ideally the diaphragm prevents the sperm from entering the uterus.

**Cervical cap** The cervical cap is a molded rubber cap that fits over the outside of the cervix. While the diaphragm covers both the cervix and the back of the vagina, the smaller cervical cap fits only over the cervix. Like a diaphragm, the cervical cap blocks sperm from entering the uterus. It must be inserted for each act of intercourse and left in place for six to eight hours afterward. Cervical caps come in different sizes and must be fitted by a physician. Effectiveness in preventing pregnancy is similar to that of the diaphragm.

**Spermicide** Spermicide is a chemical foam, cream, suppository, or jelly applied to the woman's vagina to kill sperm. Used alone, a spermicide is about 75 percent to 85 percent effective. Some disadvantages of a spermicide are that it must be applied before each individual act of sexual intercourse, it has chemical odors, and it may irritate the vagina. A chief advantage is that spermicides are readily available at drugstores without a prescription.

**Contraceptive sponge** The contraceptive sponge is a disposable, spongelike device saturated with spermicide. A woman inserts the sponge into the vagina up against the cervix, where the device works by continuously releasing spermicide for up to 24 hours. Additional applications of spermicide are not necessary, even for multiple acts of intercourse. There are other advantages as well: The sponge is available without a prescription; unlike a diaphragm, the sponge does not have to be fitted; and the sponge can be inserted ahead of time, which allows greater spontaneity in sex. The sponge has been found to be about 85 percent effective.

Some side effects are associated with the use of the sponge. Cases of local irritation or allergic reaction have been reported; however, these have been mild and infrequent. There is also concern that the sponge could become a breeding ground for infection, especially if used improperly. You should consult your doctor about the contraceptive sponge and its proper use before trying this method of birth control.

**IUD** The intrauterine device (IUD) is a small plastic device inserted into the woman's uterus by a physician. The IUD has a string attached to it that hangs into the cervix, so that the woman or her partner can check to be sure that the IUD is still in place. Most researchers believe that the IUD prevents pregnancy by causing changes in the uterine lining that disrupt the normal environment of an egg. For the woman who can use an IUD, the advantages are great, because she does not have to worry about contraception each day. The effectiveness rate is high, with only about a five percent chance of pregnancy.

However, there are several disadvantages to use of an IUD. Severe menstrual cramps and increased menstrual bleeding may follow the insertion of an IUD. Sometimes these side effects lessen after a month or two. In other cases, severe cramps and prolonged bleeding continue, and the physician may advise removal of the IUD. The IUD is also thought to increase the probability of pelvic infections and ectopic (outside the uterus) pregnancies.

**Sterilization** A woman may be sterilized by an operation that blocks the fallopian tubes (the structures through which eggs travel from the ovaries to the uterus). A man may be sterilized by a procedure called a vasectomy, in which each vas deferens (one of the two ducts through which the sperm travel from the testes to the urethra) is cut. These procedures may be reversed, but only by complicated surgery, which is not always successful. Therefore, physicians recommend sterilization only when a couple has decided, without reservation, that no further pregnancies are desired.

**Oral contraceptives** Oral contraceptives, or birth control pills, are the most effective reversible method of contraception. A woman taking the pill has less than a one percent chance of getting pregnant.

The pill—which is available by prescription only—uses synthetic female hormones (estrogen and progestin) to override the natural hormonal regulation that results in the release of an egg. The pill signals the pituitary gland, which directs hormonal activity in the body, not to release the hormones that would normally stimulate the ovary to release an egg.

Each day you take one pill, at about the same time of day, removing it from a container that has the required number of pills for one cycle (usually 21). One to three days after you take the last pill for that cycle, your menstrual period begins. Menstrual periods may be lighter in flow, and cramps are reduced or absent.

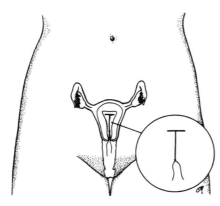

The IUD is a small plastic device that is inserted into a woman's uterus by a doctor. It is thought that the IUD prevents pregnancy by causing changes in the lining of the uterus that disrupt the normal environment of the egg.

If you forget to take one pill or more, menstrual bleeding may begin. In that case, you should continue taking the pills daily, but you should also use an additional contraceptive method, such as a condom, until after your next regular period.

Birth control pills are not recommended for women with a history of high blood pressure, blood-clotting problems, hepatitis, or cancer of the uterus or breast. A woman over age 35 who smokes heavily is advised to stop smoking if she wants to take the pill. Birth control pills should not be taken by a woman who suspects she may be pregnant. In addition, women with diabetes, epilepsy, heart disease, or thyroid disease may be advised not to take the birth control pill, depending on the nature and severity of the disease.

It is important for a woman taking birth control pills to report to her doctor if any of the following symptoms occur: blurred vision; severe chest pain; sudden shortness of breath; abdominal pain; unusual bleeding or bruising; breakthrough vaginal bleeding (spotting); changes in menstrual flow; pain in the calves; depression; difficult or painful urination; enlarged or tender breasts; hearing changes; increase or decrease in hair growth; migraine headaches; numbness or tingling; rash; skin color changes; swelling of the feet, ankles, or lower legs; vaginal itching; weight changes; or yellowing of the eyes or skin.

**Hormonal implants** With this method, five small plastic rods containing the synthetic female hormone progestin are inserted with a needle under the skin of the upper arm or forearm. The hormone is gradually and slowly released from the plastic rods, thus preventing ovulation. This method is effective for about five years from the time the implants are inserted. The major advantage of this method is that the woman does not need to remember to take birth control pills or use a spermicidal agent or diaphragm before each sexual act. Disadvantages include the high cost of the implants, possible infection at the site of insertion, irregular menstruation, and the necessity for surgical incisions on the arm when the implants need to be removed. Hormonal implants are about as effective as oral contraceptives.

**Injectable contraceptives** The newest form of contraceptive, recently approved by the FDA, is the injection of the synthetic hormone medroxyprogesterone acetate (Depo Provera). This synthetic version of the hormone progesterone is injected into a woman's muscle (usually the muscle of the upper arm) once every three months. The injection works to prevent conception in three ways: by preventing ovulation, by keeping mucus in the cervix thick so that sperm cannot pass, and by changing the lining of the uterus so that a fertilized egg could not implant and grow. The failure rate for this contraceptive is less than one percent. The advantage is that an injection is needed only once every three months, in contrast to birth control pills, which must be taken every day. The injections cost about the same as birth control pills. The disadvantages are that the injections must be made in a doctor's office exactly every three months, that some women may not resume normal menstrual periods for up to one year after stopping the injections, and that it may take up to 18 months after stopping the injections for the woman to become fertile again. Some women also experience mild headaches, skin oiliness, and water retention as side effects of the injections. These effects are normally mild and tend to disappear over a period of time.

**Natural family planning** Natural family planning is based on calculating when ovulation (release of an egg from one of the woman's ovaries each month) occurs. The couple then abstains from intercourse during the fertile period.

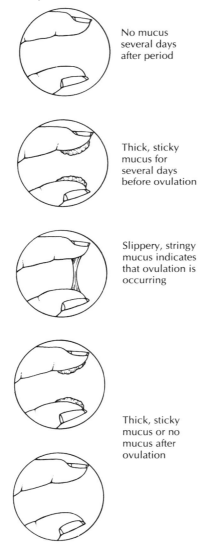

No mucus several days after period

Thick, sticky mucus for several days before ovulation

Slippery, stringy mucus indicates that ovulation is occurring

Thick, sticky mucus or no mucus after ovulation

Mucus from the cervix (neck of uterus) undergoes changes as hormone levels vary during the menstrual cycle. Testing the mucus between thumb and forefinger indicates the changes shown here.

A man's sperm can live in a woman's body for about two days. The egg can live for about 24 hours after ovulation. A few days are added to this fertile period for safety's sake because it is so difficult to determine just when ovulation occurs. All told, a couple needs to abstain from intercourse seven to ten days a month in order to have the greatest chance of preventing pregnancy.

There are three methods a woman can use to determine when she ovulates. The temperature method is one of the most reliable. Each morning on awakening and before getting out of bed, she takes her temperature with a special basal temperature thermometer (which measures temperatures only between 96°F and 100°F) and records it on graph paper. Near the middle of the menstrual cycle, the temperature may drop slightly (indicating that ovulation is about to occur) and then rise rapidly and continue to climb for the next three days. The temperature will not return to preovulation levels until the beginning of the menstrual period. The "safe" days to have sexual intercourse are from four days after the sudden rise in temperature until three or four days after the end of the period. It is important to become familiar with the menstrual cycle by recording temperature levels for several months before relying on this method of birth control.

The mucus method may also help determine the time of ovulation. Each morning the mucus from the vagina and cervix is examined. Cervical mucus undergoes changes as hormone levels vary during the course of the cycle. To detect these changes, the vaginal area is blotted each morning with a facial tissue and then the mucus is tested between the thumb and forefinger. After the menstrual period, there will be several days with no mucous discharge. This is followed by several days of a thick, sticky, yellow or white discharge. There will then be one or two days when the mucus becomes transparent and very slippery, with the consistency of raw egg whites. The mucus will form a string between the thumb and forefinger. This is when ovulation occurs. After ovulation, the mucus again becomes thick and sticky, or there may be no mucus at all. The fertile period begins with the thick, sticky, yellow or white discharge and continues until about three days after the phase when the mucus has the consistency of egg whites. Intercourse should be avoided during this time. In other words, the safe period is from three days after the slippery mucus stage to about three days after the end of the menstrual period. The use of certain medications (such as antihistamines), which alter mucus production throughout the body, will make determination of ovulation by the mucus method difficult.

The calendar method is also an option. A record of menstrual cycles is kept for one year or more. The doctor will then use the record to work out the probable day of ovulation, based on the fact that the average woman menstruates 14 days after she ovulates. However, any individual woman may vary from that average, so the calendar method is not precise.

Natural family planning does not require the use of mechanical aids or drugs. The effectiveness rate for this kind of birth control is up to about 80 percent, depending on the care with which the techniques are followed. However, even in women with regular cycles, such factors as illness, fatigue, stress, and use of certain drugs can delay ovulation or cause the techniques used to determine ovulation to become inaccurate, thereby throwing off all careful calculations.

See also Conception and Ovulation.

---

# Bladder cancer

This is the most common cancer of the urinary tract. It occurs most often between the ages of 50 and 70 and is the fourth leading cause of cancer death among men. Four times as many men as women are afflicted.

Bladder cancer has been connected with exposure to a number of carcinogens. This may be because the urinary tract comes into contact with so many foreign substances due to its excretory function. For many years it has been known that those who work with aniline dyes have a high incidence of cancer of the bladder. Bladder cancer is also associated with exposure to tar from tobacco smoke and with schistosomiasis (infestation with a tropical parasite).

Blood in the urine is usually the first symptom of bladder cancer. In addition, urination may be difficult, painful, and frequent. The appearance of blood in the urine may be intermittent, and if this symptom disappears, a doctor is sometimes not consulted. However, anyone with blood in the urine should consult a doctor, since in the early stages, this disease may be curable, and treatment is far more difficult later. If your doctor considers that the symptoms suggest bladder cancer, a cystoscopic examination may be ordered. With the patient under local or general anesthesia, a lighted tubelike instrument called a cystoscope is passed into the urinary tract through the urethra (the passageway from the bladder to the outside), so that the interior of the bladder can be examined. This instrument can also be used to obtain a biopsy specimen (a small sample of tissue for laboratory analysis) of a growth that may be of a suspicious nature. Urine cytology (the microscopic examination of urine for cancer cells) may also be of help in detecting cancer.

Treatment of bladder cancer depends on how far advanced the disease is. A small tumor can sometimes be completely removed with a cystoscope. More advanced cases are treated with surgery or radiation or a combination of the two. In certain cancers, chemotherapeutic agents are sometimes instilled directly into the bladder.

See also Cancer.

# Blepharitis

Blepharitis is an inflammation of the edges of the eyelids, with redness and thickening. Scales and crusts or shallow ulcers (eroded areas) may also appear. The disease is common, especially in children, and often affects the upper and lower eyelids of both eyes.

Infection of eyelash follicles and oil glands by *Staphylococcus* bacteria causes blepharitis with ulcers. The nonulcerous variety may be due to an allergic reaction, or it may be linked to seborrheic dermatitis, an inflammatory scaling of the scalp, eyebrows, and sometimes ears. The nonulcerous form is occasionally caused by lice, which irritate lid margins.

Symptoms of blepharitis include itching, burning, "red-rimmed" eyes; swelling of the lids; loss of eyelashes; and irritation of the underside of the lid, as if dirt or sand were underneath. The eyes may tear and be sensitive to light.

In the ulcerous configuration of blepharitis, the tough, dry crusts that form leave a bleeding surface when removed. In the nonulcerous kind of blepharitis, greasy scales that can be easily removed appear on the edges of the lids.

Blepharitis caused by a bacterial infection can be treated with an antibiotic ointment, such as erythromycin or bacitracin, that is specially formulated for use around the eyes. The medication is usually applied three times a day to the eyelash margins with a cotton-tipped swab, after the margins have been softened with warm compresses for ten minutes and the crusts have been removed. The application of medicated eyedrops may also be used in the effort to combat irritation or other types of infection.

If an allergy to a cosmetic is the cause, its use should be discontinued. If there is scaling on the eyebrows and scalp due to seborrheic dermatitis, the doctor is likely to recommend a special shampoo, such as a sulfur or tar shampoo, for control of dandruff and to prescribe a cortisone lotion or cream to be rubbed into hairy areas. Careful attention to cleanliness of hair, scalp, eyebrows, and eyelid margins is necessary during treatment.

If the blepharitis is caused by lice, the nits (lice eggs) should be carefully removed with tweezers, and steps should be taken to keep the patient free of lice.

Both of the principal varieties are difficult to cure and often recur. Nonulcerous blepharitis causes no permanent damage. However, ulcerous blepharitis, if it recurs often enough, can cause scarring of eyelids, loss of eyelashes, and even ulcers of the cornea.

Meticulous cleanliness may contribute to the effort to prevent the disease. If it is treated promptly when it occurs, permanent damage can probably be prevented.

# Blood

Blood is the fluid that courses through the blood vessels of the body. It consists of plasma (a yellowish liquid composed of water, proteins, salts, and other substances) and three formed elements—red blood cells, white blood cells, and platelets—that are visible only under a microscope. These elements are manufactured by the bone marrow (the soft tissue in the center of some bones).

Red blood cells carry oxygen from the lungs to the various body tissues. Oxygen travels attached to hemoglobin, a pigmented substance in red blood cells that contains iron. When the amount of hemoglobin in each red blood cell or the total number of red blood cells falls below a certain level, anemia is said to be present. Normally, there are about 25 billion red blood cells in one teaspoon of blood.

The job of the white blood cells is to protect the body from invasive organisms. Whenever the body becomes wounded or infected, white blood cells attack and kill disease-causing agents in the affected area. In addition, certain white blood cells produce antibodies. These substances counteract harmful agents by destroying or inactivating them. Because the body produces more white blood cells than usual in response to infection, an increase in their number signals disease. From 25 million to 45 million white blood cells are normally present in one teaspoon of blood.

Platelets are small, colorless disks numbering approximately one and a half billion in a single teaspoon of blood. They work to help the blood form clots.

See also Lymphocytes and Platelets.

# Blood vessels

Blood vessels form the network of passageways that transport blood throughout the body. The blood leaves the heart and passes through arteries of progressively smaller diameter. When the blood reaches the smallest blood vessels, called capillaries, oxygen and nutrients are exchanged for carbon dioxide and other waste products. The "used" blood then continues on its journey back toward the heart through veins of progressively greater diameter.

# Boils

A boil, or furuncle, is caused by a bacterial infection and irritation of the skin and its underlying structures. It is a painful swelling in the skin that is easily detected by touch. When a group of boils interconnects below the surface of the skin, a carbuncle forms.

Boils develop when *Staphylococcus* bacteria enter the skin through a hair follicle and multiply in its warm, moist environment. Bacteria continue to grow while producing substances that invade surrounding cells. White blood cells (which attack and kill invading organisms) travel to the infected hair follicle and enclose bacteria. As more white blood cells gather, they eventually consume the bacteria and eliminate the infection. This buildup by the white blood cells is what produces the pustule in the center of the boil. When the pustule ruptures, pus and dead skin cells killed by the bacteria drain out, and the boil heals.

*Staphylococcus* bacteria are often found in the nose and throat, where washing cannot reach them. They can

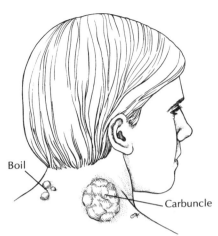

Boil

Carbuncle

A boil is a contagious bacterial infection and irritation of the skin and its underlying structures. When a group of boils interconnects below the surface of the skin, a carbuncle forms.

gresses, the pustule becomes red and hot. Excess fluid in the boil produces pressure on the nerves that are located underneath, which can result in considerable pain. When boils contain little pus, they are called blind boils; the inflammation recedes slowly without rupturing, but sometimes it leaves a scar.

If boils are large or extensive, the person may also experience fever and a general feeling of weakness. Sometimes, the infection gets into the bloodstream and spreads throughout the body. The same bacteria that cause the boil may also produce a toxin (poison) that causes blood clots, usually in the blood vessels around the boil.

Any treatment plan for boils and carbuncles emphasizes that they should *never* be squeezed, particularly if they are on the face. Squeezing may force the infection deeper into the skin and possibly into the bloodstream. Only a physician should lance a boil to encourage drainage. Afterward, the doctor may prescribe an oral antibiotic, such as penicillin or erythromycin, to fight further infection.

spread to a hair follicle from there or from another site on the body. They can also be transmitted by contact with an infected person or by contact with an infected article, such as a washcloth or towel. In most cases, however, other persons who come in contact with the bacteria do not get boils.

Persons who are run-down or who suffer diseases such as anemia (deficiency of red blood cells), diabetes, or infections that weaken their natural defenses against bacteria seem more susceptible to boils. Those who work with greasy or oily substances are more likely to develop boils because these materials trap bacteria against the skin. Poor bathing habits, especially in the summer months, when sweaty skin provides the moist climate that is conducive to bacterial growth, also invite infection.

Boils can develop anywhere on the skin. They appear most frequently on the neck, face, and back, and they can erupt in several places at once. Although boils vary in size, they characteristically form white or yellow pustules. As the infection pro-

Many boils will rupture and heal on their own. However, holding a soft cloth soaked with warm water against the boil for 15 to 20 minutes at least four times a day will speed the process. These warm compresses increase blood flow to the area and encourage pustule formation. Since bacteria from the boil are contagious, the cloth should be disinfected in boiling water or in the hot cycle of a washing machine.

When a boil bursts, the infected area should be washed thoroughly and covered with an antibiotic cream and sterile gauze to prevent infection. If the boil does not heal within a few days, or if the boil is located on or near the face, a physician should be consulted.

To prevent new eruptions, the skin needs to be kept cool and dry. Sometimes, physicians advise washing the entire body with an antiseptic (germ-fighting) soap twice a day. If boils often recur, change underclothing and bed linen daily.

See also Acne.

# Bone cancer

This rare form of cancer is most common in those between the ages of five and 20. Predisposing factors include bone diseases, bone fractures, and exposure to radiation.

Bone cancer usually develops first in the arms or legs. Pain, swelling, and brittleness of the bone may be its symptoms. It is often far advanced by the time it is discovered. The first tool in diagnosis is the X ray, which may show whether the bone is cancerous and whether the disease has spread. If cancer is suspected, an orthopedic surgeon generally performs a biopsy. Bone cancer is usually treated with a combination of surgery, radiation, and chemotherapy.

See also Cancer.

# Bones

Bones are hardened masses of living tissue that have several functions. They collect calcium for the entire body, storing 99 percent of this mineral, which is required to keep all bones firm and strong. Within some bones is a substance called marrow, which produces red and white blood cells and platelets.

There are 206 bones in the human skeleton. The skeleton maintains the body's shape and protects internal organs. For example, the bones in the skull shield the brain, and the bones

in the rib cage encircle the lungs and heart.

The place where two or more bones meet is called a joint. This juncture usually allows movement of the bones that are involved. However, movement is governed by ligaments (bands of fibrous tissue) attached to the bones and by cartilage (elastic tissue) covering the ends of the bones. Ligaments connect one bone with another. Cartilage cushions and protects bones with the aid of various joint fluids and bursae (small sacs containing lubricating fluid that encompass the joints). Other bands of connective tissue called tendons attach bones to muscles. Muscles are specific kinds of tissues that have the ability to contract. It is this contraction that pulls on the tendons and makes movement possible. To move any part of the skeleton, coordination of ligaments, tendons, and muscles is necessary.

# Brain

The brain is the control center for the entire body. The brain sends messages to and receives stimulation from all parts of the body. More than ten billion interlinked brain cells regulate the functioning of the body during sleep and wakefulness.

Different areas of the brain control different body functions. At the back of the skull is the cerebellum, which controls coordination of movements, balance, and posture. Deep inside the brain is the thalamus, which is the relay station for incoming impulses from the rest of the body, conveying sensations of pain, touch, and temperature to other parts of the brain. Around the thalamus is the hypothalamus, which governs involuntary (automatic) body operations, such as heartbeat and blood circulation. The pituitary gland is attached to the hypothalamus by a thin stalk. Because the pituitary gland controls most of the hormones in the body, the hypothalamus is considered a major influence on primary drives governed by hormones, such as sexual desire, hunger, and thirst.

Covering the inner parts of the brain is the cerebral cortex, which consists of two cerebral hemispheres. In these hemispheres are the nerve centers that regulate thought and voluntary action. Connecting the left and right cerebral hemispheres is a broad band of fibers called the corpus callosum. Because nerve fibers from the two cerebral hemispheres cross one another in a structure called the medulla at the base of the brain before progressing down the spinal cord, each hemisphere generally controls functions in the opposite side of the body. For example, a region in the left hemisphere governs movement of the right arm.

The brain is the most complex organ in the body. Although research has identified many of its capabilities in memory, reasoning, and creative thought processes, many functions of the brain remain a mystery.

# Brain cancer

Any tumor in the brain, whether cancerous or not, is very dangerous. Because the brain occupies an enclosed space within the skull, even a small tumor that weighs only a fifth of a pound can cause crowding sufficient to bring on death. Brain cancer is most often the result of metastasis from other cancer sites, particularly the breast, lung, and skin.

Symptoms of brain cancer are of two kinds. Increased pressure in the skull can cause seizures, headaches, nausea, forgetfulness, and personality changes. However, symptoms may also arise in the part of the body controlled by the affected area in the brain. For instance, coordination, vision, or strength of limbs may be affected.

In the past, brain tumors did not respond well to treatment, largely because diagnosis could not be made until late in the development of the disease. Recently, however, diagnostic techniques have improved. The computed tomography (CT) scanner produces a three-dimensional image

Corpus callosum

Cerebral cortex

Thalamus

Hypothalamus

Pituitary gland

Cerebellum

Medulla

Spinal cord

The brain is the control center for the entire body.

of the brain that can show the size and location of a tumor and can be used to monitor the progress of treatment. A new technique, magnetic resonance imaging, is also being used.

Surgery is the primary treatment for brain cancer. It is often not used, however, when cancer is present in multiple areas or when the tumor originated in another organ. Surgery in the brain is a delicate procedure; often, a tumor deep in the brain cannot be totally removed without risking impairment of body function. However, new techniques in brain surgery—sometimes with the use of a microscope—permit treatment of tumors once considered inoperable. Radiation therapy and chemotherapy are often used after surgery, although the sensitivity of brain tissue demands that these be administered cautiously. Steroid drugs may be given to reduce the dangerous swelling that a tumor can produce.

See also Cancer.

# Breast cancer

Roughly one woman in 13 will develop breast cancer at some time in her life. It is the leading cause of cancer death in women and the leading cause of all deaths in women between the ages of 40 and 44. The high-risk group for breast cancer includes women over 50, women who have never had children or who had a child for the first time after the age of 30, and women who began menstruation early or who experienced late menopause. Breast cancer also occurs more frequently in women with a family history of the disease and women who have already had breast cancer.

Self-examination of the breasts can often lead to early detection. All women should perform these examinations monthly at the end of the menstrual period. About 90 percent of all breast tumors are discovered by self-examination. The recommended technique for breast self-examination is shown in the illustration in the section on cancer.

If a lump is discovered in a breast, the doctor will probably order an X-ray examination of the breast, known as a mammogram. The doctor may also take a biopsy specimen from the lump to test for the presence of cancer. If cancer is identified, surgery will probably be performed. Women with breast cancer often dread surgery because of the disfigurement that can result; however, surgery for a breast tumor is often less extensive today than in the past. At one time, all breast cancer patients received a radical mastectomy (removal of the breast, underlying chest muscles, and lymph nodes in the armpit). Now it is known that in many cases the removal of the breast, or even the tumor alone together with removal of the lymph nodes, may be equally effective. In addition, there are techniques for reconstruction of the breast after surgery and for rehabilitation of muscle tone in an arm that has been weakened by surgery. In many cases, radiation therapy and chemotherapy will be used after surgery to destroy remaining cancer cells. Recently it has been demonstrated that the use of chemo or hormonal therapy in addition to local therapy (such as removal of the tumor) will actually prolong survival of certain groups. It also appears to delay recurrence of disease in most individuals.

See also Cancer.

# Bright's disease

See Glomerulonephritis.

# Bronchiectasis

Bronchiectasis is a lung condition in which some of the bronchi and bronchioles have lost their elasticity and have expanded and filled with fluid.

Most often, bronchiectasis follows pneumonia, whooping cough, tuberculosis, or another lung disease. (Fortunately, the use of antibiotics has reduced the number of cases due to lung infection.) Other causes include obstruction; clogging of the airways by the thick, mucous secretions of cystic fibrosis; and Kartagener syndrome, which is a condition in which the cilia (hairlike projections that line the bronchial walls and wave mucus, pus, and dirt upward) do not work properly.

Bronchiectasis is a chronic condition that persists for life. The individual almost always has some symptoms, which will worsen if an acute

Postural drainage, a way of eliminating fluid from the respiratory system, is one method of treatment for bronchiectasis. In this procedure, the patient lies head down in bed with pillows elevating the hips as a therapist strikes the back over the lungs with cupped hands to loosen mucus.

infection occurs. The most typical symptom is a chronic cough that produces thick, white or green sputum (discharge). The sputum may be foul-smelling and abundant and may also contain blood. The individual generally coughs up large amounts of sputum after changing position (for example, after rising from bed).

The doctor, listening to the chest with a stethoscope, can hear abnormal sounds inside the lungs as the patient breathes. An X ray obtained after the injection of dye into the bloodstream or directly into the bronchi will show the characteristic appearance of the disease. Chronic bronchitis must be ruled out as a cause, along with tuberculosis, certain fungal infections, a tumor, and the presence of an inhaled object that is lodged in a bronchi.

Treatment of an active case of bronchiectasis includes fighting the infection with an antibiotic, such as penicillin or tetracycline, and eliminating the fluid with postural drainage. In the latter procedure, the patient lies facedown in bed, with pillows elevating the hips, and a therapist strikes the back over the lungs with cupped hands to loosen mucus. The treatment, which can be taught to a family member, requires two to four ten-minute sessions a day. Inhaling warm mists may also help to moisten the thick mucus clogging the airways, so that it can be more easily expelled. The patient should avoid anything that can irritate the lungs, such as tobacco smoke, fumes, and dust.

In the relatively few cases in which the infection is confined to a small part of the lung and is progressing despite antibiotics and other forms of therapy, it may be best to surgically remove the affected portion of the lung.

You can prevent progression of the disease by being immunized against flu and pneumonia, avoiding anyone with a cold or cough, and stopping smoking. Prompt treatment with antibiotics can help to control new infections.

# Bronchitis

Bronchitis is a respiratory illness characterized by inflammation and swelling of the bronchi (the main airways connecting the windpipe and the lungs). When the mucous membranes lining these tubes become inflamed, the mucous glands in the membranes expand and release more mucus. The bronchi, already narrowed by the swelling, become further clogged by the excess mucus. This mucus must then be coughed up to keep the breathing tubes free for normal airflow into the lungs. This illness is characterized by frequent coughing, production of sputum (mucus), and, commonly, shortness of breath.

When the condition is of short duration, it is called acute bronchitis and is often accompanied by fever and production of thick, foul-smelling sputum. This condition is difficult to distinguish from pneumonia, and chest X rays are frequently obtained to establish diagnosis. When the symptoms linger for months or years, it is called chronic bronchitis. In either case, the coughing stops only when the source of inflammation has been removed or overcome and the inner linings of the bronchi have returned to normal.

Bronchitis alone is rarely fatal, but it may lead to another condition that proves fatal. For example, the functioning of lungs that have been severely damaged by chronic bronchitis may be so limited that the heart is deprived of adequate oxygen, ultimately resulting in death. Also, bronchitis can be very serious when com-

bined with other respiratory diseases. Such is the case for people who suffer from a category of respiratory conditions called chronic obstructive pulmonary disease (COPD). Bronchitis, emphysema, and several other diseases are included in this category. Patients may suffer from two or three of the COPD conditions, or one may lead to another.

Bronchitis occurs when the bronchial tubes are infected or irri-

Normal mucous membrane

Normal

Swollen mucous membrane with excessive mucus secretions

Bronchitis

Bronchitis is an inflammation of the mucous membranes lining the bronchial tubes. As the membranes swell, they secrete more mucus, resulting in clogged bronchial tubes and a reduced airflow into the lungs.

tated. A cold or the flu may lead to acute or, less often, chronic bronchitis. Chronic bronchitis is more commonly triggered by the constant irritation of environmental substances such as cigarette smoke, air pollutants, and occupational dusts.

Cigarette smoking is the predominant cause of chronic bronchitis. Seventy-five percent of all those who suffer from bronchitis are cigarette smokers. When tobacco smoke reaches the bronchial linings, it stops the action of the cilia (the hairlike projections that line the bronchial walls and wave mucus, pus, and dirt upward). When the cilia are stilled by smoke, particles remain trapped in the stagnant mucus, irritating the delicate bronchial tubes and eventually creating a breeding ground for infection and disease.

Some degree of bronchitis occurs in about 90 percent of all smokers who live in polluted environments or who are exposed to occupational dusts. Babies and young children with chronic bronchitis usually overcome the condition. People who are undernourished, inadequately housed, or often fatigued are more likely to contract bronchitis. This disorder tends to occur within certain families, but the reason is not yet known.

Bronchitis can be recognized by its major symptom, the persistent cough in an effort to bring up the excess mucus. Acute bronchitis may be accompanied by hoarseness, chest discomfort, slight fever, wheezing, and shortness of breath. In children, chronic bronchitis may establish itself after several short-term infections. In adults, the beginning of chronic bronchitis is signaled by regular coughing and clearing of the throat the first thing each morning; the coughing will become more persistent and the mucus more plentiful as the disease progresses, and these symptoms may be accompanied by wheezing, short-

ness of breath, chest infections, and heavy panting after exercise.

As the years pass, chronic bronchitis may cause the bronchial tubes to become severely obstructed and breathing to be irreversibly impaired. The heart sometimes becomes enlarged because it must pump harder than normal to deliver needed oxygen to the rest of the body. The nails, lips, and skin may develop a blue tinge due to lack of oxygen.

To diagnose bronchitis, the doctor will obtain the medical history, do a physical examination of the chest with a stethoscope, and perhaps order a chest X ray. Special machines can measure the amount of air flowing in and out of the lungs and can measure how well oxygen is being transported from the lungs to the bloodstream.

Bronchitis is treated by removing the irritants from the patient's surroundings, clearing the lungs of mucus, and trying to prevent infections. A patient with chronic bronchitis will need to quit smoking and to avoid constant exposure to pollutants or hazardous dusts. Humidity plays a large part in treating bronchitis; patients should drink plenty of liquids, and breathe warmed, humidified air from a vaporizer or humidifier. Humidity acts to moisten mucus trapped in the airways, allowing it to be brought up from the lungs and thereby promoting what is known as a productive cough. A bronchodilator drug, which relaxes the walls of the air passages, may be prescribed. The use of antibiotics to treat bronchitis is somewhat controversial but appears to be helpful, particularly in acute cases.

Bronchitis can best be prevented by avoiding the irritants that cause it, namely cigarette smoke, air pollutants, and dusts. Patients with chronic bronchitis can prevent further irritation by maintaining good health habits to avoid infections. Other lung disorders may precipitate the condition; therefore, antibiotics may be prescribed to treat bacterial infections, and vaccinations against influenza and pneumonia are strongly recommended in those with chronic bronchitis.

# Bulimia

Bulimia is abnormal and excessive eating, usually triggered by emotional factors. Victims of the disorder overeat far beyond the needs of their bodies. In extreme cases, they resemble alcoholics, employing food instead of drink as an escape from the problems. They may even go on food binges and eat themselves into a stupor. They often feel guilty after overeating and force themselves to vomit; overuse of laxatives is also common.

To a bulimic person, food provides a way to relieve stress. Some experts think that excessive eating is an unconscious attempt to recapture the feelings of security experienced in childhood when food was received from the mother. Psychiatrists have speculated that overeating may also represent a hunger for affection that was denied in early childhood, when the child's attention was focused on the mouth and eating. It may be a substitute for affection, attention, or sexual contact that the person is not receiving. It may be an outlet for hostile feelings, since food is being destroyed by the acts of biting and chewing. Another possibility is that the person may unconsciously seek to become more important and safer by becoming physically larger through weight gain. Bulimia is sometimes found among mental patients, especially those who have regressed to infantile behavior.

Excessive eating may also result from hyperthyroidism (overactivity of

the thyroid gland), a disorder in which great quantities of calories may be eaten without weight gain. In a very small percentage of cases, bulimia may be caused by damage to the appetite control center located in the brain.

Attempts to cure bulimia have not been very successful and have frequently caused the patient to become even more distressed. However, it is generally agreed that a logical first step is to help the patient discover the emotional causes of the disorder. This may require individual or family counseling by a psychiatrist or clinical psychologist, who also tries to help the patient gain confidence and become more sociable and self-reliant. New satisfactions are sought to replace those formerly found in overeating. Nutritional counseling by a registered dietician and a sensible exercise program may be recommended.

See also Anorexia nervosa.

# Bunion

A bunion is a swelling on the foot, usually at the joint of the big toe. Often, a bony protuberance is present at the joint of the big toe, which gives the bunion its bulging appearance.

Bunions are most often caused by wearing poorly fitting footwear, but they can also be the result of inherited deformities in bone structure. In a normal foot, the two main bones of the big toe must align to fit together. However, some people have loose joints in the foot that allow their big toes to point toward the other toes. This inherited condition causes problems when footwear encloses the foot. The shoe forces the big toe inward and the big-toe joint outward so that the joint rubs against the inner surface of the shoe. Friction from such rubbing produces a bunion. The same

Inflamed bursa

Bony protuberance

A bunion is a swelling on the foot, usually at the joint of the big toe, often accompanied by a bony protuberance and an inflamed bursa—the fluid-filled sac that acts as a cushion for the joint. A bunion is most often caused by friction or pressure on the joint.

action results when a tight or pointed-toe shoe puts pressure on the joint—regardless of whether the person has the predisposing inherited tendency to have loose joints in the foot.

A bunion is characterized by swelling at the big-toe joint, which may be accompanied by pain and tenderness. Bunion formations can be acute or chronic. Acute bunions are a type of bursitis, which is an inflammation of a bursa (a fluid-filled sac that cushions the juncture of two or more bones). With an acute bunion, the bursa covering the big-toe joint becomes inflamed from friction at the joint, often producing considerable pain. Chronic (long-term) bunions develop into inflexible bony protrusions.

Complications can occur if the bunion grows and increases pressure on the big toe. This pressure may force the other toes to overlap, encouraging the development of corns (mounds of dead skin found on toes) or other problems that could result from friction on the skin of the distorted toes.

A physician diagnoses a bunion by general physical examination. To identify bone problems, an X-ray examination may be necessary.

Surgery is the only permanent cure for bunions. It can entail simple removal of the excess bone or more complex realignment of the affected bones, muscles, and tendons. A doctor can sometimes remove a bony protrusion in the office. Local anesthetic can be used, the incision is often only about an inch long, and pain is minimal. With this treatment, the patient has full use of the foot in about six weeks.

For more extensive surgery, the patient is admitted to the hospital, and recuperation time is longer. Usually, an orthopedic surgeon performs this type of surgery.

Nonsurgical devices can often relieve the pain and discomfort of bunions. Padding can be used to shift the weight of the foot in the shoe, lessening friction. Protective shields can also prevent contact between the bunion and the inside of the shoe.

Wearing properly fitting footwear is the best preventive measure. A child's first shoes should be wide enough to accommodate all the toes without cramping, since early childhood is when many foot problems begin.

When buying shoes, the width and length of each foot need to be measured separately. If one foot is larger than the other, the shoe size should correspond to the size of the larger foot. A one-inch gap between the big toe and the tip of the shoe allows enough space for movement. Even more room is needed with pointed-toe shoes. Shoes should be comfortable from the first wearing—no breaking-in period should be necessary. People who wear high-heel or pointed-toe shoes may be damaging their feet. Heels about one inch in height are actually best for feet. However, if higher heels are chosen, open-toe styles cause fewer problems.

# Bursitis

Bursitis is an inflammation of a bursa (a fluid-filled sac that cushions the juncture of two or more bones). Bursae (the plural of bursa) contain lubricating fluid that normally eliminates friction in the area and maintains smooth muscle movement over the bones.

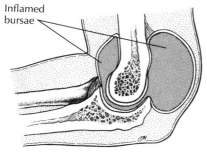

Inflamed bursae

The elbow is a common site of bursitis, an inflammation of the bursae, the fluid-filled sacs located in the joints. Bursae normally eliminate friction in the joints and maintain smooth muscle movement over the bones.

Bursitis seems to be more common in men than in women. Continual stress on a particular joint increases the probability of injury and inflammation. In advanced cases, swelling and calcium deposits within a joint may render it immobile.

The inflammation can result from either sudden extreme pressure or from continual strain. Some occupations and sports that require constant use of certain joints contribute to acute or chronic bursitis. For example, "typist's shoulder" and "baseball pitcher's elbow" are forms of chronic bursitis. Acute bursitis can develop suddenly and may be triggered by physical stress or injury.

Inflamed bursae produce tenderness and swelling near the affected joint. Pain from bursitis can be so severe that movement becomes impossible. Any joint in the body can be the site of bursitis, but shoulders, knees, and elbows are most commonly affected.

To diagnose bursitis, an X-ray examination may be ordered to determine whether there are calcium deposits in the bursa or if other problems, such as a fracture, exist. In the case of stress-related bursitis, however, such a study will show only swelling of the bursa.

Acute bursitis may heal with time if the joint is properly immobilized. Complete bed rest or use of a sling or crutches may be recommended to relieve pressure on the affected area.

Applying moist heat to the area of the inflamed joint frequently reduces the discomfort of bursitis, although some patients find cold compresses more effective. Aspirin and other over-the-counter pain relievers may also help. In some cases, anti-inflammatory corticosteroid drugs may be injected directly into the inflamed area, but they must be used judiciously since they have been known to cause adverse side effects.

For severe cases of bursitis, a doctor may recommend surgery by an orthopedic surgeon to remove calcium deposits or free the area from chronic inflammation by removing all or part of the bursa.

# Bypass surgery

See Coronary bypass surgery.

# C

# Calluses

Calluses are thickened areas of the skin. They develop most often on the balls and heels of the feet and on the hands.

Skin buildup is the result of excessive friction or pressure against the surface of the skin. As pressure mounts, dead skin cells accumulate, and the skin thickens. Wearing shoes that fit improperly or holding pencils too tightly can create the problem. Since calluses often follow blisters on the same site, they are considered to be the body's way of shielding the area against further injury.

Flat-footed persons have a greater incidence of calluses. Because of the abnormal shape of the foot, the small bones in the front portion of the foot are forced downward against the skin of the sole with great pressure during walking, creating pressure points. Those who wear high heels promote growth of calluses by increasing pressure on the balls of their feet.

Calluses vary in size and shape depending on where they grow and how much skin is affected. Sometimes, calluses grow so thick and irregular in shape that the skin becomes inflexible and cracks.

When pressure is relieved, calluses usually produce no pain. However, continued irritation, especially involving areas where the skin is split, can cause enough discomfort to interfere with physical activities.

Immediate treatment involves removal of the pressure that caused the callus in the first place. Extremely persistent or painful calluses should be examined by a doctor. In rare instances, surgery may be necessary to alleviate intense pressure. In milder cases, the pain caused by calluses can often be eased by padding the exposed area to reduce further friction.

There are over-the-counter remedies that soften the callused tissue, making it easier to remove. Salicylic acid plasters, which are sold in medicated sheets, can be placed over the callus after bathing and secured with tape. The pad should be removed just before the next bath so that the softened skin can be gently removed with a pumice stone or a special implement with a rough surface designed specifically for that purpose.

Home remedies should not be used by persons who have diabetes, atherosclerosis, or other disorders affecting circulation because their risk of infection is greater. They should consult their doctor before attempting any form of treatment.

# Cancer

Cancer is the term used to describe a broad group of diseases in which certain body cells grow out of control, invade, and spread to other tissues.

Who is most likely to develop cancer? This question is very difficult, if not impossible, to answer. There are, however, certain risk factors that increase the possibility that you may develop cancer in your lifetime. Among these are age (as a rule, the older you are, the higher your risk of getting cancer), family history (for example, if your mother or sister had breast cancer, your risk of developing breast cancer is increased), and environmental and other factors.

The rapid increase in cancer rates during this century has been blamed largely on the environment. Polluted air and water, food additives and colorings, and changes in diet from "natural" to "processed" foods all have been implicated as possible causes. Cigarette smoking has been shown conclusively to be a cause of lung and other related cancers. If you wish to reduce your risk of getting cancer, think about changing those factors that are within your control, such as diet and tobacco use.

Often a patient is the first to suspect cancer. This is why it is important to learn some of cancer's most common warning signs:

- Change in bowel or bladder habits
- A sore that does not heal
- Unusual bleeding or discharge
- Thickening or lump in the breast or elsewhere
- Indigestion or difficulty in swallowing
- Obvious change in wart or mole
- A nagging cough or hoarseness

The chances of cure are greatest if cancer is discovered at an early stage. If you are a woman, you should learn to perform the breast self-examination to detect suspicious lumps as early as possible. If you are a man, many physicians recommend self-examination for testicular cancer.

Unlike normal cells, which grow and reproduce in the orderly manner dictated by their genetic coding in their chromosomes, cancer cells grow

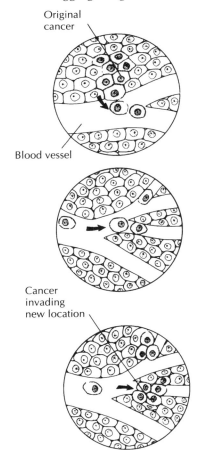

Original cancer

Blood vessel

Cancer invading new location

Benign tumor

Malignant tumor

A tumor may be either benign (noncancerous) or malignant (cancerous). A benign tumor commonly grows within a self-produced capsule and does not invade surrounding tissue nor spread itself throughout the body (metastasize). A malignant (cancerous) tumor may grow out of control and metastasize.

The spread of cancer from its original site to other locations in the body is called metastasis. As cancer progresses, cells often travel through the circulatory system to start growth in other parts of the body.

at an uncontrolled rate—taking over, causing the death of, or replacing normal cells. As the disease progresses, cancer cells often travel through the circulatory and/or lymphatic system to start growth in other parts of the body; this process is called metastasis.

A tumor is an abnormal tissue growth. A tumor may be either malignant (cancerous) or benign (noncancerous). A benign tumor commonly grows within a capsule and does not invade surrounding tissue (although it can cause trouble by pressing on surrounding tissue) or spread throughout the body. Malignant tissues usually grow out of control; quite often, they spread.

More than 200 types of cancer have been identified. There are three basic categories of cancer: carcinoma (cancer of the epithelial cells, which line organs and secrete mucus, among other functions), sarcoma (cancer of connective tissue, such as bone, fat, and muscle), and fluid cancers (for example, leukemia). Some cancers may fall into more than one category.

If you suspect you may have cancer, *do not delay* in seeing a physician. Following a physical examination, if the doctor suspects abnormal growth, he or she may order a series of tests, including special X-ray examinations (for example, computed tomography or CT scans, in which successive X rays at slightly different levels are used to create a three-dimensional image of a structure), nuclear medicine scans (in which radioactive substances are used in the imaging process), ultrasound scanning (a technique that uses sound waves to create images of internal structures), cytologic tests (microscopic examination of cells), and various laboratory evaluations. MRI, or magnetic resonance imaging, is rapidly becoming a major asset in diagnosing cancer without the use of X

rays. The doctor may also order a biopsy (removal of a small tissue sample for microscopic examination) to determine the cell type of the suspected growth and whether it is benign or malignant.

Your physician may also refer you to a specialist with expertise in treating the type of cancer that you have. This may be an oncologist (cancer specialist), a cancer surgeon, a radiation oncologist (radiologist who uses radiation to treat cancer), or a hematologist (specialist in blood diseases). These physicians are specially trained to deal with the diagnosis and treatment of cancer.

There are many places to get cancer treatment. Most cancers can be effectively treated at a well-equipped and well-staffed community hospital. There are, however, a number of large cancer centers throughout the country where specialized treatment programs (called protocols) are available. Often, diagnosis and treatment are initiated at a special center and then continued in the community by an oncologist or a family physician. If you need information or referrals, cancer hotlines and the American Cancer Society are valuable resources. They or your personal physician should be able to assist you in getting a second opinion about your case, if you want one.

There are many ways of treating cancer. Many treatment protocols have been developed that are effective in certain types of disease. Cancer therapy often includes surgery to remove the cancer, to clear obstructions of vital passageways caused by the cancer, or to cut the nerves sending pain messages to the brain; chemotherapy (use of powerful drugs to kill cancer cells); radiation therapy (use of radioactive materials in the form of energy beams or radioactive implants to destroy cancer cells); and immunotherapy (use of naturally

In front of mirror, examine breasts for changes with arms extended overhead. This position highlights bulges and indentations which may indicate a lump.

Squeeze nipples gently to inspect for any discharge. Report any suspicious findings to your doctor.

In the shower, keep one hand overhead and examine each breast with opposite hand. Wet, soapy skin may make it easier to feel lumps.

Lying in bed, place a pillow under one shoulder to elevate and flatten breast. Examine each breast, with the opposite hand, first with arm under head and again with arm at side.

In front of a mirror, stand with hands resting on hips. Examine breasts for swelling, dimpling, bulges, and changes in skin.

Make rotary motions—with flat pads, not tips, of fingers—in concentric circles inward toward nipple. Feel for knots, lumps, or indentations. Be sure to include the armpit area.

occurring substances to increase the activity of the body's immune system). Combinations of therapies are often used.

Surgery is the most commonly used method of dealing with cancers that develop into tumors. If cancer is contained in one area, surgery can sometimes completely eliminate it. New surgical techniques are continually expanding the range of tumors that can be safely removed. Furthermore, if the surgeon is able to remove only a part of the tumor, the reduced tumor can often be successfully controlled with chemotherapy or radiation therapy.

More precise surgical techniques mean that surgery today is often less disfiguring than in the past. In addition, new developments in skin grafting make it possible to begin reconstructive work on patients—for instance, those with cancer of the head and neck—simultaneously with the cancer surgery.

Sometimes surgery is performed on a patient even though it is known that surgery will not cure the cancer. The removal of a tumor may simply make the patient more comfortable. In other cases, nerve pathways to the pain center in the brain may be cut. Certain noncancerous growths may be removed because they may develop into cancer or because they are exerting pressure on adjacent anatomic structures (which may lead to functional problems).

Chemotherapy (the treatment of cancer with drugs) has gradually become much more widely used. Many kinds of cancer can be effectively treated with chemotherapy alone. Anticancer drugs are also often used as an adjuvant (supplement) to primary treatment, such as surgery. Once surgery has reduced a cancerous growth, chemotherapy can often eliminate it. Chemotherapy has proved effective against some forms

of cancer that formerly were almost always fatal, in particular, Hodgkin's disease (cancer of the lymph system), acute lymphocytic leukemia (a blood disease predominantly occurring in children), and cancer of the testes (male sex glands).

Most cancer drugs attack any rapidly reproducing cells in the body, whether they are cancerous or not, producing some of the side effects of chemotherapy. Destruction of normal cells that reproduce frequently, such as those in the digestive tract, the hair follicles, and the bone marrow, can lead to nausea, hair loss, and lowered red blood cell count.

Usually, several drugs are administered in combination. If the cancer does not respond, or if resistance to a medication develops, another combination of drugs may be tried.

Radiation destroys the ability of cells to divide. Cancer cells are far more susceptible to radiation than normal cells, although not all cancers respond to radiation. Like surgery, radiation therapy is usually a localized treatment, directed at a particular cancer site. Radiation treatment may also involve implanting a radioactive object directly into a tumor, destroying it from within. Radiation can be used before surgery to reduce a tumor to operable size, and frequently a patient receives radiation after surgery to destroy any cancer cells that might remain near the cancer site. Some tumors can be treated by radiation alone.

Radiation therapy is continually being refined. Drugs have been discovered that make cancer cells more sensitive to radiation. Different forms of radiation are being tested on resistant cancers. In addition, radiation today can be directed more precisely, and in stronger forms, with little harm to surrounding tissue. However, there are still side effects, including loss of appetite, nausea, and temporary hair loss. It is not certain how dangerous it is to be treated with radiation, which is itself carcinogenic (capable of causing cancer); however, it is generally considered that a cancer in the body is far more threatening than the future effects of radiation therapy.

The goal of immunotherapy is to enable the patient's body to produce substances that resist the growth of cancer. The basis of immunotherapy is the theory that cancer develops when, for some reason, the body fails to destroy abnormal cells. Immunotherapy for the treatment of cancer is still in the experimental stage.

Sometimes, in desperation, a patient or his or her family will seek unorthodox methods of treatment such as various forms of dietary therapy or the use of drugs of unproved value.

One such unorthodox treatment is the use of laetrile, an extract of apricot pits that some have proclaimed is a cure for cancer. This substance has been banned in the United States because it has been shown to be of no value against cancer in laboratory animals and has yet to be adequately tested in humans. Furthermore, laetrile has been shown to be poisonous.

The medical community is actively researching all known methods of treating cancer and carefully evaluating those that look most promising. Many treatments are slow, and often have severe side effects. Many quack cures offer—but do not deliver—rapid cure with fewer side effects. The harm done by quack practitioners is that they prevent a patient from seeking effective treatment until it is too late for any treatment to be of use. The best advice for someone with cancer is to trust a physician to treat the disease and not waste time, money, and hope on an unproven "cure."

If you do develop cancer, a number of prognostic factors (factors that predict length of survival) are impor-

tant. Most important are the stage and the type of the disease. The earlier the stage of the disease (that is, the earlier in its course it is diagnosed) the better the prognosis will be. The type of tumor is also important, since the various types may respond differently to treatment. Furthermore, more than one type of cancer can occur within a specific organ. For example, all lung cancers do not involve the same kind of cell. Your age and overall physical condition are also important in determining your ability to win the fight against cancer.

Cancer should no longer be considered the dreaded scourge that it was 20 years ago. It is not always fatal and is, in many instances, curable. The keys to living today should be to avoid carcinogens (cancer-causing substances, such as tobacco and asbestos), to consult your physician regularly (and discuss possible risk factors), and to perform regularly the important self-examination procedures that your doctor suggests. Early detection is extremely important.

# Candida albicans

*Candida albicans* is a fungus that is normally present on the skin and on membranes of the mouth, throat, intestines, and vagina. It becomes an infecting agent only when there is some change in the body environment that allows it to grow out of control.

The most common cause of infection may be the use of antibiotics that destroy beneficial as well as harmful microorganisms in the body and permit *Candida* to multiply in their place. The resulting condition is known as candidiasis, candidosis, moniliasis, or a "yeast" infection. In the mouth, it is thrush; on the skin, an inflamed rash such as diaper rash; in the vagina, vaginitis, moniliasis, or yeast infection; and in or next to the nails, candidal onychomycosis or paronychia, respectively. Candidal infection can also affect the esophagus (food tube) and the digestive tract. In rare instances, when body resistance is low, *Candida albicans* enters the bloodstream and causes serious infection of the vital organs.

Drug addicts, diabetics, people with AIDS, and patients receiving chemotherapy are especially at risk. So are those whose natural defenses are weakened by drugs that suppress the immune system (such as those given to recipients of organ transplants). Pregnant women are often susceptible to moniliasis, and thrush may develop in babies who passed through an infected birth canal. Babies may develop yeast infection of the diaper area because of the constant wetness.

The symptoms and treatment for the various forms of *Candida* infection are as follows:

- Vaginitis is characterized by a white or yellow discharge, with inflammation of the walls of the vagina and of the vulva (external genital area). A white, curdlike substance may cling to the walls of the vagina. Treatment is with an antifungal drug, such as nystatin, which is inserted deep in the vagina and, if necessary, applied to the entire region around the entrance to the vagina. The infection is often passed to the woman's sexual partner, causing irritation, redness, and soreness of the head of the penis and sometimes a slight discharge. Both partners should use the medication when one has a recurring infection. Otherwise, the disease may pass back and forth between them. Recurrent *Candida* vaginitis or vaginitis that does not respond to treatment may indicate that another illness, such as diabetes, is present or that a different microorganism is responsible for the infection.

- Thrush appears as creamy white or bluish-white patches on the tongue, which is inflamed and sometimes beefy red; on the lining of the mouth; or in the throat. This is especially common in young infants. Treatment is usually with nystatin oral solution or drops five times a day until a few days after all of the patches have disappeared.

- Diaper rash caused by *Candida* can be treated by keeping the baby as dry as possible with frequent diaper changes. In severe cases, an antifungal ointment may be prescribed.

- Infections of the fingernails and toenails appear as red, painful swelling around the nail; later, pus develops. After the area has been treated with hot compresses and drainage (if necessary), and the nail has been cut back, an antifungal lotion is applied. The nail itself may be involved (appearing hard, yellow, and dull), making treatment more difficult and perhaps necessitating long-term use of oral drugs. Newer oral drugs, such as ketoconazole, are reserved for more severe or resistant infections.

- Systemic infection (when infection enters the bloodstream and affects the kidneys, heart, lungs, eyes, or other organs) can result in high fever, chills, anemia, and sometimes a rash or shock. Disease in the lungs can cause bloody sputum (mucus discharge); in the kidneys, blood in the urine; in the brain, seizures; in the heart, murmurs and valve damage; in the eye, pain and blurred vision. An antifungal medicine is usually given intravenously.

In all cases, the underlying condition that caused the outbreak of *Candida* must be removed, if possible. This may mean stopping the use of antibiotics or controlling diabetes. The same approach is used to prevent future infections.

See also Onychomycosis and Vaginitis.

---

# Canker sores

Canker sores (medically known as aphthous ulcers) are inflamed tissue cavities, usually found in the mouth. They can be quite painful, often inhibiting eating ability. Even though up to one out of every four persons develops canker sores, they are not contagious.

Researchers disagree about the cause of canker sores. One unconfirmed theory suggests that the sores are the result of an autoimmune response, whereby the body develops antibodies to its own tissue. Other factors that have been said to trigger canker sores include fever, menstruation, fatigue, tension, and allergies. Some people get canker sores after eating certain foods. Poor dental hygiene, ill-fitting dentures, and injuries from stiff toothbrushes may also lead to the condition. All of the above may be contributing factors; however, the true cause of canker sores is unknown.

Canker sores may occur singly or in groups. They can be found almost anywhere in the mouth—inside the cheek and on the tongue, the lips, or the gums.

A canker sore begins as a small blister. After the blister breaks, a small ulcer develops and enlarges until there is a bright red sore surrounding the whitish-yellow cavity. This sore can last about 10 to 14 days before healing. Canker sores leave no scars. However, they often recur, sometimes as frequently as every few weeks or months.

Canker sores have no cure, but there are several treatments that may relieve pain. Some physicians prescribe the antibiotic tetracycline for canker sores. Treatment involves dissolving the capsule in an ounce of warm water and swishing the mixture in the mouth for five to ten minutes. This course of treatment is commonly followed at a frequency of three or four times a day for five to seven days. Sometimes, therapy includes soaking a cotton wad in the solution and applying it directly to the sores.

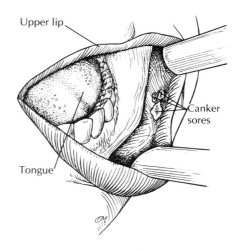

Canker sores are inflamed tissue cavities or ulcers usually found in the mouth, often inside the cheek.

There are also various over-the-counter preparations designed to reduce discomfort. However, they are of uncertain value, and you should always check with your doctor before using them.

Persons who have repeated attacks of canker sores should see a physician or dentist. Recurrence may be lessened by improving oral hygiene or by avoiding certain foods or other substances.

# Carpal tunnel syndrome

Carpal tunnel syndrome is character-ized by weakness, pain, tingling, numbness, or burning in the palm, the thumb, the index finger, the mid-dle finger, and the ring finger, caused by entrapment of the median nerve in the wrist. (This condition, like any syndrome, is not a disease in itself but rather a collection of symptoms.) The condition appears to affect women more often than men, and most often strikes people in their 30s, 40s, and 50s. It may develop or become worse because of work that requires repeat-ed grasping, twisting, or turning of the hand and wrist, especially against resistance or while using vibrating tools. Office workers, typists, and computer operators appear to be affected more frequently than the gen-eral population.

The carpal tunnel is formed by the bones of the wrist (*carpal* means wrist) and the tough band of connective tis-sue known as the transverse carpal ligament. Among the structures inside the tunnel are the median nerve and the tendons that flex the fingers and thumb. Any swelling or thickening of tissue within the tunnel can cause the median nerve to be compressed between the transverse carpal liga-ment and the tendons and other con-tents of the tunnel. The squeezed nerve, which controls the thumb, index finger, and third finger, cannot work as it should, and the symptoms of carpal tunnel syndrome result.

Pregnancy and other conditions that produce generalized swelling of body tissues may be a cause of carpal tunnel syndrome, as can localized swelling caused by a dislocation, sprain, or fracture of the wrist. Rheumatoid arthritis can cause

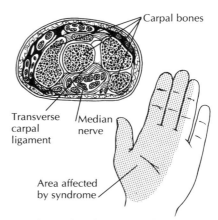

Carpal tunnel syndrome is weakness, pain, tingling, numbness, or burning in the palm, the thumb, and the index, third, and inner part of the ring fingers caused by entrapment of the median nerve within the carpal tunnel of the wrist. The carpal tunnel is formed by the carpal bones of the wrist and the tough band of connective tissue called the transverse carpal ligament.

inflammation of the sheaths (cover-ings) of the tendons, causing com-pression. Other possible causes include an inflamed wrist joint, a benign (noncancerous) tumor, myx-edema (tissue swelling due to lack of thyroid hormone), tuberculosis, amy-loidosis (a disease characterized by abnormal deposits of the protein amyloid), acromegaly (overgrowth of connective tissue), and diabetes mellitus.

Aching pain may travel up the forearm and even into the shoulder joint, neck, and chest. (This type of pain can usually be relieved by shak-ing the hand vigorously or dangling the arm loosely from its socket; occa-sionally, however, such pains are caused by compression of the median nerve in the forearm or upper arm.) Other (late) signs include an inability to make a fist, deterioration of the nails, and dryness and shininess of the skin over the involved surfaces. The pains may occur in both hands at the same time. They may be con-stant or may come and go, and are increased by manual work or movement that flexes the wrist or palm. Weakness of the fingers occurs later than other symptoms and accompanies atrophy (wasting away) of the muscles. Symptoms are usually worse at night and in the morning.

Preliminary diagnostic tests include tapping the wrist, which causes tingling in the area of pain if carpal tunnel syndrome is present, and forced flexion of the wrist, which may also reproduce the pain. An X-ray examination may reveal abnormalities of the wrist bones. Testing of the conduction of nerve impulses is the most specific means of diagnosis.

Treatment is aimed first at relieving pressure on the median nerve. If soft-tissue swelling is a cause, elevating the hand may eliminate the symptoms. It may help to place the forearm in a splint at night, which keeps the hand turned upward, extending the wrist. If an inflammation inside the wrist is at fault, cortisone may be injected into the carpal tunnel. Other causes or aggravating factors associated with carpal tunnel syndrome are treated appropriately.

If conservative forms of treatment prove ineffective, which they frequently do, surgery to release the transverse carpal ligament may be necessary to relieve the pressure on the nerve and prevent permanent damage. Usually, muscle strength gradually returns after such surgery, but if surgery has been delayed too long and muscles have severely deteriorated, full strength does not return. Symptoms usually disappear shortly after the operation, and recurrence is possible.

# Cataract

A cataract is a clouding of the lens of the eye that results in obscured vision.

People with this defect see their environment as if they were looking through a waterfall.

Normally, the lens is clear. Its function is to focus light onto the light-sensitive cells lining the back of

(1)

(2)

(3)

The main symptom of cataract is painless blurring of vision. Vision with early cataract may be close to normal (1). As cataract progresses, vision gradually blurs (2) and eventually may become extremely blurred (3).

the eye, so that objects at various distances can be seen clearly. If the lens becomes hazy, however, incoming light is scattered, and vision blurs.

The exact cause of cataracts is unknown. Aging may play a role, but the condition also occurs in newborns whose mothers contracted German measles during pregnancy and in other young persons.

Diabetes, glaucoma, and detachment of the retina (the innermost layer of the eye) may lead to cataracts. Injury to the lens, prolonged use of certain drugs, and high doses of radiation (for example, from prolonged exposure to X rays) may also trigger the condition.

Although the condition is usually curable, cataracts can cause blindness. In addition, the shadowy lens prohibits a clear view of the interior of the eye. Because of this obstruction, a physician may not be able to detect other potentially serious eye disorders, such as changes in the retina and damage to the optic nerve (which transmits information from the eye to the brain).

The main symptom of cataracts is painless blurring of vision, occurring most often in only one eye. During the initial stages of development, cataracts can cause the person to experience glare in bright light, since the clouded lens scatters, rather than focuses, incoming light. As the condition progresses, the lens becomes milky white, and vision worsens.

Successful treatment begins with surgical removal of the affected lens. With the aid of a microscope, the surgeon opens an area in the front of the eye and removes the lens. The use of local anesthetic eye drops makes the procedure relatively painless.

After the patient has recuperated for a few weeks, special eyeglasses or a contact lens can be prescribed to help correct the vision. These aids are by no means perfect and require an adjustment period. Almost all doctors now recommend the implantation of an intraocular lens in the eye after cataract removal. The lightweight artificial lens is relatively free of distortion. It affords vision that is closer to normal than cataract eyeglasses or contact lenses can provide because it occupies the exact position of the natural lens. This lens allows vision without the use of special cataract lenses, although eyeglasses or contact lenses may still be necessary. Not everyone, however, can benefit from an intraocular lens.

In the vast majority of cases, surgery for cataracts is without complications. Restoration or substantial improvement of vision results after surgery in the majority of cases. If vision remains unimproved, a disorder that was not detected due to the presence of the cataract may be the cause. Generally, however, cataracts can be removed successfully, and the patient can resume a normal life.

# Celiac disease

Celiac disease, or celiac sprue, is a chronic disorder of the small intestine caused by sensitivity to gluten, a protein found in wheat and rye and, to a lesser extent, in oats and barley. The disorder causes poor absorption by the intestine of fat, protein, carbohydrates, iron, water, and vitamins A, D, E, and K. Removal of gluten from the diet normally brings improvement.

The basic cause is probably an inherited defect found mostly in people of northwestern European ancestry. For example, celiac disease affects one person in 300 in the western part of the Republic of Ireland, and approximately one in 5,000 in the United States. It is twice as likely to affect women as men.

One theory about celiac disease holds that the body reacts to gluten and its derivative gliadin as if they were viruses or bacteria. When food containing gluten reaches the portion of the small intestine called the jejunum, antibodies in the intestinal wall are stimulated. In the process, for some unknown reason, the intestinal villi (hairlike projections through which nutrients from the intestine are absorbed into the bloodstream) are destroyed. Destruction of the villi is almost total in the jejunum, less so in the rest of the small intestine. Poor absorption of food and water is the result. Another theory states that gluten and gliadin act directly on the intestinal wall as toxins (poisons). One or both of these theories may be correct.

Symptoms of celiac disease may begin in infancy when the child starts eating wheat cereal or other foods containing gluten. The child does not thrive, suffers painful bloating in the abdomen, and passes pale, foul-smelling, bulky stools. Failure to absorb enough iron produces anemia (deficiency of oxygen-carrying red blood cells). Poor absorption of protein may cause edema (swelling of body tissues). There is little fat on the body. Growth may be stunted, signs of vitamin deficiency appear, and softening of bones may produce bone deformities and fractures. Sometimes the symptoms disappear in adolescence and reappear in adulthood.

Adults with celiac disease have many of the same symptoms, including bulky, foul-smelling stools; weight loss; vitamin deficiencies; edema; anemia; and bone pain. The disease can also cause strange sensations (burning, pricking, tickling, or tingling) in the hands and feet; dry skin; eczema; acne; cessation of menstruation; mood changes; and irritability. The disease may appear for the first time as late as age 60.

The most definitive test for celiac disease is microscopic examination of a piece of tissue taken from the wall of the small intestine. The sample is taken with the aid of a flexible tube with a cutting instrument at the tip, which is inserted through the mouth into the intestine. The specimen from a celiac patient has almost no villi, and the surface is alternately flat and bumpy, with a disorganized network of blood vessels. Various blood tests taken after the patient has eaten specific substances reveal how well the intestine has absorbed these substances. In addition, blood tests may reveal low levels of protein, calcium, potassium, and sodium. Tests of stools reveal excess fat.

The primary treatment of celiac disease is to remove all gluten from the diet, which is easier said than done. Hot dogs, ice cream, commercial soups and sauces, candy bars, and all kinds of baked goods can be sources of gluten (even small amounts of gluten must be avoided). Many doctors refer the patient to a dietitian for detailed lists of foods to avoid and for advice on following a healthful diet, which should be high in calories and protein and low in fat. Vitamin and mineral supplements are given as needed. In stubborn cases, a cortisone drug may be given. This course of treatment will often result in improvement.

The outlook is good for most patients. Recovery is most dramatic in children. In severe cases, however, complete return to normal bowel function and normal absorption may take months. Sometimes normal bowel function and absorption may never occur. For that reason, and to rule out other diseases of nutritional deficiency or poor absorption, it is best to see a doctor as soon as symptoms appear. This is one ailment that is almost completely treatable.

# Cerebral palsy

Cerebral palsy (CP) is a general term to describe various nonprogressive disorders of muscle control caused by a period of lack of oxygen to the brain.

Cerebral palsy is caused by brain or nerve damage that usually occurs before or around the time of birth. The damage may result when brain tissue becomes starved for oxygen for any reason. It may result from separation and bleeding of the placenta (the organ that anchors the fetus to the wall of the uterus and provides nourishment) in late pregnancy or from disorders caused by diabetes in the mother. It is characteristic of cerebral palsy that the neurologic problems are not progressive.

There are four major types of CP: spastic, athetoid, ataxic, and mixed. About 70 percent of cases of CP are the spastic type. Patients with spastic CP move stiffly and with great difficulty because their affected muscles are constantly tense and tight. One arm and one leg may be affected, or both arms or both legs. Affected extremities appear thin and wasted, are weak, and are likely to twist and jerk. Walking on the toes or with a scissorslike movement is typical. When all four limbs are affected, the mouth, tongue, and palate may also be affected, interfering with speech, eating, and drinking, and causing constant drooling.

Athetoid, or dyskinetic, CP accounts for about 20 percent of cases. This disorder, which is caused by damage to the basal ganglia (a mass of nerve-cell bodies at the base of the brain), is characterized by continual slow, twisting movements of the fingers and hands during waking hours. Similar movements of the upper arms or legs and trunk may

also occur. There may be sudden, jerky movements as well.

Ataxic CP results from damage to the cerebellum (a portion of the brain highly involved in muscular coordination) or the nerves leading from it. The characteristic signs of this type of CP are weakness, lack of balance and coordination, tremor, difficulty with fine or quick movements, and a clumsy way of walking, with feet wide apart.

Mixed CP occurs frequently. Often, spastic and athetoid types are combined. Ataxic and athetoid types are mixed less often.

Possible signs of CP in a baby include twitching, convulsions, back-arching muscle spasms, partial paralysis of the face, and very late development of the ability to lift the head, sit, crawl, stand, walk, and talk. Any baby who may have suffered brain damage around the time of birth should be watched carefully for signs of CP (such a baby may have been born nearly lifeless or very small and premature, or may have suffered a severe infection soon after birth). Although it is difficult to diagnose any particular form of CP in the first two years of life, parents should be on the alert to promptly report any suspicious symptoms to their doctor.

After infancy, symptoms of cerebral palsy range from simple clumsiness or slight incoordination of muscles to multiple handicaps that prevent normal movement. Frequently, the brain damage that causes CP also causes mental retardation, epilepsy, hearing problems, visual defects, and learning and behavior disorders. However, some CP children are normal in every respect except for their disordered muscle control.

Early diagnosis and treatment of CP are essential if a child is to develop as fully as possible. An important part of the diagnostic evaluation is to discover if there is any other reason for the symptoms. A wide range of medical diagnostic studies and psychological tests will be performed.

Treatment of a CP child may involve many different elements, such as speech therapy, physical therapy, special dental care, specially designed clothes, braces, corrective glasses, surgery, a hearing aid, special furniture, and special schooling. Occupational therapy can help the patient in self-care, including dressing and eating. About 25 percent of CP patients have convulsions, which usually can be controlled by anticonvulsant medicines. Ideally, a physician will work with a team of specialists in a hospital or other setting where appropriate treatments can be coordinated.

Because CP is a lifelong condition, parents need to learn as much as possible about caring for a cerebral palsy child. The parents can learn how to continue therapy at home. Every effort must be made to help the child become self-reliant. Parents can often get valuable advice and support from other parents of CP children and from professionals at the local chapter of the United Cerebral Palsy Association. Therapy for CP children and adults is provided at rehabilitation centers sponsored by the National Easter Seal Society and by various other agencies.

Expectant mothers can guard against CP with good prenatal care emphasizing adequate diet, rest, exercise, frequent checkups, and avoidance of drugs and infections. During labor and birth, the doctor can keep track of the baby's heartbeat with use of a fetal monitor and, if necessary, operate quickly to save the baby from brain damage caused by oxygen starvation. Expectant mothers with difficult pregnancies should try to have their babies delivered at a hospital with a newborn intensive care unit, directed by a certified neonatologist (a physician who specializes in the care of newborn babies). In such a unit, premature and ill babies can be watched closely and cared for by specially trained nurses and doctors using the latest methods.

# Cerebrospinal fluid

Cerebrospinal fluid (CSF) is a clear, colorless fluid that surrounds the brain and spinal cord, cushioning them against injury.

The CSF is made of water containing small amounts of minerals and organic substances (especially protein). It is continually being produced by a specialized network of capillaries (tiny blood vessels) known as the choroid plexus, located in the ventricles (chambers) of the brain. About one pint is produced every 24 hours, and approximately five ounces are circulating at any particular time. From the two lateral (side) ventricles, the CSF flows into the third and fourth ventricles of the brain. It then passes into the space between the innermost and second layers of the tissue covering the brain. By this means it bathes the entire outer surface of the brain in fluid before passing downward around the spinal cord. Eventually the fluid returns upward, is absorbed into special tissue located between the linings of the brain, and eventually passes into the blood vessels.

Samples of CSF (drawn from around the spinal cord with a needle inserted in the lower back—a procedure known as a lumbar puncture) can be valuable in diagnosing disorders of the brain and spinal cord. The samples may indicate a hemorrhage or blood clot in the brain, various types of meningitis, a brain abscess, or a tumor of the brain or spinal cord.

# Cervical cancer

The cervix is the lower part of the uterus (womb), which extends into the vagina. Cancer of the cervix is the second most common cancer among American women. The death rate from this disease has decreased 50 percent over the last 50 years, largely as a result of early diagnosis. Early cervical cancer has no symptoms but can be detected by means of a Pap smear. A Pap smear is performed routinely in a doctor's office by scraping the surface of the cervix. The collected material is then tested for indications of cancer. Today, two out of three cases of cervical cancer are detected with this test before they display symptoms.

Cervical cancer has a higher incidence among black women and poor women. In addition, this cancer also occurs more frequently among those groups of women who were sexually active at an early stage of life with many partners. Cervical cancer is also more common among women who suffer from genital herpes.

If a Pap smear indicates the possibility of cervical cancer, a biopsy of the affected area will probably be performed. Treatment depends on how far the disease has advanced; early forms are almost always curable by surgery. If a patient still hopes to bear children, and the cancer is in an early stage, this surgery can sometimes be put off until after children have been born. However, this is possible only if the disease does not seem to be progressing, and the cancer must be monitored carefully during this phase. The uterus should be removed eventually. More advanced forms of the disease are treated with radiation as well as surgery.

See also Cancer.

# Cesarean section

Cesarean section is a way of delivering a baby by cutting through the external walls of the mother's abdomen and uterus and removing the baby through these incisions. Cesarean section is performed when a vaginal delivery would cause injury to either the mother or the baby.

In the United States today, about 15 to 25 percent of births are by cesarean section. While cesarean delivery is still considered major surgery, the availability of antibiotics, improved anesthetic techniques, and blood transfusions has made cesareans much safer than in the past. Nevertheless, the indications for performing a cesarean section and the disadvantages of the procedure should be weighed carefully by the woman and her physician.

There are two main types of cesarean section.

In the *classic cesarean*, an incision is made vertically on the skin of the abdomen, extending from the navel to the pubic bone. A vertical cut is also made directly down the center of the uterus in its thick upper section. This operation is generally used only if the baby is lying in an abnormal position or if the placenta is located in an abnormally low position in the cavity of the uterus.

The *lower-segment cesarean* is the more commonly performed procedure. The incision in the uterus is made in the lower, thinner section. This incision may be either a vertical cut down the middle or a curved, smile-shaped cut near the lower part of the abdomen.

The classic cesarean produces more bleeding than the lower-segment cesarean. Also, the incision is more difficult to repair, and the uterus is more likely to rupture during a future

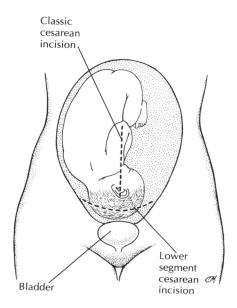

Classic cesarean incision

Bladder

Lower segment cesarean incision

A cesarean section is a way of delivering a baby by cutting through the walls of the abdomen and uterus and removing the baby through these incisions. The two main types of cesareans are the classic and the lower segment; the incisions for each are shown here.

pregnancy. For these reasons, the classic cesarean is seldom used today unless there are specific reasons.

Some of the reasons for a cesarean section include the following:

- To save the baby's life when the umbilical cord (the fetus' supply line from the placenta) is being pinched off during the birth process, or any other time that the fetus is not getting enough blood and oxygen to survive. (These conditions may be indicated by abnormal heart rate patterns during fetal monitoring.)
- To prevent infection of the baby by a dangerous vaginal infection, such as herpes.
- To prevent injury to the baby that may result from a breech birth, during which a baby emerges through the vagina buttocks or feet first rather than head first. (Many

obstetricians believe that cesarean delivery is necessary for all breech births in first-time mothers and all premature breech births.)

- To ease the birth or prevent injury when the baby is too large or the mother's pelvis is too small for a vaginal delivery.
- To deliver the baby if the mother fails to give birth after a long labor.
- To save the baby's life if problems with the placenta cause a decrease in the blood supply to the fetus.
- To facilitate delivery if immediate birth would allow more effective treatment of disease in the mother or the baby.
- To be safe if the mother has had a previous cesarean delivery. (The rule used to be that any woman who had one cesarean would have to have cesarean sections for all subsequent births; however, in recent years, many vaginal deliveries have been performed successfully on women who had previous lower-segment cesarean sections.)

Risks of a cesarean section include possible infection, bleeding, and the formation of dangerous blood clots. There is a small chance that the uterus will rupture during a subsequent pregnancy, before or during birth. The cesarean may be inconvenient for the mother, requiring her to stay in the hospital for three to five days instead of going home with her baby in two days or less. She may not be able to see the baby for a number of hours after delivery if she has undergone general anesthesia. Breastfeeding may be difficult if the mother is being given strong medications to relieve pain, which keep her asleep for long periods of time. There is pain from the abdominal incision, and the mother's activity is restricted once she arrives home. It takes up to six weeks for complete healing of the incision. The expense of the surgical procedure and the extra hospitalization is also a consideration. However, these disadvantages are relatively unimportant if they save the baby from permanent brain damage or save the life of the infant or the mother.

# Chest pain

Chest pain is a major symptom in many disorders, including heart disease and problems relating to the stomach, intestines, and lungs. It is important that you report to your doctor any chest pain, since prompt evaluation and treatment may be lifesaving.

In heart disease, chest pains may be the temporary discomfort of angina pectoris or the similar, but more severe and long-lasting, signs of a heart attack. In both cases, the discomfort is usually felt as an aching, tight, crushing sensation beneath the breastbone that may radiate to the left shoulder and arm. It may also be felt in the right arm, back, throat, jaws, and teeth, or it may spread to both arms or the abdomen. In angina, the discomfort typically is brought on by exertion and disappears in a few minutes with rest or with the taking of nitroglycerin. In a heart attack, the pain is usually much more intense and deep and is most often not relieved by nitroglycerin; in addition, the patient is restless, pale, and perspiring. Nausea and vomiting also often accompany a heart attack.

When the chest pains of angina or a heart attack spread to the abdomen, they are often mistaken for the discomfort of indigestion. Conversely, severe indigestion, ulcer pains, and gallbladder attacks can be mistaken for a heart attack. If there is any possibility that the symptoms might be those of a heart attack, the only recommended plan of action is to obtain emergency medical assistance immediately. The diagnosis must always be left to a physician.

Indigestion is a sign of failure of proper digestion and absorption of food. Among the signs of indigestion may be discomfort in the chest, whether perceived as the burning sensation of heartburn or as sharp, dull, or gnawing pains in the chest area. If chest pain or discomfort occurs only in relation to eating, it could be due to simple indigestion. Any change in severity or frequency of chest pain of any kind should always be reported to a physician.

The chest pains of pleurisy, which may be sharp and stabbing or merely uncomfortable, may occur with every breath or only when the patient breathes deeply or coughs. The pains are caused by inflammation of the pleurae (the membranes that surround the lungs and line the chest cavity). The pains may appear only over the site of the inflammation or may radiate to the lower chest and abdomen.

Among other causes of chest pain are rib injuries, pneumonia, a blood clot in the lung, pericarditis (inflammation of the sac surrounding the heart), inflammation of the nerves supplying the chest wall, and tenderness of the chest muscles after injury or exertion.

See also Angina pectoris, Heart attack, Heartburn, Indigestion, and Pleurisy.

# Chicken pox

Chicken pox is an extremely contagious disease that is characterized by a blistery rash. It occurs most frequently in children between the ages of five and eight; less than 20 percent of the cases in the United States affect people over 15 years old. Chicken pox is transmitted so easily that almost everyone gets the disease at some time.

Chicken pox is caused by infection with the varicella zoster virus.

Chicken pox is contracted by touching an infected person's blisters or anything that has been contaminated by contact with them. The virus is also thought by some researchers to be airborne, since it may be caught from an infected person before the rash develops. Another way to get chicken pox is by exposure to shingles, which is a localized rash caused by the same virus.

The incubation period (the time between exposure to the illness and the appearance of symptoms) of chicken pox is 10 to 21 days. Chicken pox is contagious for approximately six to eight days after the rash appears or until all of the blisters have dried out.

The first symptom of chicken pox is usually a rash, which can be very itchy. It begins as small, red spots on the trunk. Within hours, the spots become larger, fluid-filled blisters on a red base that begin to spread out from the trunk to the face, scalp, arms, and legs. Over the next few days, the blisters continue to fill with pus, burst, and then form a scab or crust. New spots appear periodically during a two- to six-day period. They may spread to the soles and palms. The rash may even affect the eyes, mouth, throat, vagina, and rectum.

Another main symptom is a mild fever (101°F to 103°F) that rises and disappears as the rash comes and goes. Some children have a slight fever and feel sluggish a few days before the rash begins; however, this warning is more common in adults.

Adults usually have higher fevers, a more severe rash, headaches, and muscle aches, and they take longer to recuperate than children. Recovery from all symptoms takes ten days to two weeks.

Complications of chicken pox seldom develop in otherwise healthy people. The most common complication is bacterial infection of the blisters, which may occur if the blister is scratched and the skin is broken. In some instances, the rash spreads to the eyes and causes pain and possible damage. Generally, the chicken pox rash heals without leaving scars, unless the blisters have been scratched and become infected. A rare but serious complication of chicken pox in children is Reye's syndrome (brain inflammation accompanied by liver deterioration). Aspirin should not be given to a child suffering from chicken pox because doing so may put the child at more risk for

The first symptom of chicken pox is usually an itchy rash that begins as small red spots on the trunk. Within hours the spots begin spreading out from the trunk to the face, scalp, arms, and legs.

Reye's syndrome. A doctor should be consulted if breathing problems, high fever, extreme drowsiness, severe headache, vomiting, or unsteadiness occurs within the course of the disease or within several weeks of recovery. These symptoms may indicate further complications.

Since there is no known cure for chicken pox, treatment consists of reducing the effects of the symptoms. A soothing lotion lessens itchiness. Baths in warm (not hot) water sometimes mixed with a special oatmeal solution keep the skin clean, reduce the risk of infection in the rash, and reduce itching. It is important to gently yet thoroughly dry the skin after bathing. If itching is severe, the fingernails should be trimmed and gloves should be worn at night to minimize unconscious scratching. Children may need to wear mittens and socks all day for the duration of the rash.

Since an association has been established between aspirin use during a viral infection and Reye's syndrome in children, it is recommended that aspirin not be given to a child with chicken pox. A doctor can suggest an aspirin substitute if needed for discomfort or fever. Acyclovir, an oral antiviral drug, has been advocated in early treatment of chicken pox. It may lessen the severity, course, and complication rate of the illness.

Although almost everyone contracts chicken pox once, most people do not get it again because the body manufactures antibodies to combat the virus. Nevertheless, the same virus may cause shingles later in life. Researchers are working on a vaccine against chicken pox and shingles; however, this vaccine is not yet available to the public. There is a substance known as zoster immune globulin, which is human antibody against the virus. It must be used shortly after a known exposure to the virus, and there are no guarantees of disease prevention. Because of limited supplies and possible side effects, its use is limited to special cases of exposure, such as in pregnant women or individuals for whom chicken pox could be fatal.

See also Reye's syndrome and Shingles.

# Child abuse

Child abuse encompasses all types of mistreatment—physical, emotional, and sexual—that can be inflicted on a child, particularly by a parent, guardian, or other family member. Closely related is child neglect, in which the parent or guardian chooses not to provide for the nutritional, emotional, physical, or health needs of a child.

The principal cause of child abuse is emotional inadequacy of the parent or guardian. Most parents who abuse their children were themselves abused as children. They did not learn how to give or receive affection from their parents and thus find it hard to develop a good relationship with their own children. They often use the same harsh punishment methods—threats, ridicule, and physical violence—that were used on them as children, often because they do not know any other way of managing family problems.

Some parents who neglect their children are incompetent because of drug or alcohol abuse, medical or psychological disorders, or overwhelming socioeconomic problems. Parents who do not have a support system of close friends or relatives living nearby may feel isolated and overwhelmed by the constant demands of rearing children. Others who may abuse their children are young parents with their first child, parents of ill or premature babies who are separated from them shortly after birth, and parents who did not want a child in the first place. Such parents need special attention and support in order to get their families off to a good start.

Physical symptoms of abuse (also known as the battered child syndrome) include old and new bruises; scars from cuts and burns; serious damage to the eyes, mouth, or internal organs; and X-ray evidence of bone fractures in various stages of healing. When parents cannot give reasonable explanations for the child's injuries, child abuse may be suspected.

Signs of emotional abuse are more difficult to detect. Babies who have been neglected emotionally may appear uninterested in people or even retarded. Another sign in babies is the condition known as failure to thrive, which is unexplained lack of growth even though no illness is present. Older children who are excessively well behaved and overly anxious to please adults, but who do not get along well with other children and are mistrustful may be victims of emotional abuse. At school, they may have trouble with teachers as well as with other children.

Sexual abuse by a parent or older sibling or other relative is often difficult to detect. There may be no physical symptoms, although venereal disease in a child is grounds for suspicion. The child may be too fearful or too embarrassed to reveal the situation to anyone outside the family.

When physicians, teachers, or other professionals suspect child abuse, they are required by law in all states to report it to a government social service agency or welfare department. However, punishment of the parents is not the goal of the law. Jailing a parent might injure the child as much as the original abuse if the parent is capable of being a good father or mother in the future. Removing the child from the family may be necessary to protect the youngster from future injury, but in most cases this is not done or the removal is only temporary.

The child may stay in the hospital for a few days while the case is studied and parents are interviewed. In many communities, a team made up of a social worker, a pediatrician, a psychiatrist, and other specialists talk to the child and the parents and develop a long-term treatment plan. This often involves periodic visits by a social worker to the home and psychological help for one or both parents. Practical help, such as day care for small children and household help by a trained homemaker, can ease the burdens on an overworked mother. If there is a local chapter of Parents Anonymous, an organization of parents who formerly abused their children, this may be another source of emotional support.

Parents who are afraid that they might abuse their children should talk frankly to their family doctor or a social worker. Joining a support group of other parents may be a helpful way to share child-care ideas and experiences.

If a baby is born ill or prematurely and must stay in the hospital after the mother comes home, the parents should visit the baby every day and stay as close as possible so that the baby will not be a stranger when he or she comes home.

# Chlamydia

Chlamydia is a sexually transmitted bacteria that affects the reproductive organs in both males and females. Like other venereal diseases, chlamydia is a highly contagious illness spread primarily through direct sexual contact.

Left untreated, chlamydia infection can lead to prostatitis (inflammation of the prostate gland, where seminal fluid is produced) and epididymitis (inflammation of the ducts leading from the testes) in men and to pelvic inflammatory disease (an inflammation in the pelvic cavity affecting the fallopian tubes) and infertility in women. It can be transmitted from a mother to her baby during childbirth, resulting in ear infections and pneumonia in the newborn; chlamydia has also been linked to an increased risk of stillbirths and sudden infant death syndrome (SIDS).

Chlamydia is transmitted by direct sexual contact with an infected person. It displays symptoms similar to those of gonorrhea.

Sometimes no symptoms are evident. In other cases, there is a discharge from the penis or vagina, pain and burning during urination, and other symptoms similar to those of gonorrhea. In fact, chlamydia can occur with gonorrhea, so if symptoms persist after treatment for gonorrhea, they may be due to chlamydia.

A physician can test for the presence of chlamydia infection by taking a sample of secretions from the penis or cervix. Results of this test can be obtained in as little as 30 minutes. Since gonorrhea can produce the same symptoms as a chlamydia infection, the doctor will usually test for both infections.

Penicillin has no effect on chlamydia, so this disease is treated with another antibiotic, such as doxycycline, tetracycline, or erythromycin. For this reason, treatment of gonorrhea with penicillin will not affect a coexisting case of chlamydia.

A person who has chlamydia or any other sexually transmitted disease should abstain from sexual activity until all tests have indicated that the disease is no longer present. Every sexual partner of the infected person needs to be examined and, if necessary, treated.

Chlamydia infection can be prevented by avoiding sexual contact with someone who has the disease. Because the chances of contracting chlamydia or any other sexually transmitted disease increase with the number of sexual partners a person has, limiting the number of partners is the first step toward prevention. Using condoms also helps to reduce the risk of contracting chlamydia.

# Cholecystitis

Cholecystitis is an inflammation of the gallbladder. The gallbladder is a small, pear-shaped organ that stores the bile produced by the liver and releases it as needed to help digest foods—particularly fats—in the small intestine. Cholecystitis may be either acute (sudden and severe) or chronic (recurring but less severe).

In about 90 percent of cases, acute cholecystitis results when the outlet of the gallbladder or the duct leading from it is plugged by a gallstone. A gallstone is formed in the gallbladder from cholesterol (a fatty substance), calcium, bile pigments, or a combination of these substances. Unless the stone becomes dislodged, inflammation and pressure build up behind it. In severe cases, the swollen gallbladder may not receive enough blood, resulting in tissue death. The gallbladder may become gangrenous or perforated, causing bile to spill into the abdominal cavity. An abscess (a collection of pus within a cavity) usually forms, and bacteria may colonize the region. Occasionally, the resulting leakage of infected bile causes peritonitis (an inflammation of the lining of the abdominal cavity).

However, not all gallbladder attacks progress to this extreme; they may subside only to recur later on. Cholecystitis may also result from a blockage caused by enlargement of the veins in the common bile duct, which the gallbladder shares with the liver.

Acute cholecystitis often begins following a meal rich in fats, such as one containing fried foods, chocolate, or cream. The individual may awaken in the middle of the night with indigestion, gas, and a sharp pain in the upper right quarter of the abdomen, which is often hard and tender to the touch. Pain may also be felt in the middle of the abdomen and may spread to the tip of the right shoulder blade. The pain is crampy and severe. Vomiting is likely and provides some relief. If fever is present, infection of the gallbladder or bile duct is likely. If jaundice (yellowing of the skin, caused by bile pigment in the blood) is present, the symptoms are probably due to blockage of the common bile duct by a gallstone or tumor.

Nuclear medicine scanning confirms the diagnosis of cholecystitis. In this procedure, a radioactive material is administered, and its distribution in the affected area is recorded on X-ray film. X-ray examination and ultrasonography, a technique that uses sound waves to create images of internal structures, may also be used to confirm the diagnosis and to locate gallstones.

Treatment of an acute attack may include rest, intravenous feeding, painkilling drugs, and antibiotics. Because attacks are likely to recur, however, the usual solution is surgical removal of the gallbladder. This is often done immediately. If the patient has another illness, it should be brought under control before the operation is performed. Removal of the gallbladder does not hinder the digestive process, since the liver can compensate for the lost organ.

The mere presence of gallstones found incidentally during tests for other problems does not always mean that surgery is necessary, however. In many cases, gallstones can be present for life without ever causing acute cholecystitis.

Recently, a technique for removing the gallbladder without the standard incision—via a laparoscope—has been used. A laparoscope is a periscopelike instrument inserted through a puncture in the abdominal wall. After the laparoscope is inserted, a laser is used to free the gallbladder from its bed underneath the liver. The gallbladder is then removed through the puncture by suction. This procedure has shortened hospital stays and decreased complications from surgery. In addition, instead of having a large scar, the patient usually has only four small punctures. This procedure is not for everyone with gallbladder problems, however. Individuals who have had numerous abdominal surgeries are usually not candidates. Furthermore, if the attempted laparoscope surgery is unsuccessful, the standard incision may need to be made anyway.

Other nonsurgical methods for removing gallstones, including drug and chemical therapy and lithotripsy (the use of shock waves to shatter the stones), have been tried with varying degrees of success on a select group of patients. The criteria for using these methods, however, is very strict; removal of the gallbladder is still the method of choice in most cases.

Chronic cholecystitis is a continued inflammation of the gallbladder, with repeated attacks over time that are similar to, but milder than, those of acute cholecystitis. Gallstones are usually present; whether they develop before or after the emergence of the disease is unknown. The causes of chronic cholecystitis are not entirely understood, although occasionally bacterial infection is the reason. Diet, heredity, and hormones appear to be involved, and this particular disease is more commonly found among women than men.

The pains of chronic cholecystitis commonly appear over the pit of the stomach and in the upper right quarter of the abdomen. They may range in intensity from mild to unbearable. The pains are crampy and usually come on suddenly, but they may be separated by pain-free intervals of 15 minutes to an hour. The pains may disappear after 15 minutes or continue for several hours; the average attack lasts about an hour. Although the pains may appear together with nausea, gas, and belching and may occur after eating fatty foods, these indications may not be directly related to the disease.

Diagnosis is based on the symptoms and can be confirmed by the same studies used for diagnosis of acute cholecystitis—nuclear medicine scanning and ultrasonography. The doctor must make a careful investigation of other possible causes of the symptoms, including peptic ulcer (which occurs in the stomach or in the beginning of the small intestine), inflammation of the pancreas, and bowel disease.

The ideal way to treat chronic cholecystitis is to remove the gallbladder, together with any gallstones in the duct leading from the liver to the duodenum (the first part of the small intestine). If it is not clear that the symptoms are caused by gallbladder inflammation, or if the patient cannot withstand an operation, other methods are used. These include a low-fat diet (which lowers the need for bile), weight reduction, and use of medications. The use of medication, chemicals, or lithotripsy (the use of shock waves to shatter stones) to

get rid of the stones has very strict criteria, and in most cases, removal of the gallbladder is still the method of choice.

See also Gallstones.

---

# Cholesterol

Cholesterol is a fatlike substance found in all animal fats and oils. It is manufactured by the liver from saturated fats and is a basic ingredient in the formation of normal male and female hormones, vitamin D, blood, bile, cell membranes, brain tissue, the sheaths that protect nerve fibers, and other body substances. After the first six months of life, the liver can make all the cholesterol the body needs—about 1,000 milligrams a day. However, the average American consumes an additional 400 to 600 milligrams of cholesterol a day.

Eating foods containing cholesterol and saturated fats (found in dairy products, animal fat, and coconut and palm oils) can raise the level of cholesterol in the blood. When the blood contains too much cholesterol, or when there is an inherited defect that interferes with the body's ability to use or process cholesterol and fats, the risk of heart attack and blood-vessel disease rises.

Atherosclerosis (one type of hardening of the arteries), which causes most heart attacks, may begin with an injury to an artery wall. Normally, a blood clot would form over the injury and heal it. But when there is too much cholesterol in the blood, cholesterol is also deposited at the site of the wound, which promotes the formation of a plaque. The plaque—made up of cholesterol, dead and dying cells, connective tissue, and calcium—may eventually grow to obstruct the artery. If the blockage is in one of the arteries nourishing heart muscle, it can cause a heart attack.

In the United States, levels of cholesterol in the blood are generally found to be in the range of 100 to 280 milligrams per 100 milliliters. However, dietitians and doctors recommend keeping the cholesterol level below 180, and some researchers suggest that the healthiest range is 100 to 150. Studies show that heart attack risk rises in almost direct proportion to the amount of cholesterol in the blood.

Not all people with high blood cholesterol levels develop heart disease or atherosclerosis, however. This may, in part, be due to the level of a substance called high-density lipoprotein (HDL) in their blood. HDL transports excess cholesterol to the liver, from which it is eliminated in the bile. Persons with high levels of HDL seem to have less risk of vascular (blood vessel) disease. Some people have high HDL levels because of heredity. A doctor approved exercise program will raise HDL levels. Cigarette smoking lowers HDL levels.

Diet is the mainstay of therapy to lower blood cholesterol levels. Diets rich in saturated fats and cholesterol have been proven to contribute to atherosclerosis. A diet that lowers the intake of both saturated fats and cholesterol will lower the total level of blood cholesterol more than a diet that lowers either one alone.

You can reduce the cholesterol in your blood by avoiding fatty meats, cutting back on eggs, and eating more fish and poultry, which contain less cholesterol and saturated fat than meats. Olive oil and peanut oil (monounsaturated fats) are better for cooking than is oil derived from animal fat. Reduction in the use of butter will also be helpful. Seafood, such as lobster, shrimp, crab, clams, oysters, scallops, and abalone, has little or no fat. Therefore, it can be eaten in rea-

sonable amounts. It was previously thought that seafood elevated blood levels of cholesterol. This has since been disproved. There is some evidence to suggest that increasing dietary fiber is also a good idea. Raw fruits and vegetables and whole-grain breads and cereals are all good sources of dietary fiber.

If dietary therapy alone does not lower blood cholesterol sufficiently, then drugs must be added. There are multiple drug preparations available for this purpose. Since all drugs have side effects, these must never be taken unless prescribed by a licensed physician. It must also be remembered that drugs alone will not do the job. Diet modification must be continued. Losing and keeping off excess weight, exercising regularly, and quitting smoking also help to reduce blood cholesterol levels.

# Circulatory system

See Blood, Blood vessels, and Heart.

# Circumcision

Circumcision is the surgical removal of the foreskin, the retractable sleeve of skin covering the glans (the head of the penis). In some religions, the operation is performed as a religious ritual on the eighth day following birth. In hospitals, it is usually done on the day before a baby boy goes home. In any event, if it is to be done for nonmedical reasons, it should be done in infancy and not later, when circumcision is a more serious operation and might harm the child psychologically.

During the five-minute operation, which is usually done without anesthesia, the foreskin is carefully cut away. Gauze coated with petroleum jelly is applied to the incision. In most cases, the incision heals rapidly, forming a dry scab that drops off after a few days. Although the incision should be kept as clean as possible (but not submerged in bathwater), no other special care is necessary. Other than a few drops of blood that might be produced if the diaper rubs against the cut, there is no bleeding in a normal baby.

Routine circumcision for newborns is a controversial issue. The decision about the procedure should be made by the parents after consideration of both sides of the question.

The operation has become standard in American hospitals in recent decades as a cleanliness measure. In a young boy, the foreskin completely covers the head of the penis and cannot be pulled back very far. If the penis is not kept clean, urine and other substances can cause irritation of the glans and perhaps lead to infection between the foreskin and the glans. However, normal care can prevent this problem. There is some recent evidence that uncircumcised males have a higher rate of bladder and kidney infections, but further information is needed before any strong conclusions can be drawn. Even though the foreskin at first cannot be pulled back very far because of bands of tissue that bind it to the glans, it is necessary to wash only the part of the glans that can be uncovered comfortably at any one stage (the foreskin should never be forced back). The bands of tissue gradually dissolve, and by later childhood, the foreskin can be pulled back completely.

Some researchers believe that circumcision reduces the risk of cancer of the penis in the circumcised man and cancer of the cervix (the neck of the uterus) in his sexual partner and may help prevent venereal disease.

However, there is insufficient evidence to support these views.

Very seldom is there a medical reason to perform a circumcision. It should never be done on the first day of life, or if the baby is ill or premature. Furthermore, it should be delayed indefinitely if there is any abnormality of the glans or penis, so that the foreskin can be used later as graft tissue to repair the defect. It should not be done if the mother was taking any medication that promotes bleeding, such as an anticoagulant or aspirin, during pregnancy or is taking such a medication while breast-feeding, nor should it be done if there is any family history of hemophilia or other bleeding disorders.

Risks of circumcision include local infection, which may lead to significant hemorrhage and mutilation. Many medical authorities feel that there is no absolute medical reason for routine circumcision of the newborn. Adequate hygiene offers the same advantages as routine circumcision without the risks of the operation.

Parents, therefore, should consider all factors—cultural, religious, and medical—before making a decision about circumcision.

# Cirrhosis

Cirrhosis is a disease in which cells throughout the liver are progressively destroyed. They are replaced by areas containing normal new cells but also by much scar tissue, which alters the structure of the organ. The flow of blood and lymph through the damaged liver is much less efficient, and eventually the liver fails.

Cirrhosis represents an attempt by the liver to rebuild itself and continue despite injury. The injury may be a sudden and massive infection, as in acute hepatitis, or it may occur in a less dramatic manner over a period of months or years, as in chronic active hepatitis or obstruction of the bile ducts within the liver. The process of obstruction starts with inflammation and progresses to scarring and then closure of the ducts. A similar condition is caused by obstruction of the external bile ducts by a stone, scar, inborn defect, or tumor. The damage is done over an even longer time, slowly and steadily, by alcohol abuse, which is by far the most common cause of cirrhosis. Other causes include the following:

• Use of certain medications
• Inborn errors in physical or chemical processes of the body
• Syphilis
• Passive liver congestion, due to inability of the heart to accept a normal flow of blood from the liver or to obstruction of one of the drainage systems of the liver

Frequently, cirrhosis is not suspected until it is well advanced, because it imitates many other diseases. Symptoms include general weakness, a vague feeling of being unwell, loss of appetite, loss of weight, and a loss of interest in sex. There may be a dull abdominal ache, nausea, constipation, or diarrhea. In a malnourished patient, the tongue may be inflamed. Many symptoms are the result of high blood pressure in the portal vein, which brings blood from the intestinal area to the liver. In cirrhosis, the liver cannot handle a normal flow of blood, so the pressure in the portal vein rises. One result is that fluid from the blood is lost into the abdominal cavity. The fluid may accumulate and press against the diaphragm (the muscular wall separating the abdominal and chest cavities) and interfere with breathing. Collateral blood vessels form to carry away the excess blood into the general circulation. There may be bleeding in the esophagus or stomach when these smaller collateral vessels burst under pressure. The patient may vomit blood. Serious, life-threatening hemorrhage may occur.

The liver may be enlarged and firm or, in advanced cases, shrunken. Other symptoms include an enlarged spleen, mottled redness of the mound at the base of the thumb, "spider veins" on the skin of the upper body; loss of hair from the chest and the pubic area, diminished size of the testes, and tingling sensations in the skin of the hands and feet.

Proof of cirrhosis of the liver is furnished by liver biopsy. A hollow needle is inserted through the skin and into the liver itself to obtain a tissue sample for analysis. Examination of tissue from a diseased liver reveals destruction of cells and scarring. Other diagnostic procedures include nuclear medicine scanning, in which radioactive material is administered and its distribution to the liver is recorded on X-ray film. X-ray pictures are taken of the gallbladder and of bile ducts both inside the liver and leading from it. Important clues that may be found on blood and urine tests include the presence of high levels of bile pigments in the blood, a low red blood cell count (anemia), vitamin and mineral deficiencies, and protein in the urine.

Treatment is aimed first at removing the cause of the original injury. For example, an alcoholic patient is told to stop drinking and is placed on a well-balanced diet. Often, thiamin (vitamin B1) and folic acid supplements are also given. If a stone is obstructing an external bile duct and thus causing liver damage, it can be removed. Fluids and salt are usually restricted, to prevent excess fluid buildup in the body.

Good care includes getting plenty of rest and avoiding infection, which places stress on the liver.

Avoidance of alcohol intake is paramount in the treatment of cirrhosis and most other liver diseases. All medications, including over-the-counter preparations, should be cleared by a physician.

Many of the various causes of cirrhosis of the liver cannot be predicted and guarded against, but the major one can be. Drinking moderately or not at all is the best way to reduce the risk of developing this serious disease.

See also Alcoholism.

# Cleft lip and cleft palate

Cleft lip and cleft palate, a defect in one of every 700 to 800 newborns, is characterized by a split running through all or part of the upper structure of the mouth. A cleft lip (or harelip) may be only a small notch near the center of the upper lip, or it may extend into the nostril. A cleft in the palate can be as minor as a split in the uvula (the little projection of tissue that hangs down in the back of the throat), or it may divide the entire soft palate (the muscular tissue that covers the roof of the mouth). In its most severe form, a cleft splits not only the soft palate but the entire hard palate (the bony roof of the mouth) and upper jaw, joining with a cleft lip. The cleft may even divide the palate into three parts, resulting in a split on either side of the nose and leaving the middle section of the upper jaw and gum dangling.

The formation of a cleft lip occurs in the early stage of pregnancy, soon after the fourth week, when the baby's face starts to form. Bulges of

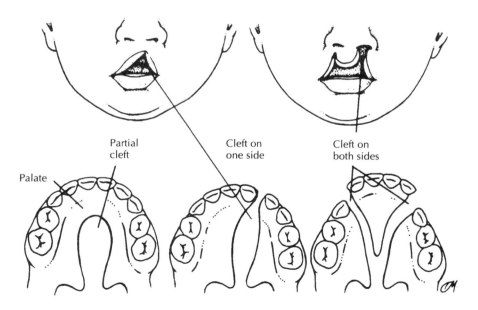

Partial cleft

Cleft on one side

Cleft on both sides

Palate

Cleft lip or cleft palate is a split running through all or part of the upper structure of the mouth. In its most severe form, the cleft may divide the palate into three parts, resulting in a split on either side of the nose and leaving a middle section of upper jaw and gum dangling, as shown on the right.

tissue on either side of the face grow toward the midline to form the nostrils and lips. At about the seventh week they normally meet and join; if they do not, a cleft lip is the result.

A failure of development in the eighth week of pregnancy causes cleft palate. The palate is formed from two plates of tissue, which originally are on either side of the developing tongue. As the head and neck grow, the tongue moves downward and the tissue plates move into position and fuse into one—unless there is an error or weakness, which results in cleft palate.

The underlying causes of cleft lip and cleft palate are not fully understood. There is an inherited tendency toward the defects. More than one-fourth of children with cleft lip also have a relative with a cleft. If parents without cleft defects have one child with a cleft, they have a five percent risk of having a second child with a cleft; if they have two children with clefts, there is a 12 percent risk of a cleft in future children. Perhaps some difference in the uterus, such as poor blood supply to the fetus, combines with an inherited weakness to produce the error of development. Certain chemicals or medications, too many vitamins or not enough, and viruses have been suggested as possible causes of cleft defects.

Cleft lip and cleft palate are often associated with other birth defects. Of every six children who have a cleft lip, with or without cleft palate, one will have one or more other birth defects. Almost 50 percent of children with cleft palate also have another defect, such as joined fingers or toes, malformed ears, spina bifida, heart disease, or clubfoot.

Treatment of a patient with a cleft lip or a cleft palate (or both) requires the services of a specialized team that includes a pediatrician, an orthodontist (a dentist who specializes in the prevention or correction of misalignment of the teeth), a speech therapist, a plastic surgeon, a psychologist, an audiologist (a specialist in communication disorders), and an otolaryngologist (a physician who specializes in the treatment of disorders of the ears, nose, and throat). Treatment may take place at a specialized clinic or hospital center or may be coordinated by a pediatrician who consults experts as needed.

Before any treatment can begin, however, steps must be taken to permit the child to eat. A cleft lip prevents normal sucking, and a cleft palate allows milk to run out of the nose, often causing choking and vomiting. Special feeding devices are used, such as a nipple with an enlarged flange to cover the cleft or a regular nipple with enlarged holes. A small syringe with a short rubber tube, like one used to baste a turkey, may be used to feed a child with a cleft lip, although sometimes such a child can be breast-fed. A few days after birth, an orthodontist skilled in cleft palate repair may be able to fashion an appliance that provides a temporary roof for the mouth, enabling regular feeding. At the same time, the appliance prevents the mouth from being distorted before the palate can be closed.

Some surgeons correct a cleft lip in the first few days of the child's life because it will make the baby more acceptable to his or her parents and make it easier to feed the baby by bottle. However, other surgeons delay the operation for two to eight months, so that surgery will not interfere with the growing bonds of affection between mother and baby (for one thing, the baby cannot breast-feed for six weeks after the operation) and to rule out other birth defects that might interfere with recovery.

Plastic surgery to correct cleft palate usually takes place in the second year of life. Some surgeons repair the soft palate first, when the child is between 6 and 18 months of age, and the hard palate much later—sometimes not until the age of five years. Although early surgery helps the child's emotional and speech development, some surgeons wait because they are concerned that early surgery may cause distortion of growth in the middle third of the face. While waiting, the child wears an appliance that acts as a roof over the mouth.

The problems created by cleft palate and cleft lip cannot be solved only by surgery. The services of an orthodontist are needed for youngsters with cleft palate, not only to make appliances but to straighten teeth that are poorly positioned. A speech therapist aids the child in developing speech, which is altered because of the missing or inadequate soft palate or artificial palate. A psychologist helps to treat emotional and social problems sometimes caused by being different in speech or appearance. An otolaryngologist should examine the child monthly for middle ear infections, which are common in young children with cleft palate. An audiologist helps those children who develop hearing loss because of middle ear infections. With proper care and encouragement and with modern plastic surgery, the average child with a cleft can make a good recovery.

# Clubfoot

Clubfoot, or talipes, is a common birth defect in which one or both feet are fixed in an awkward, twisted position. The foot resists efforts to stretch or turn it back. In *talipes equinovarus*, the most frequent form, the foot points down and turns in while the front of the foot curls toward the heel. If not corrected, the condition worsens and interferes with walking. The person seems to walk on the ankle and the outside or inside edge of the foot.

The cause of clubfoot is unknown. However, there seems to be an inherited tendency for development to be arrested around the ninth week of pregnancy, when the fetus' feet are being formed. Clubfoot may begin as a muscle abnormality. The Achilles tendon is shortened, the ankle and its muscles are deformed, and the heel bone is shortened and flattened to some extent.

Correction of clubfoot should begin as early as the first week after

Talipes equinovarus

Metatarsus varus

The most common form of clubfoot is *talipes equinovarus,* in which the foot points down and turns in with the front of the foot curling toward the heel. Related to clubfoot is *metatarsus varus,* in which the front of the foot turns inward. The condition is often called "pigeon toe."

birth, when the bones, muscles, ligaments, and tendons are soft and pliable. The correction is usually done in stages, rather than all at once. In talipes equinovarus, the first stage is to uncurl the front of the foot away from the heel. The next is to turn the foot so that the sole faces outward. The third stage is to put the foot in a cast with the toes pointing up. This may require surgery to lengthen the Achilles tendon and to free the ankle joint.

Correction generally takes place in a series of small, painless, gradual adjustments. Typically, the doctor flexes and stretches the foot by hand and then fixes it in a cast in a partially corrected position. After a week or so the cast is removed, the foot is manipulated into a better position, and a new cast is applied. Sometimes, instead of making a new cast each time, the doctor places wedges inside the existing cast to adjust the foot. The entire casting process may take three months.

Once the correction has been made, it must be followed up with exercises, devices that hold the feet in place at night while the baby is sleeping, and orthopedic shoes. A night splint (corrective shoes with soles joined by a flat metal bar that keeps the feet in exactly the right position) is often used.

Because clubfoot sometimes recurs, periodic checkups are necessary until the child becomes an adult. However, in most cases, the correction is completely successful, and the individual can walk and run in a perfectly normal way.

If early treatment has not succeeded, or if a child is not treated until the age of nine or ten years, more extensive surgery may be necessary. This is followed by several weeks with the foot in a cast. Satisfactory results are usually obtained. The foot is rather stiff, but

this does not prevent the individual from engaging in the most active sports.

Related to true clubfoot is a condition called metatarsus varus, in which the front of the foot turns inward. Also known as apparent clubfoot and pigeon toe, this is a milder deformity that may not be diagnosed in the first several weeks. Unlike a true clubfoot, the apparent clubfoot can be moved easily into a correct position. It can usually be corrected by manipulation and exercise, without the need for casts or surgery.

---

# Colic

Colic means different things to different people, but the universal characteristic is crying—not just short periods of fussiness that can be stopped by changing or feeding or cuddling—but long periods of crying with no apparent cause that defy all attempts to stop them.

It has long been assumed that colic arises from some gastrointestinal disorder. However, studies have shown no correlation between colic and poor weight gain or excessive vomiting, constipation, or diarrhea. Colicky babies are generally quite healthy, with no sign of nutritional problems. Nor does the problem appear to be hunger; the crying spells often begin after a feeding, not before one. It has been suggested that bottle-feeding is at fault, but breast-fed infants are just as likely to have colic. Lactose intolerance, food sensitivities, and allergies have also been suggested as causes of colic.

Some babies with colic seem to have no such digestive symptoms— their crying seems to be related to general irritability, possibly because of immaturity of the nervous system or exceptional sensitivity to the environment. In other cases, babies experience a combination of the two types of colic.

Colic most often begins when an infant is two to four weeks old. The baby will cry inconsolably for hours a day. These bouts of crying often occur as if on schedule (most often in the late afternoon or early evening). The colicky baby pulls his or her legs up, clenches his or her fists, screams, and turns red. The baby may nurse briefly but then stop to continue crying. The abdomen may be distended as if with gas, and the baby may even pass gas frequently. Generally, there are no other gastrointestinal symptoms; the bowel movements are normal, and the baby doesn't spit up any more than most babies. The baby's sleep pattern is often disrupted—he or she may wake frequently (every two hours or so), cry fretfully, take one to two ounces of formula or a few minutes at the mother's breast, fall into a fitful sleep, and then awaken to repeat the sequence.

Before assuming that your baby has colic, check for other possible causes of crying, such as pain from an open diaper pin or discomfort from being overheated, constipated, hungry, or wet. See whether your baby responds promptly to talking and cuddling—a baby in pain can be distracted, but only temporarily. Also check for signs of illness: colic is not associated with fever, diarrhea, vomiting, cough, a runny nose, or reddened eyes.

Your pediatrician will want to rule out more serious causes of crying before assuming that your baby has colic. Signs of illness, such as sores in the mouth or gastrointestinal or urinary tract problems, will be sought. Although conclusive scientific evidence for a dietary basis for colic is lacking, your doctor may want to investigate the possibility that something in the baby's diet (or in the mother's diet if the baby is breast-fed) may be causing the condition.

If the colic seems to be due, at least in part, to an accumulation of gas in the abdomen, be careful not to overfeed the baby and be sure to burp him or her thoroughly after feedings. If you are bottle-feeding, check the nipple hole; if it is too large or too small, the baby may be swallowing too much air. A warm hot-water bottle on the abdominal area may relieve some discomfort. The baby may be most comfortable lying on his or her stomach.

If the colic seems to be due to irritability, it might be helpful to restrict visitors and to keep the home environment as peaceful as possible. Some researchers believe that overly sensitive babies may be upset by an atmosphere charged with too much noise, too much activity, and too much emotional stress.

Your physician will probably not recommend any medical treatment for colic. Colic usually ends two or three months after it begins, with no physical or emotional consequences.

See also Crohn's disease and Ulcerative colitis.

# Colon cancer

Every year, many Americans die of cancer of the colon and rectum. About half of all cases of cancer of the colon can be cured by surgery, and early detection can greatly improve this percentage. A simple test for occult (not visible to the naked eye) blood in the stool can indicate whether further tests should be made for the presence of this type of cancer. Everyone who is over 40 or who has chronic digestive problems should have this test regularly. Cure is twice as likely if the disease is discovered before symptoms occur.

Symptoms of cancer of the colon include a change in bowel movements, bleeding from the rectum, pencil-thin stools, and abdominal discomfort not eased by bowel movement. If you have any of these symptoms, your doctor will probably perform a rectal exam, inserting a finger into the rectum to search for unusual growths. If further examination is necessary, the doctor may introduce a proctosigmoidoscope (a lighted, tubelike instrument) into the colon through the anus. This instrument permits examination of the inside of the colon and can also be used to obtain a biopsy specimen of a suspicious growth. Sometimes, a noncancerous growth called a polyp is removed with a similar instrument, because such a growth may become cancerous.

Surgery is the usual treatment for cancer of the colon. If the cancer is near or in the rectum, the surgeon may remove all of the rectum and create an artificial rectum, or colostomy, in the lower abdominal wall. A colostomy is covered with a bag to collect waste material. It is important to note that colostomy is not automatically done for any colon cancer. The type of operation performed is dictated by the size and location of the tumor along with other factors.

See also Cancer.

---

# Color blindness

Color blindness is an inability to distinguish certain colors. By far the most common type is inherited red-green color blindness, which affects eight percent of men and boys but only 0.5 percent of women and girls. Total color blindness, which is very rare, and pastel-shade blindness are believed to be inherited. Other types, including blue-yellow blindness and red-green blindness, can be either inherited or acquired. Disease or injury affecting the retina sometimes causes color blindness.

Color blindness results from a defect in the cone-shaped light-sensitive cells of the fovea (the tiny, yellowish pit in the retina, which is the center for perceiving color). The seven million cone cells differ from the 130 million rod-shaped cells in the rest of the retina in that, while the rod cells register only black and white, the cone cells contain pigments for red, green, and blue—the colors that can combine to produce all the colors of the spectrum. The pigments become more vivid or fade in response to colors that the eye sees. The changes in pigmentation produce tiny flashes of electricity, which are carried by means of the optic nerve to the visual center of the brain. There, the electrical signals are combined into a full-color picture. In the color-blind person, for unknown reasons, the cones are missing or defective. No cure is known.

Why is red-green color blindness inherited by boys more often than by girls? The reason is that the defective gene, which directs production of the defective pigment, is carried on the same pair of chromosomes that determines the sex of the child. In a female child (who has two X sex chromosomes), a defective gene on one X chromosome is almost always counteracted by a normal gene on the other X chromosome; as a result, the girl is born with normal color vision. In a male child (who has an X and a Y sex chromosome), there is no matching normal gene to block the defect on the only X chromosome the boy has; the boy is, therefore, born color-blind.

Red-green color blindness cannot be passed from a father to his sons, nor will his daughters be color-blind, unless the mother carries the defective gene. However, his daughters will all be carriers of the defective gene, and the daughters' sons will have a 50 percent chance of being color-blind.

# Colostomy

Colostomy is the creation of a stoma (opening) in the wall of the abdomen to which an opening in the colon is attached. Thereafter, the contents of the colon are eliminated through the stoma instead of through the rectum and anus (the normal opening to the outside of the body).

The opening may be permanent (as in some operations for cancer of the rectum, which eliminate the normal exit of the bowel), or it may be temporary (as in treatment of severe diverticular disease or Hirschsprung's disease).

Having a permanent colostomy does not prevent a person from leading a normal life. The patient is taught how to empty the colon once a day by using irrigations (enemas) and a special collecting device. By manip-

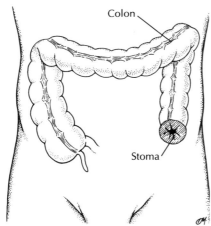

Colostomy is the creation of a stoma (opening) in the wall of the abdomen to which an opening in the colon is attached. The contents of the colon can then be eliminated through the stoma rather than through the rectum and anus.

ulating the diet, it becomes possible to anticipate bowel movements. At first, patients wear a pouch over the stoma to collect any leakage from the colon. An adhesive is used to form a tight seal around the opening of the pouch and the stoma, and a deodorant in the pouch controls odor. After a while, many patients with so-called dry colostomies need only wear a stoma cap or a small gauze patch over the stoma to absorb mucous secretions. Physical activities can be resumed, with or without a pouch, including swimming, other noncontact sports, and sexual relations. The only exceptions are heavy lifting, which could cause a hernia through the weakened abdominal muscles, and any activity that could injure the stoma or abdomen.

To avoid infection of the stoma and irritation of the skin around it, the patient needs to wash the surrounding skin area with mild soap and water each day and then rinse and dry it. Special adhesive materials that protect and soothe the skin have become available. These are applied after cleaning the skin.

Support, encouragement, and practical advice from those who have undergone the operation are available through local chapters and the national headquarters of the United Ostomy Association.

See also Ileostomy.

# Common cold

A simple common cold is a collection of familiar symptoms signaling an infection of the upper respiratory tract, which includes the nose, throat, and sinuses.

Colds are self-limiting diseases, meaning that their symptoms last a certain length of time (or "run their course") and then disappear without

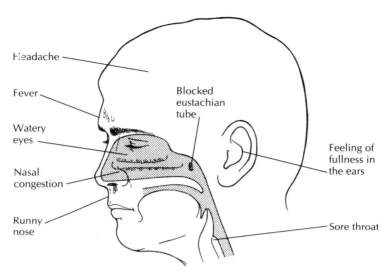

Headache

Fever

Watery
eyes

Nasal
congestion

Runny
nose

Blocked
eustachian
tube

Feeling of
fullness in
the ears

Sore throat

The symptoms of a common cold affect the upper respiratory tract, including the nose and throat.

leaving lasting ill effects. A cold is a mild but commonplace disease, contracted by adults about two to four times a year and by children about six to eight times a year. Adults with children at home are more likely to catch colds than are those who do not have children. Children are especially susceptible to colds because they have not yet developed immunity or resistance to the many viruses that can cause colds. Small children gradually build up immunity to the viruses in their homes; when they go to school and have close contact with many other children, they are exposed to new viruses. Similarly, adults who travel frequently or have a high number of close contacts outside their community are more likely to contract colds or encounter new cold viruses to which they are not immune than those leading more isolated lives.

A cold can be a minor irritation, but it can increase susceptibility to more serious conditions, especially in the very young, the very old, and the very weak. Pneumonia, an inflammation of the lungs, is probably the most serious. Ear infections, sinus infections, and bronchitis are other possible complications. A few days after a cold, children sometimes develop croup, recognized by a harsh, barking cough that signals swelling of the airways to the lungs.

At least five major categories of viruses cause colds. One of these groups, the rhinoviruses, includes a minimum of 100 different types of viruses. Various combinations of symptoms and possible complications can develop from each of these viruses. It is not known exactly how viruses spread, but it seems to be a combination of physical contact and the presence of both virus particles and moisture in the air. A virus can be spread by hand-to-hand contact, for example, or by the passage of droplets from an infected person's nasal passages and throat into the air. Colds have an incubation period of 48 to 72 hours, meaning that it takes that long after the virus enters the body for early symptoms to appear.

Early symptoms of the common cold include a stuffy or runny nose, sneezing, a sore or scratchy throat, a cough, and occasionally a mild fever. Usually, as the cold progresses, other symptoms—burning or watery eyes, loss of the senses of taste or smell, pressure in the ears or sinuses, nasal voice, and tenderness around the nose—may appear.

Symptoms vary in type and severity from one viral infection to another, so a cold can begin with any symptom or combination of symptoms. Most colds last about a week, but about 25 percent of all colds last two weeks. Smokers and those with chronic respiratory diseases tend to have more severe symptoms and longer-lasting colds and to experience complications more readily than do those who do not fall into these categories.

Since common colds are mild diseases, the physician, in diagnosing a cold, will actually be looking for symptoms indicating a condition more serious than a common cold. Material from the patient's throat or nasal passages may be tested for bacterial infections. A blood test may be recommended to check for mononucleosis, a disease characterized by a long-lasting sore throat and swollen lymph nodes. An X-ray examination of the sinuses may be necessary if sinusitis (an infection of the sinuses) is suspected.

Getting plenty of rest, drinking lots of fluids to prevent dehydration, and using a humidifier or vaporizer can help relieve the irritating symptoms of a cold. Nevertheless, the common cold cannot be cured, and no known treatment will actually hasten recovery. Many over-the-counter (nonprescription) medicines and preparations are available that will at least ease the discomfort of a cold. However, it is best to take specific medications only for the symptoms actually present and to carefully follow directions on the medication package. Overuse of an

otherwise effective remedy can backfire and actually make the symptoms worse, and treating symptoms that are not there can complicate matters. For example, the overuse of an antihistamine for nasal congestion can make a cough more uncomfortable, and the use of a nasal decongestant for more than three days can actually increase congestion (because the blood vessels tire and relax, causing rebound congestion). Anyone who is pregnant or has a chronic disease should check with a doctor before using cold preparations, even seemingly harmless over-the-counter drugs.

There is no known preventive for the common cold. Vitamin C has been said to help prevent colds, but many studies have shown that it has no measurable effect in this regard. Avoiding exposure to viruses, when possible, may be the only means of avoiding the common cold.

See also Bronchitis, Croup, Infectious mononucleosis, Pneumonia, and Sinusitis.

---

# Conception

Conception is the union of a sperm cell from the father with an egg from the mother to begin a new life.

During the course of her life, the average woman produces 350 to 400 eggs, or ova. The two organs in which the eggs are produced, known as ovaries, are located near the top and on either side of the uterus. Ducts known as fallopian tubes conduct the eggs toward the uterus. At the midpoint of the average 28-day menstrual cycle, an egg matures in one of the ovaries, is expelled from the ovary during the process called ovulation, and starts to travel through the nearby fallopian tube toward the uterus. The egg is propelled by the waving action of tiny hairlike structures, known as

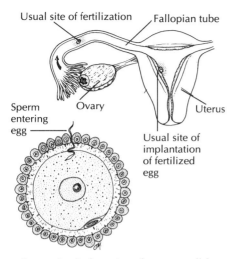

Usual site of fertilization    Fallopian tube

Sperm entering egg

Ovary    Uterus

Usual site of implantation of fertilized egg

Conception is the union of a sperm cell from the father with an egg from the mother to form a new life. Once a month one of a woman's ovaries releases an egg that travels through the nearby fallopian tube toward the uterus. If the egg meets sperm cells en route, conception may occur.

cilia, that line the tube. If the egg meets a sperm cell en route, conception may occur.

Sperm cells—which look like tadpoles through a microscope—originate in the man's testes. At the climax of sexual intercourse, an average of 300 million to 500 million sperm cells, contained in a teaspoonful of thick white fluid, spurt from the tip of the man's penis deep into the woman's vagina. Immediately the sperm start swimming forward, propelled by their long, waving tails and aided by contractions of the muscles of the woman's vagina and uterus. The goal of the sperm is to swim through the cervix, into the uterus, and up one of the fallopian tubes where it can then fertilize an egg.

Millions of sperm are killed by the acidic secretions of the vagina and the cervix or become trapped by mucus in the vagina. (During the middle of the woman's menstrual cycle, when the egg is moving along a fal-

lopian tube, the secretions are thinner, less acidic, and less of a barrier; also, there are alkaline chemicals in the fluid accompanying the sperm, which act to neutralize the woman's acidic secretions.) The vast majority of sperm fail to pass through the uterus and up one of the fallopian tubes. During most of the woman's menstrual cycle, both tubes are empty and the sperm find nothing to fertilize. Only for a few days is an egg present in one of the tubes, and then it may be reached by only a few of the millions of sperm cells that began the journey. The sperm completely surround the egg, their tails waving furiously in an attempt to force their pointed heads into the female cell. Finally, one succeeds. The tail detaches, and the head moves toward the center of the egg. In seconds, a chemical change comes about in the egg that prevents the entry of any other sperm. Conception has occurred.

Unlike all other cells in the body, the sperm and the egg each contain only 23 chromosomes (chromosomes are the chemical "blueprints" that together determine all of the inherited characteristics of an individual; all of the other cells contain twice that number). In the first 12 hours after conception, the 23 chromosomes from the mother and the 23 chromosomes from the father join to form a new nucleus of 46 chromosomes. This is the basic unit from which the new individual will develop.

During the next four or five days, as the fertilized egg, or zygote, drifts down the fallopian tube and into the uterus, the original cell divides and subdivides into anywhere from 16 to 48 cells. In another two or three days, the growing cluster of cells becomes implanted in the nourishing, blood-rich lining of the mother's uterus, which soon forms the beginning of a placenta around the baby-to-be, called an embryo at this stage. (The placenta is the structure through which oxygen and nutrients pass from the mother to the fetus and through which carbon dioxide and other waste products pass from the fetus to the mother.) Within about 17 days after conception, the placenta begins blood circulation to the embryo. In the embryo, various cells are specializing to form different parts of the baby's body. By the end of the seventh week of pregnancy, all of the basic structures of the body have been formed. The developing embryo now is called a fetus until birth.

See also Ovulation.

# Concussion

Concussion is an injury to the brain caused by a violent jar or shock, such as a blow to the head. The force of the shock causes the brain to strike against the inside of the skull, producing temporary brain swelling and malfunctioning and often loss of consciousness. The shock may even be strong enough to cause cerebral contusion (bruising of brain tissue), cerebral hemorrhage (bleeding between the covering of the brain and the skull or inside the brain covering), or formation of a hematoma (collection of clotted blood).

Unconsciousness is a common symptom of concussion. Unconsciousness may last only a few minutes or as long as a few hours, but rarely more than 24 hours (a longer period of unconsciousness or a deep coma indicates more serious brain damage). The patient may then feel nauseated, irritable, "dragged out," or dizzy, or may have a severe headache; these symptoms may continue for days or weeks (or longer) after the accident. Frequently, the individual cannot remember what happened just before the injury and later may not be able to recall anything that happened in the first few hours or on the day following the concussion.

A person who suffers an accident serious enough to cause a cerebral contusion; laceration (cutting and tearing) of nerve tissue, blood vessels, and brain covering; or edema (fluid buildup) within or around the brain often shows symptoms other than those accompanying a simple concussion. Some major signs of serious damage to the brain include partial paralysis of the body, posture with the limbs extended and with the jaws clenched, and unequal or pinpoint pupils of the eye.

A simple concussion usually requires no special care. The purpose of the doctor's examination is to determine if any more serious injury may have occurred. The patient is

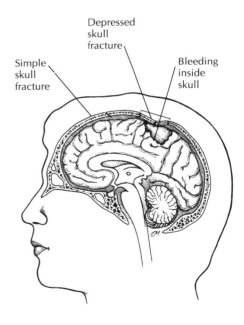

A simple or depressed skull fracture and bleeding between the covering of the brain and the skull should always be ruled out in a person who appears to have suffered a concussion.

observed for level of consciousness, mental sharpness (if awake), and proper nerve and muscle functions and reflexes. An X-ray study of the head may be performed to rule out a skull fracture (although most simple undepressed skull fractures are allowed to heal without treatment). If the patient acts strange or out of character or does not respond correctly to the tests, hospitalization and evaluation by a neurologist or neurosurgeon may be necessary.

Once a doctor has determined that a patient has had only a simple concussion, the patient may be allowed to return home without hospitalization. For the next 24 hours, the person is advised to relax and to take no medication stronger than an aspirin substitute (acetaminophen). It is best not to eat solid foods following any vomiting. Someone is usually asked to wake the patient every two hours during the night and ask three questions: What is your name? Where are you? What is my name? If the patient cannot answer these questions, will not awaken, or has convulsions, he should be rushed to the hospital. The patient should return to the hospital immediately if any of the following danger signals is noted: a continuing or worsening headache, blurring vision, extreme or constant vomiting, unusual eye movements, twitching, a staggering way of walking, or any change in personality. If none of these symptoms develops, normal activities can be resumed after a day or so of rest.

---

# Congenital hypothyroidism

Congenital (present at birth) hypothyroidism is a condition that leads to defective physical and mental development because of a deficiency of thyroid hormone. If untreated, a person born with congenital hypothyroidism grows to a maximum height of three or four feet and has a large, flat, broad head; short forehead; puffy, wide-set eyes; broad, short, upturned nose; thick lips; large tongue protruding from a drooling mouth; narrow chest; potbelly; swayback; rough skin; dry hair; and severe mental retardation.

Iodine is necessary in order to allow the body to produce thyroid hormone, and foods that are obtained from the ocean constitute the best sources of iodine. Before the widespread use of iodized salt became the norm, hypothyroidism was much more common in inland areas, where foods naturally contain little iodine.

Congenital hypothyroidism can result from a defect in the development of a child before birth. The thyroid gland may be missing or underdeveloped, possibly because of a severe deficiency of iodine in the mother's diet during pregnancy. In rare cases, congenital hypothyroidism is caused by an inherited absence of a body chemical needed to produce thyroid hormone.

When hypothyroidism first appears in children over the age of two years, it is usually due to an inflammation of the thyroid gland, a condition that comes about due to an immune disorder. It can also be caused by certain diseases of the pituitary gland or hypothalamus.

The first symptoms of untreated congenital hypothyroidism usually appear between the ages of three and six months or whenever the mother stops breast-feeding (breast milk contains tiny quantities of thyroid hormone). The baby is "too good," in the sense that he or she seldom cries (when the baby does cry, it is a strange, hoarse cry), sleeps more than normal, is inactive, and thus is easy to care for. This behavior is a result of the baby's lack of thyroid hormone, which regulates the rate of body processes, and increasing mental retardation. The baby's movements are slow and awkward, and the child has feeding difficulties, is constipated, and develops jaundice. The stomach protrudes, and a hernia may develop at the navel.

These symptoms are followed by the appearance of the characteristic facial features: the thick tongue, which interferes with breathing; the wide-set eyes; the turned-up nose; and the dull expression, indicating mental deficiency. The baby's heart beats slowly, resulting in poor circulation and cold skin. The hair is dry and dull. Teeth come in late and decay easily.

The child in whom symptoms of hypothyroidism first appear after the age of two is typically short and fat, with short legs and arms and a head that appears too large. Sexual development in an older child may be delayed.

Early diagnosis is now much more common since all states began to require that every newborn be tested for thyroid hormone level.

Diagnosis of congenital hypothyroidism may require not only a blood test to determine thyroid hormone levels, but also a nuclear medicine study after the administration of radioactive iodine to evaluate thyroid function. Special X-ray studies may also be used to detect delayed development of the skeleton, and an electrocardiogram (which measures the electrical impulses generated in the heart) may be ordered to reveal heartbeat patterns.

Treatment for congenital hypothyroidism is lifelong replacement of thyroid hormone with a synthetic substitute, ideally starting at birth. Those who receive the hormone before the age of three months usually develop normally. Children born without a thyroid gland are more at risk than those whose thyroid gland works poorly; if not treated by three months of age, the individuals will be mentally retarded even though their growth is corrected.

Pregnant women can help prevent congenital hypothyroidism in their offspring by eating a well-balanced diet that includes iodine-rich foods, such as fish and seafood, and by using iodized salt. At birth, every child's blood should be tested for thyroid hormone level.

See also Hypothyroidism.

# Congestive heart failure

Congestive heart failure (also called left ventricular failure or, simply, heart failure) is a condition in which the heart weakens and fails to keep the blood moving adequately. As a result, the supply of blood to the body's tissues decreases, lowering efficiency and endurance. With poor circulation, the kidneys fail to remove enough water, salt, and wastes from the blood. In addition, the kidneys, because of the decreased blood flow presented to them, retain even more salt and water in an effort to increase blood volume. The increased blood volume makes more work for the already overworked heart, which may enlarge and beat faster in an attempt to satisfy the body's hunger for oxygen-rich blood. The veins distend with fluid, and the balance of pressures between fluids inside and outside the veins shifts, which causes fluid that normally stays in the bloodstream to leak into surrounding tissue. This fluid leakage, the reduction of forward blood flow, and the backflow of blood are primary factors responsible for the pulmonary edema (accumulation of fluid in the lungs) and the swelling of the abdomen and legs that often accompany this condition.

The usual cause of congestive heart failure is a diseased heart that cannot pump enough blood. The most common reason is severe coronary artery disease, which decreases blood flow to the heart muscle. If the person has suffered a heart attack, the resultant nonworking scar tissue further reduces the efficiency of the heart as a pump. Leaky or narrowed heart valves, due to a birth defect or rheumatic fever, are another cause of heart failure. A large cardiac aneurysm (a bulge caused by the thinning of the wall of the left ventricle of the heart) may also decrease the pumping ability of the heart.

Less frequently, the root of the problem is one of several heart muscle diseases; some are caused by poisons like excessive alcohol, some by a viral infection, and others by the deposition in the heart tissue of iron or a protein called amyloid. Cardiac arrhythmias (disturbances of the normal rhythm of the heart) can also lead to heart failure or palpitations.

Early signs of congestive heart failure include unexplained rapid heartbeat, unusual fatigue during exertion, shortness of breath during stair climbing or other mild exercise, and inability to withstand cold. Attacks of shortness of breath and coughing when lying in bed that are relieved by sleeping with pillows under the back to tilt the chest are also early symptoms. Sometimes, a person is actually awakened by a sensation of "air hunger" and must sit or stand to breathe more easily. These symptoms are caused by increased fluid pressure in the lung circulation. The relief obtained by assuming a more erect position is due to a shift of blood volume to the lower half of the body, easing the burden of the heart. In advanced congestive heart failure, shortness of breath and a severe cough with reddish-brown or brownish sputum are common. There may also be swelling of the legs and ankles and a feeling of fullness in the neck or abdomen.

Usually, congestive heart failure can be diagnosed after a physical examination, on the basis of symptoms. However, a chest X ray is commonly taken to determine how much the heart has become enlarged by its overload and to see if fluid has accumulated within the lungs. An electrocardiogram (a recording of the electrical impulses generated in the heart) may reveal damage due to a previous heart attack and irregularities in the heart rhythm.

Treatment for congestive heart failure includes rest, oxygen, medication (such as digitalis) to strengthen the pumping ability of the heart, and medication to prevent irregular heart rhythms. Diuretic medications are given to help the kidneys remove more salt and water from the blood and thus decrease the volume of blood the heart must pump. A low-salt diet is prescribed to prevent water buildup in the blood and tissues (salt tends to cause fluid to accumulate in the body). In more severe or chronic cases, a drug may be given to expand the blood vessels and thus make it easier for the heart to pump blood through them. Newer drugs known as angiotensin converting enzyme (ACE) inhibitors have been especially effective in treating congestive heart failure.

In some cases, the original cause of the congestive heart failure can be corrected. For example, bypass surgery may be performed on the coronary arteries to improve blood supply to the heart muscle. Surgery may also be done to replace or correct a faulty heart valve or to repair an aneurysm. Contributing factors to be controlled or eliminated include high blood pressure, anemia, excess salt or alcohol intake, fever, an overactive thyroid gland, and stress due to overexertion.

The prevention of congestive heart failure rests on those good health habits that help prevent heart disease in general: choosing a well-balanced diet with moderate or low intake of fats; maintaining appropriate body weight; getting plenty of exercise, rest, and sleep; avoiding tobacco and excess alcohol intake; and having periodic medical checkups to detect conditions, such as high blood pressure, that might eventually overload or injure the heart and thus lead to congestive heart failure. Salt restriction in those suffering from mild congestive heart failure is also very important.

See also Aneurysm, Coronary bypass surgery, Heart attack, Heartbeat irregularities, Heart disease, Hypertension, and Rheumatic fever.

---

# Conjunctivitis

Conjunctivitis, or pinkeye, is an inflammation of the conjunctiva. The conjunctiva is a delicate membrane that lines the inner surface of the eyelid and covers the exposed surface of the eye.

Most cases of conjunctivitis result from disease-causing microorganisms such as bacteria and viruses. Allergies, chemicals, dust, smoke, and foreign objects that irritate the conjunctiva may also lead to conjunctivitis. Swimming may also be associated with conjunctivitis, due to exposure to chlorine in a pool or to contaminated water. Occasionally, a sexually transmitted disease can cause pinkeye if the eyes are rubbed after the hands have touched infected genital organs.

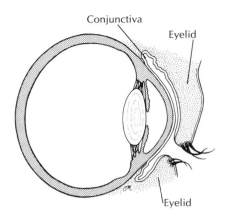

The conjunctiva is a delicate membrane lining the inner surface of the eyelid and covering the exposed surface of the eye.

Children are most often affected by conjunctivitis. Measles, a viral disease, may be accompanied by this eye inflammation. In addition, those people, both children and adults, who have allergies, such as hay fever, or who work and live in areas where they are exposed to chemicals or other irritants are more susceptible to noninfectious conjunctivitis.

Conjunctivitis may cause redness, a grating sensation, burning, itching, and light sensitivity. Occasionally, tearing occurs, or a discharge containing pus will be present. Symptoms can last a few days or up to two weeks.

Conjunctivitis usually produces no permanent damage. However, if left untreated, the infection may lead to more serious eye problems. Ulcers (eroded areas) may form on the cornea (the clear "window" in front of the iris and pupil of the eye). If these ulcers persist, they can scar the eye and interfere with vision.

Treatment depends on the cause and resulting symptoms of the conjunctivitis. If the inflammation is environmentally caused, simply removing the irritant may be sufficient to eliminate the condition. For more difficult cases, a physician may prescribe antibiotic, steroid, or combination eyedrops to be used several times a day as directed. Frequent use is necessary because the drops tend to be washed away by the natural cleansing action of the tears.

Sensitive eyes should be rested and shielded from bright lights. When the discharge glues the eyelids closed, bathing them with warm water and wiping with a clean cloth will loosen them.

A most important fact about conjunctivitis is that its infectious form is highly contagious. Individuals with infectious conjunctivitis should not share handkerchiefs, towels, or washcloths and should be careful to avoid touching the unaffected eye after contact with the infected eye.

# Constipation

Constipation is a condition in which the stool (feces) is hard and its elimination from the bowels is infrequent and difficult. This condition is often more uncomfortable than harmful, although occasionally a change in the bowel movements (for example, prolonged constipation or extreme discomfort when eliminating) may be a symptom of a serious illness, such as cancer, intestinal obstruction, or a nervous system or endocrine gland disorder.

It is important to remember, however, that it is not necessary to have a bowel movement every day. From three bowel movements per day to three per week is considered in the normal range.

Common causes of constipation are physical inactivity; lack of fiber or roughage in the diet; inadequate fluid intake; emotional stress, particularly depression; drug side effects;

and the habit of postponing bowel movements.

Conditions that often accompany constipation are difficulty and strain in producing a bowel movement, a bloated feeling, abdominal cramps, headache, gassiness, and hemorrhoids.

The treatment of constipation usually depends on its cause. In mild cases that are not related to other disorders, simple methods of recommended treatment include adding more fiber-rich foods (such as bran, whole-grain breads and cereals, fruits, vegetables, and other forms of roughage) to the diet; drinking eight to ten glasses of water daily; increasing exercise; and developing good bathroom habits. This last recommendation may involve an attempt to have a bowel movement at the same time every day, usually 30 to 60 minutes after breakfast. Early morning is a good time, because the entry of food into an empty stomach activates and increases normal intestinal contractions; also, residue from the previous day's meals has moved by this time to the rectal area for elimination.

Laxatives and enemas are usually not recommended for treating simple constipation. Laxatives, in particular, should be used only when absolutely necessary; overuse can lead to irritation of the lining of the rectum, and the intestine can become so dependent on the stimulation of laxatives that it cannot function properly without them. Frequent enemas can also lead to dependence.

Drinking plenty of water, getting adequate exercise, eating fiber-rich foods, and recognizing the urge for a bowel movement as soon as it is felt should be beneficial in promoting regular elimination and preventing constipation.

# Contact dermatitis

Contact dermatitis is a type of allergy in which the skin becomes inflamed in the area where it has come in contact with an irritating substance.

Contact dermatitis can be caused by a virtually limitless array of substances, among them soaps, detergents, metals, shaving materials, shampoos, hair colorings or sprays, solvents in household cleaners, chemicals in foods and cosmetics, dyes in household products, and certain plants, such as poison ivy and poison oak. Photodermatitis (a skin inflammation caused by light) is a type of dermatitis that develops when certain ingested drugs, such as some antibiotics, sensitize the skin so that a rash develops on skin that is exposed to the sun.

The major symptoms of contact dermatitis are burning, swelling, severe itching, and stinging sensations on the area of the skin that has been exposed to the allergen. Blisters that ooze a clear fluid may form (a cloudy or yellow, foul-smelling fluid indicates that a bacterial infection, rather than contact dermatitis, is present).

Contact dermatitis is diagnosed by first identifying the allergen causing the trouble. The location of the rash often gives an important clue to the identity of the allergen. For instance, if the inflammation is on the scalp, the disorder may be assumed to be triggered by a shampoo, hair spray, or hair coloring. More specific identification of the allergen may be obtained with one of several available tests, including scratch tests, in which a small amount of the suspected allergen is applied to a scratch on the skin; intracutaneous tests, in which a small amount of the allergen is injected into or under the skin; and radioallergosorbent testing, a blood test in which antibodies produced in response to the allergen are measured.

Once the allergen has been identified, the best treatment for contact dermatitis is for the patient to avoid the allergen or to remove it from his or her environment. It is often possible to do this by switching brands of soaps or shampoos, wearing rubber gloves when using harsh detergents, and using unscented or hypoallergenic cosmetics. If the use of a drug cannot be discontinued despite a case of photodermatitis, sunscreens should be used and adequate clothing should be worn to shield the skin when outdoors.

Oral steroid drugs (such as cortisone) help to relieve the itching of contact dermatitis; however, these are reserved only for the most serious cases. Topical (applied directly to the skin) steroids and antihistamines are more commonly used.

There is no preventive treatment for contact dermatitis, but those susceptible to one or more contactant allergens can usually prevent outbreaks by avoiding exposure as much as possible.

See also Dermatitis.

# Contraception

See Birth control.

# Corns

Corns are small, round mounds of firm, dead skin that form on or between the toes. Their hard, waxy core, which bores down into the skin and presses on the underlying tissue and nerves, can cause extreme pain. Corns sometimes are associated with bursae (fluid-filled sacs), which can become irritated, resulting in bursitis.

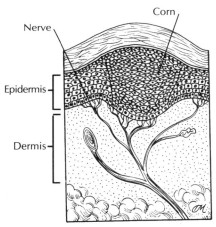

Corns are small mounds of dead skin that form on or between the toes. Their cores, formed in the epidermis layer of the skin, bore down into underlying tissue and nerves in the dermis layer, causing pain.

Corns are caused by a great deal of pressure or friction on the toes (as are calluses, their basis), usually from ill-fitting shoes or high heels. Since the skin acts as the body's protector from the outside environment, corns form when the body attempts to protect the troubled area by building up a mass of dead skin cells and secreting a hard substance called keratin. Persons who have abnormal bone structure in their feet or certain types of arthritis tend to develop corns. Generally, those who avoid wearing high heeled or tight-fitting shoes should be able to avoid the problem.

Corns are usually regular in shape, and can be white, gray, or yellow. They most often form on the outside of the first or fifth toe, since that is where pressure most often occurs. Corns that form between the toes are called soft corns; they are not as firm as other corns because of the moistness between the toes, which tends to soften them.

Corns are best treated by first eliminating the cause of the pressure. Over-the-counter preparations are available. These include padding to reduce the friction on the area, ointments, and medicated pads, which will soften and blister the skin layers, making them easier to remove and reducing the pain. Severe or persistent corns must be treated by a doctor, but only rarely do they necessitate surgery. Persons with diabetes, atherosclerosis, or other circulatory diseases should *never* treat a corn themselves, as the risk of infection is much greater for them.

See also Calluses.

# Coronary bypass surgery

Coronary bypass surgery is performed on one or more of the coronary arteries, which lie on the outer surface of the heart and supply the heart muscle with the oxygen and nutrients it needs. In coronary artery disease, a section or sections of the arteries gradually become obstructed by a buildup of cholesterol, calcium, and scar tissue. The purpose of the operation is to bypass the obstructed area to permit free blood flow. Without the procedure, heart muscle beyond the obstruction is starved for blood and oxygen, especially during exercise. This condition causes the chest pains known as angina. If one or more of the coronary arteries become completely obstructed, the result may be a heart attack, in which a portion of heart muscle becomes so starved for blood that it dies.

Bypass surgery is usually considered when a person suffers frequent, severe chest pains from angina. However, not all persons with angina need bypass surgery. Advances are being made in using medication to control angina. Furthermore, some angina is caused by spasms (sudden, violent contractions) of the coronary arteries, which bypass surgery may not prevent or ease.

Obstructions in the coronary arteries can now sometimes be eliminated by methods that do not require cutting open the chest, such as percutaneous transluminal coronary angioplasty (also called balloon angioplasty), which consists of threading a long, balloon-tipped catheter (tube) through the arteries to the site of obstruction and inflating the balloon to open a clogged vessel (the balloon is then deflated and removed). Even without outside help, and given enough time, the heart may create its own partial bypass via collateral circulation (a system of smaller blood vessels that bypass a blocked artery and increase the blood supply to the area served by that artery).

If a patient often has severe chest pains that cannot be controlled by medication, the doctor may decide to order coronary angiography (also called coronary arteriography or cardiac catheterization). Through a thin, woven plastic catheter inserted into an artery in the arm or leg and passed through large blood vessels to the heart, X-ray contrast medium is injected so that it flows into the coronary arteries, outlining them on an X-ray screen. The pictures show exactly where and to what extent the blood vessels are narrowed or blocked. Thus, the doctor can determine whether bypasses are needed and, if so, where. The most urgent reason to operate is significant obstruction of the left main coronary artery, which supplies blood to about forty percent or more of the left ventricle.

First, the surgeon makes several incisions in one leg to obtain a long section of a large vein for use as bypass tubing. Next, the surgeon makes an incision down the middle of the chest, divides the breastbone with an electric saw, and separates the two sides of the rib cage enough to expose the beating heart. The heartbeat is then stopped using electric shock, ice water, or certain drugs. A heart-lung machine is connected to the large vessels that carry blood to and from the heart and takes over the job of adding oxygen, removing carbon dioxide, and pumping the blood through the patient's body.

The surgeon then cuts through the pericardial sac (a thin bag of tissue that surrounds the heart) to expose the coronary arteries, which lie on the surface of the heart. A small hole is made in the aorta, and one end of the vein segment to be used as bypass tubing is sewn to it. The other end is attached to the affected vessel beyond the obstruction. The internal mammary artery in the chest is commonly used as a bypass graft in addition to vein segments. Thereafter, blood will flow freely around the obstructed portion of the artery to nourish the heart muscle. This procedure should decrease the patient's chest pains and risk of heart attack.

The bypass surgery operation takes about four or five hours, depending on the number of bypasses. A double bypass operation is one in which portions of two vessels are bypassed, a triple bypass involves three vessels, and so forth. Usually the patient can walk about three or four days following the operation and return home in about a week.

Considering that the procedure is such a major operation, the death rate is very low—less than one percent in most hospitals in which it is performed. In 80 percent of cases, angina pains are eliminated, and the patient can return to a normal life. There has been much controversy surrounding coronary bypass surgery, mainly centering on the question of whether this procedure can increase life expectancy for those with coronary artery disease and angina. At present, there is no question that the surgery relieves pain and allows for greater exercise tolerance in the majority of patients who undergo it for severe angina. In certain patterns of disease, such as obstruction of the left main coronary artery, the operation definitely prolongs life expectancy. In other patterns, such as triple vessel disease, in which branches of the coronary arteries (except for the left main coronary artery) are involved, the procedure most likely allows a longer life. In still other patterns, the question remains unsettled. Whether coronary bypass surgery will prevent a heart attack, however, is another matter that has not been determined.

# Cor pulmonale

See Emphysema.

# Corticosteroids

Corticosteroids are hormones produced in the cortex of the adrenal glands in response to stimulation by adrenocorticotropic hormone (ACTH), which is secreted by the pituitary gland. There are more than 30 corticosteroids, which regulate essential processes throughout the body. They are divided into three groups: mineralocorticoids, glucocorticoids, and androgens (male sex hormones).

Mineralocorticoids are involved in maintaining salt and water balance in the body. Without these hormones, the tissues and blood would become depleted of salt and water; the resultant decrease in blood volume would cause a drop in blood pressure that could lead to shock (collapse of the circulatory system).

Glucocorticoids help regulate the body's use and reserves of sugars and proteins, among other complex metabolic processes. They also participate in the inflammatory response and the body's reaction to stress. The most important of these hormones is cortisol, which plays a major role in protein breakdown and formation, blood sugar control, and reduction of inflammation. Cortisol is also necessary to mount an effective response against severe stress due to disease or injury.

Androgens (which are also produced in the testes) stimulate the development of the male secondary sex characteristics, such as beard growth and increased muscle mass.

Pharmacologic preparations of both ACTH and corticosteroids are used to treat disease in the same way that the natural hormones would or as substitute or supplemental hormones for patients who have lost the ability to manufacture their own. The primary difference is that ACTH acts less directly and more generally than corticosteroid drugs. ACTH stimulates the adrenal glands to enlarge and secrete more of all the steroids that they produce, rather than any one specific hormone. Corticosteroid drugs can be administered to the part of the body that needs them most. For example, a dab of hydrocortisone cream will eliminate a rash, and a hydrocortisone injection will diminish the swelling of a painful knee joint, generally with little effect on the rest of the body. Sometimes, however, corticosteroids are considered for generalized use throughout the body. Corticosteroids have an advantage over ACTH in that they can be taken by mouth and may be given in doses that far exceed what the adrenal glands can produce. ACTH must be injected because it would otherwise be destroyed by digestive enzymes, which do not affect the corticosteroids.

See also Adrenal glands and Pituitary gland.

# Cough

A cough is a normal reflex of the body to clear the airways. Coughing can result from inhaling dust, dirt, or irritating fumes; from breathing icy air; or from drawing food into the airways. It can also be caused by mucus and other secretions from such respiratory disorders as the common cold, influenza, pneumonia, and tuberculosis. Persistent coughs (those that last several weeks) without other respiratory symptoms may, on occasion, suggest diseases of other organs, such as the heart. For example, a cough may be an early sign of congestive heart failure.

The type of cough—productive or nonproductive—partially determines how it should be treated. Productive coughs (those that produce fluid or mucus) are often caused by a lung infection. When microorganisms attack the lungs, the lung tissue produces large amounts of secretions in defense. These accumulated secretions irritate the lungs, resulting in coughing that brings up fluid or mucus. A yellowish or reddish fluid in particular may indicate infection or other serious problems that require a doctor's attention.

Nonproductive coughing does not bring up fluid. It occurs when secretions from nasal passages drip into the throat or when smoke, dust, pollen, or other irritants enter the respiratory tract. Irritations and tumors may also cause a nonproductive cough, as can any inflammation of the airways or lung tissue. Another cause is insufficient moisture in the air. This is particularly common in winter, when humidity is lowest. A humidifier or vaporizer may provide more relief than cough-suppressing drugs.

Because coughing has the vital function of clearing the airways, it should never be totally suppressed. In fact, suppressing a cough in an individual with chronic lung disease may be dangerous. Furthermore, indiscriminate use of cough suppressants may mask important symptoms. However, controlling a cough that disrupts sleep or aggravates other conditions may sometimes be necessary. This may be accomplished by using a cough suppressant or an expectorant. A suppressant helps to inhibit the cough by depressing the coughing center in the brain. An expectorant promotes the discharge of mucus from the respiratory tract.

For all but the mildest coughs with obvious causes, and certainly for persistent coughs, a doctor should be consulted to determine the cause and to suggest appropriate treatment.

# Coxsackie viruses

See Enteroviral infections.

# Crohn's disease

Crohn's disease (also known as regional enteritis and ileitis) is characterized by inflammation of a section or sections of any part of the digestive tract—most often, the ileum (the last third of the small intestine). The disease may begin as patches of tiny ulcers in the innermost lining of the intestine, with swelling of nearby tissues. The inflammation eventually extends through all layers of the intestine, which becomes thickened, hard, and brittle. Deepening ulcers, scarring, and swelling may obstruct the intestinal tract.

The cause of Crohn's disease is unknown. However, research indicates that infection, immune disorders, or an inherited defect may play a part. There is some evidence of an increased incidence of Crohn's disease in Jews; black persons are least likely to have the disease. The disease usually begins between the ages of 15 and 35, but it can occur at virtually any age.

Symptoms usually develop gradually, with spells of diarrhea (four to six stools a day, frequently bloody), low fever, weight loss, loss of appetite, general weakness, and steady or colicky pains in the abdomen, commonly on the right side. Milk, milk products, and coarse foods contain ingredients that may make symptoms worse.

Occasionally an acute (sudden and severe) case resembles appendicitis, with sharp pain in the lower right portion of the abdomen, cramping, nausea, fever, and diarrhea. There may or may not be bloody stools. An acute case of Crohn's disease can resemble infectious diarrhea.

While probing the abdomen and pelvis, the doctor may detect a tender mass of thickened or matted loops of intestine. The chronic form of the disease can occasionally be mistaken for other problems, such as irritable bowel syndrome. However, an X ray of the small intestine taken after administration of the contrast medium barium may reveal the charac-

teristic pattern of narrowed portions of the bowel sharply differentiated from healthy portions. The doctor may use a proctosigmoidoscope (a lighted, hollow instrument inserted through the anus) to inspect the lower intestinal lining for patchy areas of inflammation or to perform a biopsy (obtain a sample of tissue from the lining of the intestine for microscopic examination).

Complications include abscesses (pus-filled cavities) and fistulas. Fistulas are abnormal connecting channels that originate from inflamed portions of the bowel and commonly extend into and around adjacent tissue. In the anorectal area, they may sometimes be seen as openings in the skin. They can also extend from one section of the bowel to another, from the bowel to the bladder or vagina, and from the bowel to the abdominal wall. Fistulas are often infected and discharge pus.

Perforation of the intestine can also occur, leading to peritonitis (inflammation of the lining of the abdominal cavity). This is marked by severe abdominal pain and rigidity of the abdomen, and is most often a surgical emergency. On occasion, a small perforation may become walled off, creating an abscess.

Malnutrition is a very common complication of Crohn's disease because areas of inflamed intestine cannot properly absorb nutrients. The risk of cancer of the colon and rectum is also increased. Arthritis, eye disorders, kidney stones, and certain skin disorders may also accompany this illness.

At present, there is no cure for Crohn's disease. Surgery is sometimes necessary to remove an entire section of diseased bowel, drain an abscess, or eliminate a fistula. This relieves the condition for a time, but symptoms almost always recur, and then another operation may be necessary.

Treatment of the disease is directed at making the patient as comfortable and functional as possible by reducing the severity of his or her symptoms.

A diet rich in calories and vitamins with adequate protein is desirable, to compensate for the patient's poor absorption of nutrients from the intestines. Individuals with severely inflamed or obstructed bowels may be placed temporarily on intravenous feeding or a special diet. Patients with anemia may need supplements of vitamins and minerals (such as iron, folic acid, and vitamin $B_{12}$) and sometimes blood transfusions; those with severe diarrhea or dehydration (loss of body fluids) may need intravenous fluids.

Cramps and diarrhea are frequently controlled by various medications that relax the bowel wall, while preparations such as psyllium may help to firm stools.

Antibiotics are used on a short-term basis to treat abscesses and infected fistulas. Sulfasalicylate combination drugs may be used on a long-term basis to curb inflammation and prevent acute episodes, particularly in disease involving the large intestine. The steroid drug prednisone is a mainstay in treating flare-ups of symptoms. Newer salicylate (aspirin-like) drugs, either in enema or oral form, are quite effective in relieving symptoms even in small intestinal disease.

# Croup

Croup is a condition marked by a hoarse, barking cough that sometimes follows a cold or fever in very young children, most commonly those under the age of two years. A croup attack may occur on only a single occassion, or it may linger or reappear after it seems to have gone.

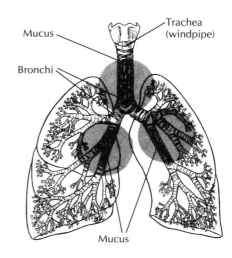

Croup can be complicated by mucus blocking the windpipe and the bronchi leading into lungs. This may lead to serious breathing problems and become a medical emergency.

Croup is usually caused by a viral infection of the larynx (voice box). The characteristic barking cough is produced when air forces its way through the child's swollen larynx. The air passageways in a child's throat are very narrow; when an infection causes swelling, little room is left for air to pass through, and breathing can be severely hampered. Also, the windpipe and the bronchi (the main breathing tubes that connect the windpipe and the lungs) may become blocked with mucus, further impairing breathing.

The identifying symptoms of croup are a deep, barking cough and breathing difficulties, especially when inhaling. Sometimes a fever and hoarseness are also present. The child may gag while coughing, causing vomiting, which usually relieves the cough somewhat. The coughing attack often occurs in the evening and usually lasts less than an hour.

Symptoms that indicate a worsening condition include blue skin and lips, drooling, and extreme exhaustion. When the croaking sound continues while the child is inhaling, a condition called stridor has developed. If any of these symptoms occurs or if there are severe breathing difficulties, medical help should be obtained *immediately.*

The emphasis in diagnostic evaluation is on establishing that the difficulty in breathing is actually due to croup and not to epiglottitis, a life-threatening emergency condition in which the inflamed epiglottis (the lid-like structure covering the opening to the windpipe) rapidly becomes completely obstructed. Epiglottitis is usually caused by bacteria, most often *Hemophilus influenza,* and is associated with sudden onset of high fever (up to 104°F). This is an important diagnostic clue to help doctors differentiate between epiglottitis and viral croup.

Choking on a foreign object may also resemble croup, since both conditions share the symptom of frantic efforts to breathe. An X-ray examination may be performed to rule out this possibility.

Croup can usually be treated at home. The first step is calming the child. The barking cough, especially when accompanied by difficulty in breathing, can frighten the child, and this fear can only aggravate the symptoms. Sometimes the child can be told to imagine a relaxing scene or can listen to a calming bedtime story; a relaxed child will respond much better to home remedies.

The goal is to relieve the cough by reducing the inflammation and swelling in the larynx. This can be accomplished by breathing in moist air from a humidifier or vaporizer, by leaning over a pan of hot water with a towel draped over the head, or by sitting in a steamy bathroom with a hot shower running. Moist air reduces the swelling and makes breathing eas-

ier. Of course, precautions should be taken to protect a young child from being scalded while taking part in these treatments, and the child should never be left alone.

Drinking extra fluids (not milk or orange juice) at room temperature is also recommended. Cough medicine will not help (and may even harm) a child with croup, nor is it advisable to put a spoon or any other object into the mouth in an attempt to aid the breathing. In a severe case, a physician may administer drugs to control the inflammation in the throat; also, antibiotics can sometimes control the infections connected with croup.

It is not known why some children develop croup after a cold or fever and others do not; therefore, there is really no way to prevent croup.

# Cushing's syndrome

Cushing's syndrome is a group of abnormalities resulting from an excess of the hormones produced by the cortex of the adrenal glands. The hormones produced in excess are chiefly cortisol, which has many complex functions; various hormones that regulate the body's use of sugars and proteins; male sex hormones; and a hormone that controls the distribution of fluids and salts in the body.

In most cases, Cushing's syndrome is caused by excess production of adrenocorticotropic hormone (ACTH), which is normally manufactured by the pituitary gland to stimulate production of hormones by the adrenal glands. This excess of ACTH can be caused by an ACTH-producing tumor in another organ, such as the lung or pancreas; by overmedication with ACTH or corticosteroid drugs; by tiny, nonmalignant ACTH-producing tumors on the pituitary gland; or by a tumor (usually nonmalignant) on the adrenal gland. The effect of too much ACTH, for whatever reason, is overgrowth of tissue in the adrenal cortex, resulting in overproduction of all its hormones. Since these hormones regulate essential processes throughout the body, excess production causes widespread disorders.

One of the most obvious signs of Cushing's syndrome is the moon-shaped face, caused by excess fluid in the tissues. Because of deposition of excess fat, the trunk of the body is obese (although the arms and legs are thin), and there are fat pads over the shoulders and neck, producing a "buffalo hump." Purple "stretch marks" on the skin (usually of the abdomen), poor wound healing, easy bruising, muscle weakness, fractures in weakened bones, and emotional instability may also be part of the syndrome. Hairiness, acne, and decreased or absent menstruation may occur in women, due to the increase in male hormones. Diabetes and high blood pressure are also very commonly seen.

Diagnosis of Cushing's syndrome requires measurement of adrenal cortex hormones in the blood and urine. In normal persons, cortisol levels in the blood are high on awakening but decrease during the day; in the person with Cushing's syndrome, cortisol levels are high all of the time. Various tests can determine whether the cause of the syndrome is a tumor of the pituitary gland (in which case the disorder is known as Cushing's disease) or a tumor on the adrenal gland or elsewhere. Tumors on the adrenal glands may be identified by X rays, ultrasound, and computed tomography, or CT scans. CT scans and other special X rays of the head can often locate tumors of the pituitary gland.

Cushing's syndrome is treated by restoring a normal balance of hormones. This may involve surgery, radiation treatments, or drugs. Tumors on the adrenal glands are removed by surgery. If there is a tumor on just one adrenal gland, the other gland usually shrinks and ceases normal productivity. Hormone supplements are usually given before surgery and must be taken for weeks or months after surgery until the second gland recovers normal function. In a rapidly worsening case of Cushing's syndrome in which the cortex is greatly enlarged on both sides, one treatment is to remove both adrenal glands. This is usually a last-resort measure, however; more commonly, another method, such as chemotherapy (drug treatments), radiation treatments of the pituitary gland (to weaken it and lower its output of ACTH), or removal of any adenomas (nonmalignant growths) on the pituitary gland, is tried first. If other measures fail, the adrenal glands are removed, and the patient must take daily supplements of adrenal cortex hormones for the rest of his or her life.

If Cushing's syndrome is being caused by production of ACTH by a cancerous tumor in a part of the body other than the adrenal glands, the cancer is removed, if possible. However, in many cases it is inoperable, so drugs to suppress production of the adrenal glands are given.

Cushing's syndrome is a very serious, possibly fatal, disease unless it is detected and treated early. The outlook is best for those whose condition is caused by noncancerous growths and who receive early treatment.

Those who must take replacement hormones after treatment should carry a medical identification card and immediately tell their doctor about any infections, injuries, or stressful situations that might require an increase in hormone dosage. They should also report signs of under-dosage, such as weakness, dizziness, or fatigue, as well as signs of over-dosage, such as swollen tissues and rapid weight gain. Anyone whose adrenal glands have been removed must always take replacement hormones; stopping these medications for any length of time is fatal.

See also Adrenal glands, Corticosteroids, and Pituitary gland.

# Cyanosis

Cyanosis is a bluish discoloration of the skin and mucous membranes due to inadequate oxygenation of the blood. The abnormal coloration is easily seen in these areas because of both their rich blood supply and their relative transparency.

Blood rich in oxygen from the lungs is bright red. This is because of the red, iron-containing pigment known as hemoglobin, which is found in the erythrocytes (the disk-shaped red blood cells). When blood passes through the blood vessels of the lungs, oxygen from the air in the lungs combines with the hemoglobin, which causes it (and consequently the blood) to turn a very bright red. After the blood releases its oxygen to the cells of the body and picks up carbon dioxide and other waste products, the hemoglobin fades and the blood turns dark. However, if the lungs are not working well or if for some other reason the red blood cells are not being oxygenated, the blood appears bluish.

Cyanosis can be due to asthma, choking, pneumonia, or lung collapse. It can also be a sign of certain inborn heart defects, of severe cor pulmonale (right heart failure), or of abnormally excessive production of red blood cells. It is seen most frequently in cold weather when lips, toes, and fingers turn blue from extreme cold, the result of sluggish surface circulation of the blood (in this case, it may be a normal phenomenon and does not necessarily indicate disease).

# Cyst

A cyst is an abnormal sac or membrane containing a fluid or semisolid material.

Cysts may develop virtually anywhere in the body. They may form around a foreign body, such as a particle in the lung or beneath the skin, or around a parasite. Cysts may also develop from the entrapment of an escaping body liquid, such as blood hemorrhaging into tissue or fluid leaking from a bursa (a sac containing lubricant for a joint).

Perhaps the most common cysts are those of the skin and mucous membranes.

A *sebaceous cyst* occurs when a sebaceous gland (the tiny oil gland at the base of each hair root) becomes plugged. Ordinarily, this plugging results in a blackhead or, if the blackhead becomes infected, a pus-filled pimple. Occasionally, however, the pimple does not break, and the swelling becomes entrapped beneath the surface of the skin. Sebum (oil from the sebaceous gland) continues to flow into the sac that forms in the cavity, and the cyst grows to the size of a marble or larger. Sebaceous cysts—which can occur in any part of the body where there is hair, including the neck, scalp, and back—can easily be removed surgically if bothersome; if they become infected, they must be drained and removed. A type of tiny cyst known as milium, which usually occurs on the face and scrotum, can simply be opened and drained. Larger cysts must be removed completely, or they will recur.

*Mucous cysts* that occur in the mouth, on the tongue, or on the lower lip are caused by plugged mucous glands and may grow to the size of a pea or larger. They may be removed in the same manner as sebaceous cysts.

*Traumatic epithelial cysts* usually result from the trapping of a piece of skin, a blood clot, or foreign material beneath the skin because of some injury. In some cases, they may not need to be removed.

# Cystic fibrosis

Cystic fibrosis is a serious hereditary disease characterized by abnormal secretions that affect many parts of the body, but primarily the lungs, pancreas, and digestive tract.

Cystic fibrosis is caused by an inherited defective gene. This defective gene is recessive, meaning that it must be inherited from both parents. If the gene is received from only one parent, the child is a carrier but will not get the disease. About five percent of the white population in the United States are carriers; the incidence in the black and Oriental populations is much lower. Approximately one in every 400 marriages involves two carriers. A child of two carriers has a 25 percent chance of getting the disease, a 50 percent chance of being a carrier, and a 25 percent chance of being completely free of the defective gene.

The effect of the defective gene is to cause the exocrine glands to release abnormal mucus, sweat, and other secretions. (Exocrine glands are those that release their secretions through ducts, rather than directly into the bloodstream.) The most serious effects of cystic fibrosis occur when the mucous glands release thick, gummy mucus rather than the

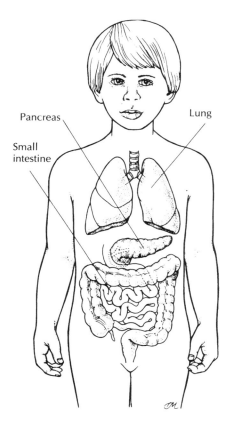

Cystic fibrosis is a disease characterized by abnormal secretions that affect many body parts, particularly the lungs, the pancreas, and the intestinal tract. In the lungs thick mucus hampers breathing and promotes infection. Thickened secretions can obstruct the ducts in the pancreas and block the passage of pancreatic digestive enzymes into the small intestine.

normal clear, free-flowing fluid. This thick mucus accumulates in the glands, causing swelling, forming cysts, and, most important, blocking various ducts throughout the body. One of the more serious complications of cystic fibrosis occurs when the mucus in the lungs, which normally sweeps bacteria and foreign particles from the lungs, becomes thick and sticky, accumulating in the airways and creating a breeding ground for infection, rather than preventing it. Consequent infections cause still more mucus to be produced, and the airways, already narrowed from the swelling, become even more clogged. Recurrent infections can lead to long-term breathing difficulties. Most deaths from cystic fibrosis are due to respiratory failure caused by obstruction of the airways and by persistent infections.

Also affected by this disorder is the pancreas, the organ that normally secretes digestive enzymes through a series of ducts into the small intestine. These ducts become blocked by abnormally thickened mucous secretions, preventing important digestive enzymes from reaching the small intestine, where they are needed to digest fats.

Reproductive tract secretions are also thickened. In women, an overabundance of mucus in the cervix may block the passage of sperm, making it difficult to become pregnant. About 98 percent of male patients are sterile because the ducts through which the sperm normally travel are blocked by thickened mucus.

Heat exhaustion is another problem related to this disease, because of the large salt loss due to excessive sweating.

The symptoms of cystic fibrosis may show up at birth or may not appear until adolescence. About ten percent of babies with cystic fibrosis are born with a mucous plug in their intestinal tract, which must be corrected surgically.

Because the pancreas is prevented from releasing the enzymes necessary to digest fat, digestive problems are common, and stools are large and foul-smelling. Typically, children afflicted with the disease eat well but gain weight slowly and show signs of malnutrition because the fat in their food is excreted from the body without being used. In addition, the patient usually has excessively salty sweat, a chronic cough accompanied by mucous discharge, and rapid and difficult breathing, and frequently experiences fatigue and muscle cramps from salt loss. Sinusitis (inflammation of the air-filled cavities in the facial bones), nasal polyps (growths in the nose), and a barrel-shaped chest from overinflated lungs may also develop.

Because many of these symptoms are also indications of less serious disorders, cystic fibrosis often remains undiagnosed or undetected for some time while the disease progresses.

Diagnostic evaluation usually includes a physical examination, medical history, chest X ray, and a sweat test. (Most cystic fibrosis patients have excessively salty sweat, although the salt level does not indicate the severity of the condition.) Tests of the stool and digestive juices can show how well the pancreas is functioning.

Although cystic fibrosis cannot be cured, its symptoms can be relieved to some extent. Dietary management is extremely important; patients are advised to reduce the fat in their diets, to eat nutritious foods with high amounts of essential minerals and vitamins, to take salt tablets, and to take pancreatic enzyme tablets to aid digestion of fats. The risk of respiratory infections can be reduced by means of antibiotics, aerosol mists, appropriate vaccinations, and postural drainage (in which the patient is positioned so that gravity can be used to help clear mucus from clogged lungs). Regular exercise may also be useful.

There is no means of preventing cystic fibrosis today. Researchers continue to look for a reason why the defective gene causes mucus to become abnormal, as well as for a way to identify carriers of the gene. One new test measures certain chemicals present in the amniotic fluid (the liquid that surrounds a fetus in the womb), so that an unborn baby with the gene can be identified. Meanwhile, scientific advances in this area have at least helped those with the disease to live more comfortably. Until the 1960s, few patients lived beyond the age of 10, but today those with cystic fibrosis can live to age 25 or beyond because of medical advances in managing this particular condition.

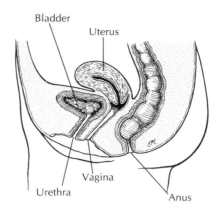

The female urethra is about one inch long, making it easier for infecting bacteria to invade the bladder.

# Cystitis

Cystitis is an inflammation of the urinary bladder; the term, however, is commonly used to mean bladder infection.

Cystitis is usually caused by bacteria that have invaded the urethra and entered the urinary bladder. Women are more susceptible than men because their urethras are shorter (approximately one and a half inches long, compared with about eight inches in men), thus presenting less distance for the bacteria to travel. Also, in women, the anus and the external openings of the urethra and the vagina (birth canal) are so close together that bacteria can easily migrate from one to another. Almost always the bacteria responsible are types that normally live harmlessly in the human intestine but that can cause infection if they invade the area around the opening of the urethra and enter the bladder.

Obstruction is also a common cause of urinary tract infection. When obstruction occurs, the bladder may not empty properly. The urine remaining in the bladder can then create a breeding ground for bacteria to multiply. Causes of obstruction include tumors, kidney stones, and an enlarged prostate gland.

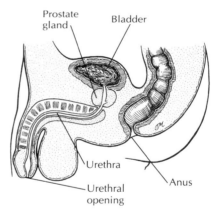

The male urethra is about seven or eight inches long, making a bacterial invasion of the bladder less likely than in a woman.

The urethral lining may have a defect that allows bacteria to enter the urinary tract. For example, frequent intercourse may traumatize the urethra, disrupting or tearing its lining and making it more susceptible to infection.

Cystitis in men is uncommon. When it does occur, the usual cause is an infection that has spread from an inflamed prostate gland or that has developed in the bladder because of an enlarged prostate.

Urethritis, an infection or inflammation of the urethra, often sets the stage for the development of cystitis. Urethritis occurs in both men and women and is usually acquired through sexual intercourse with an infected individual. Gonorrheal and nongonococcal urethritis are the two most common types.

The symptoms of cystitis include a painful sensation or burning on urination, a frequent and often urgent need to urinate (sometimes causing nighttime awakening), and, occasionally, low back pain. These symptoms, along with bloody urine, indicate hemorrhagic cystitis, which is relatively common in women. Although quite frightening, this is most often a minor, easily treatable condition. However, repeated episodes or persistent bleeding, either visible or microscopic, requires further investigation. In men, however, bloody urine is not usually attributable to hemorrhagic cystitis and demands immediate investigation.

With the exception of visibly bloody urine, all of the symptoms mentioned can be present in urethritis, which is also commonly accompanied by a discharge. High fever, chills, and back pain (usually one-sided), with or without any other symptoms, usually indicate pyelonephritis (kidney infection), which demands the immediate attention of a doctor.

The diagnosis of urinary infection rests on the urinalysis and urine culture results. The presence of moderate to large numbers of white blood cells, along with at least 100,000 colonies of any one type of bacterium in a culture, provides conclusive evidence of infection.

Not infrequently, it is difficult to determine which part of the urinary tract is infected, or if there is infection at all. In women, some white blood cells and bacteria are usually present at the opening of the urethra. Therefore, in order to keep the urine specimen free of these contaminants, a midstream specimen is usually requested. The first spurt of urine is thought to wash away the urethral contaminants, and the rest of the urine sample is then normally uncontaminated. For the vast majority of cases of simple cystitis, this procedure is adequate; however, if a question exists as to the validity of the specimen or if for some reason the specimen must be absolutely free of contaminants, a catheter (thin, flexible tube) may be inserted into the bladder through the urethra. In women, this is an easy procedure and eliminates vaginal and anal contaminants. If the catheterized specimen is free of pus and bacteria, the symptoms are the result of another condition—commonly vaginitis or urethritis. In a man, the procedure is somewhat more difficult and often not necessary. If prostatitis is the suspected cause of the infection, the physician can insert a gloved finger into the anus and feel the gland directly. A specimen of prostatic fluid is usually obtained (by massaging the gland at the time of examination) through the urethra for culture.

Appropriate treatment is dependent on correct identification of the site of infection of the urinary tract. The experience of the physician, the patient's history of signs and symptoms (such as discharge, back pain, or fever), and the findings obtained with more sophisticated diagnostic techniques are all important in making the correct diagnosis of the patient.

In difficult chronic cases of cystitis in both men and women, in which the cause of recurring infection may be an obstruction or a drainage problem, special X-ray studies are necessary; contrast material is placed in the bladder by means of a catheter, and

X-ray pictures are taken of the bladder and the urethra during urination. With such studies, narrowing of a portion of the urethra, the presence of kidney stones, and incomplete emptying of the bladder (which promotes cystitis) may be detected. The bladder may also be examined through cystoscopy (examination by means of a flexible, lighted, tubelike instrument called a cystoscope, which is inserted through the urethra). Most often, these procedures are preceded by an intravenous pyelogram, in which contrast material injected through a vein is eliminated by the kidneys, providing an X-ray picture of the kidneys, ureters, and bladder.

Treatment of first-time cystitis is usually by means of antibiotics taken by mouth. Occasionally, large single doses of drugs are used. Recurrences may be treated in the same way if they are due to a different organism. If the same organism is causing the trouble, the condition may require larger doses of medication or long-term treatment (for up to four to six weeks). If cystitis persists, daily doses of medications may be necessary for up to six months. It is important that dosage instructions be followed exactly, because a person is vulnerable to a new infection or reinfection if the entire course of recommended drug therapy is not completed.

Some individuals are prone to repeated episodes of cystitis or upper urinary tract infection. If there is an anatomic defect, such as a narrowed urethra, dilation (enlarging) may be needed. If stones are present, they may have to be removed. If an infected prostate is the source of infection, antibiotics are usually tried first; surgery is a last resort. If no obvious cause of recurrent cystitis is found, low doses of antibiotics may be prescribed for long periods of time (this is called prophylactic, or preventive, therapy).

Women may be able to guard against recurrent cystitis by front-to-back wiping with toilet tissue and by cleansing with soap and water after each bowel movement. They should also try to urinate immediately after sexual intercourse to wash away infecting bacteria that might enter the urethra. Loose, absorbent underclothes allow evaporation and absorption of body fluids and thus help prevent infection. Both men and women should drink plenty of fluids and urinate frequently, completely emptying the bladder each time.

---

# Cystocele

A cystocele is a protrusion into the vagina of a portion of the urinary bladder.

Cystocele is usually the result of damage to the wall of fibrous tissue that normally separates the vagina and the bladder. Such an injury often occurs during childbirth and may happen with the birth of a baby of

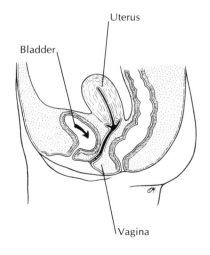

A cystocele is a protrusion of a portion of the urinary bladder into the vagina.

any size. However, women who have never given birth may also develop a cystocele. A cystocele may not appear until menopause, when the damaged area is weakened further, permitting the rear and base portions of the bladder to protrude into the vagina. A portion of the rectum (the final part of the large intestine), the small intestine, or the urethra (the tube through which urine leaves the body) may also bulge into the vagina, or prolapse of the uterus (in which the uterus drops through the vagina and in very severe cases protrudes through the vaginal opening) may occur.

The protrusion of the bladder into the vagina creates a pool of stale urine in the bladder, which cannot be easily emptied and as a result, becomes a breeding ground for bacteria. Cystitis (inflammation of the bladder), signaled by painful and difficult urination, often results.

A woman with a cystocele may feel a fullness in the vagina and may find it difficult to empty her bladder completely. However, many women with a cystocele have no symptoms at all.

Diagnosis is made by examining the inside of the vagina. If a bulge can be seen in front of the cervix, a cystocele is suspected. Also, if a catheter inserted into the bladder after urination can draw out more than two ounces of leftover urine, the diagnosis is even more likely. If a special X-ray study in which dye is injected into the bladder reveals a bulged-out section of the bladder, the diagnosis is confirmed.

The preferred treatment for cystocele is surgery to repair the damaged wall and put the protruding section of bladder back in its original place. A pessary (a device inserted into the vagina to support the vagina and reduce the cystocele) may be used in women who cannot or do not wish to undergo surgery. A cystocele does not require treatment in every case. However, if frequent bouts of cystitis occur, some form of treatment will be necessary.

See also Cystitis, Prolapse, and Rectocele.

# D

## D and C

See Dilatation and curettage.

## Deafness

Deafness is a term used to describe complete or partial loss or absence of the ability to hear.

There are three major types of deafness:

**Conductive deafness** This is caused by a defect in the outer or middle ear, which prevents normal transmission of sound. It may be present at birth as the result of an inherited defect, an abnormality in development, or an infection of the fetus in the womb. It may be produced by an injury that perforates the eardrum or that breaks up the linkage of the three tiny bones—hammer, anvil, and stirrup—that normally transmit sound from the eardrum through the middle ear to the inner ear. Inflammation of the middle ear, a condition known as otitis media, is another important cause of conductive deafness. Infection from an upper respiratory tract ailment, such as strep throat or the flu, can produce a buildup of pus in the middle ear so great that it ruptures the eardrum. Also, a plugged eustachian tube (the tube leading from the back of the throat to the ear) may trap fluid in the middle ear, creating temporary deafness. Conductive deafness in the middle and later years is most often caused by otosclerosis. In this inherited condition, new spongy bone grows over the stirrup bone, preventing it from vibrating when sound travels to it through the hammer and anvil bones.

**Sensorineural deafness** This is a type of hearing loss that occurs because of damage to the structures of the inner ear, to the auditory nerve carrying sound messages to the brain, or to the hearing center of the brain itself, which is located in the temporal lobe. It may be due to a head injury during birth, the effects of a woman's rubella infection on her unborn baby, a skull fracture affecting the inner ear or the auditory nerve, fever, bacterial or viral infections (such as mumps or meningitis), tertiary (final stage) syphilis, Meniere's disease, tumors, multiple sclerosis, a hemorrhage or blood clot in the inner ear, drug side effects, normal aging, prolonged or repeated exposure to intense noise, or edema (fluid buildup) caused by a thyroid deficiency. Most sensorineural deafness is not nerve deafness, the popular term for it. It is usually sensory deafness, caused by defects in the structure of the inner ear, especially in the fluid-filled cochlea and its organ of Corti. The cochlea contains sensory cells that convert sound waves into electrical impulses, which can then be transmitted via the auditory nerve to the brain.

**Mixed deafness** This is a relatively common condition. It is a combination of conductive and sensorineural deafness.

People with pure conductive deafness simply need louder volume to hear all sounds. Those with defects in the inner ear usually can hear low-pitched sounds more easily than high-pitched sounds, and some sounds may be distorted. When there is damage to the hearing center in the brain, the person may be able to hear sounds, but has trouble recognizing them and understanding words (this problem can also occur with the other types of deafness).

When hearing loss is suspected, a complete examination of the ears, nose, and throat is necessary to identify infections or abnormalities that may be present. Infections of the adenoids or tonsils, as well as sinus or nasal infections, may be linked to ear infections.

Testing of hearing is important for all ages, but especially for infants. Many times, partial deafness in a baby is not discovered until the child fails to learn to talk, a direct result of the hearing loss. Babies who were born prematurely or ill or whose mothers had certain viral infections, such as rubella, during pregnancy are in special need of testing.

Although inborn hearing defects usually cannot be corrected, deaf children can be helped to deal with their handicap. Starting very early, they can be fitted with hearing aids and can be instructed in lipreading, speaking, and sign language.

Surgery to correct conductive hearing loss includes operations to replace the stirrup bone or all three tiny bones with tissue or synthetic material, to repair a punctured eardrum, and to clean a middle ear that has been chronically infected.

A hearing aid can often help to restore hearing. However, one should be purchased only after thorough testing by a specialist in audiometry, who can suggest the most appropriate type. Classes in lipreading and listening can also be helpful.

It is far easier to prevent deafness than to cure it. Antibiotics have made it possible to eradicate most of the middle ear infections that have been the major source of conductive hearing loss in children. Middle ear problems are sometimes eliminated by treating allergies that cause the eustachian tubes to close up or by removing infected adenoids. Nerve deafness caused by continued exposure to intense industrial noise, gunshots, rock music, or aircraft engines may be avoided by wearing earplugs or other ear protectors. Some lost hearing may return after several months of relief from intense sound. Drugs that can cause hearing loss, including some antibiotics and certain diuretics (drugs that stimulate production of urine), need to be used with care, and signs of hearing loss should be brought to a doctor's attention.

See also Ear, nose, and throat.

# Defibrillation

Defibrillation is a technique to correct fibrillation of the heart, an abnormal condition marked by very rapid, disorganized twitching or trembling of the heart muscle in place of the normal rhythmic beat. Ventricular fibrillation produces a condition called cardiac arrest, in which no heartbeat, pulse, or blood pressure can be detected. Death or permanent brain damage follows within a few minutes unless this condition is corrected or unless first-aid measures maintain blood circulation and breathing until emergency treatment is available.

The most common cause of fibrillation is a heart attack. When this happens, certain parts of the heart will start contracting independently of the normal heartbeat. Other causes of fibrillation are severe electrical shock and prolonged exposure to cold temperatures.

An electrical device called a defibrillator is used to correct fibrillation. A pair of metal paddles are placed on the patient's chest, and a jolt of direct-current electricity from the defibrillator is directed through them into the heart to shock it back into its regular rhythm. The shock stops the independent action of individual muscle fibers and allows the natural pacemaker function of the heart to take over again.

Once the normal heartbeat has been restored, other measures are taken. A drug such as lidocaine is injected to prevent further fibrillation. An intravenous tube is inserted to administer sodium bicarbonate (to neutralize acids in the blood) and other medication. A breathing tube may be passed into the trachea (windpipe); it is attached to a mechanical pump that forces air in and out of the lungs. Then the patient is taken to a

To correct fibrillation—the disorganized twitching or trembling of the heart muscle in place of its normal beat—a pair of metal paddles is placed on the chest, and a jolt of electricity from the defibrillator is directed into the heart to shock it back into its normal rhythm.

hospital cardiac intensive care unit, where monitoring devices constantly keep track of the patient's condition and sound an alarm if danger threatens. An electrical defibrillator is close at hand if needed in an emergency.

Electrical defibrillation is also used to restart a heart that has been stopped for purposes of heart surgery.

# Dehydration

Dehydration is a condition in which the body in general or certain body tissues in particular suffer from lack of fluid.

Tissue dehydration may occur in dry climates and during the winter heating season: extremely dry air causes rapid evaporation of water from the skin and from the mucous linings of the respiratory (breathing) system. The results are discomfort and sometimes cracking of the skin, unless it is protected by lotions, and increased susceptibility of the respiratory system to infections.

Dehydration of the entire body can be life-threatening. Illnesses that produce diarrhea and vomiting are common causes of dehydration, since both of these conditions cause loss of body fluids. Cholera, which results in extreme diarrhea and vomiting, can kill through dehydration. Other causes of dehydration include diabetes, kidney disease, excessive use of diuretics (drugs or other substances that stimulate production of urine), liver disease, and inflammation of the abdominal cavity.

Burns may also be a cause of dehydration. Tissue beneath a burn swells with body fluid. If the burn covers much of the body, the buildup of fluid in burn tissue draws considerable water from the blood. This can decrease the blood volume so much

that shock (general collapse of the circulatory system) occurs.

Symptoms of dehydration include thirst; sudden weight loss; rough, dry skin; dry mucous membranes; rapid heartbeat and low blood pressure; lack of energy; and weakness. In an extreme case, the patient goes into shock, which is characterized by pale skin; bluish lips and fingertips; rapid, shallow breathing; and a weak, rapid, irregular pulse. Blood tests reveal thickening of the blood because of decreased water content.

The treatment of mild to moderate dehydration is to have the patient drink water with some salts added. However, if the individual has been vomiting, suffers from diarrhea, or is unconscious, it may be necessary to administer saline (saltwater) solution intravenously. The intravenous method is always used in severe cases of dehydration. The goal is to stabilize vital signs such as blood pressure, temperature, and pulse as soon as possible and to replace the lost fluid within 48 to 72 hours, together with the valuable mineral salts that have also been lost.

# Delirium

Delirium is a confused mental state marked by disorganized or incoherent speech and hallucinations (imagined perceptions). Often, the person is unaware of time or place; is fearful, excited, and restless; and suffers from delusions. The heartbeat is rapid, the pupils of the eyes are dilated (enlarged), and sweating is common.

Delirium can occur because of fever, disease, injury, poisoning, or mental disease. It may result from the sudden withdrawal of alcohol or another drug on which the individual has become dependent; from liver, kidney, or heart failure; or from deficiencies of certain B vitamins or thyroid hormone. It can also be caused by bruising of brain tissue or by pressure on brain tissue, which may be caused by fluid, inflammation, hemorrhage, a tumor, or an abscess.

Delirium often develops rapidly and fluctuates in severity. The patient usually cannot remember what happened during the episode of delirium and does not recall past events well. Depending on its cause, delirium may last from hours to weeks.

Treating the underlying disease or condition is the first step in treating delirium. In the meantime, the patient should be cared for patiently and sympathetically in a quiet, relaxed environment. Every effort should be made to answer questions, remove fears, and keep the patient in touch with reality.

Partial or complete recovery depends on the nature, severity, and treatability of the underlying cause.

# Deoxyribonucleic acid

See Genes.

# Depression

Depression, the most common form of emotional disorder, is characterized by prolonged sadness, combined with other negative mood symptoms, such as indecisiveness, inability to concentrate, anxiety, apathy, loneliness, lowered self-esteem, self-blame, and loss of interest in others, in work, and in recreation.

Deep sadness or depression is a normal reaction of an emotionally healthy person to discouraging life events such as loss, separation, death of a family member, and disappointment. It is probably a protective reaction, possibly enabling a person to withdraw from everyday concerns long enough to sort out his or her feelings and prepare for a new approach to life.

Temporary depression can also occur because of normal chemical changes in the body. Two examples are premenstrual depression and postpartum (after childbirth) depression— both of which are thought to be linked to female hormonal activity. In addition, alcohol and certain drugs, including oral contraceptives, reserpine (formerly used to lower high blood pressure), and some sedatives, may cause depression as a side effect in some people. Certain infections (including influenza, viral hepatitis, infectious mononucleosis, and tuberculosis) can depress a person's mood, as can deficiency of vitamin $B_{12}$, overproduction or underproduction of hormones by the outer layer of the adrenal gland, and various diseases of the nervous system.

Temporary depression can be eased by the support of family and friends or simply by the passage of time and by steps the person takes to change his or her life situation. Medication is not usually necessary, nor is any other treatment. However, a visit to a physician can provide valuable reassurance that the depression is not abnormal.

Unlike temporary depression, which is sometimes called reactive depression because it is a reaction to a specific circumstance, severe depression does not always have an obvious cause. Even if there is an apparent cause, the reaction is out of proportion, and it may continue for weeks or months.

The causes of severe depression are unclear. Loss of a parent at an early age or growing up in a cold, critical, unstable, or unfriendly family setting may make a person susceptible to depression. There is also an inherited tendency to suffer certain forms of depression.

The symptoms of severe depression include crying spells, slowing of speech and thought processes, agitation, feelings of hopelessness and helplessness, withdrawal from usual activities, recurring thoughts of death and suicide, and irritability. (Some of these symptoms also occur in temporary depression, to a lesser degree.) Early awakening, insomnia, fatigue, loss of appetite, weight loss or gain, loss of sexual desire, and imagined pains are also common. Depressed patients with certain mental diseases may hear voices accusing them of unpardonable crimes, see visions of coffins or dead relatives, believe that others are watching or persecuting them, or suffer delusions that they are worthless, sinful, or ill with some incurable disease.

Sometimes periods of deep depression alternate with periods of elation, high hopes, grandiose ideas, and overactivity. This is known as manic-depressive disorder. When in the manic phase, the person is overwhelmingly confident and inexhaustible, racing from thought to thought. Eventually, however, the mood cycles to bleakest despair.

Diagnosis of severe depression can be complicated. Some depression is masked—the person is "smiling on the outside, crying on the inside" and may not even be aware of his or her depressed mental state. Instead, the depression is expressed in symptoms, such as headaches and backaches, that have no physical cause. In addition, the person may seem to have lost all emotion, including the ability to take pleasure in anything.

The physician needs to rule out physical causes of depression, such as nutritional deficiencies and the side effects of certain medications. Drug abuse and alcoholism may be involved (however, they may be the result, rather than the cause, of the depression). Schizophrenia and other mental disorders must be considered.

With appropriate treatment, the symptoms of severe depression can often be reduced or eliminated. Hospitalization is not usually necessary, unless the patient is suicidal, in a stupor, agitated and out of touch with reality, or physically deteriorated as a result of the depression. Hospital treatment for the first three types of cases may involve treatment with antidepressant drugs or electroconvulsive therapy.

Most severe depression, however, can be managed with a combination of drugs and psychotherapy (counseling by a psychiatrist or psychologist, with office visits once or twice a week at the beginning of treatment and less often as improvement occurs). It is extremely important to find a professional who is not only knowledgeable but also reassuring and encouraging, and who is trusted by the patient. An extended course of psychotherapy is usually not called for unless there is a serious personality disorder. If depression is a result of a serious physical illness, individual reassurance and support groups may provide the most help.

Lithium carbonate is used to treat manic-depressive illness both in its extreme form and in its moderate form, known as cyclothymia. In the latter condition, the person alternates between brief periods (usually days) of gloom and elation.

Suicide is a major risk in depression and should be guarded against, especially when the person seems to be recovering from the depression but is still feeling "low," when anniversaries of landmarks in the person's life occur, and in the days preceding menstruation.

See also Electroconvulsive therapy.

---

# Dermatitis

Dermatitis is an inflammation of the skin. There are many different kinds of dermatitis and a great variety of causes. Some of the more common varieties include the following.

**Chronic dermatitis** This often occurs on the hands or feet, and may simply be the result of continued irritation, especially by contact dermatitis. It is marked by thickened skin, inflammation, and scaling. It is sometimes caused by excessive hand washing or by accumulation of soaps or detergents under rings. Occasionally, a fungal infection is the cause.

**Contact dermatitis** This is a skin inflammation caused by a substance that has touched the skin. This may be a harsh chemical or a detergent or soap that irritates directly, or it may be a substance that produces an allergic reaction that does not appear until five or six days after the contact. Less commonly, the reaction appears only after years of repeated use. Common causes of allergic contact dermatitis are poison ivy, chemicals in shoes and clothing, metal watchbands and rings, antibiotic salves, and cosmetics. There are also cases in which a substance, such as a shaving lotion or cosmetic, produces a "photoallergic" reaction—that is, a rash develops when the skin under the substance is exposed to sunlight.

**Eczema** This inflammation of the skin is marked by small blisters (when severe), redness, fluid in the tissue, oozing, scales, crusts or scabs, burning or itching, and sometimes dryness. The skin of flexor surfaces (those subject to bending movements, such as the back of the knee and the top of the elbow) is most commonly affected. There are several different forms of eczema. One of the more common types is atopic dermatitis, which is an itching skin inflammation due to an allergy. Susceptible persons often have a family history of allergic diseases, such as asthma or hay fever. Typically, it begins in infancy, subsides by age three, and may reappear by age 10 or 12. Certain foods (such as wheat, milk, and eggs) and other substances (such as pollen and fur) often bring on symptoms; if so, they must be avoided.

**Exfoliative dermatitis** This condition produces shedding of skin all over the body, together with hair loss. The entire skin surface is red, scaly, and thickened. The cause is unknown in most cases, but it sometimes occurs following a less severe case of dermatitis or as a side effect of a drug. Hospitalization is frequently necessary because the condition can be life-threatening. A first step is to consult a doctor about any medications and to ask about stopping or changing them.

**Localized neurodermatitis** This condition is characterized by thick, sharp-bordered, scaly breaks in the skin, occasionally with little blisters. This condition is caused by habitual scratching of an insect bite or other real or imagined irritation of the skin and is corrected by covering the area and stopping the scratching. In the case of an itch in the area around the openings of the vagina and colon, however, warts, pinworms, hemorrhoids, infections, or certain diseases may be the cause.

**Nummular dermatitis** Coin-shaped patches of blisters that later ooze and crust over mark this condition, which usually is accompanied by dry skin and itching. Most often, it appears on the legs and sometimes the buttocks and trunk of middle-aged persons.

**Seborrheic dermatitis** This is a scaling and inflammation of the scalp and sometimes the face and other parts of the body. This is the cause of dandruff in adults and cradle cap in infants.

**Stasis dermatitis** This stubborn skin inflammation of the lower legs is usually the result of poor blood return from the area. There is redness, mild scaling, and brown discoloration of the skin. If the condition is neglected, the skin swells and may become infected, or ulcers (eroded skin sores) may develop.

Because there is such a bewildering variety of skin diseases and because some can be dangerous if neglected, it is important to seek medical care for any dermatitis. In general, this care usually begins with very simple measures. Dry skin needs lubricating agents, while moist or oily skin may require powders or other drying substances. Inflamed skin is commonly treated with cortisone-type creams; cool, wet dressings; or baths.

Hardened, dried skin may be peeled off with strong substances available only by prescription. If possible, the cause of the dermatitis is sought (with the patient's help) and eliminated. Cortisone creams are often used to make the patient more comfortable by reducing inflammation, although continuous use is not usually recommended. Antibiotics are employed promptly to eliminate any infections before they can spread to other parts of the body. Patients must resist the constant temptation to scratch itchy areas or remove scabs, because that will simply prolong and even worsen the problem. In addition, while cleanliness is desirable, some patients need to be told to reduce hand washing and the number of baths they take, because they may be washing away natural oils that protect the skin. Along the same lines, patients should not use any medication that has not been recommended by a doctor or use it more frequently than directed. Overmedication of skin dis-

eases may be worse than undermedication in some cases.

See also Contact dermatitis.

---

# DES

Diethylstilbestrol (DES) is an artificial estrogen (female sex hormone) used to treat a variety of disorders. For nearly three decades, this drug was frequently prescribed to prevent miscarriage. In 1971, however, the Food and Drug Administration banned its use for this purpose because it had been found ineffective in preventing miscarriages.

Use of DES has been linked to an increased incidence of adenocarcinoma (a rare cancer of the glandular cells of the reproductive organs) in the daughters of the several million women who took it to prevent miscarriage and other complications of pregnancy. Testicular cancer in male offspring has also been associated with maternal DES use. Persons exposed to DES before birth also have a higher than average incidence of benign (noncancerous) growths, structural changes involving the reproductive organs, and infertility problems. These abnormalities usually appear in the late teens to early 30s. Although the incidence of serious complications is small, physicians strongly advise that persons who were exposed to DES before birth be routinely examined to detect any abnormalities.

Because of the potential problems, DES should not be taken by a woman who is pregnant or suspects that she is pregnant. DES may be used safely by nonpregnant women to treat a variety of disorders, including certain vaginal conditions and estrogen deficiency that may occur at menopause or after the surgical removal of the ovaries. Recently, DES has also been shown to be effective in some male patients in reducing the growth of advanced prostate cancer. Since DES is a hormone that may produce a variety of effects in the body, its use must always be supervised by a physician.

# Detached retina

Normally, the retina is firmly attached to the choroid, an underlying layer of tissue that is rich in blood vessels. If blood or other fluid collects between the retina and the choroid, the retina may become partially or totally detached. Fluid from the vitreous cav-

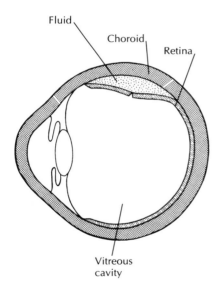

Fluid
Choroid
Retina
Vitreous cavity

A detached retina is a condition in which the retina separates from its attachment to underlying tissues in the eye. Normally, the retina—the light-sensitive lining of the inner eyeball—is firmly attached to an underlying structure called the choroid. If fluid collects between the retina and the choroid, the retina may partially or totally detach. Fluid from the vitreous cavity may penetrate beneath the retina because of a small hole in the retina. Fluid leaking out of certain blood vessels in the eye may also penetrate beneath the retina to cause detachment.

ity (the fluid-filled space within the eye) may penetrate beneath the retina because of a small hole in the retina. Fluid leaking out of certain blood vessels in the eye may also penetrate beneath the retina to cause detachment.

Cataract surgery, severe myopia (nearsightedness), and injury can cause retinal detachment. Although injury can be the primary cause of this condition, it is more likely to accelerate a detachment that has already begun. Conditions that increase susceptibility to retinal detachment are inflammation or tumors of the eye, high blood pressure, and vitreous hemorrhaging.

Initial symptoms include seeing floating dark spots or flashes or streaks of light and experiencing blurring of vision. As the condition progresses, a curtain or veil seems to fall over part or all of the field of vision.

A detached retina can be treated by using a laser to fuse the retina to the choroid. It can also be treated by diathermy (repair using heat), cryotherapy (repair using extreme cold), or microsurgery (surgery using a microscope). Left untreated, the detachment may increase and lead to the loss of sight.

# Diabetes mellitus

Diabetes mellitus, often called sugar diabetes, is a condition in which the body is unable to properly utilize glucose, which is the body's major source of energy.

Normally, digestion of food causes the release of a form of sugar called glucose into the blood. As the blood glucose level rises, the pancreas is stimulated to secrete the hormone insulin. Insulin allows the body to utilize glucose in the blood by transporting glucose from the blood into

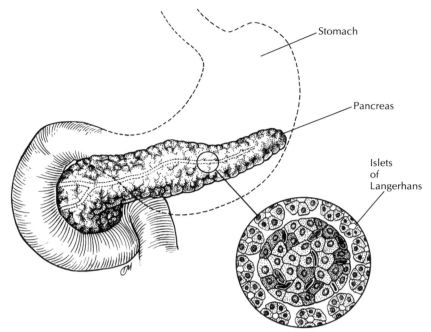

Stomach

Pancreas

Islets
of
Langerhans

The islets of Langerhans in the pancreas secretes insulin, the hormone that helps the cells utilize sugar as fuel. One type of diabetes results from a defect in the islets of Langerhans, causing decreased production of insulin.

body cells, where it is used for fuel. Glucose not immediately needed is transported to the liver, where it is stored until needed for fuel.

When the pancreas produces insufficient insulin or the body cannot use the insulin it manufactures, diabetes mellitus results. The glucose concentration in the blood increases because glucose circulates throughout the body without being used. When the amount of glucose presented to the kidneys exceeds its ability to process it, glucose spills into the urine and can be measured by various techniques.

There are two major forms of diabetes mellitus. Type I (or insulin-dependent) diabetes results from a defect of unknown origin in the islets of Langerhans (the specialized cells in the pancreas where insulin is produced). This form of diabetes usual-ly develops in children and young adults.

With Type II (or non-insulin-dependent) diabetes, either the specialized area of the pancreas functions inadequately or the body is unable to use insulin efficiently. A shortage of insulin-receptors (sites on body cells where the interaction of glucose and insulin occurs) allows the insulin to be present in the bloodstream without working properly. Obesity often contributes to the problem because the presence of excess fat cells leads to increased resistance to insulin. Type II diabetes, which appears most often in adults over the age of 40, may evolve from a gradual slowing of insulin production within the pancreas. In addition, other disorders of the endocrine system may cause hormonal imbalances that disturb glucose regulation.

Research shows that people who have a family history of Type II diabetes may have a greater tendency to acquire the condition. Women are more likely to be affected, but for all adults, the risk of developing Type II diabetes doubles with every decade after the age of 40.

In some women, pregnancy triggers diabetes. The condition usually subsides after childbirth. However, women who show signs of diabetes during pregnancy and deliver babies weighing over ten pounds have a greater risk of diabetes later in life.

Although patients with diabetes can usually control the condition, uncontrolled diabetes can lead to serious complications. Extremely high blood sugar levels place great strain on other organs. Diabetes may accelerate atherosclerosis (clogging of the arteries). Insufficient blood supply contributes to heart attack, stroke, kidney disease, eye disorders, impotence, gangrene (death of tissue due to inadequate blood circulation), and even death. Diabetes is also associated with impaired response to infection.

Symptoms of Type I diabetes are excessive thirst and urination, fatigue, altered vision, fainting, irritability, and weight loss despite constant hunger and voracious eating.

Type II diabetes may present the same symptoms, though weight loss is uncommon and slow healing of cuts and scrapes is often noticed. Sometimes symptoms appear very gradually, and sometimes no symptoms appear at all. Physicians frequently detect diabetes Type II when performing routine examinations or tests.

In addition to evaluating symptoms, doctors can diagnose diabetes by analyzing blood samples for elevated glucose concentrations. They may also test blood and urine for excess ketones, the chemical by-products of the breakdown of fat for energy. Since people with diabetes do not use glucose normally, their bodies burn fat for fuel, and as a result, ketones are eliminated in the urine. Ketones are acidic, and their overabundance in the blood causes serious imbalances in body fluids and electrolytes.

Type I diabetes requires injections of insulin to maintain blood sugar levels as close to normal as possible. If the blood glucose concentration rises, weakness, fatigue, and thirst will result. These symptoms mean that more insulin is needed. However, if blood glucose concentration falls too low, an insulin reaction occurs, causing dizziness, hunger, fatigue, headache, sweating, trembling, and (in severe cases) unconsciousness. A quick remedy for this problem is to give the person simple sugar, such as is found in orange juice and hard candies. This should be done only if the person is conscious and alert; however, nothing should be given by mouth to an unconscious or semiconscious person, because of the risk of choking. In this case, emergency professional help is required.

Ideally, these fluctuations of blood sugar levels can be prevented by coordinating the type and timing of insulin injections with meal content and activity. A special diet is important to balance daily insulin injections. Insulin requirements for persons with Type I diabetes differ greatly. Some patients may maintain balanced blood sugar levels with one insulin injection taken daily. Most patients require two or more insulin injections per day. Insulin requirements may change as the patient grows older, undergoes surgery, becomes pregnant, or develops an unrelated illness such as an infection. Recently, an insulin pump has become available. So far, it has been limited to use in individuals with very erratic blood sugars, but with the advantage of meticulous control now clearly evident, it may become more commonplace. The pump consists of a small machine that is worn on a belt or in a pocket. It contains a reservoir into which regular insulin is loaded, usually enough for three days. A tube from the pump leads to a catheter or needle that is inserted into the subcutaneous fat of the abdomen. Regular insulin is infused at a constant rate throughout a 24-hour period along with increased doses before meals. Blood sugars must be checked often, and the pump must only be used under the close supervision of professionals.

Many people with Type II diabetes can regulate their condition with proper diet and exercise. Sometimes oral antidiabetic drugs may be prescribed. These drugs work by stimulating the pancreas to produce more insulin and by increasing the number of insulin receptors.

Special attention to diet is critical for diabetes control. A diet should be prescribed by a physician, then implemented and monitored by a nutritionist. Overweight individuals need to lose weight. Thereafter, emphasis is on eating balanced meals that will sustain the recommended weight. A diabetic diet usually consists of about 60 percent carbohydrate, 20 percent protein, and 20 percent fat. Portion control and meal timing are important.

With either type of diabetes, professional follow-up is important to plan diet and exercise, determine changes in medication, and monitor blood glucose levels. Testing urine for sugar has been shown to be inaccurate, and the availability of home blood glucose machines has replaced urine sugar testing.

The use of home blood glucose monitoring has revolutionized diabetic care. A fingertip is pricked with a tiny needle, and a drop of blood is then placed on a special strip that is inserted into a meter. Within a minute, a blood glucose reading is displayed. Multiple daily readings are often required to achieve optimum control. The technique is easily learned. Glycosylated or "glyco" hemoglobin is a blood test done to determine the degree of control of blood glucose over a period of about three months. A doctor will order this test at intervals to determine the effectiveness of the overall treatment plan. Urine testing for ketones, however, remains important, particularly during periods of illness.

There is no cure for diabetes, but the disease can be controlled through a treatment plan of diet, exercise, and, if needed, medication. The goal of treatment is to maintain blood glucose levels as close to normal as possible. With a good treatment plan, a person with diabetes can lead a very normal life. A team approach, consisting of a diabetes nurse educator, a dietician, and a physician has proven most beneficial in controlling the disease and preventing complications.

See also Ketosis and Retinopathy.

# Dialysis

Dialysis is the removal of wastes and other undesirable substances from the blood by means of a special membrane that is selective in what it allows to cross. In the healthy body, this task is performed by the kidneys.

In a patient suffering from temporary or permanent kidney failure, cleansing of the blood can be done with an artificial kidney machine; this is known as hemodialysis. Two plastic tubes, one connected to an artery and one to a vein, are implanted in the patient's arm or leg. During dialysis, which can take three to five hours per treatment, blood from the artery tube enters the machine and comes into contact with a thin membrane. Wastes from the blood pass through the membrane into circulating fluid on the other side of the membrane. The blood cells themselves, along with other protein elements, cannot cross the membrane. The cleansed blood is then piped back into the patient through the vein tube.

In peritoneal dialysis, the patient's own peritoneum (lining of the abdominal cavity) is used as the dialysis membrane. A sterile plastic catheter (tube) is passed into the abdominal cavity, and a solution of glucose (a form of sugar) and mineral salts is periodically injected into and withdrawn from the cavity. The fluid comes into contact with delicate blood vessels in the peritoneum. Because of the difference in concentration of certain chemical elements in the blood and the solution, wastes from the blood are forced through the membrane of the peritoneal wall. The dialysis liquid is periodically withdrawn and replaced with fresh solution.

A new method called continuous ambulatory peritoneal dialysis has greatly lowered the cost of dialysis and made it more convenient. It can be done at home by the patient without the complex equipment and the skilled supervision that has made machine dialysis so expensive. A tube is surgically implanted in the patient, just below the navel. About every four to five hours and just before bedtime, the patient drains out the old fluid and empties a bag of fresh dialysis fluid into the abdominal cavity through a tube. The fluid remains in the cavity, soaking up wastes from the blood, while the patient sleeps or goes about his or her usual daily activities. The procedure takes only about 30 minutes each time and

enables the patient to be independent and mobile.

See also Kidney failure.

# Diaphragmatic hernia

See Hiatal hernia.

# Diarrhea

Diarrhea is abnormally frequent and excessively liquid bowel movements. This is often the body's defensive attempt to rid itself of irritating or toxic substances. It is a symptom that accompanies many disorders, both mild and serious.

There are two basic types of diarrhea, acute (short-term) and chronic (long-term). Acute diarrhea, the more common form, comes on quickly and usually lasts no more than two or three days, although it can last as long as two weeks. Chronic diarrhea may also appear suddenly, but it lingers for many weeks or months, either being constantly present or alternately appearing and disappearing.

Both acute and chronic diarrhea can become a serious problem because of the danger of dehydration (excessive loss of body fluids and salts), as well as loss of nutrients. Diarrhea may also be a symptom of an inflammatory bowel disease (for example, Crohn's disease or ulcerative colitis).

The reasons for the consistency of the stool (feces) in diarrhea are complex. In an infection, the intestine may pour out massive quantities of fluids and salts in response to a bacterial toxin (poison) or other irritant. In inflammatory bowel disease, protein, blood, and mucus are lost through the inflamed lining of the bowel, taking large quantities of water with them. Other disorders speed up the normal movement of the colon, thereby not allowing time for absorption of fluids. Yet another type of diarrhea is caused by poor absorption of a type of sugar called lactose, which draws fluid out of the colon. In many cases, diarrhea is caused by a combination of these mechanisms.

Other causes of diarrhea include changes in the diet, drugs taken for other disorders (particularly antibiotics, which upset the bacterial balance in the intestines), stress, infection, and food allergies.

The symptoms often experienced with the characteristic loose and frequent stools are nausea, cramps or pain in the abdomen, gassiness, fatigue, and fever.

Diagnostic evaluation will include assessment of the patient's normal diet and emotional state, as well as recent changes in daily habits. In addition, a sample of the stool may be examined for color, consistency, odor, chemical content, and presence of blood. Stool cultures are often done to identify the causative microorganism if infection is suspected.

Treatment for diarrhea usually involves removing or correcting the cause of the condition. If diarrhea lasts for more than three days or is a recurring problem, a doctor should be consulted, as this may be a warning sign of a more serious illness. Antidiarrheal medications can be prescribed for particularly bothersome or persistent diarrhea, but these should be used only with caution; in the case of some infections, they may actually prolong the course of the illness.

The discomfort of occasional bouts of acute diarrhea, however, is usually treated with simple remedies, such as adequate rest and increased intake of liquids to replace lost fluids. The diet should consist of light meals, perhaps soup or broth at first; as solid food is added to the diet, irritating substances, such as bran, fruits and vegetables, fried foods, coffee, and alcoholic beverages should be avoided at mealtime.

See also Crohn's disease, Dehydration, and Ulceratice colitis.

# Diethylstilbestrol

See DES.

# Digestion

Digestion is the process by which the body converts food into basic substances that can be either absorbed in the bloodstream as nutrients or passed out of the body as waste. This process of breakdown and assimilation occurs within the digestive tract, a convoluted tube more than 30 feet long that is lined with a mucous membrane. The tract includes several hollow organs—the mouth, esophagus, stomach, small intestine, and large intestine (colon)—each of which has a specific function in digestion. The muscles of these organs move the food through the system, while mucus lubricates the tract and prevents irritation. The liver and pancreas are also critical organs in the process of digestion. While not considered an essential organ, the gallbladder is involved in digestion as well.

Food first enters the digestive tract through the mouth. Movement of the jaws allows the teeth to cut and grind the food into smaller pieces, which are mixed with saliva (a secretion of the glands in the mouth). Saliva moistens food for easier swallowing and contains an enzyme (a special type of protein) that begins the chemical breakdown of starches.

From the mouth, food passes down the throat and into the esophagus, the muscular tube through which the food is conducted to the stomach. The stomach is a large pouch in the abdominal cavity, where food is combined with acid- and enzyme-containing digestive juices secreted by glands within the stomach walls. The food becomes semifluid, which allows it to pass easily into the small intestine, which consists of three portions—the upper section, or duodenum; the middle section, or jejunum; and the lower section, or the ileum.

In the duodenum, the first ten inches of the small intestine, digestive juices from the liver and pancreas continue the process of breaking down the food into its constituent nutrients, which can then be absorbed into the bloodstream in the remainder of the small intestine.

Aiding digestion is the liver, an accessory organ of digestion. The liver produces bile, which is necessary for absorption of fat in the small intestine. The liver also removes some wastes from the blood, produces and stores glucose (a form of sugar), and processes many drugs.

The gallbladder, located on the underside of the liver, is another organ that performs an indirect digestive function. The gallbladder stores the bile manufactured by the liver. As bile is needed, the gallbladder contracts and releases the fluid into the duodenum. If the gallbladder needs to be removed for medical reasons

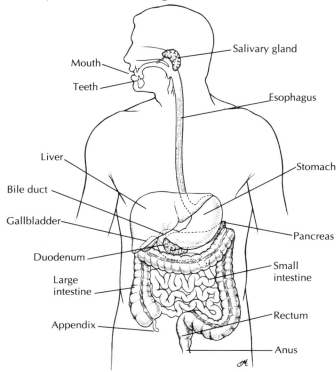

Mouth
Teeth
Salivary gland
Esophagus
Liver
Bile duct
Gallbladder
Duodenum
Large intestine
Appendix
Stomach
Pancreas
Small intestine
Rectum
Anus

The digestive system includes the mouth, esophagus, stomach, small intestine, large intestine, liver, gallbladder, and pancreas—each of which plays a specific role in digestion.

(such as in severe gallbladder disease), however, the liver can compensate for its role, and digestion is not hindered.

Other digestive juices required by the small intestine to digest and absorb food, particularly fats and starches, come from the pancreas, an organ located just behind the stomach. The pancreas also secretes insulin and other hormones into the blood. Insulin is the hormone responsible for aiding absorption and use of glucose.

Whatever substances are not assimilated into the bloodstream through the small intestine move into the large intestine. Within the large intestine, waste material is processed into stool (feces), and water and certain chemicals are absorbed into the bloodstream to preserve the body's fluid balance.

The fecal matter continues to move through the colon to the rectum (the lower part of the large intestine). Once in the rectum, waste is ready to be passed out of the body through the anus (the opening at the end of the digestive tract), thus completing the process of digestion.

# Dilatation and curettage

Dilatation and curettage, also called a D&C, is a surgical procedure in which the cervix of the uterus is dilated (expanded) and the endometrial lining of the uterus is scraped with a curette (a loop-, ring-, or scoop-shaped instrument with a long, rodlike handle).

This procedure is often used in the diagnosis of diseases of the uterus (such as cancer) and to halt excessive bleeding. It is also used to perform an abortion and may be employed after a miscarriage (involuntary expulsion

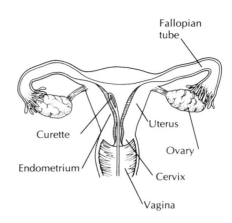

Dilatation and curettage is a surgical procedure in which the cervix is dilated (expanded) and the endometrium (uterine lining) is scraped with a curette (a loop-, ring-, or scoop-shaped instrument with a rodlike handle).

of a fetus before it is able to live on its own) to remove any remains of tissue and thereby lower the risk of hemorrhage and infection.

Dilatation alone may be performed to enlarge the passageway out of the uterus. This might be done if a severely narrowed cervix is causing painful menstruation because of restricted flow of menstrual fluid. For treatment of this problem, multiple dilatations may be necessary since the cervix will often become narrow again after several months.

Although a D&C is a relatively minor procedure, hospital admission is sometimes recommended. Because the large intestine should be empty before the procedure, an enema is often given; the urinary bladder should also be emptied.

The procedure is performed in an operating room under sterile conditions. Anesthesia may be general (the patient is put to sleep) or local. The patient rests on her back with her feet in stirrups. The surgeon inserts metal dilators of progressively larger sizes into the cervix until it is open enough to permit the insertion of the surgical instruments. (An alternative method of cervical dilatation employs a small tube of dried seaweed that is left in the cervical canal for 8 to 12 hours. As the seaweed absorbs moisture from the cervical canal, it expands and enlarges the canal.)

A curette is used to remove endometrial tissue. Special forceps may also be used to remove tissue. When the operation is finished, an absorbent pad is placed over the entrance to the vagina. The pad is checked every 15 minutes for two hours, and excessive bleeding is reported to the physician.

Mild painkillers should be enough to control discomfort from the operation. If there is pain in the abdomen that cannot be relieved in this way or that is continuous or sharp, it should be reported immediately. Some difficulty in urinating is to be expected immediately after the procedure.

In most cases, the patient stays in bed for one to two hours following surgery. Most women return home several hours after the procedure or the next day. A return to many daily activities is possible immediately, and in a week all normal physical activities may be resumed. Sexual intercourse and use of tampons should not be attempted, however, until after the follow-up visit to the doctor (usually about two weeks after the procedure).

The principal risks of a D&C are hemorrhage, infection, and perforation (puncture) of the uterus. The latter is more likely during pregnancy, when the uterine walls are especially soft and thin.

# Diphtheria

Diphtheria is a sudden, severe, and highly contagious disease that primarily affects the tonsils, upper airways, and larynx (voice box). Diph-

theria bacteria destroy the outer layer of the mucous membrane of the throat or larynx; the slush of dead cells, bacteria, and white blood cells that remains forms the grayish membrane covering the tonsils and throat that is the chief sign of the disease. Complications may include inflammation of the heart muscle (myocarditis), which sometimes results in heart failure, and temporary neuritis (nerve inflammation). Diphtheria bacteria also infect skin wounds but cannot invade intact skin.

Diphtheria is caused by the bacterium known as *Corynebacterium diphtheriae*, which is transmitted via droplets of moisture from the throat and nose of an infected person. It is most common during the colder months, when schools are in session and people are in closer contact. Frequently, the bacteria are transmitted by carriers—people who have no symptoms and do not even know that they harbor the disease. The incubation period (the time between exposure to the infection and appearance of the first symptom) is one to seven days.

Early symptoms include a mild sore throat, hoarseness, a rasping croupy cough, pain when swallowing, and a mild fever. Children may be nauseated, may vomit, and may have chills and headache as well as fever and other symptoms. The membrane that forms typically is tough, adheres tightly, and causes bleeding if removed. It appears in patches and can vary from yellowish to grayish green or dirty gray (the most common color). Some people have little or no characteristic membrane. If the membrane extends from the throat to the trachea (windpipe), larynx, or bronchi (air tubes in the lungs), it can become detached and obstruct the passage partially or completely, choking off the air supply. Signs of this life-threatening emergency are rapid breathing, high-pitched breathing sounds, and blue lips and fingertips. Narrowing of the air passage may also be caused by edema (swelling of fluid-filled tissue) of the lining of the larynx and throat.

Treatment is with diphtheria antitoxin (a solution of refined and concentrated protective antibodies obtained from the blood of horses that have been immunized against the poisons created by the diphtheria bacteria). This should be done at once, after a skin test to determine that the patient is not allergic to horse serum (blood fluid). (A patient who is found to be allergic is desensitized with a series of diluted doses of antitoxin.) After the antitoxin has been administered, antibiotics, such as penicillin or erythromycin, are given for at least a week to eliminate the diphtheria organisms. The patient is isolated until two cultures obtained 24 hours apart indicate that the infection is gone.

Because of the possible severe or even fatal complications of diphtheria, patients with symptoms need to be placed in a hospital intensive care unit for complete rest and careful observation. If signs of airway obstruction occur, a tracheotomy (surgical creation of a hole in the neck) will be performed immediately so that a tube can be passed into the lungs to supply oxygen. Frequent checking of the heart and nervous system is needed to identify complications. In severe cases, these can include heart irregularities, cardiac arrest (heart stoppage), and nervous system disorders, such as swallowing difficulty caused by paralysis of swallowing muscles.

Those who have been in close contact with the patient and who have not been immunized should receive throat cultures and be immunized with vaccine. These people should be watched carefully for the development of symptoms and be given antitoxin should symptoms occur. Another approach is to give antitoxin immediately (after allergy has been ruled out). In people who have been immunized, a booster of vaccine will be sufficient. Cultures of the nose, throat, and any open wounds should be obtained from all contacts of patients with diphtheria. Carriers of diphtheria should be given seven to ten days of treatment with an appropriate antibiotic (usually erythromycin). If the organism is still present, another course of drug therapy should be given. If this fails, tonsillectomy may be needed.

Fortunately, widespread immunization has made diphtheria a rare disease. To maintain this status, children should be immunized beginning in infancy. The diphtheria vaccine is usually given in combination with the vaccines against tetanus and pertussis (whooping cough)—the DTP immunization.

See also Immunizations.

# Diverticulosis and diverticulitis

Diverticulosis is the occurrence of diverticula (little pouches) that form when the inner lining of the colon (large intestine) is forced, under pressure, through weak spots in the muscular outer layer of the colon. Diverticulosis may be present in about one third of persons over the age of 60 in the United States, and both its incidence and the frequency of complications increase with age. Diverticulitis is inflammation and/or infection of the diverticula.

One theory about the cause of diverticulosis is that abnormal movement of the colon (possibly because of too little bulk in the diet) produces

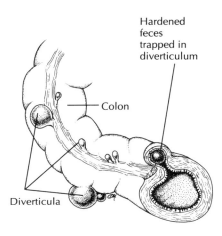

Hardened
feces
trapped in
diverticulum

Colon

Diverticula

Diverticulitis is the inflammation of diverticula (small pouches that balloon out from the colon wall when the inner lining is forced through weak spots in the muscular lining). Inflammation often develops when a mass of hardened feces becomes trapped in a diverticulum, reducing the blood supply to the pouch wall and making it more susceptible to infection by bacteria in the colon.

intense pressure, which forces the intestinal lining through weak spots in the muscular layer. Most people with simple diverticulosis have no symptoms. Occasionally, however, a pouch next to a blood vessel may ulcerate, causing it to bleed. If the vessel is an artery, severe bleeding can result, seen as bleeding from the anus. Shock and even death may result if the condition is not treated.

It has been estimated that about one-fifth to one-fourth of the persons who have diverticulosis will suffer from diverticulitis. Diverticulitis develops when a mass of hardened waste matter (called a fecalith) forms in a pouch and reduces the blood supply to the thin walls of the pouch (by means of pressure against the wall), making them more susceptible to infection by the bacteria of the colon. The inflammation that follows can lead to perforation, formation of an

abscess (an enclosed sac of pus around the perforation), or peritonitis (infection of the lining of the abdominal cavity). Not infrequently, the inflamed section of bowel becomes attached to the urinary bladder or vagina, burrowing out from the colon to create a fistula (abnormal channel), which leaks infectious material into the other organ. Repeated inflammation can cause thickening of the wall of the colon, thus narrowing the colon and causing partial or sometimes total obstruction.

Symptoms of diverticulitis include intermittent crampy abdominal pains and tenderness, usually on the lower left side, but sometimes in other areas of the lower abdomen, in which case the pains may resemble those of appendicitis. Pain that worsens during urination may indicate that the inflamed colon has become attached to the bladder. Stool (feces) or air in the urine may indicate a colon-to-bladder fistula. Constipation or constipation alternating with diarrhea is common. Fever is usually present with acute attacks.

The diagnosis of diverticulitis usually is made if there is a history of pain in the left lower section of the abdomen, accompanied by fever and a change in bowel habits. A physical examination may reveal a mass in that area, along with extreme tenderness. After the acute episode has subsided, the doctor may insert a proctosigmoidoscope (a lighted, tubelike instrument) through the anus and into the lower part of the colon to see if there is any evidence of cancer that might be causing the symptoms. X-ray studies with a contrast medium such as barium are usually done to further rule out cancer of the colon and to locate diverticula, obstructions, and fistulas.

Treatment of severe diverticulitis begins with bed rest in a hospital and intravenous feeding; no food is given by mouth, to give the intestines a rest. Antibiotics are given if there is fever or other evidence of infection. If peritonitis develops, it may be necessary to operate. The inflamed section of the colon may simply be cut out, and the remaining sections joined. More often, a temporary colostomy (a surgically created opening in the abdominal wall, which allows the colon to empty to the outside of the body) is necessary. Later, after all inflammation and infection have subsided, the redirected portion of the colon is reconnected to the remaining portion of the colon or to the rectum.

Choosing a diet with plenty of bulk appears to be a way to avoid diverticulosis. Persons who have diverticulosis should eat a relatively high-fiber diet. Supplements, such as psyllium, that increase bulk may be recommended to move the stool through the colon at a normal rate.

See also Colostomy.

# Dizziness and vertigo

Dizziness and vertigo are similar but distinct sensations of disorientation and distorted perception. Recurrent dizziness or vertigo can be a symptom of a variety of disorders, particularly those involving the eyes, ears, or nervous system.

Dizziness and vertigo are sometimes confused with each other. Dizziness is characterized by unsteadiness and a distorted sense of the environment; the word *dizziness* is often used to describe a sensation of light-headedness or faintness. Vertigo is a false sense of movement, often the perception that one is spinning or that one's environment is whirling around. Vertigo is often accompanied by nausea. It is important to be able to describe these different symptoms to your doctor.

Dizziness and vertigo can be caused by a malfunction in one of the parts of the body that is responsible for giving the brain information on balance, position, and movement. These parts include the eye, the inner ear, and certain areas of the brain. Thus, balance can be disturbed by any injury, impairment, or disorder involving the eyes, ears, and certain areas of the brain, as well as the nerves leading to and from these areas. A wide variety of problems, such as injury to the head, ear infections, and migraine headaches, can include dizziness or vertigo as a symptom. Also, occasional mild upsets to the body can cause dizziness (but usually not vertigo), including such harmless factors as being overheated, overtired, or tense. Standing up too quickly after reclining or sitting for some time is another cause of dizziness.

Dizziness is characterized by feelings of unsteadiness, swaying, light-headedness, weakness, and faintness and may be accompanied by nausea and vomiting. Vertigo is marked by a feeling of spinning and may be associated with unsteady walking, a tendency to fall or to veer to one side while walking, paleness, sweating, nausea and vomiting, and continuous rapid eye movement. Recurrent light-headedness or feeling faint can be a symptom of heart irregularities as well as a neurologic problem.

Simple dizziness can easily be avoided. Getting up slowly after reclining or sitting, leaving overheated rooms to get some fresh air, eating a balanced diet, and getting adequate rest should all help to prevent common episodes of dizziness. Recurrent dizziness, however, should be brought to a doctor's attention.

True vertigo, on the other hand, may be a sign of physical disease, such as labyrinthitis (inflammation of the inner ear) or a brain disorder. Frequently, however, no cause is found, and the vertigo is treated symptomatically with drugs. In all cases, any episode of true vertigo should be reported to a physician.

# DNA

See Genes.

# Down's syndrome

Down's syndrome is a congenital (present at birth) disorder characterized by varying degrees of mental retardation and a variety of physical abnormalities.

Normally, each cell in the human body has 46 chromosomes; the cells in someone with Down's syndrome, however, have 47. In ways that are as yet unknown, the presence of the extra chromosome causes all of the unusual characteristics of Down's syndrome. In 95 percent of cases, the condition is called trisomy 21 (because the extra chromosome is attached to the twenty-first pair of chromosomes), and the mistake in genetic coding is one that apparently could happen to anyone. In five percent of cases, the syndrome is caused by a defect that is believed to run in families.

Down's syndrome is marked by a number of physical characteristics: somewhat slanted eyes in small sockets (which is why it used to be called mongolism); a small, short head, flattened in back and front; a nose flattened at the bridge; a thick tongue; short hands, feet, neck, trunk, arms, and legs; a single, rather than a double, crease across the top of the palm; flabby arms and legs with poor mus-cle tone; a wide gap between the first and second toes; and generally retarded physical development. A child with Down's syndrome may have a poorly functioning thyroid gland (which regulates metabolism, the rate at which the body uses energy) and pituitary gland (which regulates other glands, including those responsible for growth, maturation, and reproduction). About one third are born with heart defects, and both the skin and mucous membranes are especially susceptible to infection.

Characteristically slower than other children to walk, talk, and learn, youngsters with Down's syndrome benefit from "early intervention" programs designed to help them develop their abilities as much as possible. Such programs are frequently available from the time the mother and baby leave the hospital after the birth. A number of organizations exist to promote such programs and assist parents in developing their child's

The normal human cell contains 23 pairs of chromosomes, one of which is a pair of sex chromosomes (either two X chromosomes or one X chromosome and one Y chromosome), for a total of 46 chromosomes. In Down's syndrome (also called trisomy 21), however, there are three number 21 chromosomes, rather than two; the presence of this extra chromosome is responsible for the collection of symptoms that characterize Down's syndrome.

potential. The degree of retardation that accompanies Down's syndrome ranges from mild to severe (the average IQ is about 50), and the extent to which an individual will be affected is not predictable at birth. Some children with Down's syndrome can attend special education classes in public schools; others can attend special schools for the mentally retarded. As adults, some may be able to live independently or semi-independently and work in the community. Depending on the degree of retardation that is present, others will require more supervised living arrangements and may be able to hold simple, routine jobs, perhaps in what is called a "sheltered workshop."

Prospective parents can reduce their chances of having a child with Down's syndrome by starting their families early. At age 20 a woman's risk of giving birth to a child with Down's syndrome is only one in 2,000 live births, but at age 35 the risk is one in 300, at age 40 it is one in 100, and at age 45 it is one in 40 live births. The age of the father also has some bearing on the risk, but not as much as the age of the mother. Diagnosis of Down's syndrome can be made between the fourteenth and sixteenth weeks of pregnancy through a procedure called amniocentesis. During an amniocentesis, the doctor will insert a needle through the mother's abdominal wall and into the uterus. A sample of the amniotic fluid is then drawn into a syringe, grown on a special culture plate, and analyzed to see if there are abnormal chromosomes. A newer technique used to check the chromosomes of the growing fetus is called chorionic villus biopsy. This procedure, performed during the eighth or ninth week of pregnancy, involves the removal of a small portion of the placenta by a small instrument inserted through the woman's cervix. Tissue that is obtained can be immediately evaluated for the presence of chromosome abnormalities.

# Dysmenorrhea

Dysmenorrhea is the term for painful menstruation. This condition occurs most commonly in teenagers and in women who have never been pregnant.

There are two types of dysmenorrhea. Primary dysmenorrhea is a recurring condition, usually beginning shortly after the onset of menstruation in a young girl. Secondary dysmenorrhea develops later in life, after a woman has been menstruating for some time.

Dysmenorrhea is not a serious condition, but it can be annoying, uncomfortable, and even incapacitating. Since secondary dysmenorrhea usually indicates that another disorder is present, treatment should always be sought for this condition.

The cause of primary dysmenorrhea is thought to be the release of prostaglandins from the lining of the uterus shortly before the beginning of a menstrual period. (Prostaglandins are substances that, among other functions, stimulate uterine contractions.) The resulting contractions constrict blood vessels in the uterus, causing pain in the same way that a decrease in blood supply to the heart causes chest pain. The reason for this excessive production of prostaglandins is not known. Secondary dysmenorrhea is usually a result of another reproductive problem, such as fibroid tumors, a narrow cervix, or endometriosis (the displacement of tissue from the uterine lining to areas elsewhere in the body).

The major symptoms of dysmenorrhea are cramps and pain in the lower abdomen, possibly extending around to the back. Nausea, vomiting, diarrhea, headache, fatigue, and nervousness are mainly associated with primary dysmenorrhea. These symptoms usually appear at the beginning of, or slightly before, the menstrual period, and may last several hours or several days.

Diagnostic evaluation will include a complete physical examination as well as medical and menstrual histories. If the symptoms have been present from the onset of menstruation at puberty, primary dysmenorrhea is usually the diagnosis. If the symptoms appeared suddenly in a woman who has been menstruating for some years, secondary dysmenorrhea can be assumed. In that case, further diagnostic evaluation of the reproductive organs will be necessary to identify the underlying disorder. Ultrasound examinations (in which the echoes of sound waves are used to create images of internal structures) or X-ray studies often prove useful.

Primary dysmenorrhea has been treated successfully with nonsteroidal anti-inflammatory drugs (such as ibuprofen, naproxen, meclofenamate, diflunisal, and mefenamic acid), which, when taken just before a period is to begin, act to suppress the release of prostaglandins and thereby reduce the intensity of the contractions that cause pain.

Secondary dysmenorrhea is treated by correcting the problem that is causing it. For instance, if endometriosis is the underlying problem, it may be treated with hormone therapy or surgery, thereby relieving the dysmenorrhea as well.

Home remedies often help to ease menstrual pain and relieve pressure. These include placing a hot-water bottle or heating pad on the abdomen, taking hot baths, and lying on the back with the knees bent. A woman who experienced dysmenorrhea before pregnancy may find that the problem is lessened after childbirth, possibly because of enlargement of the cervix or destruction of some nerve fibers in the uterus.

See also Premenstrual tension and Prostaglandins.

# Dyspareunia

Dyspareunia is difficulty or pain for a woman during sexual intercourse.

Dyspareunia may be caused by a resistant hymen (the membrane that usually covers the opening to the vagina in virgins) or by inflammation of or injury to the vagina, the urethra (the tube that carries urine from the bladder to the outside), the vulva (the structures around the opening to the vagina), or the anus. It can be the result of formation of scar tissue around an episiotomy (a surgical cut to enlarge the opening of the vagina immediately before childbirth) or surgery to repair the vagina. Other physical causes include tight muscles in the area around the vagina, an "hourglass" contraction of the vagina, a divided vagina, inflammation of the cervix, prolapsed (fallen) uterus, infected fallopian tubes, and endometriosis.

Inadequate lubrication of the vagina is a common cause of dyspareunia. This deficiency may be due to inadequate arousal of the woman before insertion of the penis or to menopause, which is accompanied by a decrease in vaginal secretions and thinning of the vaginal lining. Unconscious tightening of the vaginal muscles, called vaginismus, is another possible cause—perhaps the result of fear, unreadiness or unwillingness to perform the sex act, or other psychological reasons. Improperly fitted or improperly lubricated birth control devices (condoms or diaphragms) and an allergy to contraceptive spermicides are other causes of dyspareunia.

Pain during or following sexual intercourse is the primary symptom.

Diagnosis is made on the basis of both a physical and an emotional evaluation. In some cases, physical abnormalities can be detected during the physical examination. In other cases, careful inquiry into the patient's emotional state and sexual history may reveal factors that account for the discomfort.

Treatment for dyspareunia is correction of any underlying disease, injury, or structural defect, if such a problem exists. For some couples, counseling by a psychiatrist or sex therapist is helpful in removing psychological barriers to sexual closeness that may result in dyspareunia.

Water-soluble lubricating jelly (not petroleum jelly), obtainable in any drugstore, provides a good vaginal lubricant. Estrogen creams can be used along with water-soluble jelly to restore lubrication to a dry vagina after menopause. Soothing creams and temporary avoidance of intercourse can relieve the soreness of dyspareunia.

# Dyspepsia

See Indigestion.

# Dyspnea

Dyspnea is a sensation of "air hunger." It is usually accompanied by difficult, labored breathing and discomfort. Dyspnea is a symptom that may occur in a variety of diseases and conditions, from congestive heart failure to emotional upset.

Dyspnea may be caused by inadequate delivery of oxygen to the tis-sues, as in severe anemia; by failure of the heart to keep up with the needs of the body, as in congestive heart failure; by overexertion; by obstruction of the airways; by narrowing of air passages, as in asthma; or by restriction of lung capacity. Emphysema is commonly associated with dyspnea. It can also occur if there is fluid in the lungs, as in pneumonia or congestive heart failure, because the entry of oxygen into the alveoli is blocked by the fluid, preventing oxygenation of the blood.

In a nighttime form of dyspnea called paroxysmal nocturnal dyspnea, the patient awakens gasping for breath and can breathe only by sitting up or standing. Usually this is caused by congestive heart failure.

Another type of dyspnea, called psychogenic or hysterical hyperventilation, is a physical response to stress, anxiety, or emotional upset. In this condition, excessive breathing results in exhalation of too much carbon dioxide, which causes light-headedness, numbness and tingling of the hands and toes, and fainting.

Signs of dyspnea include noisy breathing; an anxious, distressed expression; dilated nostrils; gasping; a protruding abdomen; an expanded chest; and a blue coloration of the lips and fingertips.

Treatment involves controlling the contributing causes.

See also Anemia, Congestive heart failure, Emphysema, and Pneumonia.

# E

# Ear infection

See Middle ear infection.

# Ear, nose, and throat

The ear, nose, and throat are interconnected, and for this reason they are usually grouped together. Because they are joined, infection in one structure will often spread into one of the others.

**Ear** The ear consists of three parts: the outer ear, the middle ear, and the inner ear.

The outer ear consists of the pinna, or external ear, which captures sound waves and directs them inward, and the ear canal, which leads to the eardrum. In the middle ear, sound waves vibrate through three tiny bones commonly called the hammer (malleus), the anvil (incus), and the stirrup (stapes). The vibrations continue into the inner ear, where a spiral structure called the cochlea transforms them into nerve impulses. These impulses are conveyed to the brain via the auditory nerve.

The eustachian tube in the middle ear connects the ear with the nasopharynx (the upper part of the throat). This tube allows the air pressure in the middle ear to equalize with the pressure outside the body, thus helping to prevent rupture of the eardrum. However, the eustachian tube also provides a passageway that makes it possible for infecting microorganisms to enter the middle ear from the nose or throat.

The semicircular canals (also called the labyrinth) within the inner ear serve as the organ of balance by detecting motion of the head and conveying this information to the brain.

**Nose** The nose is a specialized structure that serves dual functions as the organ for the sense of smell and as an entry to the respiratory tract.

Nerve receptor cells within the nose detect odors that enter via the nostrils and transmit signals to the brain through the olfactory nerve. The sense of smell also enhances the sense of taste. The ability to smell is

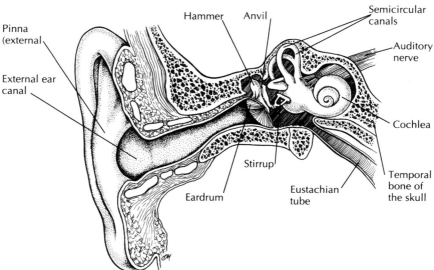

The ear is a complex structure that is responsible for the sense of hearing and for the sense of balance.

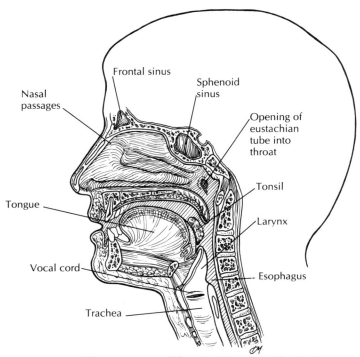

The ear, nose, and throat are interconnecting structures.

more refined than the ability to taste; therefore, when a cold blocks nasal passages, food may seem bland and tasteless.

As part of the respiratory tract, the nose moisturizes and warms incoming air and filters out foreign materials. Small glands within the lining of the nose secrete mucus, a sticky substance that lubricates the walls of the nose and throat. Mucus humidifies the incoming air and traps bacteria, dust, and other particles entering the nose. Many bacteria are either dissolved by chemical elements in the mucus or transported to the entrance of the throat by tiny, hairlike structures called cilia. In the throat, bacteria are then swallowed and killed by acids and other chemicals produced in the stomach. This efficient line of defense protects the body against the billions of bacteria that continually enter the nose.

Connected to the nose are the sinuses—air-filled cavities lined with mucus-secreting glands that are located within certain facial bones. There are four groups of sinuses—frontal, sphenoidal, ethmoidal, and maxillary.

**Throat**  The throat, or pharynx, is a passageway connecting the back of the mouth and nose to the esophagus (the tube between the mouth and the stomach) and to the trachea, or windpipe. Because air and food pass through the throat, the throat is considered to be a part of both the respiratory and the digestive systems.

Three sections make up the five-inch throat tube. The nasopharynx is the upper part of the throat, which opens into the nose. The oropharynx is the middle portion, which opens into the mouth. The lower section of the throat, or laryngopharynx, connects the other sections with the larynx, or voice box.

Within the throat are two small, almond-shaped masses of lymphoid tissue called tonsils. Tonsils help fight disease by destroying bacteria that enter the throat.

# Echoviruses

See Enteroviral infections.

# ECT

See Electroconvulsive therapy.

# Ectopic pregnancy

An ectopic pregnancy is one in which the fertilized egg develops outside the uterus. Usually it occurs in one of the two fallopian tubes, through which the egg travels from the ovary to the uterus. (In that case, it is also known as a tubal pregnancy.) However, on rare occasions, the fertilized egg starts to develop in the ovary, on the cervix (neck of the uterus), or attached to the outside of a nearby organ in the abdominal cavity. (The ovary is not directly connected to the fallopian tube. There is a slight gap between the two, and this gap sometimes permits an egg to enter the abdominal cavity.)

The usual cause of an ectopic pregnancy is an obstruction or narrowing of the fallopian tube that prevents the egg from passing through the tube to the uterus. The obstruction or narrowing is usually the result of inflammation or scarring from an infection, such as gonorrhea, but it may also develop after abdominal surgery or because of a growth, such as a pelvic tumor. Tubal infections can occur after miscarriage or childbirth or during the use of an intrauter-

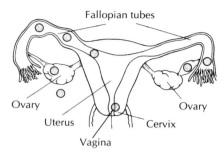

The circles indicate some of the possible sites of an ectopic pregnancy, in which the fertilized egg develops outside the uterus. The most common site is in one of the fallopian tubes, but development in an ovary, on the cervix, or attached to another organ in the abdominal cavity can also occur.

ine contraceptive device (IUD). If these infections are severe, blockage of the tube may result.

An ectopic pregnancy may be fatal unless it is promptly treated. The danger of a tubal pregnancy is that it will not be detected until the tube enclosing the egg has ruptured (broken), causing massive bleeding into the abdomen. When a fertilized egg begins to develop in an area other than the uterus, such as the ovary or the cervix, nearby large blood vessels may be invaded, causing massive bleeding.

Symptoms of ectopic pregnancy usually begin two to four weeks after a woman misses her menstrual period. She may be bothered by sharp, continuous pains on one side of her lower abdomen and by slight bleeding from her vagina. When rapid bleeding into the abdomen occurs, which is usually not until after the sixth week of the pregnancy, she may experience sudden sharp pains in the lower abdomen, backache, low blood pressure, fainting, and even shock (collapse of the circulatory system).

The examining doctor may discover a tender swelling on one side of the pelvis. Movement of the uterus during a pelvic examination may cause pain. When ectopic pregnancy is suspected, the patient is hospitalized immediately. An ultrasound study may reveal the outline of the expanding mass. In most cases, there is slow bleeding from the end of the fallopian tube into the abdominal cavity, which may be detected by inserting a hollow needle through the wall of the vagina beneath the cervix. The diagnosis is confirmed by inserting a laparoscope (a lighted tubelike instrument) through a small incision into the abdominal cavity to inspect the area directly.

Treatment for ectopic pregnancy is surgical removal of the embryo and surrounding tissues. When the condition occurs in a fallopian tube, the entire tube and sometimes the ovary must be removed. It is sometimes possible to reconstruct the tube.

A woman who has had one ectopic pregnancy has about a 15 percent chance of having a second one. This does not mean that she should not try to become pregnant again; however, when she does try, she should be especially watchful for symptoms of ectopic pregnancy, and when she suspects that conception has occurred, she should see her physician immediately so that the location of the embryo can be determined.

# Eczema

See Dermatitis.

# Edema

Edema is the accumulation of excessive amounts of fluid within the body's tissues. It is a symptom of both minor and serious conditions.

The fluid that accumulates comes from the blood. Normally, there is a constant exchange of fluid between the blood vessels and other body tissues. The blood removes any extra fluids and carries them to the kidneys, from which they are excreted via the urinary tract. Edema occurs when that exchange does not take place in the proper fashion, either allowing too much liquid to leave the blood vessels or too little fluid to enter the blood vessels.

A change in pressure within the blood vessels because of heart disease, high blood pressure, blocked or damaged vessels, or a kidney disorder can cause an imbalance in fluid exchange.

Mild edema is common before menstruation and during pregnancy, when the blood volume increases. Being overweight, wearing tight clothing, and becoming overheated can also lead to edema.

Edema can be confined to a small area of the body or can become generalized. Some forms are more noticeable than others. For example, the swelling that appears around a splinter in the skin is edema. However, generalized edema results in widespread swelling and puffiness, usually first noticed in the fingers and feet. The most serious forms of edema occur within the internal organs of the body. Heart disease, for example, may result in internal edema of the lungs, causing them to fill with fluid and thereby creating severe difficulty in breathing.

Simple or temporary edema can be relieved by decreasing salt intake, since the sodium in salt causes the body to retain fluid. Elevation of the legs or removal of tight socks may also help. More severe or internal edema can be treated with a diuretic (a drug that stimulates production of urine). Edema that is symptomatic of an underlying disorder will often disappear with management of that condition.

Controlling weight gain, eating a balanced low-salt diet, and wearing loose clothing may prevent milder forms of edema. Any prolonged edema not attributable to causes such as hot weather or menstruation should be investigated by a physician to determine the cause.

# Electroconvulsive therapy

Electroconvulsive therapy (ECT) is a procedure in which an electric current is passed through the brain to create a convulsion of the central nervous system, like an epileptic seizure, after which the patient is often in a clearer state of mind. Also referred to as electroshock therapy and shock treatment, ECT is used chiefly in cases of severe depression and manic-depressive illness. Occasionally, it is employed to arouse a schizophrenic patient from catatonia (an unresponsive state).

Prior to treatment, the patient is examined and given appropriate tests, which may include an electroencephalogram (brain wave test) to detect brain injury that might be related to the patient's condition. Such an injury would rule out the use of ECT.

Usually, ECT is given early in the morning, because the patient must not have had anything to eat or drink for eight hours before treatment. The patient is put to sleep with an anesthetic given intravenously. Electrodes are placed on one or both sides of the head, and electric current is administered. The seizure that results lasts from 5 to 20 seconds. Recovery is rapid; after half an hour or an hour of drowsiness, most patients are alert and willing to talk. Some temporary memory loss is common, and headaches also sometimes occur. However, the use of general anesthesia prevents the anxiety and spinal injuries that used to occur occasionally during ECT treatments. The incidence of serious complications of ECT has been reported to be less than one case in a thousand.

A usual course of ECT treatments is two or three times a week for three to four weeks. A faster method, in which the patient's heart rate is monitored with an electrocardiograph, employs repeated surges of electric current in one to three sessions.

See also Depression and Schizophrenia.

# Embolism

An embolism occurs when some part of the circulatory system is either partially or completely blocked by some obstructing mass that has traveled through the system. The occurrence

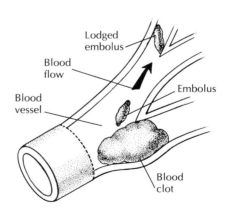

Lodged embolus
Blood flow
Blood vessel
Embolus
Blood clot

An embolus may be a piece of a blood clot that has traveled through the circulatory system and become lodged in a small blood vessel, causing loss of blood flow and death of tissue in the area nourished by that vessel.

of such an obstruction is called an embolism, while the mass causing the embolism is called an embolus.

Emboli (the plural of embolus) are classified into three major groups:
- Solid emboli, which are made up of a variety of substances, such as clumps of tissue, tumor cells, or pieces of blood clots
- Liquid emboli, which are made up of globules of fat or amniotic fluid (fluid that surrounds the fetus in the uterus)
- Gaseous emboli, which are made up of the various constituent components of air

Emboli may be further categorized according to their origin and the location of the blockage that they cause:
- Arterial emboli, which originate either from the heart or the artery itself, travel downstream, and become lodged in a smaller blood vessel, preventing the flow of fresh blood to whatever area or organ is normally supplied
- Paradoxical emboli, which originate in the venous system, pass into the arterial system (usually through a defect in the walls separating the chambers of the heart), and block an artery anywhere in the body
- Pulmonary emboli, which block vessels in the lungs.
- Coronary artery emboli, which block the coronary arteries of the heart
- Cerebral emboli, which block vessels in the brain but usually originate in the heart or the carotid arteries in the neck, which lead to the brain

The most common cause of emboli is blood clots from within the heart or blood vessels. Arterial emboli also commonly originate from plaques or other accumulations on the valves of the heart, from aneurysms, and from plaques or clots within arteries. Fat emboli can result from injury to the bones (particularly the long bones of the legs) or from damage to cells in fat tissue. Air emboli can develop if a very large amount of air is admitted during an intravenous infusion or during surgery, especially in operations on the neck or chest (in the latter cases, air enters vessels that are open because of the surgery). However, the oxygen in air is not the only gas involved in gaseous emboli. When divers ascend from high-pressure levels in deep water to normal-pressure levels too quickly, or when pilots in planes without cabin pressurization climb from normal-pressure levels to low-pressure levels, there is always the possibility that nitrogen bubbles will arise in the bloodstream because of too-rapid decompression. If any of these gaseous emboli find their way into the central nervous system, the results can be catastrophic.

The symptoms produced by an embolism vary according to the site at which the embolism occurs. An embolism deprives the affected area of its blood supply, which can cause damage or death of tissue in the area. An embolism in a brain artery may produce the symptoms of a stroke, such as unsteadiness, slurring of speech, and numbness or weakness in the face, arm, or leg on one side. If an embolism occurs in the leg, the area beyond the blockage may become white and painful. Pain may be the first symptom of embolism in other areas.

Emboli resulting from blood clots are often treated with a variety of anticoagulants (agents that inhibit normal clotting mechanisms in the blood). Common anticoagulants, such as heparin and warfarin, do not dissolve clots, but instead prevent additional clots from forming and embolizing. There are newer drugs that do dissolve clots, but their use is restricted to special situations. If an embolism is in an accessible location, such as an artery in a limb, and tissue is threatened, surgery to remove the clot is the preferred method of treatment to save the limb. In cases of massive embolism in the lung in which life is threatened, surgery can also be attempted. If an individual has clots in the deep venous system of the lower half of the body and anticoagulants cannot be prescribed (for example, because of a recent hemorrhage in the brain or other vital organ), blocking devices, such as clips, can be placed on or in the inferior vena cava (the main vein receiving blood from the lower part of the body) to prevent emboli from reaching the lungs.

See also Pulmonary embolism and Stroke.

# Emphysema

Emphysema is a chronic, progressive lung disease. Emphysema develops when the small air passages leading to the alveoli (the tiny air sacs in the lungs, where gas exchange takes place) become distended and the walls dividing the alveoli are injured or destroyed. Spaces form where alveoli had been, and lung tissue becomes nonfunctional and stiff rather than elastic. Emphysema is commonly associated with chronic bronchitis, in which the airways become inflamed, causing specialized cells within them to secrete abnormally large amounts of mucus. The inflammation, swelling, and excessive mucus production result in obstruction to airflow and entrapment of air within the lungs.

As the disease progresses, many complex changes take place, ultimately leading to diminishment of the amount of oxygen in the blood, frequently associated with an increased amount of carbon dioxide. As the lung tissue deteriorates and loses its elasticity, changes also occur in the blood vessels carrying deoxygenated blood to the lungs for a fresh supply of oxygen. The net effect is that the right side of the heart, which is responsible for collecting deoxygenated blood from the veins of the body and pumping it through the lungs, must work much harder. As the process continues, the muscle of the right side of the heart is weakened by this extra work and becomes less able to pump blood into the lungs. The blood "backs up," causing increased pressure in the veins. This, in turn, causes fluid to recede into the tissues, resulting in severe swelling of the feet, ankles, and legs. If this right-sided heart failure (also known as cor pulmonale) is very severe, the abdomen will become distended with fluid.

External factors that irritate the lungs, such as tobacco smoke and air pollutants, are commonly linked to emphysema. Unlike many respiratory diseases, emphysema is not caused

Bronchi

Overinflated alveolus

Normal alveoli        Emphysematous alveoli

Emphysema is a chronic disease in which the alveoli (tiny air sacs in the lungs) become overinflated with trapped air.

by a viral or bacterial infection. However, it is often aggravated by a case of bronchitis or another lung infection.

In a minority of cases, emphysema is a result of a genetic deficiency or an inherited lack of a specific blood protein, which leads to loss of elasticity in the alveoli.

Those afflicted with emphysema are most likely to be white men over the age of 50, although women are becoming equally susceptible because of an increase in smoking among women during recent years. The overwhelming majority of emphysema cases are directly linked to cigarette smoking.

Emphysema is characterized by one major symptom—shortness of breath. Patients may also have a persistent, racking cough, which either brings up mucus or is overly dry. Patients experience difficulty in breathing, often taking twice as many breaths as others to get enough oxygen. It has been found that advanced emphysema sufferers exert tremendous amounts of energy just to breathe. They also tire quite easily and require more calories to maintain their weight than healthy individuals do. An enlarged, rounded "barrel" chest often develops due to overinflation of the lungs and excessive growth of the chest muscles due to the increased stress placed upon them to inflate stiff lungs. Lips, ear lobes, skin, and fingernails may be tinged blue from lack of oxygen in the blood.

With the exception of the minority of cases caused by genetic disorder, there is no single test that can pinpoint the condition. Breathing tests to measure the amount of air being inhaled and exhaled will not reveal the disease in its early stages. A blood test may be performed to determine the red blood cell count (when emphysema causes diminished oxygenation of the blood, more red blood cells are produced in an effort to increase oxygen transport; because of this compensation, the red blood cell count is elevated). A chest X ray may be taken to search for specific changes in the lungs that may point to advanced stages of the disease; however, a chest X ray is not diagnostic of early emphysema. Thus, emphysema is diagnosed by putting together a collection of findings.

There is no known cure for emphysema, nor is it reversible. However, the progress of the disease can be checked by removing irritants, particularly tobacco smoke, from the patient's environment. Patients are encouraged to drink large amounts of fluids to help thin out the mucus that may block the airways. Adequate rest, a balanced diet, and moderate regular exercise are recommended. Vaporizers, humidifiers, and air conditioners help to moisturize and filter the air. A respiratory therapist can teach an emphysema patient how to use his chest and abdominal muscles to breathe more efficiently.

Several drugs may aid the emphysema patient. They act to loosen mucus or to relax and expand the air passages. Antibiotics are sometimes prescribed if an infection exists. Cortisone drugs (corticosteroids) are often prescribed chronically. Drugs such as albuterol and terbutaline are also used both in inhalation aerosol and oral forms. In advanced cases, oxygen may have to be administered continuously. However, an emphysema patient must be particularly careful to use only the amount of oxygen prescribed. Too much oxygen can suppress the drive to breathe, thereby causing respiratory failure and possibly death. In addition, sedatives and sleeping medications should be avoided by patients with severe emphysema, as these can also lead to a dangerous slowing of breathing.

Emphysema is a very serious condition. However, with the help of modern treatments, breathing aids, and medications, patients can lead a reasonably comfortable life. It is, however, necessary for these individuals to stop smoking and avoid air pollutants as much as possible.

See also Bronchitis.

# Encephalitis

Encephalitis is an inflammation of the brain. The term is usually used to describe an infectious process caused by bacteria, parasites, vaccines, or, most often, viruses. Noninfectious agents such as poisons, metabolic abnormalities due to liver or kidney failure, and tumors can also cause conditions that closely resemble encephalitis.

Viruses may cause encephalitis either as a primary disease or as a complication of an infection. Some of these viruses are mosquito-borne and afflict humans only in warm weather, when mosquitoes are in season. Many cases of encephalitis occur as complications of viral infections, such as measles, mumps, chicken pox, and rubella (German measles). These cases usually develop five to ten days after the onset of the original illness, but can develop as long as six weeks afterward.

Encephalitis may be associated with meningitis (infection of the layers of tissue that cover the brain and spinal cord). There may be evidence of brain disturbances, such as alterations in mental state, personality changes, seizures, and paralysis. Edema (fluid buildup) in the brain is present, and there may be petechial hemorrhages (small, red spots that indicate bleeding) scattered throughout parts of the brain and spinal cord. Fever, headache, vomiting, a gener-

al feeling of illness, and a stiff neck may be the first symptoms to appear.

Prompt diagnosis and supportive treatment are essential in any case of encephalitis or suspected encephalitis. Even patients who have been seriously or critically ill with encephalitis often recover. One diagnostic problem is differentiating encephalitis from bacterial meningitis and other similar ailments. Even with ideal circumstances for diagnosis, the encephalitis virus is often not identified. Viruses can sometimes be isolated directly from cerebrospinal fluid or from the tissues. Since many forms of encephalitis, such as the mosquito-borne forms, have important public health implications, blood is often drawn whenever encephalitis is suspected; the sample is sent to the local department of health, which can provide a more precise diagnosis.

With a form of encephalitis called herpes simplex encephalitis, early recognition and treatment with a medication that inhibits the reproduction of viruses reduce the chances of death and neurologic impairment significantly. However, for maximal effectiveness, the drug should be given before coma or paralysis occurs. Supportive therapy involves bed rest and maintaining fluid bal-

Encephalitis is characterized by fever, a severe headache, and sometimes a stiff neck.

ance to avoid dehydration (loss of body fluids).

See also Meningitis.

# Endocarditis

The heart is made up of three cellular layers: the epicardium (outermost layer), the myocardium (middle, muscular layer), and the endocardium (innermost layer). The endocardium lines all of the chambers and valves of the heart, and its cells are continuous with those of blood vessels leaving the heart. Endocarditis is an inflammation of the endocardial layer of the heart.

The most common form of endocarditis, infectious endocarditis, is caused by microorganisms. *Staphylococcus* and *Streptococcus* bacteria are most often the infectious agents, but viruses, fungi, and other bacteria may also be responsible.

Infective endocarditis usually occurs in persons with congenital (inborn) or acquired defects in the walls or valves of the heart. An example of a congenital defect would be a hole in the wall between two chambers of the heart. An example of an acquired defect would be damage of the heart valves caused by rheumatic fever or calcium deposition. Such abnormalities make the heart more susceptible to infection.

Bacteria probably circulate through the bloodstream of all people at some time or another. However, certain procedures, such as dental work and surgery, may lead to bacteremia (the presence of large numbers of bacteria in the bloodstream). The bacteria accumulate on these abnormal areas in the heart and cause inflammation or infection that serves as a foundation for the collection of platelets, strands of fibrin (clotting material), and other debris of the circulatory sys-

tem. The clump of material that forms is referred to as a vegetation.

Infectious endocarditis is a serious systemic disease with a wide spectrum of symptoms and signs. Patients may complain of fevers, weakness, and weight loss. Anemia (deficiency of red blood cells) may also be present. Pieces of vegetations may break off and travel through the bloodstream to other areas of the body, causing symptoms of obstruction (for example, a stroke if the brain is affected, or microscopic blood in the urine if a kidney is affected).

The diagnosis is made on the basis of the history, the physical examination, and the results of laboratory studies, such as blood cultures, to identify the microorganisms present.

Once the infectious agent has been isolated, appropriate antibiotics can be administered. Antibiotic administration is by the intravenous route, at least at first, and usually continues for long periods (up to eight weeks).

If infection of a heart valve is particularly severe or if a prosthetic (artificial) valve is involved, the valve may have to be replaced.

Persons with abnormal heart valves, prosthetic valves, and other structural abnormalities must be given antibiotics before and after any procedure likely to disperse bacteria (for example, dental work, surgery of the urogenital tract or large intestine, or opening of an abscess). The antibiotics serve either to prevent the passage of microorganisms through the bloodstream or to lessen their number, thereby decreasing the chance that endocarditis will develop.

# Endocrine system

The endocrine system comprises a number of glands that produce hormones with a varied array of vital functions. Hormones are chemical substances that are secreted by organs or by cells of organs in one part of the body and are carried by the bloodstream to other organs or tissues, where they control or regulate the development or function of those structures.

Endocrine glands are also called ductless glands because they secrete hormones directly into the bloodstream. In contrast, exocrine glands release their secretions through ducts (for example, the sweat glands produce fluid that flows to the skin's surface through tiny tubelike sweat ducts).

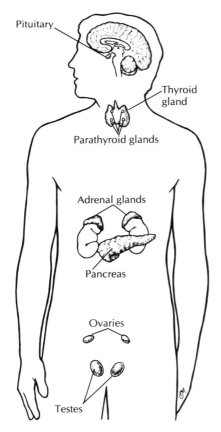

The endocrine system is composed of glands that release vital hormones into the blood. (Ovaries are shown here only to indicate placement.)

Hormones can be considered chemical messengers. They are targeted at specific cells in the body, and their arrival in those cells causes specific activities to occur. One of the major tasks of hormones is to coordinate the activities of organ systems. For example, when a person has to run or do other physical exercise, the hormone epinephrine acts on the heart to increase its rate and force of contraction and on the blood vessels to increase blood flow to the muscles and decrease blood flow to the gastrointestinal tract (so that more blood will reach the muscles, where the need is temporarily greater). Hormones also help control the type and rate of body growth and metabolism, and they help the body maintain a consistent internal environment.

The endocrine system has a large influence on the way we feel and act. In turn, our energy and other needs in any given situation set the activity of the endocrine system. This feedback relationship is crucial in maintaining our general well-being.

The adrenal glands are critical to normal body functions, such as maintenance of fluid balance, reaction to stress, and reproduction. There are two adrenal glands, each of which lies above a kidney. The adrenal glands have two distinct parts: the cortex (outer layer), which secretes steroid hormones, and the medulla (inner part), which secretes epinephrine and norepinephrine. The more than 30 steroid hormones regulate a wide array of processes throughout the body. Epinephrine and norepinephrine are responsible for the changes in heart rate, blood pressure, and level of usable glucose (a form of sugar) needed to cope with stress.

The pancreas is located in the rear center of the abdominal cavity, behind the stomach. Specialized cells in the pancreas produce two hormones, insulin and glucagon, needed to maintain stable blood sugar levels in the body. Insulin helps body cells utilize glucose for energy, thereby reducing the amount of sugar in the bloodstream. To balance this action, the hormone glucagon stimulates the liver to release its stored sugar into the blood, thereby raising the blood sugar levels.

The pancreas also functions in digestion. Nonendocrine cells in the pancreas produce special chemicals called enzymes, which are secreted directly into the small intestine through ducts. These enzymes help break down proteins, carbohydrates (sugars and starches), and fats in the small intestine.

This dual activity of the pancreas means that it functions as both an endocrine organ and an exocrine organ.

The pituitary gland is a small organ located just beneath the base of the brain, between the two frontal lobes and directly above a cavity called the sphenoid sinus. It is sometimes called the master gland because all other endocrine glands come under its control. Its job is to receive messages about the need for a particular hormone and to secrete either the hormone or substances that cause the manufacture and release of the hormone.

The anterior (front) lobe of the pituitary gland secretes somatotropin (also known as growth hormone), which affects the body's general growth; thyrotropic hormone (also known as thyroid-stimulating hormone), which acts on the thyroid gland to stimulate production of thyroid hormones; adrenocorticotropic hormone (ACTH), which stimulates the adrenal cortex; follicle-stimulating hormone and luteinizing hormone, which are necessary for maturation and release of egg and sperm cells; and prolactin, which acts on the mammary glands to promote the secretion of milk.

The posterior lobe of the pituitary gland secretes oxytocin, which stimulates smooth muscle tissue to contract and is of critical importance during childbirth, and vasopressin, which regulates kidney function with respect to water balance in the body.

The primary responsibility for hormone production for the reproductive system lies with the testes (male sex glands) and ovaries (female sex glands).

The testes are two oval organs in the scrotum (the pouch of skin behind the penis). They produce sperm and sex hormones that govern the male secondary sex characteristics, such as facial hair growth.

The two ovaries are located in the pelvis. They secrete the hormones estrogen and progesterone, which govern ovulation (monthly release of an egg from an ovary) and the female secondary sex characteristics.

The thyroid gland is located at the front of the neck above the top of the breastbone. It consists of two main lobes on either side of the trachea (windpipe) that are connected by a narrow band of tissue called the isthmus. The hormones secreted by the thyroid influence the rate of metabolism (the chemical processes in the body having to do with energy production).

The four parathyroid glands are located on the back and side of each lobe of the thyroid gland. Their secretion, parathyroid hormone, controls calcium levels in the blood.

See also Adrenal glands, Diabetes mellitus, Pituitary gland, and Reproduction.

---

# Endometriosis

Endometriosis is a condition in which tissue from the endometrial lining of the uterus becomes detached and

Displaced endometrial tissue

Fallopian tube

Backflow of menstrual blood into abdominal cavity

Ovary

Uterus

Chocolate cyst

Vagina

Endometriosis is a condition in which tissue from the endometrium (uterine lining) becomes detached and grows outside the uterus, usually elsewhere in the abdominal cavity. One possible cause may be backflow of menstrual blood through one of the fallopian tubes into the abdominal cavity. Blood-filled pockets called "chocolate cysts" sometimes form when scar tissue surrounds accumulations of blood and displaced endometrial tissue.

grows in the abdominal cavity outside the uterus. It occurs only in women of childbearing age, especially in women between the ages of 30 and 40.

During each menstrual cycle, the endometrium normally thickens and swells in preparation for possible pregnancy. If no pregnancy occurs, portions of endometrial tissue break down and pass out of the uterus as part of the menstrual flow. When endometriosis develops, displaced endometrial tissue continues to swell and bleed each month in an abnormal location, but the blood has no outlet. The body responds to the presence of this accumulated blood by surrounding it with scar tissue, which builds up month after month, until blood-filled pockets, or cysts (often called "chocolate cysts"), are formed on the affected organs.

The exact cause of endometriosis is not known, but several conditions are thought to lead to its development: menstrual blood may flow backward through the fallopian tubes and into the abdominal cavity; the cervix or vagina may be blocked, so that the menstrual blood cannot flow out normally; or surgery or another condition may lead to the displacement of some tissue from the uterus.

The symptoms of endometriosis are pain immediately before, during, or immediately after the menstrual period; pain during intercourse; discomfort in the lower urinary tract or intestine; irregular or excessively heavy menstrual flow; bleeding from the rectum; blood in the urine; and infertility. Some women may experience all of these symptoms; others may experience only one or two.

Diagnostic evaluation begins with a complete medical and menstrual history. Pelvic examinations may be performed—once during menstruation and once between periods—to investigate the changes in the reproductive organs during the cycle. The doctor may also perform a laparoscopy, in which a small, lighted, tubelike instrument is inserted into the lower abdomen through a tiny incision, allowing visualization of displaced tissues.

Treatment of this disorder consists of halting the condition, reducing the pain, and restoring normal menstruation and fertility. The best way to halt endometriosis is to modify the body's natural hormonal secretions with drugs in order to stop menstruation and ovulation for some time, thus allowing the endometrial tissue to shrink. Naturally, the patient will be unable to become pregnant during this type of drug therapy, but since endometriosis often causes infertility, many patients are already unable to conceive.

Three types of drugs are usually used in this treatment. Birth control pills, as well as several other medications that modify female hormonal secretions, are sometimes prescribed in doses high enough to stop menstruation and ovulation. However, an excessive dosage often brings with it undesirable side effects, such as nausea, fluid retention, and blood clotting.

A synthetic hormone called danazol creates a condition similar to menopause, causing menstruation and ovulation to stop and the endometrial tissue to shrink almost immediately. Danazol does not have some of the side effects of other hormonal drugs but it is relatively expensive and not always effective.

The newest form of treatment of endometriosis is a nasal spray that causes the brain to stop producing hormones that cause ovulation and menstruation. Like danazol, the spray shrinks endometrial tissues quickly.

If drug therapy is unsuccessful, surgery may be necessary, involving either the removal of scar tissue and endometrial tissue or, in advanced cases, the removal of the uterus and ovaries, rendering the patient sterile. In certain cases, endometriosis may be destroyed by using very precise medical lasers. This form of therapy has been used to successfully dissolve areas of endometriosis while leaving surrounding normal tissue unharmed.

---

# Enteroviral infections

The enteroviruses are a group of viruses that cause a wide variety of usually brief, but occasionally serious, illnesses that are particularly common in children. Included in the group are the coxsackieviruses, the echoviruses, and the polioviruses.

Enteroviral infections occur most often in the summer and fall and can be spread by contact with infected human feces or respiratory secretions. Although they produce a great deal of temporary discomfort, most of the enteroviral infections generally do not cause lasting illness. Often, the only treatment possible is to make the patient comfortable, with plenty of liquids, bed rest, lukewarm sponge baths, and nonaspirin pain relievers, such as acetaminophen, to control fever until the illness has passed. Careful hand washing along with the proper disposal of human wastes are additional steps that can help prevent the spread of infection.

The following diseases are among those caused by the enteroviruses.

**Aseptic meningitis** This inflammation of the membrane covering the brain causes headache, pain and stiffness in the neck and back, fever, nausea, vomiting, drowsiness, and a general sick feeling. Most patients recover in a week or so, but the disease may be fatal for newborns.

**Hand, foot, and mouth disease** In this disease, which is common in young children, little blisters erupt all over the mucous membranes in the mouth, on the hands and feet (including the palms and soles), and sometimes in the diaper area. A low-grade fever is common.

**Herpangina** An epidemic disease in infants and young children, herpangina is marked by sudden high fever, headache, sore throat, vomiting, and the appearance of grayish spots on the soft palate (rear roof of the mouth), tonsils, or throat. The spots become shallow ulcers and heal in three to six days.

**Myocarditis and pericarditis** Possibly fatal heart failure in newborns may result from myocarditis (inflammation of the heart muscle) caused by cox-sackieviruses or echoviruses transmitted to the baby by the mother. Myocarditis and pericarditis (inflammation of the sac around the heart) in older children and in adults may also be caused by a coxsackievirus; patients usually make a complete recovery, although congestive heart failure can occur.

**Paralytic disease** Various echoviruses, coxsackieviruses, and polioviruses produce muscle weakness or paralysis that is similar to the paralysis of poliomyelitis and is treated in the same manner.

**Pleurodynia (Bornholm disease)** Sudden, recurrent pains in the lower chest or abdomen signal the onset of this illness, which is often accompanied by fever, headache, nausea, abdominal tenderness, and sore throat. The disease may spread to cause pleuritis (inflammation of the membrane sac surrounding the lungs and the lining of the chest cavity), pericarditis, or aseptic meningitis.

**Poliomyelitis** Poliomyelitis (also known as polio and infantile paralysis), caused by the three types of polioviruses, is a serious infection of the spinal cord which can result in paralysis of all of the muscles. The symptoms include muscle soreness and stiffness of the neck and spine. With the development of the polio vaccine, polio has been virtually eradicated in the United States, but the threat of polio epidemics remains if children are not routinely immunized.

**Respiratory disease** The enteroviruses cause respiratory illnesses accompanied by head cold, fever, sore throat, and sometimes vomiting and diarrhea.

**Rubellalike rash** A mild rash like that of rubella (German measles), but lasting longer, this usually occurs in epidemic form and only on the face, neck, and chest. Fever is common, and meningitis can develop, but usually this is a mild disease.

# Epilepsy

Epilepsy is a disorder characterized by sudden surges of disorganized electrical impulses in the brain which lead to seizures (attacks).

There are several categories of seizures; they can be so mild as to go almost unnoticed or so severe that, if untreated, they can cause serious harm.

Epilepsy is usually divided into two categories: idiopathic (of unknown cause) and acquired (caused by some known factor, such as a brain tumor or an injury). Until the age of 25, idiopathic epilepsy is a very common cause of seizures. Seizures beginning after the age of 25 are more often a sign of acquired epilepsy due to injury, tumors, or other brain disorders (such as cerebral palsy, infection, or malformations of blood vessels).

Idiopathic epilepsy, although by definition of unknown cause, has several consistent attributes. It occurs with highest frequency between the ages of two and five years and again at puberty and tends to run in families.

The symptoms of epilepsy vary according to the type of seizure experienced. Not all seizures are convulsions. A convulsion involves the nerves that control movement and is characterized by jerking, spastic muscle movements. It is also marked by alterations in sensation and consciousness; loss of consciousness is common.

Seizures are classified according to the symptoms present. In the past, classifications were grand mal (French for "big sickness"), petit mal (French for "little sickness"), psychomotor, and focal. The current classification separates epileptic seizures into partial and generalized types, depending on the extent to which the brain is involved.

The four currently used categories (and their symptoms) are as follows:

- Simple partial seizures, confined to small areas of the brain, may be accompanied by feeling a tingling sensation in the arm, finger, or foot; perceiving a bad odor; seeing flashing lights; or speaking unintelligibly. The patient remains conscious.

- Complex partial seizures include episodes of "automatic behavior," in which the patient remains conscious but sits motionless or moves or behaves in a strange, repetitive, or somehow inappropriate way.

- Generalized convulsive seizures have a number of symptoms: the patient may cry out, stiffen, and fall to the ground unconscious, lose urinary and bowel control, and have muscle spasms or thrashing movements that cause the limbs to jerk. Spasms of the jaw muscles can cause the victim to bite his tongue. After the convulsion, the patient falls into a deep sleep and then awakens dazed, often with a headache and no recollection of the seizure. A warning sensation, called an aura, may precede the seizure; this may be a headache, sleepiness, yawning, or tingling in the arms or legs.

- Generalized nonconvulsive, or absence, seizures are characterized by periods of staring into space, rhythmic blinking, and what appears to be daydreaming. The patient remains conscious but is totally unaware of the seizure. This type of seizure, which is most common in children, may be mistaken for a short attention span or a learning disability.

Epilepsy is diagnosed by observing the symptoms and by obtaining an electroencephalogram (EEG), which is a visual record of the electrical activity of the brain. Abnormal electrical discharges can be detected if they are present in the brain. However, an abnormal EEG in the absence of symptoms is by no means proof of epilepsy, nor does a normal EEG rule it out.

Nonmedical treatment of an epileptic seizure should be limited to preventing injury and keeping the patient comfortable by loosening clothing or placing a pillow under the head. The patient should not be left in any position in which vomit can be swallowed or inhaled or in any position in which he might suffocate. *Never* should an attempt be made to pry open the mouth or insert any object into the mouth of a person who is having a convulsion.

Epilepsy cannot be cured, but it can usually be controlled with a program of anticonvulsant drug therapy. Patients who tend to have seizures following emotional or physical stress may also benefit from tranquilizers. After two to five years of drug control of idiopathic epilepsy, the dosage is sometimes decreased and, occasionally, when enough time has elapsed during which no seizures have occurred, medication can cease.

Epilepsy cannot be prevented, but once the seizures have been controlled by medication, epileptic persons can lead normal lives.

# Episiotomy

An episiotomy is a surgical incision into the tissues surrounding the opening of the vagina during childbirth in order to make the delivery easier and to avoid extensive tearing of the tissues. The advantage of the procedure

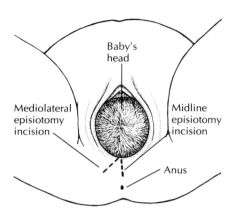

An episiotomy is done to make childbirth easier and to avoid extensive tearing of tissues. The most common type of episiotomy is a midline incision from the midpoint of the vaginal opening directly downward toward the anus. Some doctors, however, prefer an incision at an angle, called a mediolateral episiotomy.

is that it substitutes a controlled surgical incision for excessive stretching and tearing of all the tissues. The incision itself is easier to repair later than a tear or break in the tissues would be.

Episiotomy is often performed in women who are having their first baby. With subsequent pregnancies, episiotomy may not be necessary, since the tissues surrounding the vagina have often been stretched sufficiently by the first delivery to allow an easy second delivery.

The most common type of episiotomy is an incision made with surgical scissors from the midpoint of the vaginal opening directly down toward the anus. An important risk with this type of incision is that during the birth, the opening might further extend into the anal sphincter (the ring of muscle surrounding the opening from the rectum) or the rectum itself; however, such a tear can be repaired relatively easily and will eventually heal itself. To avoid the

risks of entering the rectum, some physicians prefer the mediolateral episiotomy, in which the incision is made at an angle, thus avoiding the rectum and anus.

# Extrasystole

An extrasystole is a contraction of the heart caused by a stimulus or impulse somewhere in the heart other than in the sinoatrial node, the natural pacemaker of the heart. In some ways, the condition is like static in an electrical circuit.

While physicians have for years debated the importance of extrasystoles, recent thought on the subject has led to a reassessment of the seriousness of the phenomenon. In many cases of sudden death attributed to severe cardiac arrhythmia (a disturbance of the normal rhythm of the heartbeat) in patients with severe underlying heart disease, the arrhythmia may have actually been triggered by ventricular extrasystoles.

While the immediate cause of an extrasystole is an accidental signal telling the heart muscle to contract, the real causes lie elsewhere. For example, strenuous activity, especially if there are existing heart problems, can trigger extrasystoles, which, in turn, may trigger an episode of heart arrhythmia that leads to more serious complications. Coffee, nicotine, and certain drugs, as well as anxiety and sudden shocks or frights, are thought to play a role in extrasystoles. It is important to note, however, that extrasystoles also occur in normal hearts and, in these cases, are quite harmless and do not necessarily indicate underlying heart disease.

The symptoms of extrasystoles are familiar to anyone who has ever been startled and felt his or her heart had "skipped a beat." The extrasystole sometimes presents itself as one or two extra heartbeats. On other occasions, there will be a beat followed by a long silence, then a couple of quick beats. Some people experience a feeling of giddiness, shortness of breath, and weakness, with momentary feelings of blacking out. These symptoms, if prolonged (particularly if associated with loss of consciousness), usually indicate that a sustained arrhythmia is occurring, which should be reported to a doctor.

The primary diagnostic tool is the electrocardiograph (an instrument that records the electrical impulses generated in the heart). One method of documenting the occurrence and nature of extrasystoles is continuous ambulatory electrocardiographic monitoring with a device called a Holter monitor. The monitor, which is like a combination tape recorder-electrocardiograph, is worn by the patient for as long as 24 hours. A diary is furnished so that the patient can record his or her activities and symptoms. The patient goes about his or her routine during the test. After the specified time period, the monitor is taken off, and the tape is translated into a continuous electrocardiographic record. Comparison of this record with the diary allows a diagnosis to be made as to the presence and type of arrhythmia.

Any treatment program must be based on the underlying cause of the extrasystoles, as revealed by electrocardiographic studies. Treatment may involve medications to regulate the heartbeat, lifestyle changes (such as restriction of tobacco use and caffeine intake), or implantation of an artificial cardiac pacemaker. If the electrocardiographic studies indicate that the extrasystoles do not reflect any disease process, no medical treatment is necessary.

See also Heartbeat irregularities.

# Eye

The eye is the organ of sight. This complex structure works by capturing light and transforming it into impulses that the brain can interpret as images.

To understand visual perception, it is important to know the functions of the parts of the eye. The eye includes the eyeball and all structures within and surrounding its almost spherical mass. This delicate organ is nestled within the bony socket of the skull. A layer of fat cushions the socket; and the eyebrow, eyelashes, and eyelid provide a barrier against incoming irritants. Lining the inside of the eyelid and continuing over the exposed surface of the eyeball is the conjunctiva, a thin protective membrane. Tears released from the lacrimal glands in the upper eyelid moisten the conjunctiva and keep the eye clean. The sclera is the tough, white, outer layer of the eyeball. The sclera covers the entire eyeball, except for the circular area in front that admits light, which is covered by the transparent cornea. The choroid layer contains blood vessels that nourish the eye.

Light enters the eye through the cornea. The curved cornea helps to focus the light inward. Behind the cornea is a pigmented (colored) structure called the iris. The iris surrounds an opening known as the pupil. The iris changes the size of the pupil, depending on the amount of light present in the environment: if the surroundings are relatively dark, the pupil is enlarged to admit more light; if the environment is bright, the pupil is made smaller. Behind the iris is the lens, a transparent structure held in place by elastic, muscular-type tissue. The tissue can change the shape of the lens to accommodate the

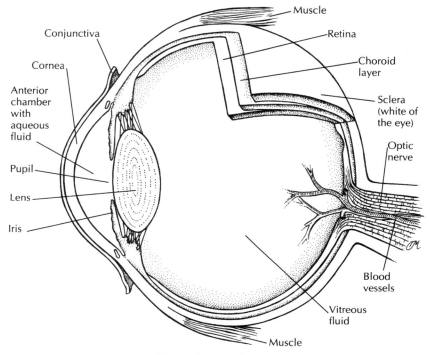

Muscle
Conjunctiva
Retina
Cornea
Choroid
layer
Anterior
chamber
with
aqueous
fluid
Sclera
(white of
the eye)
Optic
nerve
Pupil
Lens
Iris
Blood
vessels
Vitreous
fluid
Muscle

The eye is a complex structure.

available light and to finely focus the incoming light rays onto the light-sensitive cells that line the rear surface of the eye.

Between the cornea and the lens is a space, the anterior chamber, which is filled with a fluid called aqueous humor. Aqueous humor contains nutrients that nourish the cornea and the lens. The fluid also allows light rays to pass through with ease.

The chamber of the eyeball behind the lens holds a clear jelly called vitreous humor. In the retina (the layer of light-sensitive cells that lines the back of the eyeball) are the specialized cells, called rods and cones, that convert light focused from the cornea and lens into electrical impulses. Sensitive nerve endings then transmit these electrical impulses to the brain via the optic nerve, which extends

from the rear portion of the eyeball to the brain.

# F

# Fainting

Fainting is a brief loss of consciousness often resulting from the body's attempts to supply extra blood to the brain. Fainting can be a symptom of a relatively mild condition, such as hunger, or a serious disorder, such as heartbeat irregularity.

When the brain experiences a temporary reduction of its blood supply, the body reacts defensively; in effect, it causes itself to fall down, bringing the head to the level of the heart and thereby minimizing the effect of gravity, which favors pooling of blood in the legs. The net effect of fainting is an increase in the amount of blood coming back to the heart, which allows the heart to pump blood to the brain more easily.

Fainting can be caused by interference with any one of several internal mechanisms that protect and maintain the brain's blood supply. These mechanisms work against gravity and its tendency to allow blood to pool in the lower parts of the body. One of these mechanisms is the "muscle pump." The muscles of the legs act to squeeze the veins in the legs, thereby forcing blood up toward the heart. If a person stands motionless for a long period of time without using these muscles, blood pools in the legs, reducing the amount available to the brain. This reduction frequently causes fainting or loss of consciousness. The ability of the heart to increase its rate and force of contraction when under stress is another built-in protective mechanism.

These protective functions can be impaired by a variety of conditions, such as an overheated or crowded environment, emotional stress, hunger, extreme fatigue, various drugs (particularly some high blood pressure medications), as well as certain circulatory disorders.

The symptoms that usually precede fainting are light-headedness, confusion, spots before the eyes, white or grayish coloring of the face, and cold, moist skin. Nausea and vomiting may also be present.

Fainting is treated by taking several simple steps to make the person more comfortable. The patient should be lying down, preferably with the feet higher than the head (to help blood return to the brain), and the clothing should be loosened. The patient should have plenty of fresh air

to breathe. Recovery should occur within a few seconds of fainting, but a sense of disorientation may linger for several minutes. Spirits of ammonia and smelling salts are not usually recommended for fainting, as they may be ineffective or may cause vomiting. Fainting should be reported to a doctor.

Fainting can often be prevented by lying down, preferably with the legs up, as soon as any of the warning symptoms are noticed. This precaution lowers the brain to the level of the heart, increasing the blood supply to the brain. The head should be turned sideways in case the person vomits.

# Fatigue

Fatigue may be physical or mental exhaustion, an overwhelming feeling of weariness, or a lack of energy and enthusiasm for even pleasant activities. It is a symptom of a vast number of diseases and disorders.

Fatigue should not be confused with weakness, which is an actual loss of physical strength.

Feeling fatigued and tiring rapidly with minimal activity are often among the early signs of an approaching illness. Fatigue is a warning signal of a variety of diseases and disorders, among them the common cold, influenza, hepatitis, infectious mononucleosis, and other infectious diseases; heart disease; lung disorders, such as emphysema; some glandular diseases, such as diabetes; anemia and nutritional deficiencies; and some diseases of the nervous system. Overwork, either physical or mental, can also cause fatigue, as can psychological disorders or emotional stress.

In addition to the general feeling of being more tired than usual, fatigue can be accompanied by nervousness, anxiety, depression, and feelings of irritability, as well as by headache, diminished sexual function, and difficulty in concentrating. When fatigue is due to psychological problems, sleep disorders, including insomnia, and a pattern of frequent nighttime and early morning awakening are often present as well.

Fatigue is best dealt with by treating the physical disorder or psychological problem that is causing it. Some types of fatigue, particularly those due to physical overexertion, can probably be prevented by getting adequate exercise and rest, as well as by eating well-balanced meals and reducing stress, tension, and overwork.

# Fertilization

See Conception.

# Fever

Fever is an abnormally high body temperature. A fever is present when the body temperature rises above the normal range of 98.6°F to 99.6°F. Generally, if the body temperature is more than 101.5°F when measured with a rectal thermometer, 100.5°F when measured with an oral thermometer, or 99.5°F when measured under the arm, it is considered to be abnormal.

Fever is a symptom of illness and often appears to be an undesirable condition, but many researchers believe that fever acts as a defense mechanism for the body when it is being attacked by bacteria or viruses. There is a regulatory center in the brain that acts to maintain a constant body temperature regardless of the surrounding environment. Fever occurs when this center responds to an illness or infection, such as a common cold or influenza, by setting the body temperature higher. This mechanism is thought to work because infectious microorganisms cannot survive the higher-than-normal temperatures.

Infections are the most common cause of fever, but a fever can also be a symptom of heart attack, some forms of cancer, and disorders in the portion of the brain that regulates temperature (such as stroke, brain tumor, or brain injury).

The early signs of fever include chills or hot flashes, flushed skin, increased pulse and breathing rates, headache, and aching of muscles or joints. A slight fever, however, may produce none of these symptoms. A high fever may result in delirium or convulsions, and a prolonged fever may cause weakness and dehydration (excess loss of body fluids).

Treatment of fever depends on its severity, duration, and cause. Immediate emergency medical treatment should be sought if the temperature is near 105°F (even though fevers tend to be high in very young children) or if convulsions have occurred. A doctor should be consulted if a high fever (103°F to 104°F) lasts for 12 to 24 hours; if a moderate fever (101°F to 102°F) lasts for several days; if the body temperature fluctuates widely; or if the fever disappears and then returns several days later, which usually signals a new or resistant infection.

The goal in treating a patient with a fever is actually to diagnose and treat the cause of the fever, rather than the fever itself. Merely lowering a mild fever may do more harm than good, because it reduces the protection that the fever may be providing in fighting off the infection; it may also mask the underlying cause or disturb the natural course that the disease would have taken, thus hindering diagnosis. Therefore, treating a fever should never be confused with treating its cause.

At times, however, fever should be lowered to keep the patient comfortable and to prevent the weakness and dehydration that can result from prolonged fever. Increasing fluid intake and taking aspirin or an aspirin substitute (such as acetaminophen) will usually lower a fever; taking tepid, not cold, baths and using comfortable, but not overly warm, clothing and blankets will help to lower the fever and also keep the patient from feeling chilled.

It should be noted that any drug treatment for fever, especially for children, should be undertaken only after consulting with a doctor. An association between the use of aspirin in children with viral illnesses (particularly chicken pox and influenza) and the often fatal Reye's syndrome (a condition characterized by severe, sudden deterioration of liver and brain function) has been demonstrated. It is therefore recommended that the use of aspirin be avoided in children with viral illnesses unless the aspirin has been prescribed by a physician.

See also Reye's syndrome.

---

# Fever blisters

Fever blisters, also called cold sores, are fluid-filled blisters that appear on the border of the lips and on or around the nose. They are the result of a very contagious virus that affects most of the population at one time or another.

Fever blisters are caused by a type of herpes simplex virus. It enters the body most often through the mouth or nose areas, where the skin is easier to penetrate.

At first, characteristic blisters may not result. Antibodies (protective substances) in the body defend against the invading virus. The inactivated virus withdraws to a nearby nerve, where it remains until stress to the body or a diminished capacity to fight off infection triggers a recurrence. When the virus is reactivated, it overruns the body's protective system and progresses back along the nerve to the general area of original infection. Factors that seem to favor the appearance of blisters include fever, colds, menstruation, skin injury from dental work, excessive sun and wind exposure, and emotional stress. Cold sores can return every few weeks for several weeks or not at all.

Initially, the virus may present no symptoms, so some people are unaware of infection. For others, the infection begins with numbness or tenderness in the affected area. Then small, fluid-filled blisters appear. These blisters break, encrust, and heal within one to two weeks.

Occasionally, excessive pain or swelling of lymph nodes develops. These symptoms may indicate a secondary bacterial infection that needs a doctor's attention.

Other complications can be more serious. *Herpes simplex keratitis* is a painful viral infection of the cornea (transparent covering of the eye) that can result in blindness if not treated. When inflammation of the eyes accompanies fever blisters, a physician should be consulted immediately. Steroid (cortisone-type) medications should not be used near the eyes during a herpes attack without first consulting a doctor, since these preparations can encourage the spread of the virus to the eye.

Other serious complications can occur in infants and extremely ill patients who contract herpes virus if the infection travels to the lungs, brain, or other internal organs.

Treatment involves relieving symptoms, since there is no known cure for fever blisters. Some over-the-counter remedies may relieve pain and help dry blisters. Topical corticosteroid creams, however, should not be applied unless prescribed by a physician; the possibility of spreading infection increases because the corticosteroid can depress the immune response.

Healing time may be shortened by certain newer prescription drugs, such as acyclovir, but these drugs should not be used for routine fever blisters.

# Fibrillation

See Defibrillation.

# Fibrocystic disease of the breast

Fibrocystic disease is a condition in which benign (noncancerous) lumps form in the breast, either temporarily or for the duration of the childbearing years.

This condition is not dangerous in itself, but it has been found that women with certain forms of fibrocystic disease may be two to four times more likely to develop breast cancer than are other women. To complicate matters, the presence of these benign lumps makes it difficult to detect any new, possibly dangerous growths.

The exact cause of fibrocystic disease is not known. However, the tendency to develop it may be inherited. Also, it is seen more often in women who have never breast-fed a child; the reason is unknown.

The most noticeable symptom of this disorder is the presence of the

lumps, which may take the form of either solid masses or fluid-filled sacs called cysts. Large cystic lumps near the surface can be moved about freely, unlike cancerous lumps, which are usually firmly attached to surrounding tissue. Changes in hormonal secretions during the menstrual period tend to slightly increase the size of the lumps, which causes additional pain, but the size of the cysts decreases following the period. Other symptoms may include a slight discharge from the nipple, as well as persistently heavy and tender breasts,

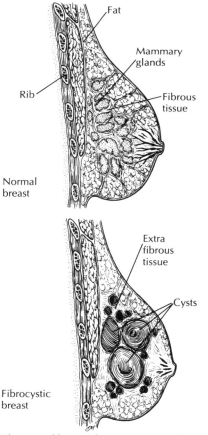

The normal breast (shown at top) contains some fibrous tissue, which supports the mammary (milk) glands. The fibrocystic breast (shown at bottom) is characterized by the presence of extra fibrous tissue and solid masses or fluid-filled sacs (cysts).

not only before and during menstruation (as is commonly seen in healthy breasts) but all the time.

Diagnostic evaluation of fibrocystic breasts will begin with a physical examination. Mammography (a special X-ray study of the breasts) is often done to determine whether the lumps are fluid-filled cysts or solid masses. If they are found to be solid, a biopsy (the removal of a small piece of tissue for analysis) may be performed to detect the presence of cancerous cells in the breast.

Fibrocystic disease often requires no treatment. In some cases, the lumps may disappear in a few months. However, cysts that are unusually large or particularly bothersome may be drained of their fluid by the insertion of a hollow needle in a procedure called aspiration. If there are many small lumps or if there is continuous development of new ones, other forms of treatment may be necessary to prevent the formation of cysts. Birth control pills may be prescribed, since they act to equalize the concentration of hormones in the body throughout the monthly cycle; however, birth control pills have also been found to cause cysts in some women. Large doses of vitamin E (taken under a doctor's supervision) have also been reportedly effective in treating this disorder.

Relieving or preventing fibrocystic disease may be promoted by discontinuing or drastically limiting the intake of nicotine and a chemical called methylxanthine, found most commonly in coffee, tea, cola, chocolate, and some cold medications. It is thought that both nicotine and methylxanthine may promote the growth of fibrocystic tissue.

Because certain forms of this disorder carry a greater risk of breast cancer, women with fibrocystic disease should have an examination at least twice a year, report any new growths or enlargements of existing lumps, and perform self-examination of their breasts each month following the menstrual period.

See also Cancer and Mastitis.

# Fibroid tumors

Fibroid tumors are solid, noncancerous growths composed of smooth muscle fibers and connective tissue that grow in the walls of the uterus or out from the uterus. Only rarely do fibroid tumors appear on the cervix. Occasionally they fill the entire uterus, push through the cervix, and appear in the vagina. These tumors usually grow slowly and vary in size and shape.

Fibroid tumors are thought to be the most common type of abdominal tumor, found in about 25 percent of all women over the age of 30 (more frequently in black women). Cancer rarely develops in fibroid tumors;

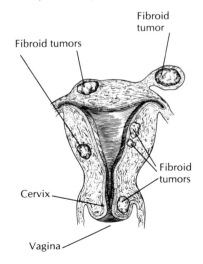

Fibroid tumors are solid, noncancerous growths that grow within the walls of the uterus or out from the uterine wall on a stalk.

however, they do sometimes cause problems. For example, the tumors tend to enlarge during pregnancy, which can cause complications as the fetus grows.

The cause of fibroid tumors is not known, but their growth seems to be related to the female hormone estrogen, since these tumors rarely appear before puberty and tend to recede by the menopause years. They most commonly appear in the middle to late reproductive years, when the estrogen level in the body is at its peak.

Fibroid tumors may occur along with other disorders, such as endometriosis (the displacement of tissue from the uterine lining to areas elsewhere in the body) or pelvic inflammatory disease (an infection of the fallopian tubes).

Common symptoms of fibroid tumors are dysmenorrhea (pain during menstruation) and gushing or flooding of the menstrual flow. Occasionally, there is abdominal pain; however, pain is not usually a symptom unless a complication develops (for example, if the tumor becomes twisted, cutting off its blood supply). If fibroid tumors become very large, they may press on surrounding organs, such as the intestines and bladder, which may result in constipation or frequent urination. If they extend into the uterus, heavy and prolonged menstrual periods may result. If the tumor is advanced, the abdomen may be noticeably enlarged. Sometimes, however, these tumors cause no symptoms at all and are simply discovered during a routine physical examination.

Diagnostic evaluation begins with a physical examination and may include curettage (scraping the uterus walls) or endometrial biopsy (removal of some tissue from the lining of the uterus) to test for cancer. X rays and ultrasound (a technique that uses sound waves to create an image of internal structures) may also be used to establish the location, size, and nature of the tumor.

Fibroid tumors may require no treatment at all, other than regular checkups with the doctor. Those that are causing complications may require one of two types of surgery: removal of the tumor (called a myomectomy), which is usually recommended for women in their early reproductive years whose symptoms are somewhat mild and who desire a future pregnancy, or removal of the uterus (called a hysterectomy), which is usually recommended for older women and for those who do not want to become pregnant, since this operation makes pregnancy impossible.

Two new drugs used in the treatment of fibroid tumors are Lupron and Syneral; both are gonadotropin-releasing hormone antagonists. These drugs are used—for a maximum of six months only—to shrink fibroid tumors prior to myomectomy. They prevent secretion of FSH and LH from the pituitary gland and therefore stop the production of estrogen; when the estrogen is eliminated, the tumors will shrink, making surgical removal easier. The side effects are similar to menopause: hot flashes, sweats, vaginal dryness, and irreversible calcium loss from bones. These symptoms go away when the drug is halted. However, while no further loss of calcium will take place, the calcium lost from bones does not reappear. It's for this reason that the drugs cannot be taken for more than six months. So these drugs are not intended as a medical cure for fibroids, but they are a common presurgical treatment. Once the drug is stopped, the tumors will grow back to their original size.

See also Dysmenorrhea, Endometriosis, and Pelvic inflammatory disease.

# Fistula

See Crohn's disease.

# Fluoride

Fluoride is a compound of the chemical element fluorine. Fluoride is found in soil and is necessary to plant life and to the formation of teeth and bones in animals, including humans. In the human body, traces of fluoride are found in the bones, the teeth, the thyroid gland, and the skin.

It has been found that fluoride can help prevent or reduce tooth decay when taken in somewhat larger amounts than are naturally present in the teeth. The best source of fluoride for prevention of tooth decay is fluoridated drinking water. Water with a fluoride content of one part per million is considered safe and effective, especially if given to children while their teeth are developing. The maximum benefit is obtained when the child drinks fluoridated water daily until the permanent teeth are complete (between the ages of 10 and 13). However, if fluoride intake is excessive before the permanent teeth erupt (while the tooth enamel is still forming), the enamel may become stained and mottled. If the teeth have erupted, this staining and mottling cannot occur.

There is evidence that fluoridation prevents dental problems other than cavities, such as periodontal diseases (diseases of the gums and the bones supporting the teeth) and abnormal positioning of the teeth. Many physicians and researchers have found that fluoride also may play a significant role in the treatment and prevention of osteoporosis (abnormal thinness and brittleness of the bones, common in women after menopause and in both men and women over the age of 65).

Fluoridation of drinking water has been a controversial issue. Opponents of fluoridation are concerned about the unknown long-range effects of adding fluoride to the water supply and about what they see as the infringement on freedom of choice inherent in imposing this "compulsory medication" on the population. Supporters of fluoridation counter these charges by pointing out that fluoride is not a medication but a preventive, used in the same way that chlorine is used to kill bacteria in water supplies. They also assert that fluorides are normally found in teeth and bones as well as in water and that other methods of obtaining fluoride are more costly and less effective in the long run than fluoridation of the water supply. Most health scientists today believe that a fluoride level of about one part per million does not damage either teeth or other body tissues.

See also Minerals and Tooth decay.

# Fontanelles

Fontanelles are the gaps between the bony plates of an infant's skull. The largest and most noticeable of these gaps is the "soft spot" on top of the head, toward the front. There is also a groove that runs like a center part toward the back of the head, where a much smaller soft spot is located. The fontanelles serve two purposes. During birth, they permit the head to adapt without injury to being squeezed as it passes through the birth canal. After birth, they permit the brain to grow.

During the first two or three years of a child's life, the skull plates grow

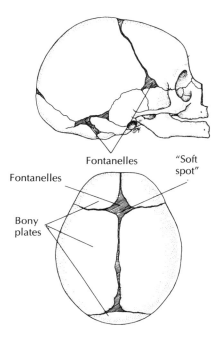

Fontanelles

Fontanelles

"Soft spot"

Bony plates

Fontanelles are the gaps between the bony plates of an infant's skull. Fontanelles permit the head to adapt without injury to being squeezed during birth, and after birth they allow room for the brain to grow.

toward each other until they meet, thereby covering the soft spots. However, the plates do not completely knit together until shortly before adolescence, at which time the brain stops growing.

The baby's soft spot is supported by a tough membrane and therefore does not have to be treated more delicately than any other part of the baby's head. It is perfectly normal for the soft spot to be slightly depressed, to tense up when the baby cries, and to pulsate in rhythm with the heartbeat. (The pulsation is not that of an artery directly beneath the soft spot. Instead, it is caused by fluctuations in the pressure of the cerebrospinal fluid, which surrounds and protects the brain and spinal cord.)

# Food allergy

A food allergy is an unusual sensitivity to a specific food. A food allergy is not a food intolerance, which exists when the body lacks the enzymes that are needed to digest a certain food. A food allergy exists when the body's immune system manufactures antibodies as a reaction to the food. This food then becomes an ingestant allergen (an allergy-causing substance that is swallowed or eaten). Any food has the potential to become an allergen, but the foods most commonly found to cause allergic reactions are milk, eggs, shellfish, fish, peanuts, chocolate, tomatoes, strawberries, and citrus fruits.

The symptoms of a food allergy most commonly arise in the digestive tract and include cramps, nausea, vomiting, and diarrhea. Other signs that may also be present include hives, rash, headache, nasal congestion, and anaphylactic shock (a very serious reaction that can be fatal, characterized by breathing problems due to swelling of the larynx and collapse of blood vessels). Food allergies occur more often in children than in adults.

Food allergy is diagnosed by having the patient maintain a detailed record of all foods eaten, as well as of the times when symptoms appear. Elimination trials may also help identify the allergen; the patient eliminates one food at a time from the diet to see if the symptoms disappear. In addition, several tests are used to detect various types of allergens: scratch tests, in which a small amount of the suspected allergen is applied to a scratch on the skin; intracutaneous tests, in which a small amount of the allergen is injected in or under the skin; and radioallergosorbent testing, in which the level of antibodies developed in response to specific allergens are measured in a blood sample.

There is no way to treat a food allergy other than to avoid eating the food and to treat the symptoms of a reaction should one develop. Fortunately, children usually outgrow these allergies.

Some doctors feel that infants who are breast-fed for up to a year are less likely to develop food allergies than babies who are formula-fed or who are breast-fed for only a couple of months. This continues to be a controversial issue.

# Fracture

A fracture is a break in a bone or a cartilage. Among the possible conse-

Impacted          Composite          Greenstick

Artery          Complicated

Open

Closed

There are several major categories of fractures, depending on the site and extent of injury.

quences of a fracture are infection and damage to nearby nerves, blood vessels, and internal organs.

Most often, fractures are caused by direct stress, such as a blow from a heavy object, or a severe strain, such as a violent twist. They can, however, be the result of an indirect cause. A fall on a hand, for example, may result in a fracture of the collarbone. There are also pathological fractures, in which disease softens the bone, making it more vulnerable to a break.

There are many types of fractures, among them the following:

- Closed fracture—one in which the skin is not broken
- Comminuted fracture—one in which the bone is broken into several pieces
- Complicated fracture—one in which significant injury has been done to internal organs, blood vessels, or nerves
- Green-stick fracture—one in which only one side of the bone is broken and the bone is not severed
- Impacted fracture—one in which the ends or fragments of bone are jammed together
- Open fracture—one in which one or more of the broken ends of the bone pierce the skin (this is also referred to as a compound fracture)
- Stress fracture—one in which there is a tiny crack (or cracks) in a bone; the crack causes severe pain but may be undetectable by conventional X ray. This type of fracture is commonly seen in the small bones of the foot due to athletic activity.

Fractures are common among children and the elderly. Children have relatively soft, elastic bones; breaks in their bones are often incomplete, affecting only one side of the bone. Elderly persons have brittle bones that tend to break easily; hip fractures are particularly common.

Among the symptoms of a fracture are pain, swelling, loss of strength, abnormal movement, and a grating sound when the pieces of broken bone rub together. Shock is likely to occur with a severe fracture if large amounts of blood have been lost.

Bone fractures are treated by closed (nonsurgical) or open (surgical) reduction. Reduction is a procedure in which the broken bone is manipulated (for example, by pulling or bending) so that its ends will be in the best position for healing. Most fractures are treated through closed reduction. However, open reduction may be necessary when damage to bones, joints, ligaments, tendons, or other internal parts is severe or extensive. In open reduction, the pieces of bone are often held together by pins, metal plates, or rods; some are left in the body, and others are removed after healing has taken place.

# Frostbite

Frostbite is damage to skin tissue resulting from exposure to low environmental temperatures. The condition can affect any part of the body, but the areas most often involved (such as the face, hands, and feet) are those with the poorest blood circulation and the greatest exposure to cold.

When exposed to cold, the body naturally tries to protect vital organs. Blood vessels near the surface of the skin constrict to preserve internal body heat. This tightening causes blood to be diverted from the outside of the body, thereby reducing the supply of blood to skin tissues. As a result, skin tissue freezes from the lack of a warm blood supply and dies. Frequently, frostbite develops after prolonged exposure to the cold. Extremely low temperatures or forceful winds can also cause the condition. Wearing insufficient or improper clothing increases susceptibility to frostbite. Skin can freeze to the surface of a metal object and block circulation to the area. In addition, any health problem that weakens the body or reduces circulation increases the likelihood of frostbite.

Frostbite develops in three stages, and each stage can produce varying degrees of pain. First-degree frostbite appears as whiteness or slight yellowness of the skin accompanied by burning or itching sensations. In this stage, symptoms can be reversed if the affected area is gradually rewarmed.

Should exposure to cold continue, sensation in the affected area ceases. Disappearance of pain and reddening and swelling of the tissue signals second-degree frostbite. At this stage, warming the area may produce blisters and skin peeling. The blisters may persist for weeks, and tenderness may linger for months.

Skin with third-degree frostbite becomes waxy and hard. At this stage, skin tissue dies and edema (excess fluid retention in the tissues) may occur. Severe frostbite can damage muscles, tendons, and nerves. Blood clots may form in small blood vessels and inhibit or block circulation, which can lead to gangrene.

Initial treatment focuses on what not to do, since there are many misconceptions about the proper course of action. Frostbitten tissue should not be rubbed with snow. In fact, the affected part should not be rubbed at all, because further damage to tissue can result. Exercising the frostbitten area will aggravate the condition.

To reduce tissue loss and avoid complications, frostbitten tissue should be immersed in lukewarm water rather than exposed to the extreme heat of a radiator, stove, or fire. Ideally, water temperature should be between 100°F and 110°F. Any temperature above 110°F can burn skin that lacks sensation, and thawing that is too rapid may produce pain, redness, and blisters. Gently patting (but not rubbing) the skin dry helps prevent additional injury.

If the patient remains outdoors, affected areas can be warmed by placing them in contact with warm portions of the body, such as under the armpits or between the thighs. The area can also be wrapped in a warm, dry blanket. Frozen areas should be kept clean to prevent infection. Warm, nonalcoholic drinks aid circulation. Smoking should be avoided because it causes constriction of blood vessels.

Once frozen tissue has been rewarmed, the affected area should be elevated to promote increased blood circulation and maintain the skin at room temperature. All cases of frostbite should be examined by a physician, who may prescribe medication to prevent infection or formation of clots in blood vessels.

The best prevention is to wear adequate clothing to protect the skin. Feet, hands, and parts of the face need covering since these areas are likely to have the poorest blood circulation and are the most exposed. When weather is unusually cold or windy, remaining indoors or keeping outside trips short is recommended.

See also Gangrene.

# G

## Gallstones

Gallstones are hardened masses that consist mainly of cholesterol (a fatlike substance found only in animal products), blood, bile (fluid produced

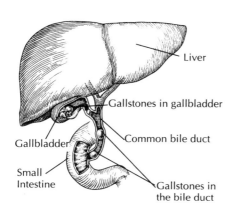

Liver

Gallstones in gallbladder

Common bile duct

Gallbladder

Small Intestine

Gallstones in the bile duct

Gallstones can form in the gallbladder or bile duct and cause inflammation of the gallbladder or liver damage if they block the flow of bile from the gallbladder to the small intestine.

in the liver and stored in the gallbladder, which is required for fat absorption in the small intestine), calcium, and other substances. The development of gallstones takes place in the gallbladder or in the bile duct leading from the gallbladder into the small intestine.

When bile contains excessive amounts of cholesterol, the unnecessary cholesterol separates from the solution and forms stonelike masses. Unfortunately, since the body itself produces cholesterol, formation of these types of stones cannot always be prevented merely by controlling cholesterol intake in the diet.

Pregnancy, obesity, diabetes, liver disease, and certain forms of anemia can increase the risk of gallstones. Overweight people who frequently lose and gain large amounts of weight seem more susceptible to gallstones, as do women who have had two or more children. Although the reasons are unclear, twice as many women as men over age 40 develop gallstones.

By themselves, gallstones often produce no signs of disease. About half the people with gallstones have no symptoms. Symptoms that do appear are usually chronic (long-term) in nature, including discomfort and pain in the upper abdomen, indigestion, nausea, and intolerance of fatty foods. Sometimes stones pass through the bile duct into the intestines to be excreted naturally.

However, symptoms can occur if the stones lodge in the bile duct. In an acute gallbladder attack, a sharp pain (often on the right side of the upper abdomen) may travel to the back and under the right shoulder blade. Frequently, the pain develops suddenly after a meal and leads to fever, chills, vomiting, and possibly jaundice (yellowing of the skin and whites of the eyes caused by the presence of excess bile pigment in the bloodstream). These symptoms occur when a stone that had been floating in the gallbladder becomes trapped in the bile duct.

Serious complications of liver damage may develop if stones block the flow of bile. When gallstones remain in the gallbladder, the organ may become inflamed. This condition, which is called chronic cholecystitis, may not cause any symptoms, but repeated attacks of pain will ordinarily occur.

Gallstones that cause no symptoms may be detected by an X-ray study of the gallbladder, called a cholecystogram. A cholecystogram is performed after the patient has swallowed a tablet containing dye that outlines the gallbladder and any stones that may be present. Nowadays, most physicians prefer to use ultrasound (a technique that uses sound waves to create images of internal structures). Some studies using radioactive isotopes can be used to differentiate between acute and chronic cholecystitis.

For acute gallbladder attacks due to gallstones with severe and prolonged symptoms, doctors generally recommend a cholecystectomy (surgical removal of the gallbladder). This treatment is one of the most common forms of abdominal surgery. Recently, a technique for removing the gallbladder without a standard incision—via a laparoscope—has been used. Other nonsurgical methods for removing gallstones, including drug and chemical therapy and lithotripsy (the use of shock waves to shatter the stones), have been tried with varying degrees of success on a select group of patients. The criteria for using these methods, however, are very strict; removal of the gallbladder is still the method of choice in most cases. Since the gallbladder is not necessary to maintain life, some doctors suggest removing a gallbladder containing stones even if they are not causing symptoms. However, unless there are extenuating circumstances, this is becoming a less common practice.

See also Bile and Cholecystitis.

# Gamma globulin

Gamma globulin preparations are derived from the blood of a person or animal and contain antibodies made by that person or animal in response to invasion by harmful agents, such as bacteria and viruses. These preparations are widely used for the prevention, modification, diagnosis, and treatment of many kinds of infectious diseases.

Gamma globulin is usually injected. Since it contains almost all the antibodies in the blood, it can provide passive (borrowed) immunity that lasts for about six weeks.

Gamma globulin injections may be useful in preventing infectious hepatitis when given—within about two weeks of exposure—to individuals who have been in intimate contact with someone with hepatitis. Many physicians recommend that persons traveling to underdeveloped countries, particularly rural areas, receive doses of gamma globulin before departure and during an extended stay.

Measles can often be prevented by the administration of gamma globulin injections within five days of exposure. The injections are especially important for children under three years of age, for pregnant women, for tuberculosis patients, and for those with impaired immune mechanisms. Even if measles is not prevented, a less serious case may result; however, gamma globulin is of no use once the symptoms have appeared.

Gamma globulin level in the body can also be used as a diagnostic tool. For example, one sign of multiple sclerosis is an elevated level of gamma globulin in the cerebrospinal fluid.

# Gangrene

Gangrene is a term that refers to the death of body tissue due to diminishment or loss of blood supply, leading to nutrient and oxygen deprivation. There are three major types of gangrene: moist, dry, and gas gangrene. Although gangrene usually affects the extremities of the body, it can sometimes affect the internal organs.

Moist gangrene is generally caused by a sudden stoppage of blood flow to a body site, usually resulting from burning by heat or by acid, from severe freezing, from a physical accident that destroys the tissues, from keeping a tourniquet in place too long, or from a blood clot or other blockage. The tissue death that results

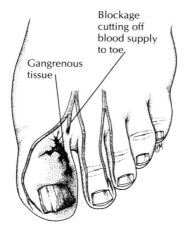

Gangrene is the death of tissue due to lack of blood circulation to an area, often in one of the extremities.

from loss of blood supply is accompanied by decomposition due to bacterial action. The gangrenous infection is likely to spread rapidly as toxins (poisons) are formed in the affected tissues and absorbed.

Dry gangrene usually occurs gradually and results from a slow, progressive reduction of blood flow in the arteries. There is generally no bacterial decomposition; the tissues simply become dry and shriveled. This type of gangrene occurs only in the extremities. It may occur as a secondary effect of arteriosclerosis in the elderly, of advanced stages of diabetes, or of Buerger's disease (an inflammatory condition that affects the blood vessels of the limbs, primarily the legs).

Gas gangrene is often caused by infection of a wound by anaerobic (able to live without air) bacteria, which are commonly found in soil. It can follow rapidly after contamination of deep wounds. The bacteria break down tissues, giving off gas and toxic by-products.

Gangrene in an internal organ can be caused by any condition that cuts off blood supply to an area. For example, if a loop of intestine is caught in an opening in the abdominal wall, the blood supply to that part of the intestine may be cut off (causing what is called a strangulated hernia), and gangrene may then occur in that section of the tissue. In acute appendicitis, areas of gangrene may occur in the walls of the appendix, with rupture of the appendix through the gangrenous area. In severe cholecystitis (inflammation of the gallbladder, usually associated with gallstones), gangrene can develop in areas where the stones compress the mucous membrane, cutting off the blood supply.

Moist gangrene is characterized by a purplish-red, bruised appearance; by swelling; and, often, by blisters.

Dry gangrene is marked by gradual shrinking of the tissues, which first grow cold and lack a pulse, then turn brown, then black. Usually there is a sharp line of demarcation where the gangrene stops because the unaffected tissue nearby is continuing to receive blood. This type of gangrene is sometimes called mummification of tissue because of the dry, shriveled, and dark appearance.

The initial symptoms of gas gangrene are swelling, paleness of skin, and a thin, bloody (but not foul) discharge. The characteristic foul smell comes later in the progression of this form of the disorder. It is an acute, painful condition in which the muscles and tissues under the skin become filled with gas and a thin, brownish-black fluid.

Symptoms of gangrene in an internal organ may include pain, tenderness over the organ, and fever.

The appearance of the affected area usually suggests the diagnosis to the physician. Laboratory analysis of a tissue specimen will allow the identification of the infective microorganism, which is necessary for selection of an appropriate antibiotic.

Areas of gas gangrene may be seen on X-ray studies.

Treatment of gangrene generally involves cleaning of the area and administration of antibiotics. The effectiveness of antibiotic therapy seems to depend on the time elapsed between injury or infection and the beginning of treatment.

In the case of gangrene caused by deterioration in the blood supply of the elderly or gangrene associated with appendicitis, hernia, diabetes, or Buerger's disease, the treatment begins with the diagnosis and treatment of the underlying condition.

Preventing gangrene in an open wound begins with cleanliness. All dirt and particles in an open wound should be removed as soon as possible, and the wound should be cleansed with a soap solution and water. Burned skin requires careful, antiseptic handling to avoid infection. Frostbite also is dangerous because freezing impairs the circulation of the skin, making it tender and easily damaged. Frostbitten skin, especially on the fingers, toes, and earlobes, must be handled with great care to avoid gangrenous infections.

See also Frostbite.

---

# Gastric bypass

See Coronary bypass surgury.

---

# Gastroenteritis

Gastroenteritis is an inflammation of the lining of the stomach and the intestines.

Gastroenteritis can be caused by bacteria or viruses; by allergic reactions to certain foods or drinks; by infectious diseases, such as typhoid fever and influenza; by food poison-ing; by overconsumption of alcohol; or by certain drugs.

Symptoms include headache, nausea, vomiting, diarrhea, and gas pains in the stomach and the intestines. Often, the individual will feel that gas is "caught" in certain portions of the intestine. On occasion, cramps can possibly produce severe pain.

The first task in treating gastroenteritis is to identify the cause or causes of the inflammation. Blood tests and cultures for viruses or bacteria may be done. If the problem is caused by an allergic reaction, the source of the reaction may sometimes be identified by allergy tests.

Antibiotics can be used to treat bacterial infections. A variety of medicines (many of them nonprescription) can ease the effects of stomach cramps and gas pains. Diarrhea may necessitate replacement of lost fluids. Elderly or extremely ill persons may have to be hospitalized for intravenous replacement of fluids.

Maintaining a clean kitchen, eating in restaurants where the kitchens are kept clean, washing fresh foods thoroughly, and cooking foods carefully are all safeguards against bacterial and viral infections. Identification of allergy-causing foods and moderation in alcohol consumption also help prevent gastroenteritis, if these are the causes of the problem.

---

# Genes

The genes are the basic units that determine the hereditary (inborn) characteristics of an organism. Genes, which are composed of molecules of deoxyribonucleic acid (DNA), can be thought of as chemical instructions. Each gene, by virtue of the particular structure of its DNA molecule, contains the code for a specific trait, determining both what a cell is and how it works (as if a computer program not only told the computer what to do but helped to form the machine itself).

Within each cell, thousands of genes are linked in a specific order, like beads on a necklace, to form structures called chromosomes, which are, in effect, continuous strands of DNA. It has been estimated that each cell contains about five feet of coiled DNA strands and that each strand is made of about 100,000 genes.

The particular composition of the genes and their arrangement on the chromosomes are what constitute the genetic blueprint for each individual. Cells that develop into liver tissue, rather than blood cells or nerve fibers, for example, do so because that is what their genetic coding dictates. In this way, the cells of the body are programmed to create a person with a certain color of eyes and hair, as well as the hundreds of thousands of other characteristics that make each human being unique.

Each cell in the human body contains 46 chromosomes. The only exceptions are the sex cells—the ovum (egg) and the sperm—each of which contains only 23 chromosomes. When these sex cells unite in the fertilization of the ovum by a sperm, the result is a full complement of 46 chromosomes, with genes donated by both parents. Since each parent contributes only 23 chromosomes (half of the genetic coding that makes each parent a unique individual), the genetic makeup of their offspring is a blend of components of the genetic material derived from both parents.

The traits that genes give rise to may be either dominant or recessive. A recessive gene is one that produces a certain trait only if its effects are not overridden by those of a dominant gene.

Eye color provides a relatively straightforward illustration of how inheritance of traits works. The gene for brown eyes is dominant; the gene for blue eyes is recessive. The child of a brown-eyed parent who has two brown-eye genes and a blue-eyed parent (who must have two blue-eye genes) will have brown eyes because the brown-eyed parent has only dominant brown-eye genes. However, if the brown-eyed parent has a dominant brown-eye gene and a recessive blue-eye gene, the child has a fifty-fifty chance of receiving a blue-eye gene from each parent and thereby having blue eyes. (Actually, inheritance does not always work with such textbook simplicity—sometimes the child of a brown-eyed parent and a blue-eyed parent will have green or hazel eyes.) The union of two blue-eyed persons, because it involves only recessive blue-eye genes, will always produce blue-eyed offspring. The offspring of two brown-eyed persons who each have a recessive blue-eye gene have a one-in-four chance of receiving a blue-eye gene from each parent and, as a result, having blue eyes. (This final combination illustrates how recessive genes can be present but unsuspected, allowing a trait to appear unexpectedly after skipping generations.)

Genes are normally transmitted unchanged from one generation to the next. Sometimes, however, mutations occur—that is, the structure of the gene itself is changed, perhaps due to the effect of a toxic substance, an infection, or exposure to radiation. Offspring that receive a mutated gene will exhibit a characteristic that is not present in either parent.

The discovery of the structure of the DNA molecule opened a new era in medical research. Scientists in the new field of genetic engineering are exploring ways of artificially creating mutations in genes so that someday it may be possible to correct the errors in genetic coding that cause various disorders.

As the medical profession has learned more about inherited diseases, it has been able to offer genetic counseling to couples concerned about the possibility of having a child with an inherited disease or abnormality. A genetic counselor or specialist in genetic disorders can estimate the likelihood that a couple's offspring will be afflicted with a problem due to an inherited trait or to the age of the parents. For some genetic disorders, tests can determine whether one or both parents are carriers or can detect whether a defect is present in a fetus. However, genetic counseling cannot guarantee the health of a child; it can only be a source of advice.

# Genital warts

Genital warts (known medically as condylomata acuminata) are viral growths that appear on the external genital organs. The condition is considered to be a sexually transmitted disease.

If left untreated, genital warts can grow quite large, causing discomfort during sexual intercourse, urination, and bowel movements. They are seen more frequently in uncircumcised men than in those who have been circumcised. Scientists now believe that some viruses that cause genital warts may, over a period of several years, lead to the development of certain genital tumors such as cancer of the cervix and cancer of the penis.

Pregnancy may make genital warts grow faster, but they usually shrink after the baby is born. They may even become large enough during pregnancy to block the birth canal, making a cesarean (through an incision in the walls of the uterus and abdomen) delivery necessary. The wart virus can be transmitted from a mother to her child during birth, sometimes causing the development of warts within the throat of the baby.

Genital warts are caused by direct sexual contact with an infected person. About 60 percent of all those exposed to genital warts will develop the condition. However, the warts will not appear until six weeks to eight months after the initial exposure.

The only symptom of genital warts is the warts themselves, which appear most frequently on the penis, vagina, vulva (the structure surrounding the vagina), and anus. They may also be found in the mouth or on the cervix. They are soft, moist, and pink, occurring alone or in clusters; cluster formations tend to resemble cauliflower in their uneven, puffy appearance. They are seldom painful, but they can be irritated by sexual intercourse; in fact, they often grow on the parts of the sex organs that receive the most friction during sexual intercourse.

Genital warts can usually be diagnosed by a simple physical examination because their appearance is so distinctive. If there is any doubt, a sample of tissue from the wart can be tested to rule out other disorders, such as cancerous growths or the warts that often accompany syphilis (another sexually transmitted disease). Sometimes a magnifying instrument called a colposcope is used to detect small warts that are not visible to the naked eye.

Small genital warts are treated with a drug called podophyllin, which is applied directly to the warts and then washed off several hours later. More than one application may be necessary. Podophyllin, however, is toxic in large doses. Another agent used to treat genital warts is trichloroacetic acid. Like podophyllin, it is applied directly to the wart. Trichloroacetic acid, however, does not need to be washed off after application. It is not toxic, but care must be used in application because chemical burns of normal skin may occur. Very large or persistent warts are often removed by cryotherapy (a process in which liquid nitrogen is used to freeze the growths, which then fall off); by heat treatments, which dry out and destroy the warts; or by laser therapy, which literally vaporizes the growths.

A person who has genital warts or any other sexually transmitted disease should abstain from sexual activity until all tests have indicated that the disease is no longer present. As is the case with all other sexually transmitted diseases, every sexual partner of the infected person needs to be examined and, if necessary, treated.

Genital warts can be prevented by avoiding sexual contact with someone who has the condition. Because the chances of contracting this and other venereal diseases increase with the number of sexual partners a person has, limiting the number of partners is the first step in prevention. Using condoms also helps to reduce the risk of contracting genital warts.

# Gilles de la Tourette's syndrome

Gilles de la Tourette's syndrome is a neuromuscular disorder marked by intense tics (twitchy, repetitive movements of certain muscles). It occurs most often in boys. It generally begins around the age of seven or eight years. At first the tics are simple: facial twisting, blinking, grimacing, shoulder shrugging, or twitching. Later the tics progress to vocal tics accompanied by psychological involvement.

The causes of Gilles de la Tourette's syndrome are unknown. It is still disputed whether the disorder is of physical or psychological origin.

The symptoms of Gilles de la Tourette's syndrome are at first limited to the muscles in the face, head, neck, and shoulders. Often, the first symptom is a characteristic breathing noise from the larynx (voice box), as if the patient were barking, wheezing, or gasping for air. As the tics spread to the shoulders and arms, there are shoulder shrugs and twitches, as well as twisting of the neck and arms. Vocal tics, such as grunting, snuffing, shouting, and barking sounds, then begin to develop. As the vocal symptoms worsen, the patient begins to exclaim in a loud voice words or phrases with obscene meanings or "swear words." Echolalia (repetition by the patient of words that have been said to him or her) is common. The patient will seem to fixate on a word or phrase and repeat it over and over with increasing speed. Often, too, the individual will spasmodically and automatically repeat or mimic the actions of those nearby.

The symptoms of Gilles de la Tourette's syndrome tend to come and go, especially as the patient approaches puberty and adulthood. Tics that are very violent during waking hours often stop during sleep. Some tics are intensified by emotional upheavals. The tics of Gilles de la Tourette's syndrome, unlike those of most neuromuscular disorders, are often suppressed in school or social settings and expressed more often when the patient is alone or with family members. In some cases, the tics can be controlled voluntarily. The excessive swearing, however, occurs only in the presence of others; some patients attempt to cover it up by coughing, thus developing another tic. Often symptoms decrease in adult life and disappear, only to return during a period of stress. Mental activity remains normal.

Diagnosing Gilles de la Tourette's syndrome is often difficult, since symptoms in the early stages often resemble common childhood tics seen in many young school-age children. Also, early- and middle-stage symptoms are difficult to distinguish from those of certain brain conditions. However, Gilles de la Tourette's syndrome can often be diagnosed with some assurance as the course of the illness unfolds.

Gilles de la Tourette's syndrome can be treated with medications starting with small doses and increasing the dosage until the tics are controlled. Often a combination of drugs is used. Group psychotherapy can be helpful in some cases. In extreme cases, leukotomy (surgical interruption of white nerve fibers of the frontal lobe of the brain) is considered. There are no known preventive measures.

# Glaucoma

Glaucoma is an eye disorder caused by increased pressure within the eyeball, which builds up because fluids are unable to drain normally.

Although glaucoma is understood to be a problem with the fluid-regulating mechanism of the eye, its precise cause is unknown. In the healthy eye, aqueous fluid in the anterior chamber of the eyeball (between the lens and the cornea) is under a slight degree of pressure. If the delicate fluid balance changes, internal pressure rises in the eye. This buildup produces damage to the sensitive structures and the nerve endings within the eye.

Depending on the type of defect in the fluid-regulating system, one of

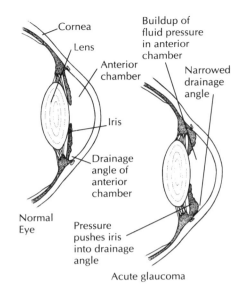

Acute glaucoma

In acute glaucoma, normal drainage of aqueous fluid may be obstructed by a sudden elevation of pressure within the anterior chamber of the eye, which pushes the iris into the angle where the iris meets the cornea.

two primary forms of glaucoma results. *Chronic*, or *open angle*, *glaucoma* develops when pressure is elevated gradually, and normal fluid drainage slows but is not obstructed at the drainage angle (the network of tissue between the iris and the cornea, through which fluid can normally pass). *Acute*, or *closed angle*, *glaucoma* occurs when pressure mounts suddenly and forces the iris into contact with the cornea, thereby blocking fluid drainage from the anterior chamber of the eye.

Both forms of glaucoma are more common in adults over 40 years of age. Statistics indicate that people with a family history of glaucoma have a greater risk of acquiring the condition, but inheritance has not been proved. Some evidence suggests that glaucoma may be linked to long-term use of certain drugs, especially steroids, which can alter body fluid levels. Glaucoma can also follow other eye disorders, such as infections and cataracts.

Chronic glaucoma begins with no noticeable symptoms. Vision deterioration is so gradual and painless that this form of glaucoma has been termed the "sneak thief of sight." Sometimes, loss of peripheral vision slowly progresses as central vision remains normal. As the disorder advances, other symptoms (which may be intermittent or constant) include foggy or blurred vision, difficulty in adjusting to brightness and darkness, and slight pain in or around

Untreated glaucoma can cause progressive loss of vision. View 1 is what is seen if glaucoma is properly treated and there is no vision loss. View 2 shows some loss of side vision that occurs with untreated glaucoma. View 3 shows serious loss of side vision with advanced untreated glaucoma.

the eye, usually on one side. The one symptom indicative of chronic glaucoma is the perception of a faint white circle or halo surrounding a light, which is most easily visible when looking at a distant light while in the dark.

Acute glaucoma brings sudden and severe symptoms of extreme eye pain and abrupt vision blurring. Frequently, the pain can be so intense that it causes nausea and vomiting. Fortunately, acute glaucoma is rare, but when it does occur, medical attention is needed immediately in order to prevent permanent blindness. Usually, the symptoms are so severe that medical help is promptly sought.

If left untreated, glaucoma can lead to partial or complete vision loss. However, if diagnosed early, treatment can usually halt the process. Because chronic glaucoma has no warning signs, it is particularly important that persons over the age of 40 be tested for glaucoma every two or three years. In addition, physicians recommend that persons with a family history of the disease be screened for glaucoma every year beginning even before the age of 40.

Glaucoma testing is a relatively simple office procedure. The doctor uses a special device called a tonometer to measure the amount of pressure within the eyeball. The doctor also inspects the interior of the eye through an instrument that allows a view of the angle where the iris and the cornea meet. This part of the examination shows whether there is blockage in the drainage system or damage to the optic nerve. Peripheral vision is also tested by measuring the point at which objects enter the patient's field of vision.

Glaucoma treatment is usually effective if started early in the course of the disease. Oral drugs work by decreasing production of eye fluid, while daily applications of eyedrops promote fluid drainage. Because some medications cause constriction of the pupils of the eyes, which can be misconstrued as a symptom of drug overdose, many glaucoma patients carry an identification card that describes their medical history in case of emergency.

Beta-blocker eyedrops reduce production of eye fluid without altering the size of the pupil. However, beta blockers can affect the heart rate and cause narrowing of the breathing passages, which may make these drugs unsuitable for patients with heart or respiratory disease. Other antiglaucoma medications are available.

Although chronic glaucoma responds to medication, some patients (fewer than five percent) require surgery to open new pathways for fluid drainage. Laser therapy is a relatively new surgical technique under investigation. The laser uses an intense light beam to slightly modify tissues in the region in order to allow better fluid drainage.

The best way to prevent serious complications of glaucoma is to undergo periodic screening for early diagnosis.

# Glomerulonephritis

Each kidney contains more than a million filtering units called nephrons, in which wastes are drawn from the blood to form urine. In each nephron is a network of capillaries (tiny blood vessels) called a glomerulus. Glomerulitis is an inflammation of the glomeruli (the plural of glomerulus), which interferes with the normal functioning of the kidney. First described in 1827 by the English physician Richard Bright, the condition used to be called Bright's disease, but doctors today are more likely to refer to it as glomerulonephritis (from *glomerulus; nephro*, referring to the kidney; and *itis*, meaning inflammation).

Glomerulonephritis can be caused by an infection in the kidneys, but most often it is due to an allergic or immune response to infections in other parts of the body. Although many different kinds of infections can lead to glomerulonephritis, including pneumonia, bacterial infection of the heart, syphilis, malaria, hepatitis, and measles, the most common cause is infection of the throat, tonsils, or skin by certain types of *Streptococcus* bacteria. The immune response to the infection occurs as an inflammation of the capillaries in the glomeruli. The capillaries become congested and surrounded by blood cells and pus. Fluid builds up in surrounding tissues, sometimes causing the kidneys to enlarge. Protein, which should remain in the blood, is discharged into the urine through the diseased glomeruli, and there is edema (fluid buildup) in

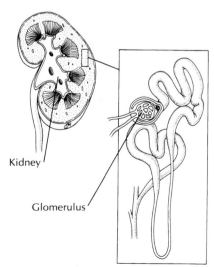

Glomerulonephritis is an inflammation of the tiny blood vessels of the glomeruli, the kidney's filtering units that draw wastes from the blood to form urine.

body tissues. These two signs—edema and the presence of albumin (a type of protein) in the urine—are the chief indicators of the disease.

If the disease continues to progress, the tiny arteries in the kidneys become thickened and scarred so that some can no longer carry blood. The parts of the kidneys that they serve shrink. The eventual result of this process over many years may be total kidney failure. The disease affects both kidneys.

Symptoms of glomerulonephritis usually begin one to three weeks after an initial infection, such as strep throat. The patient has headaches, a mild fever, a puffy face, pain in the area between the ribs and the hips, and decreased urine output. The urine may be bloody, smoky, or coffee-colored. Shortness of breath may occur, together with increased heartbeat and a rise in blood pressure. Detection of protein and red blood cells in the urine confirms the diagnosis. In extreme cases, bloating due to accumulation of fluids can cause the symptoms of heart failure, including rapid heartbeat, heart enlargement, and congestion of the lungs.

Treatment consists of antibiotics if strep are still present, and rest and symptomatic treatment until one to two weeks after tests of blood, blood pressure, and urine indicate that the kidneys are back to normal. Sodium and protein may be restricted or even forbidden for a time. Fluids are restricted until the output of urine returns to normal. Heart failure is treated with restriction of salt and water and with use of oxygen and medications. Any infection is treated promptly with antibiotics. The overwhelming majority of patients with glomerulonephritis due to streptococcal infection recover fully.

Guarding against infection, injury, and fatigue can help prevent flare-ups of the disease. Intake of protein may have to be limited, depending on how well the kidneys are working. A return to normal activity is desirable, but strenuous exercise should be avoided, to prevent fatigue.

If the disease is still present after one to two years, it may be considered chronic. This occurs in five percent to 20 percent of patients. Typically, the damage to the kidneys continues to progress, but so slowly that the patient is without symptoms; the only evidence may be the presence of protein and red and white blood cells in the urine. A normal life may be possible for 20 or 30 years, until the kidneys can no longer function. At that time, replacement with a kidney transplant or dialysis is necessary.

There are also many types of glomerulonephritis other than that due to strep; their treatment and prognosis vary significantly.

# Glossitis

Glossitis is an acute (short-term) or chronic (long-term) inflammation of the tongue. It may exist either as a primary disease or as a symptom of another disease or disorder.

The causes of glossitis can be either local or systemic (affecting the entire body). Local causes include immediate irritants, such as jagged or broken teeth, badly fitting dentures, poor oral hygiene habits, biting of the tongue (such as during convulsions), and external irritants, such as alcohol, tobacco, hot or spicy foods, and even mouthwashes, toothpastes, and breath fresheners. Local infections, burns, and injuries may also produce symptoms of glossitis. Systemic causes may include certain vitamin deficiencies (especially vitamin B deficiencies, such as pellagra), anemia, syphilis, and generalized skin diseases.

Symptoms vary widely, ranging from simple redness of the tip and edges of the tongue (if the cause is pellagra, anemia, or irritation from smoking or a tooth with a rough surface) to painful ulcers and whitish patches. In the later stages of pellagra, the entire tongue may be fiery red, swollen, and ulcerated. In iron deficiency and pernicious anemia, the tongue is pale and smooth. Painful ulcers on the tongue may indicate a number of diseases, including herpes, tuberculosis, and streptococcal infection. White patches suggest candidiasis (a type of yeast infection), syphilis, or simple mouth breathing (which dries out the mucous membrane of the tongue). Very smooth and painless areas may be what is called geographic tongue, or benign (harmless) glossitis. So-called hairy tongue often follows antibiotic therapy, a high fever, excessive use of certain mouthwashes, or a simple reduction in saliva secretion.

Severe acute glossitis, which can result from local infection, burns, and injury, can cause tenderness, pain, and swelling sufficient to make the tongue protrude from the mouth into the back of the throat—creating the danger of airway obstruction and even suffocation. In severe cases, the patient may not be able to chew, swallow, or speak. Steroid drug treatment usually reduces the swelling and helps relieve symptoms.

Patients may also complain of a painful burning tongue without other symptoms of inflammation. This is a common complaint among postmenopausal women. Diabetes, anemia, nutritional deficiencies, and malignant conditions should all be considered as possible underlying causes.

The patient should be reassured that redness and most lesions of the tongue are usually harmless and respond well to treatment. Such complaints as ulcers and hairy tongue often recur periodically; however, if an ulcer does not respond to treatment after several weeks, a biopsy (removal of a tissue sample for examination under a microscope) may be performed.

In treating glossitis, specific causes, such as jagged teeth and ill-fitting dentures, should be corrected. Irritants, including hot or spicy foods, tobacco, alcohol, mouthwashes, and toothpastes, should be avoided once they have been identified as the source of the trouble. A bland or liquid diet, preferably one that is cool or cold, will often have a soothing effect. Good oral hygiene is necessary in all cases.

Tiny brown growths on the tongue are usually caused by contact with tobacco or certain bacteria; the treatment is to stop smoking or otherwise correct the underlying cause and also to brush the tongue with a toothbrush.

Symptomatic relief for large lesions includes rinsing the mouth with a medicated mouthwash before meals. Application of topical anesthetics, such as lidocaine and benzocaine, can also bring relief. Patients with complaints of painful burning should be tested to rule out vitamin $B_{12}$ deficiency, diabetes, and some types of anemia.

Prevention of glossitis involves avoiding irritants, correcting nutritional and vitamin deficiencies, and treating any primary infections that produce glossitis as a secondary symptom.

# Goiter

A goiter is an enlargement of the thyroid gland, which appears as a swelling at the front of the neck.

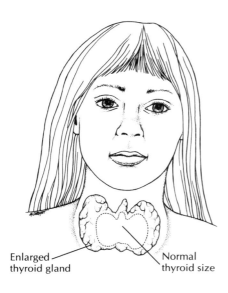

Enlarged thyroid gland

Normal thyroid size

A goiter is an enlargement of the thyroid gland, which appears as a swelling at the front of the neck.

Goiter may be caused by a lack of dietary iodine, which is necessary for the production of thyroid hormone. In this case, the thyroid gland enlarges in an attempt to satisfy the body's demand for more hormone. When this happens, the cells in the gland enlarge but they do not increase in number.

At one time, goiter was common in areas where there is a lack of iodine in the soil and water. Since the ocean is the basic source of iodine, inland areas were the most deficient (in the United States, the Great Lakes region was such an area; in Europe, inhabitants of mountainous inland regions in the Alps often had an iodine deficiency). In recent times, however, the use of iodized table salt has solved this problem to a great extent.

Some forms of goiter are associated with an overactive thyroid gland, that is, one that produces more hormone than the body needs.

Often, the only symptom is the swelling in the neck. If the thyroid is active, nervousness, weight loss, bulging eyes, rapid heartbeat, and high blood pressure may be noted. If the thyroid is underactive, sluggishness, weight gain, dry skin and hair, and fatigue may be present.

The diagnosis is made primarily on the basis of the classic appearance and the dietary history of the patient. Blood tests to determine the concentration of thyroid hormones and a nuclear medicine study of the thyroid may be performed to rule out more serious thyroid disorders.

The chief objective of goiter treatment is reduction of the swelling. The first step is usually to suppress the overfunctioning of the thyroid gland. If the goiter is caused by simple iodine deficiency, small doses of iodine can be given. Sometimes, administering synthetic thyroid hormone, in an attempt to halt the increased efforts by the gland to produce the natural hormone, will reduce the enlargement. If treatment is started early enough, surgery to remove portions of the enlarged gland can possibly be avoided. Surgery may be necessary if the size of the goiter interferes with normal breathing.

See also Hyperthyroidism and Hypothyroidism.

# Gonorrhea

Gonorrhea is one of the most frequently reported sexually transmitted diseases. It is a highly contagious bacterial infection, spread primarily through direct sexual contact between individuals.

Gonorrhea predominantly affects the penis in men, the vagina in women, and the throat and anus in both sexes. Left untreated, it can lead to a generalized blood infection, sterility (inability to conceive children), arthritis, and heart trouble. Additionally, in men it can spread throughout the prostate gland and the ducts of the reproductive system, causing painful inflammation.

Gonorrhea can also lead to eye infections if the genital secretions come in contact with the eyes—for instance, if a person rubs his or her eyes after handling infected genital organs. Because the infant passes through the potentially infected birth canal during the birth process, every state requires that a few drops of silver nitrate or penicillin be placed in the eyes of all newborns to prevent infection and possible blindness.

In females, this disease may exist entirely without symptoms, but in many cases it is marked by a discharge from the vagina and urethra and by frequent, painful urination. Gonorrhea often leads to pelvic inflammatory disease (PID), which results when the infection extends to the fallopian tubes; scar tissue that forms may block the tubes, preventing conception and often

causing sterility. The symptoms of PID include the following: lower abdominal pain, fever, chills, vaginal discharge, and vomiting.

The primary symptom of gonorrhea in men is a yellowish discharge from the penis within two to ten days of exposure to the disease, accompanied by painful and burning urination.

Gonorrhea of the anus is marked by an often bloody or mucus-filled discharge from the anus and pain during bowel movements. Gonorrhea of the throat may have no noticeable symptoms or may reveal itself only as a scratchy, sore throat or a severe, flame-red, sore throat.

Diagnosis is accomplished by taking a sample of the discharge, examining it under a microscope to identify the gonorrhea bacterium, and confirming the diagnosis by performing a culture (a technique in which the sample of the discharge is placed in a special substance that encourages the growth of bacteria).

Gonorrhea is usually treated with penicillin or tetracycline, either injected or taken orally.

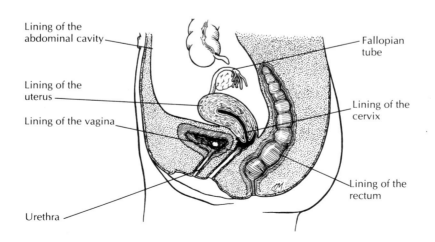

In females, untreated gonorrhea may spread to various sites in the pelvic area, causing pelvic inflammatory disease and perhaps sterility.

Vas deferens

Bladder

Urethra

Testis

Prostate gland

Epididymis

In males untreated gonorrhea may involve the prostate gland, the male duct system (including the epididymis, which connects each testis to its vas deferens, and the vas deferens, which conducts the sperm cells to the urethra), the bladder, and the urethra.

Men being treated for gonorrhea should avoid alcoholic beverages. This is due to the fact that recent studies have shown that drinking may increase the chances of developing an inflammation of the urethra (the canal leading from the bladder through the penis).

While under treatment, the patient should abstain from sexual activity until further tests have confirmed that gonorrhea is no longer present. This testing is usually done two weeks after the beginning of treatment. If signs of the disease are still present at that time, a different antibiotic can be administered.

A culture to detect a chlamydia infection is usually performed along with the culture to detect gonorrhea (since symptoms of the two infections are the same). If chlamydia is found, it will be treated with the antibiotic tetracycline.

Every sexual partner of the infected person should be examined and, if necessary, treated.

Gonorrhea can be prevented by avoiding sexual contact with someone who has the disease. Because the chance of contracting this and other venereal diseases increases with the number of sexual partners, limiting the number of partners is the first step in prevention. Using condoms helps to reduce the risk of contracting gonorrhea.

See also Nongonococcal urethritis and Pelvic inflammatory disease.

# Gout

Gout is a form of recurrent acute arthritis. Most gout victims are middle-aged men. Women are also affected by gout, but usually this occurs only after menopause.

The underlying cause of gout is a defect in the body's processing of uric acid, a chemical normally found in the blood and urine. If the body does not properly process uric acid, the level of uric acid in the blood becomes elevated. The excess uric acid may crystallize and become deposited in and around the joints

Degenerative joint changes

Uric acid deposits

Gout is an extremely painful condition caused by an excess of uric acid in the blood that leads to deposits of uric acid crystals in the joints. The big toe joint is commonly affected, and changes within the joint can occur if the condition is not treated.

and their tendons. An acute attack of gout is caused by the body's inflammatory response to the deposits of uric acid crystals.

The high levels of uric acid can also lead to deposition of crystals in areas of the body other than the joints. Most notably the skin and the kidneys could be affected. Uric acid deposits in the kidneys may form kidney stones. About 20 percent of patients with chronic gout also have kidney stones. In the event that the kidneys become blocked by stones, kidney failure may result.

Gout usually first appears as a sudden and extremely painful attack in a single joint, usually the big toe. Later attacks can involve several joints, such as the ankle, knee, wrist, and elbow. The pain, which commonly begins at night during sleep, may occur without warning or may be preceded by excessive alcohol consumption or unusual exercise ear-

lier in the day. The pain grows in intensity and is often described as throbbing or crushing. Inflammation follows, with swelling, warmth, redness, and tenderness over the affected joint. The pain is sometimes so severe that the individual cannot even tolerate a weight as slight as that of a bed sheet over the joint. Other symptoms that may accompany the joint pain and swelling include fever, rapid heartbeat, chills, and an overall feeling of being unwell. Uric acid deposits in the skin may be observed as white lumps under the skin; these lumps most often appear in the hands, the feet, the elbows, and the rims of the outer ears.

The first attacks usually last only a few days, but if the disorder goes untreated, later attacks may last for weeks. Symptoms eventually disappear, and joint function returns to normal between attacks. As the course of the disease progresses, the periods of remission become shorter and shorter as more and more attacks occur each year.

The treatment of gout is twofold—to relieve the symptoms of an acute attack and to prevent recurrences. The drug colchicine has traditionally been used to relieve a gout attack, but nonsteroidal anti-inflammatory drugs are now more often prescribed to relieve the inflammation and pain. These drugs are quite effective. However, they do have side effects, so they should be used only under close and continuous medical supervision.

Once the acute attack is under control, prevention of future attacks is the main goal. This can be done with the drug allopurinol, which interferes with the production of uric acid and thus prevents the deposition of uric acid crystals in the body. Allopurinol usually has to be taken for long periods of time to maintain normal blood levels of uric acid.

There are also other drugs, called uricosurics, that speed up the excretion of uric acid by the kidneys. These drugs, however, may not be used if there is known kidney damage or if the uric acid content of the urine is high.

# Gynecomastia

Gynecomastia is excessive development of the breasts in a male. Breast enlargement is a normal, short-term occurrence in some newborn boys, whose breasts enlarge in response to female hormones they receive from their mother during pregnancy. The condition may also appear at puberty, when a boy's body is undergoing normal hormonal changes.

In most cases, gynecomastia is the result of too much estrogen (a female sex hormone) in the male's body. Breast enlargement at birth and at puberty usually occurs because the estrogen level has not yet adjusted to normal (both females and males normally have estrogen in their bodies). Abnormal gynecomastia occurs when some condition, such as a tumor of one of the testes or an estrogen-secreting tumor of one of the adrenal glands, results in abnormally high levels of estrogen. Medications are also a frequent cause.

In addition to the obvious enlargement of the breasts, symptoms may include tenderness in the breasts and, in extreme cases, secretion of milk.

Gynecomastia should always be brought to the attention of a doctor. It is especially important that tumors of the adrenal glands or testes be ruled out or treated. Such tumors are usually removed surgically. In severe or prolonged cases, the excess breast tissue can be removed by plastic surgery, with little visible scarring. In most cases, patients can be reassured that the condition is normal and temporary. Especially in need of such reassurance are teenage boys, who are often embarrassed and fearful that they are abnormal.

# H

# Hay fever

Hay fever is the name for acute (short-lived), seasonal attacks that are the result of allergic reactions to pollen. Most often, spring attacks are reactions to tree pollen; summer attacks are reactions to grass pollen; and autumn attacks are reactions to weed pollen.

The symptoms of hay fever are usually the same, regardless of the allergen (irritating substance). Common symptoms include itching of the nose and roof of the mouth; a thin, watery discharge constantly draining from the nose; itchy, watery eyes; sneezing; headache; irritability; a feeling of exhaustion; insomnia; loss of appetite; and, in advanced cases, coughing and wheezing.

Hay fever, as with other allergies, is diagnosed by identifying the allergen. This is done by taking a medical history and reviewing the patient's environment, daily habits, and recent changes in lifestyle. Skin tests and blood tests may also be performed. These include scratch tests, in which a small amount of the suspected allergen is applied to a scratch on the skin. There are also intracutaneous tests, in which a small amount of the allergen is injected in or under the skin. Finally, there is radioallergosorbent testing, a procedure by which antibodies developed in response to specific allergens are measured in a blood sample.

A severe case of hay fever may be best treated by changing the environment, that is, by removing the allergen causing the trouble or reducing the patient's exposure to it. Those who react to weed pollen may need to move to a more urban location with a lower concentration of pollen in the air. Many hay fever sufferers will benefit from using an air conditioner, which filters the air and thus keeps pollen levels in the home to a minimum.

Several medications are available for the hay fever sufferer: oral antihistamines, which counteract the histamine that is released by the body in reaction to the allergen; corticosteroids, which reduce inflammation; eyedrops, which relieve itching and redness; and desensitization shots, which cause the body to develop tolerance to the allergen.

There is no way to prevent hay fever, but avoiding the allergen as much as possible may at least help to relieve some of the discomfort.

See also Headaches.

---

# Headaches

A headache is a symptom, not a disease. A headache is rarely the symptom of a serious illness, but severe or frequent headaches can be exhausting and can affect daily life.

There are three basic types of headaches. The *vascular headache* occurs when blood vessels in the head enlarge and press on nerves, causing pain. The most common vascular headache is the migraine. The second type of headache is the *muscle contraction headache*, which results when the muscles of the face, neck, or scalp contract and tighten. A tension headache is an example of a muscle contraction headache. The third kind of headache is the *inflammatory headache*. Such a headache is the result of pressure within the head. The causes range from relatively minor conditions, such as sinusitis, to more serious problems, such as brain tumors.

A more detailed description of each type of headache follows.

**Vascular headache (migraine)** One theory about migraine headaches is that they occur when the blood vessels in the head expand and press on the nerves, causing pain. Another theory states that they result when the blood vessels first overreact to outside stimuli by constricting and thus blocking blood flow to parts of the brain; this may cause the visual impairment and numbness that often accompany or precede a migraine headache. The blood vessels then become full of blood and press on surrounding nerves, causing pain.

Women are more prone to migraines than are men, and a certain personality type—compulsive, perfectionist, excessively neat, and very success-oriented—seems to be more susceptible to this kind of headache.

A migraine headache occurs when the blood vessels in the head expand and press on the nerves, causing pain.

A number of physical and emotional factors may contribute to migraine headaches. Migraines may be triggered by a sharp reduction in caffeine intake or by allergies to certain foods or food additives (among them chocolate, coffee, fatty foods, alcohol, citrus fruits, monosodium glutamate, and nitrates). Emotional stress can also cause migraine headaches, as can drinking, smoking, or an interruption in routine eating and sleeping habits (all of which may be responsible for "weekend" headaches suffered by some patients). Cyclical, seasonal, or emotional factors, such as menstruation, for instance, may be associated with migraine. A tendency toward having this type of headache may also be inherited.

The predominant symptom of a migraine headache is a sharp, pulsating, incapacitating pain on one or both sides of the head. Paleness, sweating, nausea, and sensitivity to light may accompany the pain.

A warning sensation (called an aura) may indicate an approaching migraine headache. Before the pain begins, some individuals may see flashing lights or "shooting stars," hear noises, smell fragrances or odors, or feel a tingling sensation in the arms or legs.

Cluster headaches, a form of migraine most commonly experienced by men, occur in groups of up to six a day, lasting for weeks or months. Their chief symptom is intense pain on one side of the head, accompanied by tearing of the eye and a runny nose on the same side. Drinking and smoking may aggravate these headaches.

Vascular headaches are diagnosed by a careful review of the circumstances surrounding the headaches as well as by a physical examination to rule out any other disorder that might be causing them. Elimination tests may be done to identify the exact cause of migraines suffered by people who seem to react to certain foods or changes in eating and sleeping habits. In an elimination test, all the substances that are suspected of causing the trouble are eliminated and then reintroduced one at a time in order to identify the cause of the headaches.

Treatment of a migraine already in progress usually consists of a drug therapy program chosen from a variety of painkillers, sedatives, and special drugs to combat migraine. For the occasional migraine sufferer, tranquilizers and sedatives may relieve some of the symptoms experienced during an attack.

Prevention of migraines is possible with several types of medication. One commonly prescribed is ergotamine, which constricts the blood vessels and thus prevents the swelling that causes pressure on the surrounding nerves. This drug is usually taken to stop an approaching migraine; it may have no effect on the aura symptoms some patients experience. Ergotamine has many potential side effects, including aggravation of preexisting vascular and coronary artery disease. Antidepressant drugs, taken in small doses, may prevent migraines in a patient who experiences them regularly.

A recent development in migraine treatment is the use of the beta-blocking drugs. These drugs work in the body to block what are called the beta effects, one of which is dilation (enlargement) of the blood vessels. Because these drugs block the dilation of blood vessels, they have been used to prevent, but not treat, acute attacks of migraine headaches. New drugs known as calcium-channel blockers, such as verapamil, nifedipine, and diltiazem, are also effective in prevention of migraine. They probably act by preventing the initial constriction of blood vessels. Newer injectable drugs to constrict blood vessels appear to be helpful in acute resistant cases.

**Muscle contraction headache** A muscle contraction headache occurs when muscles of the face, neck, or scalp remain contracted (tightened) for long periods. These muscles are then said to be in spasm.

A muscular contraction headache occurs when muscles of the face, neck, or scalp contract (tighten) for long periods.

A muscle contraction headache usually occurs following a specific event that has caused the muscles to tense. The tension turns into physical discomfort in the form of a clenched jaw, aching neck, and tightened muscles of the face and head.

Muscle contraction headaches can also be brought about by abnormalities in the eyes, neck, teeth, or jaws, or they may be caused by poor posture—especially by holding the head awkwardly while reading, driving, or watching television, for example.

The major symptom of these headaches is a tight, squeezing pain in the forehead or jaws or around the back of the head or neck. This constant, dull pain usually occurs on both sides of the head.

Diagnostic evaluation involves a review of the events that usually precede the headaches, as well as a physical examination to rule out any other disorder that might be causing them. A psychological examination may also be conducted to detect any emotional problems that may be contributing to the headaches.

Eliminating the tension or correcting the physical problem that is causing the headaches is a good start in treating them. Painkillers, muscle relaxants, and tranquilizers may be used occasionally (although not on an everyday basis). Antidepressant drugs may also be effective for those individuals who suffer from them regularly.

**Inflammatory headache** An inflammatory, or traction, headache is caused by pressure within the head, due to any of a variety of disorders.

Clogged sinuses and sinus infections are probably the chief cause of this type of headache. The sinuses are the cavities, lined with mucous membranes, within the facial bones. When mucus, which normally flows freely through the sinuses and drains down the nasopharynx or out the nose, cannot drain properly, it collects in the sinuses and causes excess pressure on the surrounding tissues, leading to headache.

Other causes of inflammatory headaches include an aneurysm (a bulge in a blood vessel) in the head and a brain tumor. Aneurysms may not cause pain until they rupture or enlarge rapidly. Brain tumors are usually associated with swelling in the surrounding tissues, which causes increased pressure within the skull and, as a result, a dull, constant headache and sensation of pressing.

High blood pressure, which causes blood to rush through the vessels with too great a force; infections, which inflame sensitive tissue; and fever, which may enlarge the blood vessels, can also cause headache due to excess pressure within the skull.

The symptoms of an inflammatory headache are a dull, aching pain, often occurring early in the day, accompanied by a feeling of pressure in the head. The pain is heightened by sneezing, coughing, bending over, or doing anything that increases the amount of blood in the head.

This type of headache is diagnosed by determining first whether sinus problems are causing it. If not, the doctor may order an electroencephalogram (EEG), which is a visual record of electrical activity in the brain; X-ray studies; a computed tomographic (CT) scan, which provides a cross-sectional picture of the brain; or a magnetic resonance imaging (MRI) study, which yields images comparable to those obtained with CT but without the use of X rays. These tests may detect the presence of a tumor, an aneurysm, or another abnormality in the brain.

Inflammatory headaches are treated according to their cause. Those triggered by a sinus infection can be treated with painkillers; antibiotics, which fight the infection; or antihistamines and decongestants, which dry out and help drain the sinuses. Headaches resulting from more serious disorders, such as a brain tumor, brain abnormality, or aneurysm, will almost certainly require surgery.

Prevention of these headaches is possible if the cause is as simple as a sinus infection. Of course, the correction of a more serious disorder that has caused the pain should also prevent future problems with inflammatory headaches.

# Head lice

Infestation with head lice (or pediculosis capitis, as it is known medically) has become a relatively common occurrence among school-age children; however, persons in all age groups are susceptible. Sometimes erroneously thought to be an indication of an unsanitary lifestyle, lice infestation can actually afflict anyone, without regard for distinctions related to social status or personal hygiene.

Head lice are tiny parasites, less than one-eighth inch long. They are grayish-white, almost transparent, six-legged creatures that live exclusively on humans. Lice can be passed easily from one person to another (for example, by using the comb or wearing the hat of an infested person). Head lice live on or close to the scalp, where they bite and suck blood. Their eggs, which are called nits, are milk-white and about the size of a flake of dandruff.

Head lice cause itching of the scalp, and sometimes they are responsible for a red, scaly rash on the back of the neck at the hairline. Scratching may cause sores on the scalp. The lymph nodes at the base of the skull may be enlarged.

Unless hundreds are present, it is difficult to see lice in the hair. However, the nits attached to the shafts of the hairs are usually clearly visible. Although nits are about the same color and size as flakes of dandruff, they can be easily distinguished from dandruff: flakes of dandruff can be blown or brushed away; nits can be removed with the fingernails only with difficulty.

Both prescription and nonprescription medicated shampoos (called pediculicides) are used to combat lice infestations. It is important to remember that these substances can be poisonous if swallowed or absorbed through the skin or if they come in contact with the eyes. Care must be taken to use them exactly as directed and neither more nor less often than recommended, especially in pregnant women and young children. Sometimes a vinegar rinse is recommended to loosen the nits after using the special shampoo. The nits can then be removed with a fine-tooth comb.

If infected sores on the scalp or enlarged lymph nodes at the base of the skull accompany a lice infestation, this must be called to the attention of a physician.

The best preventive measure is to avoid sharing combs, brushes, towels, and hats with others.

If one member of the family has head lice, it is usually necessary to treat the rest of the family as well (a physician may have special recommendations for infants and pregnant women). Lice cannot be transmitted by pets, however. Combs and hairbrushes should be discarded or thoroughly cleaned in boiling water. Pillowcases, hats, and clothing that may have been in contact with an infested person should be cleaned by washing in very hot water.

# Heart

The heart is a hollow, muscular organ that maintains blood circulation throughout the body. It lies behind the sternum (breastbone), between the lungs. Its size in most adults approximates that of the clenched fist. A heartbeat is a rhythmic contraction of the heart muscle as it pumps blood. A normal heart usually beats 60 to 90 times per minute when the person is at rest.

The heart has four chambers through which the blood passes. Valves control the movement of blood between these compartments. The blood flows from two large veins (the superior vena cava and the inferior vena cava) into the right atrium (upper chamber). The blood continues down to the right ventricle (lower chamber). From this chamber, the blood is pumped to the lungs, where carbon dioxide (a waste product from the cells) is exchanged for oxygen (an

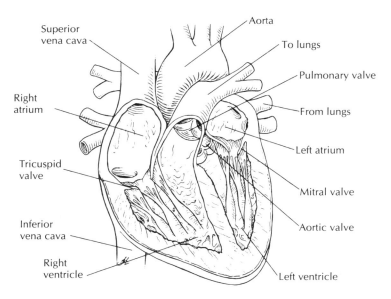

The heart is a hollow, muscular organ that acts as a pump to maintain the circulation of the blood. One-way valves direct the movement of blood through the four chambers of the heart.

element necessary for cell life). The rejuvenated blood then returns to the left atrium. From there, the blood passes to the left ventricle, which forces the blood away from the heart through the aorta (the main artery of the body, which extends through the chest and abdomen) to the other arteries, which carry the blood to all the tissues of the body.

---

# Heart attack

A heart attack, or myocardial infarction, occurs when an area of the heart muscle is damaged or dies because a coronary artery (an artery that delivers blood to the heart muscle itself) has been blocked and the oxygen-rich blood supply to that area of the heart has been drastically reduced. The damaged muscle tissue of the heart is replaced with scar tissue, which does not function as muscle, but rather as a kind of patch. If the area of damage is large enough, the ability of the heart to pump blood is seriously diminished.

Although the chances of surviving a heart attack are now better than ever and complete recovery is common, heart attack is still the number one cause of death in the United States. Heart attacks that do not result in death may lead to serious complications, including shock, cardiac arrhythmia (irregularity of the heartbeat), and congestive heart failure, in which the heart cannot pump enough blood to meet the body's needs.

Heart attack is caused by the blockage of a coronary artery by a thrombus (blood clot) or by atherosclerosis, a disease in which the arteries become clogged by fatty deposits. Damage to the heart muscle occurs when the narrowed coronary arteries are unable to deliver the extra oxygenated blood needed by the heart

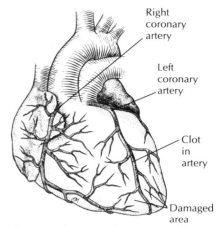

Right coronary artery

Left coronary artery

Clot in artery

Damaged area

A heart attack occurs when an area of the heart is damaged or dies because the coronary artery supplying the area has been blocked by a blood clot or advanced atherosclerosis.

during emotional stress or physical exertion.

A number of factors have been associated with an increased risk of heart attack. Hypertension (high blood pressure) increases the resistance in the blood vessels, forcing the heart to pump harder to push blood through the body. Smoking acts to constrict and damage the arteries and reduce blood flow to the heart muscle. Use of birth control pills, especially by women over the age of 35 and by women who smoke, has been linked to an increased incidence of heart attack. Stress increases the oxygen requirement of the heart muscle. A diet high in saturated fats (fats that are usually solid at room temperature, including those animal fats found in butter and meats) has been found to increase the serum cholesterol level in the blood and thus the chances of developing atherosclerosis. The lack of moderate, regular exercise results in poor tone of the heart muscle and may also prevent the development of collateral circulation (a system of smaller blood vessels that bypass a blocked artery and increase the blood supply to the area served by that artery).

The major symptom of a heart attack is a crushing pain in the middle of the chest, behind the breastbone; the pain can also extend down one or both arms and into the neck, back, teeth, or jaws. Fatigue, heavy perspiration, dizziness, difficulty in breathing, and fever may accompany this pain. The pain may be somewhat similar to that due to angina pectoris, but the pain of a heart attack is more intense, will not be relieved by nitroglycerin, and will not go away within a few minutes, as angina pain will. Also, a heart attack may take place during sleep, which is uncommon for angina pain.

Heart attacks may be very mild, signaled only by slight discomfort, faintness, and nausea. In very serious cases, a heart attack may be accompanied by cardiac arrest (cessation of the heartbeat) or ventricular fibrillation (degeneration of the normal, steady heartbeat to a useless quivering that prevents blood from being pumped through the body).

Heart attack is diagnosed on the basis of the medical history, the physical examination, and test results. The electrocardiograph (an instrument that records the electrical impulses generated in the heart) will show disturbed patterns of heart activity because the impulses must travel around the damaged area. The white blood cell count may also be elevated because the body's immune system increases the number of white blood cells to remove damaged tissue from the heart. Measurements of certain enzymes (special proteins) in the blood may signal that heart muscle has been damaged, although these tests may not confirm that a heart attack has taken place until 24 to 72 hours after the event.

There is no home treatment for a heart attack other than emergency first-aid resuscitative measures—cardiopulmonary resuscitation (CPR)— if the patient loses consciousness. The only recommended plan of action is to summon emergency medical assistance as soon as a heart attack is suspected. Until help arrives, keep the patient warm and comfortable.

Many deaths could be prevented if heart attack victims or their families, acting on their behalf, did not delay seeking medical attention. Studies have shown that, on the average, heart attack victims wait three hours before seeing a doctor.

In almost every case, hospitalization will be necessary following a heart attack. Treatment in the hospital will probably begin in the cardiac care unit, with limited physical activity at first and a gradual return to normal activities.

A variety of medications are used to treat heart attack patients: antiarrhythmics, which inhibit irregularities in the heartbeat; diuretics, which reduce strain on the heart by removing excess water from the blood; antianginals, which diminish chest pain; sedatives, which relax the body; and beta blockers, which ease the strain on the heart by decreasing its work. Another category of drugs, calcium-channel blockers, also appear to be effective in reducing injury to the heart muscle and risk of death due to a heart attack.

Interventional therapy during the first few hours following a heart attack has become common. Usually, an angiogram (also called an arteriogram or cardiac catheterization) is performed first. In this procedure, a thin catheter is inserted into an artery in the arm or leg and advanced through the large blood vessels to the heart; a special dye is then injected through the catheter into the coronary arteries, outlining them on an X-ray screen. Once the area of obstruction has been localized, it may be possible to inject drugs to dissolve an obstruction. In other cases, percutaneous transluminal coronary angioplasty (also called balloon angioplasty) may be performed. In this procedure, a long tube with a balloon tip is threaded through the arteries to the site of the obstruction, and the balloon is inflated to open a clogged vessel (the balloon is then deflated and removed).

In recent years, if the individual is presented to the emergency room within the first six hours following a heart attack, intravenous clot-dissolving drugs may be given in an attempt to restore blood flow. The timing of this procedure is crucial: The sooner given, the greater the chance of saving heart tissue. A complete medical history must also be available as these drugs can cause serious bleeding. Those particularly at risk are patients that have had recent surgical procedures or strokes.

Prevention of heart attack begins with sensible health and dietary habits. Those who do not smoke and do not overeat or overindulge in saturated fats, and who exercise regularly and eliminate as much stress as possible from their lives, are much less likely to become heart attack victims. Those who have already suffered one or more heart attacks may be able to prevent further attacks by changing their living habits.

See also Angina pectoris, Beta-adrenergic blockers, and Coronary bypass surgery.

# Heartbeat irregularities

Heartbeat irregularities (also called cardiac arrhythmias) are deviations from the normal, steady beating of the heart.

Minor irregularities in the heartbeat are common, but more serious arrhythmias can lead to fainting, angina pectoris, or heart attack. The most devastating heartbeat irregularity is called ventricular fibrillation, which occurs when the normally steady pumping action of the heart is reduced to a useless quivering.

Serious arrhythmias are usually caused by damage to the heart muscle or to specialized heart tissue called the conduction system. The first part of the conduction system, called the sinus node, serves as the natural pacemaker of the heart; it is responsible for establishing and maintaining a healthy, steady heartbeat.

Heartbeat irregularities can also be caused by improper use of certain drugs (among them, drugs prescribed for arrhythmia, which can actually cause arrhythmia if the dosage is too high), excessive smoking (the nicotine in cigarettes alters the heartbeat), or consumption of large quantities of caffeine (the amounts found in coffee, tea, chocolate, cola, and some cold medicines may overstimulate the heart).

Heartbeat irregularities may also develop as a result of congenital (present at birth) damage to the heart, a poorly functioning left ventricle, high blood pressure, or a previous heart attack (because the resulting scar tissue may interfere with transmission of the nerve impulses governing the heartbeat).

Ventricular fibrillation often occurs after a myocardial infarction (heart attack) or some other serious injury, such as a severe electrical shock.

Some heartbeat irregularities have no noticeable symptoms. Others will be signaled by light-headedness, fainting, pounding of the heart, dizziness, and chest pain.

Arrhythmias are diagnosed primarily with the electrocardiograph (an instrument that records the electrical impulses generated in the heart). A normal heart will produce a record of regular peaks and valleys; an arrhythmic heart will show an uneven pattern. Continuous recording of the heartbeat can be done on an outpatient basis with a Holter monitor, which is like a combination tape recorder-electrocardiograph. This small device can be worn by the patient for as long as 24 hours. Electrocardiographic wires are taped to the patient's chest, and recordings of the heartbeat are made on magnetic tape. The patient makes a note of his or her activities and of any symptoms he or she experiences during the testing period, and these reports are later correlated with the recorded heartbeat rhythm.

Occasionally, cardiac arrhythmias are so mild that no treatment is required. However, more serious irregularities are treated with medication, defibrillation, or implantation of an artificial pacemaker. All of these methods act to steady the heart rhythm and to maintain a healthy, steady heartbeat.

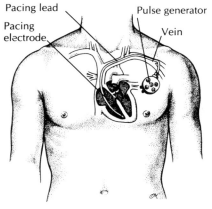

Pacing lead    Pulse generator

Pacing electrode    Vein

An artificial cardiac pacemaker can be used to correct heartbeat irregularites in persons whose natural conduction system is defective. The pacing lead is threaded through a vein until the pacing electrode at the tip of the lead rests within the heart. The electrical pulse generator is then sewn in place under the skin.

Medications commonly used include digitalis, beta blockers, and antiarrhythmics, such as quinidine.

A defibrillator is a device applied to the chest that electrically jolts a quivering heart in a state of ventricular fibrillation back into a normal pattern of beating.

For those whose arrhythmia is caused by a faulty conduction system, an artificial cardiac pacemaker may be implanted in the chest. The pacemaker incorporates a small electrical generator, which causes the heart to beat when its own conduction system fails and steadies an abnormal heartbeat by sending out electrical impulses similar to those emitted by the heart.

Lifestyle changes will probably be recommended to patients suffering from heartbeat irregularities; they may need to quit smoking, lose weight, exercise more regularly, and reduce their caffeine intake. These precautions may also be taken in an effort to prevent arrhythmias.

See also Defibrillation and Extrasystole.

# Heartburn

Heartburn is an uncomfortable, burning sensation felt behind the lower part of the breastbone, sometimes extending up into the upper chest or lower neck. Despite its name, it is not caused by pain in the heart or by a heart attack. In fact, heartburn is often triggered by simple digestive upsets, although occasionally a severe case of heartburn may be a symptom of a more serious disorder.

Heartburn occurs when the acidic digestive juices and partially digested food from the stomach back up into the lower esophagus (the passageway between the mouth and the stomach) and irritate its tissues.

Heartburn most often develops ten minutes to one hour after eating. It may be caused by overeating, smoking, lying down or bending over after eating (which allows the backup of stomach acids and food into the esophagus), taking aspirin, or consuming alcoholic drinks, coffee, spicy or highly seasoned foods, or acidic fruits or fruit juices. Heartburn is a common problem during pregnancy for many reasons, one of which is the pressure exerted by the expanding uterus on the organs within the abdomen; this disappears after childbirth.

The major symptom of heartburn is the characteristic burning sensation behind the breastbone and up toward the throat. It may be accompanied by gassiness, belching, and an uncomfortable, tight feeling in the chest.

Heartburn can usually be relieved by merely standing or sitting upright or by drinking milk or something soothing and nonacidic. Nonprescription antacids may also be helpful in more severe cases. Any case of persistent, uncontrollable, or severe heartburn should be reported to a doctor because it may be a sign of a more severe condition, such as peptic ulcer.

Heartburn can often be prevented by avoiding spicy, acidic, or other troublesome foods, as well as coffee and alcoholic beverages, if they seem to trigger it. Eating smaller meals more frequently and refraining from smoking at mealtimes are also beneficial in avoiding heartburn. Sleeping with the back and head propped up on pillows may prevent the stomach contents from flowing upward and into the esophagus.

# Heart failure

See Congestive heart failure.

# Heart murmurs

Heart murmurs are extra whishing sounds—in addition to the regular "lub-dub" sounds of the heartbeat—that are made as blood flows through the chambers and valves of the heart. In most cases, heart murmurs are quite harmless and represent no cause for concern. In other cases, however, heart murmurs can be a sign that first alerts a doctor to the presence of heart disease or a structural abnormality in the heart.

Heart murmurs can be heard in many healthy persons, especially children, teenagers, and pregnant women. These murmurs are normal sounds caused by the blood rushing through the heart and do not indicate a heart condition. They are called innocent, functional, or insignificant heart murmurs.

In contrast, organic, or structural, heart murmurs are caused by narrowing or obstruction of the heart valves or by incomplete closure of the valves, which allows blood to seep back into the upper or lower heart chambers. Such heart murmurs can be congenital (existing at birth) or acquired, due to damage to the heart valves caused by rheumatic fever, atherosclerosis, syphilis, or other ailments. Heart murmurs also occur when there are holes in the walls separating the chambers of the heart.

Heart murmurs can be detected only by physical examination. By listening to the heart through a stethoscope, a doctor can usually distinguish any extra sounds and judge (by their quality, intensity, location, and timing) whether they signify a serious problem.

If the heart murmur is considered to be organic, the doctor will order special studies—for example, chest

X ray, electrocardiography, and angiography—to evaluate the cause and extent of the condition. Echocardiography, or ultrasound of the heart, gives a relatively clear picture of the heart valves and chambers without the use of X rays and contrast agents. This test is frequently done when a murmur is detected.

An innocent heart murmur does not require any medical treatment or special care, and a person with such a murmur can live a completely normal life. In fact, it is very important that a child with an innocent murmur be treated as the normal, healthy child that he or she is. Parents are sometimes frightened by the idea of a heart murmur and overprotect a child unnecessarily, which is not good for the child's emotional well-being. Most innocent murmurs detected in children disappear or become undetectable by adolescence; only 15 percent to 20 percent of such murmurs continue into adulthood.

If a murmur is organic, the underlying condition can usually be corrected surgically. In cases of heart murmur due to actual diseased valves, it is important to discuss with your physician or dentist the taking of antibiotics prior to dental work or surgery. This simple technique may prevent bacterial endocarditis.

---

# Heat rash

Heat rash, or prickly heat, is a mild skin condition that produces an itchy, burning sensation. It is found most frequently in infants and in overweight individuals who have overlapping folds of fat.

The sweat glands in the skin normally work along with blood vessels to regulate the body's heat. When the blood temperature rises, the brain triggers a reflex in the sweat glands to encourage secretion of sweat. Sweating reduces body temperature by releasing sweat to the surface of the skin, where it evaporates and cools the skin. However, when skin surfaces press together, the sweat ducts, which carry secretions from the sweat glands to the skin's surface, become temporarily blocked. If sweat cannot reach the skin's surface, it may break through the duct wall and remain trapped in an inner layer of the skin, where it can cause inflammation and a rash.

Heat rash can result any time the body is unable to perspire adequately. Most often, hot weather or exertion triggers the reaction. Wearing tight clothing or overdressing, even in cold weather, may compound the problem.

Heat rash in infants occurs primarily because their sweat glands cannot transport large amounts of perspiration to the surface of the skin. The sweat remains trapped within the skin, which causes the characteristic inflammation and irritation.

Usually, heat rash (known medically as miliaria) appears on moist parts of the body where skin surfaces can touch, such as on the neck, under the arms, and between the legs. An infant can have the rash under a tight-fitting diaper. The rash looks like tiny, pinhead-sized red pimples, and it can cause itching and a prickling or burning sensation.

Heat rash is sometimes confused with a condition called chafing because the symptoms are similar. However, chafing is caused by friction between two skin surfaces rubbing together and not by obstructed sweat ducts. Under extreme conditions, the warm, moist areas where heat rash develops can become breeding grounds for microorganisms that cause secondary infection.

Treatment and prevention of heat rash involve reducing or eliminating

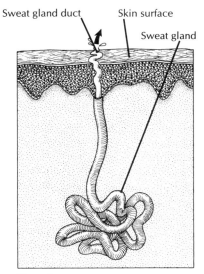

Sweat gland duct     Skin surface

Sweat gland

Normal

Heat rash

A sweat gland normally releases sweat through its duct onto the skin's surface. When perspiration cannot reach the surface, the sweat may break through the duct wall and become trapped beneath the skin, causing inflammation and a rash.

the stimulus for sweating. The affected person needs to stay in a cool environment and refrain from exertion. Cool showers followed by thorough drying can also help, as can wearing light, loose-fitting clothes. Once sweating stops, the rash may disappear in a few hours.

Babies who suffer from heat rash should be bathed in clear water and dried thoroughly. Cloth diapers are more likely to allow the natural evaporation process to occur than are disposable diapers. If the discomfort becomes prolonged or extreme, a doctor should be consulted in order to rule out the possibility that some other disorder could possibly be causing the symptoms.

# Hemoglobin

The role of the red blood cells is to carry oxygen throughout the body. The red blood cells can perform this task because of the presence of hemoglobin, the pigment (coloring agent) that is formed when the red blood cells develop within the bone marrow.

Each hemoglobin molecule is made up of a protein molecule called globin and four pigmented molecules of a compound called heme. Each heme molecule has one atom of iron, and there are four heme molecules in a single molecule of hemoglobin; hence, a single molecule of hemoglobin has four atoms of iron. This structure makes it possible for one hemoglobin molecule to join with four oxygen molecules to form a substance called oxyhemoglobin. This reaction is reversible, enabling hemoglobin to pick up oxygen when the blood is in the lungs and to release oxygen in the cells when the blood is pumped to the tissues.

In general, the blood of men usually has a greater concentration of hemoglobin than that of women. Men have about 14 to 16 grams of hemoglobin per 100 milliliters of blood, whereas women have only about 12 to 14 grams per 100 milliliters of blood. (100 milliliters is approximately equal to 3.5 ounces.)

A number of blood disorders have to do with hemoglobin abnormalities. In many forms of anemia, there is not enough hemoglobin in the red blood cells. In polycythemia, there is too much hemoglobin in the blood. In other conditions, such as thalassemia, the abnormal chemical composition or production of hemoglobin molecules reduces the oxygen-carrying or oxygen-releasing capability of the red blood cells.

See also Anemia and Polycythemia.

# Hemophilia

Hemophilia is a sex-linked hereditary bleeding disorder in which the clotting mechanism of the blood does not function properly. Blood normally contains several factors that enable clotting to occur. These are designated coagulation factors I through XIII. In the most common form of hemophilia—classic hemophilia, or hemophilia A—factor VIII is deficient. In this case, factors I through VII function adequately, but the clotting process is interrupted by a lack of sufficient amounts of factor VIII. Hemophilia B is the other common form of hemophilia, although it occurs significantly less often than hemophilia A. Hemophilia B is caused by a deficiency of factor IX. Hemophilia B is also known as Christmas disease.

Hemophilia is inherited as a sex-linked recessive trait—a woman can pass on the defective gene for the trait without being affected herself. The gene that causes the disorder appears on the X chromosome, which is the female sex chromosome. (Males have one X chromosome and one Y chromosome, while females have two X chromosomes.) If a woman has one defective X chromosome, the presence of her other, normal X chromosome ensures that she will not suffer from the disease herself. However, she can pass on her defective X chromosome to her sons, who will have the disease because they do not have a normal X chromosome to counteract the defect. If she passes the defective chromosome to her daughters, they, too, will be carriers but will not have the disease. A male hemophiliac passes his defective X chromosome to his daughters, making them carriers. However, he passes on only his normal Y chromosome to his sons, who therefore will not have the disease (unless their mother is a carrier). Although the condition appears almost exclusively in males, a woman can be a hemophiliac if her mother is a carrier and her father is a hemophiliac (in such a case, she inherits two defective X chromosomes).

Although affected individuals are born with the disease, the onset of symptoms is variable. Milder cases may not be readily apparent. The symptoms of hemophilia usually appear during early childhood. When a cut in the skin occurs or an injury is suffered, the bleeding may be substantial and prolonged. In severe cases, spontaneous internal bleeding may occur without any obvious cause. Blood may appear in the urine due to internal bleeding. Pain is also a symptom when the bleeding occurs internally, between muscles and into joints. The course of the disease may result in irreversible damage to the joints, which, in turn, results in greater pain and in limitation of movement.

If a child has any of the symptoms of hemophilia, or if there is a family history of hemophilia, a physician should be consulted. The physician will order laboratory tests to establish the diagnosis. The most common test for hemophilia is determination of the partial thromboplastin time (PTT), which indicates how long it takes for the blood to clot. Additional laboratory tests may be ordered in certain cases.

Treatment of hemophilia has recently undergone dramatic changes. One important breakthrough has been the development of factor VIII replacement therapy. One factor VIII replacement, cryoprecipitate, is prepared from donated blood plasma (the fluid portion of blood, which contains more factor VIII than whole blood does). The plasma of an individual donor is quickly frozen by a special process and then slowly thawed, so that the portion rich in factor VIII can be separated out. This portion can then be prepared later for intravenous administration. Cryoprecipitate has the disadvantage of having to be stored and prepared in a hospital.

Treatment of hemophilia A has been further advanced by the development of a process of rapid freezing and dehydration (removal of water) of plasma, called lyophilization. Freeze-dried concentrates are prepared and packaged so that they can be readily dissolved by a simple mixing procedure. (This process is similar in concept to the preparation and use of freeze-dried coffee.) This concentrate, which quickly stops bleeding, is particularly efficient for home use in comparison with cryoprecipitate.

There is a risk of transmission of diseases such as hepatitis and AIDS through the use of human blood products. New methods of purification of factors are being developed, including heating to destroy viruses. The use of recombinant DNA to actually create factors is becoming more common, as is the use of monoclonal antibody purification. These techniques will lessen or eliminate the risk of viral contamination.

Treatment of hemophilia B usually involves the use of fresh or frozen plasma. Concentrate is also available for hemophilia B and is known as prothrombin complex concentrate.

There is no preventive for hemophilia. Genetic testing can now identify carriers of hemophilia with considerable accuracy, however, and this allows affected individuals to decide whether they wish to risk transmitting the disorder to their offspring.

# Hemorrhage

Hemorrhage is the technical term for bleeding, often referring to substantial blood loss or uncontrollable bleeding, either externally or internally. The effects of hemorrhage depend on the part of the body that is bleeding and the total amount of blood that is lost. Hemorrhage can be a symptom of a number of serious, sometimes fatal, disorders.

Hemorrhage occurs when blood vessels are torn or broken. Normally, blood will clot within seconds or minutes, stopping the blood flow. However, when serious injuries or other disorders (such as hemophilia, peptic ulcer, or cancer) are involved, the body's normal blood-clotting mechanism may be inadequate or may malfunction. If blood loss is not quickly stopped, death may result.

Severe external hemorrhage is associated with the following symptoms: rapid pulse; dizziness or faintness; collapse; a drop in blood pressure; a rise in pulse rate; and pale, cold, clammy, or sweaty skin.

Internal hemorrhage may also show symptoms, even if the bleeding is slight. Black, tarry stools may signal bleeding in the intestinal tract from a peptic ulcer; blood in the vomitus indicates bleeding in the stomach; and blood in the urine means that bleeding is occurring in the kidneys or urinary tract.

Blood in the stool, urine, or vomitus should always be reported to a doctor at once, as should external bleeding that occurs frequently or that cannot be stopped within a matter of minutes.

Treatment for internal hemorrhage involves correcting the cause of the bleeding, possibly with surgery. External hemorrhage is treated by applying pressure to the wound with a sterile bandage (or, in an emergency, just pressing it with the fingers) until the bleeding stops. If bleeding cannot be stopped, the patient will almost certainly have to be hospitalized, so that lost blood can be replaced with transfusions of blood products and, in some cases, so that damaged blood vessels can be surgically tied off and sealed.

# Hemorrhoids

Hemorrhoids (often called piles) are enlarged veins inside or just outside the anal canal, which is the opening at the end of the large intestine. As veins swell, they cause severe inflammation and discomfort.

In some cases, hemorrhoids are the result of poor toilet habits. Habitual postponement of bowel movements can lead to loss of rectal function and undesirable straining during elimination. Straining puts increased pressure on veins and slows the flow of blood, thereby contributing to swelling and inflammation of veins. If bowel movements are postponed, the stools retained in the bowels may lose moisture. When feces becomes dry and hard, the added strain of constipation favors the development of hemorrhoids.

Another source of hemorrhoid irritation comes from pressure on the veins due to diseases of the liver or heart or from a tumor. Pregnancy may also contribute to the development of hemorrhoids because the enlarged uterus increases pressure on the veins.

Moreover, prolonged pressure from pushing during labor and delivery can lead to hemorrhoids.

Diet plays a major role in the development of hemorrhoids. A diet containing a high proportion of refined foods rather than foods with natural roughage increases the likelihood of constipation and, therefore, the likelihood of hemorrhoids.

Hemorrhoids seem to be more prevalent in some families. However, this tendency has been attributed to similar dietary and personal habits.

Hemorrhoids may take years to develop and almost always cause irritating symptoms. The first signs of hemorrhoids include itching and discomfort during and after bowel movements. Continued straining during elimination will eventually produce slight swelling of the lining of the anal canal. This swelling may not be noticed until hard stools scrape the anal lining and cause bleeding—an early clue that a hemorrhoid has developed.

With prolonged straining, a portion of the anal canal may jut out of the anus during a bowel movement. As long as the elastic connective tissue is still strong enough to pull the hemorrhoid back into the anal canal unassisted, the individual may not be aware of the growing problem. However, with persistent pressure, the protruding tissue may remain outside the anus after a bowel movement and need to be manually returned to the anal canal. Once outside the anal canal, the hemorrhoid creates a dull aching sensation or ulcerates and bleeds.

A more involved problem develops when the hemorrhoid is difficult or impossible to return within the anal canal, and permanent swelling at the anal opening interferes with elimination. The patient may then postpone bowel movements in an effort to avoid pain. Instead of helping, this intensifies the problem because it leads to constipation.

To diagnose a hemorrhoid, a physician inspects the anal canal, often with special instruments. An anoscope (a short, lighted, tubelike instrument) inserted into the anus can reveal the presence of hemorrhoids. The proctosigmoidoscope, a longer instrument that provides a view of the lower portion of the large intestine, may be used to rule out other causes of rectal bleeding or pain.

Painful hemorrhoids can be treated at home by taking warm sitz baths (sitting in a tub of warm water). Over-the-counter preparations cannot cure hemorrhoids, but they can help relieve itching and swelling. Should symptoms worsen after application of any remedy, its use should be suspended and a doctor consulted. Chemicals in these preparations may produce an allergic reaction. Non-irritating laxatives may be useful in softening stools and easing bowel movements.

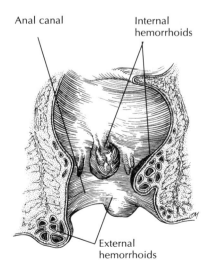

Anal canal

Internal hemorrhoids

External hemorrhoids

Hemorrhoids are enlarged veins inside or protruding from the anal canal. These swollen veins cause itching and pain, which may be accompanied by bleeding.

In the early stages of hemorrhoid development, adjustment of personal habits may prevent progression of the condition. A bowel movement should never be delayed once the urge is felt. During bowel movements, straining should be avoided. A diet including plenty of roughage—natural grains, fresh fruits, and vegetables—also softens stools. Fiber supplements are also quite helpful.

For severe cases of hemorrhoids, a doctor may recommend a surgical procedure called hemorrhoidectomy to remove dilated portions of the affected veins and to tie off the remaining parts of the vein. Newer procedures, such as cryosurgery and laser surgery, remove the hemorrhoid, but with less pain and fewer postoperative complications. Laser surgery uses an intensified beam of light to burn off the hemorrhoid. With cryosurgery, the hemorrhoid is frozen with an extremely cold probe. The frozen tissue dies, and the hemorrhoid falls off within several days. Physicians can perform cryosurgery in their offices in a matter of minutes. Frequently, the only postoperative complaint from patients concerns a slight watery discharge from the anal canal for a few days.

Another technique used to eliminate hemorrhoids is rubber-band ligation. With this procedure, which can be performed in the physician's office, the blood supply of the hemorrhoid is cut off by tying a rubber band around the swollen tissue. The hemorrhoid drops off within three to nine days. Unfortunately, as is the case with the nonsurgical procedures, this procedure is not suitable for all patients. Rubber-band ligation is often done only in the presence of internal hemorrhoids.

Recurrence of hemorrhoids after treatment is not uncommon.

# Hepatitis

Hepatitis is an inflammation of the liver, usually caused by a viral infection, which is characterized by jaundice (yellowing of the skin and the whites of the eyes).

The disease is caused by several viruses, but the most common are those that cause hepatitis A (infectious hepatitis) and hepatitis B (serum hepatitis). The hepatitis A virus and the hepatitis B virus both attack cells in the liver.

Hepatitis A is transmitted from person to person via contaminated food or water or direct or indirect contact with the stools of an infected person. This disease may occur in epidemics where sanitation is poor and the water supply is contaminated. The incubation period (the time between exposure to the disease and the appearance of symptoms) is between 14 and 40 days. Sometimes, cases of hepatitis A are so mild that symptoms never appear, but the infected person can still be a carrier and can transmit the disease to others.

In hepatitis B, the virus enters the bloodstream through contact with contaminated blood or other body fluids, such as semen, or with stool or through the use of contaminated hypodermic needles. Hepatitis B begins more gradually than does hepatitis A, so the disease may be present 40 to 180 days before the onset of symptoms. Because the virus can live in almost all body fluids, including saliva, semen, stool, and tears, hepatitis B can be transmitted by sexual contact or, rarely, by casual contact.

Recently, a hepatitis C virus has been characterized. The virus is presumed to be a major cause of what was previously known as "non-A, non-B hepatitis." Its incubation peri-

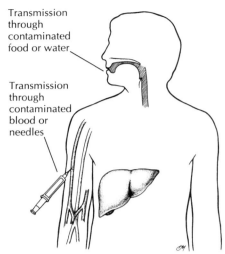

Transmission through contaminated food or water

Transmission through contaminated blood or needles

Hepatitis A can be transmitted through he digestive system by contaminated water or food. Hepatitis B is transmitted most often through contaminated blood or needles, although it is also thought to be passed by intimate person-to-person contact.

od is somewhere between that of A and B, and its mode of transmission is similar to type B hepatitis.

Hepatitis that is not due to any of the above may also result as a complication of the viral infection called infectious mononucleosis.

Early signs of hepatitis include general fatigue, joint and muscle pain, and loss of appetite. Nausea, vomiting, and diarrhea or constipation may follow, with a low-grade fever of 101°F or less. As the disease develops, the liver enlarges and becomes tender. Chills, weight loss, and distaste for smoking appear along with the characteristic jaundice. Jaundice results from an accumulation of yellow bile pigment in the blood, which turns the skin and whites of the eyes yellow.

In hepatitis A, the disappearance of jaundice generally signals the beginning of recovery. However, in hepatitis B or C, the virus may persist for years or even a lifetime.

Any sudden rise in fever, extreme drowsiness, or severe prolonged pain requires immediate medical attention to avoid permanent liver damage. Chronic (long-term) active hepatitis can lead to irreversible liver failure or cirrhosis (a condition in which normal cells of the liver are replaced by fibrous scar tissue that inhibits normal function of the liver).

To determine the extent and severity of hepatitis, a physician analyzes blood and urine specimens from the patient. If the disease has progressed, the patient may have yellow skin and soreness in the upper abdomen over the liver.

More severe acute or chronic hepatitis may necessitate a liver biopsy—a diagnostic procedure in which a needle is inserted into the liver to obtain a sample of liver tissue. A local anesthetic is first injected into the upper abdomen to reduce discomfort from the test.

There is no cure for viral hepatitis. Even treatment is limited, especially for acute hepatitis. Once the virus attacks, recovery is usually up to the body's natural defense mechanisms.

To encourage the healing process, physicians advise patients to avoid strenuous activity. Bed rest is important during the acute phase of hepatitis. More serious cases may require hospitalization to ensure adequate nutrition. All hepatitis patients must avoid alcoholic beverages, because processing alcohol puts a tremendous strain on the liver. All drugs taken, including over-the-counter preparations, must first be cleared by the physician since the liver is responsible for clearing most drugs from the body. Inflammation of the liver may lessen its ability to do this and thus lead to increased levels of the drugs in the body, which can cause toxic effects.

Persons exposed to hepatitis A may prevent or minimize the severity of the disease by obtaining an injection of gamma globulin, a disease-fighting substance derived from blood. Gamma globulin usually defends against hepatitis A virus and may offer modest protection against hepatitis B virus.

A hepatitis B vaccine is now available. (A vaccine is a preparation of a disease-causing agent that stimulates the body to produce antibodies to fight the disease.) Hepatitis B vaccine is recommended for persons who are in direct contact with hepatitis carriers, for health-care workers, and for persons in certain other high-risk groups (for example, travelers to regions where hepatitis is prevalent and hemophiliacs who receive pooled blood products). Newer recommendations include children and teenagers among those to be considered for vaccination. Hepatitis B immune globulin (or HBIG) prepartion containing antibody to hepatitis B is useful for prevention of hepatitis B if given soon after known exposure along with hepatitis B vaccine.

See also Cirrhosis, Gamma globulin, and Jaundice.

# Hernia

A hernia is an abnormal protrusion of part of an organ through the tissues that normally contain it. In this condition, a weak spot or opening in a body wall, often due to laxity of the muscles, allows part of the organ to protrude. A hernia may develop in almost any part of the body; however, the muscles of the abdominal wall are most commonly affected.

A hernia can be congenital (present at birth) or acquired (often the result of some stress or strain on the body wall involved). Although there are a wide variety of types of hernias, the following are some of the most common:

• Umbilical hernia—protrusion of part of the intestine at the umbilicus (navel). This type is seen mostly in infants.

- Inguinal hernia—protrusion of a loop of intestine into the groin (where the folds of abdominal flesh meet the thighs). This type of hernia, which accounts for about 75 percent of all abdominal hernias, is often the result of increased pressure in the abdomen because of lifting, coughing, or straining.
- Scrotal hernia—an inguinal hernia that has passed into the scrotum (the sac containing the testes).
- Femoral hernia—protrusion of a loop of tissue into the femoral canal, which carries nerves and blood vessels from the abdomen into the upper thigh/groin area. This type of hernia is more common in women than in men.
- Incisional hernia—a hernia that occurs at the site of a surgical incision. This type of hernia is often due to strain on healing tissues due to excessive muscular effort, lifting, coughing, or extreme pressure.

A hernia can develop in almost any part of the body, but the more common locations are shown here.

- Hiatal hernia—protrusion of part of the stomach through the diaphragm and into the chest.

The symptoms vary slightly, depending on the cause and the structures involved. Most hernias begin as small breakthroughs that are hardly noticeable. At first, they may be soft lumps under the skin, a little larger than a marble; there is usually no pain. As time goes by, the pressure of the internal contents against the weak wall increases, and the size of the lump increases.

In the early stages, the hernia may be reducible, that is, the protruding structures can be pushed gently back into their normal places. If those structures cannot be returned to their normal locations by manipulation, the hernia is said to be irreducible, or incarcerated.

If an incarcerated hernia progresses, bulging out farther through the weakest points in its containing wall, the opening in the wall will close behind it, forming a narrow neck. If the neck is pinched enough to cut off the blood supply to the protruding tissue, the hernia will swell quickly and become strangulated—that is, the blood supply will be totally cut off. Unless treated, a strangulated hernia can cause tissue death. Fortunately, the symptoms of strangulation of a hernia are usually detectable. When a hernia suddenly grows larger, becomes tense, will not go back into place, and is accompanied by pain and nausea, the hernia is most likely strangulated. Sometimes, however, there is no pain or tenderness when this happens, especially in elderly patients.

Diagnosis of a hernia can usually be made by thorough examination and by studying the patient's medical history and symptoms.

For small nonstrangulated and nonincarcerated hernias, various supports and trusses may offer temporary, symptomatic relief. However, the best treatment is herniorrhaphy (surgical closure or repair of the muscle wall through which the hernia protrudes). When the weakened area is very large, some strong synthetic material may be sewn over the defect to reinforce the weakened area. Postoperative care involves protecting the patient from respiratory infections that might cause coughing or sneezing, which would strain the suture line. Recovery is usually quick and complete.

Avoiding strain or pressure on any body wall, especially the abdominal wall in men, is the only real preventive measure against hernias.

---

# Herpes

Herpes is a sexually transmitted disease—a highly contagious illness spread primarily through direct sexual contact.

Herpes can be treated but not cured. Its symptoms appear briefly and then disappear; the disease lies dormant in nerve cells, but it may be reactivated by stress or illness. It is believed to be contagious only during active periods, when blisters are present. Persons taking drugs that suppress the body's immune system (for instance, cancer or organ transplant patients) are at a higher risk of contracting herpes because their bodies are in a weakened state.

Herpes is spread primarily by direct sexual contact. It can also be transmitted to an infant during childbirth, causing brain damage or death. Therefore, if a woman shows signs of the active disease while in labor, the baby will be delivered by cesarean section (through an incision in the walls of the uterus and abdomen), rather than through the vagina, where the herpes blisters may be present.

Herpes is caused by herpes simplex virus type 2, which is similar to the virus (herpes simplex virus type 1) that causes cold sores and fever blisters on the lips.

The predominant symptom of herpes is the outbreak of painful, itching

Skin surface    Nerve

Herpes blister

Dormant herpes virus    Active herpes virus

Herpes simplex type 2 virus causes painful, itching blisters. The blisters eventually disappear, but the herpes virus lies dormant within nerve cells until stress or illness reactivates the virus, triggering a new outbreak of active herpes blisters.

blisters filled with fluid on and around the external sexual organs. Females may have a vaginal discharge. Symptoms vaguely similar to those of the flu may accompany these outbreaks, including fever and fatigue.

The blisters will disappear without treatment in about two to ten days, but the virus will remain, lying dormant among clusters of nerve cells until another outbreak is triggered by such factors as stress, a cold, fever, or menstruation. Many patients are able to anticipate an outbreak—they notice a warning sign, a tingling sensation called a prodrome, of the approaching illness. Herpes is thought to be contagious only during actual outbreaks, so sexual activity should be avoided while blisters or other symptoms are present.

Diagnosis of herpes is accomplished by microscopic examination and culture of the fluid contained in the blisters.

Unlike other sexually transmitted diseases, herpes cannot be cured, because any medication that will attack the virus while it lies dormant in the nerve cells will also damage the nerve cells. However, there is treatment for acute outbreaks now available that involves the use of either the antiviral drug acyclovir or laser therapy, both of which will heal blisters, reduce pain, and, most important, kill large numbers of the herpes virus organisms. Acyclovir has also been found to reduce the reproduction of the virus in initial outbreaks, thus possibly lessening the number of subsequent outbreaks. It should be noted, however, that to be effective, therapy must be started immediately after the first sores appear. Every sexual partner of the infected person needs to be examined and, if necessary, treated.

Herpes can be prevented by avoiding sexual contact with an infected person whose disease is in its active period. Because the chances of contracting this or any other sexually transmitted disease increase with the number of sexual partners a person has, limiting the number of partners is the first step toward prevention. Using condoms also helps to reduce the risk.

# Hiatal hernia

A hernia is a protrusion of a body part through the structures that surround it. A hiatal hernia (also called a hiatus or diaphragmatic hernia) occurs when a portion of the stomach protrudes above the diaphragm (the muscular wall separating the chest and abdominal cavities) into the chest.

Normally, the esophagus (the passageway from the throat to the stomach) passes through a tight muscular collar, called a hiatus, that prevents the stomach from squeezing up into the chest cavity. However, if the collar is too large or if it relaxes, a sliding hiatal hernia may occur. Pressure in the abdominal cavity (such as may be caused by obesity, pregnancy,

tight clothing, bending or other changes in position, coughing, or straining) causes the top part of the stomach to herniate (slide through the opening) along with the gastroesophageal junction (the junction of the stomach and the esophagus). This condition is very common, especially in women and older persons. It is often without symptoms. Surgical treatment is recommended in only the most severe cases.

Until recently it was believed that the mere presence of a sliding hiatal hernia causes regurgitation (backward flow) of food and harsh stomach acid into the esophagus, which produces the burning sensation of heartburn. Current thinking, however, is that regurgitation and heartburn are the result of the functional ability of the esophageal sphincter.

A relatively uncommon but quite dangerous type of hiatal hernia is the paraesophageal, or rolling, hiatal hernia. In this type, the gastroesophageal junction retains its normal position while a portion of the stomach and part of its peritoneum (covering membrane) rolls up through the opening in the diaphragm, alongside the junction. The danger is that the herniated section may become trapped in the chest with its blood supply choked off, thereby causing death of stomach tissue. Bleeding is also a common complication. Although dangerous, this condition may have no symptoms and is usually found accidentally on an X ray taken for another purpose. The only common symptom is a sense of fullness in the chest after eating.

Because of the potential complications of the paraesophageal hernia, many authorities recommend surgery, even in the absence of symptoms. Surgery for the paraesophageal hernia involves entering the abdomen and pushing the herniated portion of the stomach back into its proper position while removing the sac of peritoneum around it. The next step is to tighten the muscular collar of the diaphragm with stitches.

# Hirsutism

Hirsutism is excessive hair growth or hair growth in areas that are not usually hairy. In general, this condition is due to a hormonal imbalance in the body.

Some degree of hirsutism is present in about 30 percent of women, and it may be a symptom of some other disorder. Family and racial tendencies, however, account for a large percentage of cases of hirsutism in women. Many cases have no known cause. It is thought, though, that hirsute women may have hair follicles that are hypersensitive to normal female androgen levels. (Androgen is a male sex hormone, but it is present to a lesser extent in women as well.)

In some cases, hirsutism is only one sign of virilization (masculinization), which is characterized by acne, balding, and increased muscle mass, as well as by hirsutism. This condition may be due to overactive adrenal glands (which secrete some sex hormones), ovarian tumors, adrenal tumors, or use of steroid medications. However, the majority of hirsute women are not masculinized.

A common cause of hirsutism is polycystic ovaries; in this condition, the presence of numerous cysts on the ovaries leads to infrequent menstruation or absence of menstruation, absence of ovulation, obesity, and enlarged ovaries. Hirsutism is also seen in Cushing's syndrome, a condition that in women is characterized by excessive fat tissue in the face, neck, and trunk; absence of menstruation; convex (outward) curvature of the spine; high blood pressure; and muscular weakness. Mild hirsutism also appears in young girls with underactive thyroid glands. Absence of or damage to the pituitary gland, anorexia nervosa (self-inflicted starvation), and use of some drugs can also cause hirsutism.

The only symptom of hirsutism is excessive growth of hair in men or women or growth of hair in normally hairless areas in women (for example, on the face, neck, breasts, chest, and abdomen). The hair may be soft and fine or coarse, depending on many factors.

Diagnosis is usually confirmed through visual examination and medical history.

The treatment of hirsutism is based on removing the cause. For example, adrenal hyperplasia (an abnormal increase in the number of cells in the adrenal gland) can be suppressed by corticosteroid drugs. Patients with polycystic ovaries can be treated with low-dose estrogen birth control pills or with other drugs.

Removing the cause does not always diminish the hair growth, however, and hair removal may be desired for cosmetic reasons. The only safe, permanent local treatment is electrolysis (destruction of individual hair follicles with an electric current). Other measures, such as plucking, shaving, waxing, or using a depilatory wax or chemical, will mask the problem only temporarily.

Other than prompt diagnosis and treatment of the primary cause or underlying disorder (provided there is one), there are no known preventive measures against hirsutism.

# Histoplasmosis

Histoplasmosis is an infection that follows the inhalation of spores from the fungus *Histoplasma capsulatum*. The parts of the body principally affected are the lungs, the liver, and the spleen.

The *Histoplasma capsulatum* spore is found in soil and in the air. There is no practical defense against breathing the spores. Development of symptoms seems to be a matter of individual immune system response.

In most instances, histoplasmosis does not reach the point at which symptoms appear. People may have the disease but, because of the action of their immune system, never have enough damage to make the symptoms noticeable, much less to create an acute condition. However, if symptoms do appear, they can be serious, especially when left untreated. The most common symptoms are as follows:

- Acute pneumonia (inflammation of the lungs)
- Influenzalike illnesses, with lethargy, cough, and fever, along with lung involvement
- Enlargement of the liver and the spleen, with accompanying interruption of normal function
- The development of fibrous scar tissue in affected organs, particularly the lungs

Histoplasmosis can become inactive and then be reactivated at a later date. In cases of reactivated histoplasmosis, the lungs, meninges (coverings of the brain and spinal cord), heart, peritoneum (lining of the abdominal cavity), and adrenal glands can be involved.

Most affected people probably have histoplasmosis in a dormant form (present within their bodies, but not at the stage at which symptoms are evident). Fatalities occur only in cases of massive infection (which also implies a massive breakdown or malfunctioning of the body's immune system).

Treatment for histoplasmosis begins with diagnosis. The best procedure is to cultivate growths of *Histoplasma capsulatum* organisms from tissue or fluid samples. Another method is to note the rise in the body's production of antibodies (the protective substances produced by the body).

An antifungal medication, such as ketoconazole or amphotericin B, is usually used to treat chronic cases. These drugs help control the disease but appear to have little effect on the fibrous scarring that often occurs in advanced cases.

# Hives

Hives (also called urticaria) is a reaction of the skin marked by intense itching and, most noticeably, by the rapid development of raised, smooth patches, or welts (also called wheals). Hives is most often a sign of an allergic reaction.

Hives is often caused by an allergy to certain foods, particularly shellfish, tomatoes, strawberries, eggs, milk, and chocolate. It can also be a reaction to drugs, food dyes, molds, bacteria, and animal skin or hair. In a susceptible person, cold, the rays of the sun, and vigorous exercise have also been known to cause hives.

Hives is characterized by an outbreak of red and white welts that vary in size and appear suddenly either in small areas or all over the body. They often appear and disappear, lasting anywhere from a few minutes to a day or two, but the outbreak can last for weeks. Accompanying symptoms may include intense itching, fatigue, fever, nausea, and difficulty in breathing if the allergic reaction has led to swelling of the mucous membrane lining the respiratory tract.

Diagnosing the allergy and pinpointing the allergen that is causing the trouble can require extensive testing, especially when a food may be involved. Eliminating many suspected foods and then reintroducing them one at a time sometimes helps to diagnose the cause of hives. This should always be done under professional supervision and with caution.

Hives can be treated immediately by taking antihistamines. When taken several times a day at a prescribed dosage, the correct type of antihistamine will help control swelling by preventing the released histamine from triggering the hives. Drowsiness and dry mouth are common side effects of antihistamines, so the type and dosage may need to be adjusted from time to time. Concurrent medical problems, such as glaucoma, enlarged prostate, or heart disease, may preclude the use of antihistamines. It is best to consult your doctor before taking an antihistamine. Other drugs (such as corticosteroids, which reduce inflammation) may be used to treat serious hives.

Hives can be prevented by avoiding contact with the allergen or stimulus once it has been identified. Sometimes, no stimulus or disease process can be identified, and the hives are called idiopathic (of unknown cause). This condition can result in chronic episodes of hives and may require chronic treatment with antihistamines and/or corticosteroids.

# Hodgkin's disease

See Lymphoma.

# Huntington's chorea

Huntington's chorea is an inherited degenerative nerve disorder that seldom becomes apparent before early middle age. It is characterized by disorganized body movements (the word *chorea* comes from a Greek word meaning dance) and mental deterioration. It is thought that Huntington's chorea is the result of a disturbance in the part of the brain that automatically regulates voluntary movements.

The condition is transmitted as a dominant genetic trait from a parent who has the disease. There is about a 50 percent chance of a child's inheriting the disease from an affected parent. Since the symptoms of Huntington's chorea usually do not appear until the victim is between 30 and 50 years of age, a person with a family history of Huntington's chorea lives through the years of adolescence and early adulthood in dread of reaching the middle years, when the symptoms may begin. Even more tragic, a person who is unaware of a family history of Huntington's chorea may have children before discovering that he or she has the disease.

The first symptoms of mental deterioration are usually personality changes—obstinacy, moodiness, lack of interest in surroundings, and inappropriate behavior may be displayed. It should be noted, however, that all of these symptoms can also be due to psychological or other disorders that have nothing to do with Huntington's chorea.

These symptoms are accompanied by irregular, jerky movements that begin in the arms, the neck, and the face. They may start as "fidgeting" and gradually develop into facial grimaces, halting speech, irregular movements of the torso, and muscle contractions in the neck that cause the head to be held to one side.

In advanced cases, a wide stance will be adopted in an attempt to maintain balance. The gait will become prancing, as control of the legs deteriorates. As the disease progresses, the victims usually become paranoid, walking ability is lost, swallowing becomes difficult, and dementia (loss of intellectual capabilities) increases.

No treatment has yet been found to control the symptoms or halt the disease. However, the body movements may be controlled somewhat by drugs, most notably haloperidol and chlorpromazine. There is no known treatment for the mental degeneration that accompanies the physical symptoms.

There is no known preventive for Huntington's chorea, other than advising affected patients not to have children.

# Hyaline membrane disease

Hyaline membrane disease (HMD) is a respiratory distress syndrome that occurs in premature infants who do not have fully functioning lungs. It is the leading cause of illness and death in premature infants.

The cause of HMD is the inability of the immature lungs to produce enough pulmonary surfactant, which is a chemical in the alveoli (the tiny air sacs in the lungs) that keeps them expanded. Without adequate surfactant, the alveoli tend to collapse when the infant exhales. As a result, the infant's lungs do not expand completely, and the blood passing through them cannot obtain enough oxygen to sustain life.

The symptoms of HMD are easily observable. The skin is bluish due to lack of oxygenation of the blood, and there are other symptoms of oxygen deprivation—irregular heartbeat; rapid, labored, and shallow breathing; flaring of the nostrils; grunting when breathing out; and edema

(swelling of tissues due to fluid accumulation).

Treatment of HMD is aimed at maintaining adequate oxygen levels. Until the lungs can sufficiently oxygenate the blood, oxygen must be provided in such a way as to prevent damage to the infant. An oxygen face mask is often used to provide warmed, moisturized oxygen. In more severe cases, a ventilator is necessary to "breathe" for the infant.

Great strides in the treatment of HMD have been made in the last few years. An artificial surfactant (a lubricant for the lungs), has been produced that, when administered via the baby's trachea (windpipe), markedly relieves the baby's respiratory distress. Because of the availability of surfactant, the rate of death of newborns from HMD has dropped dramatically in the last few years.

Fluids, glucose (a form of sugar), and electrolytes (certain chemicals needed by the body) are provided intravenously.

Either the condition will clear up as the lungs develop and begin to produce their own natural surfactant or the infant will not survive.

The best preventive measure is to guard against premature birth. Women should be carefully monitored during the last weeks of pregnancy for any signs of premature labor.

If the mother is diabetic, the fetal lungs may not be fully formed until the fortieth week of pregnancy, and HMD is possible until then.

# Hydrocele

A hydrocele is an abnormal collection of fluid around a testis, which is noticeable as a soft mass in the scrotum. The term hydrocele literally means a sac of water.

There is normally a double-layered covering around each testis. Within these two layers there is usually just enough fluid for lubrication. Occasionally, however, the amount of fluid is increased, causing the swelling around the testis. As a rule, hydroceles are harmless. They are also relatively common, especially in older men.

If the hydrocele is caused by an injury or inflammation in the scrotum, it is called a secondary hydrocele. If there is no apparent cause, it is called a primary hydrocele.

The most obvious symptom is the swelling. Although hydroceles are usually painless, pain may also be present.

A small, painless hydrocele often requires no treatment. However, care must be taken not to dismiss something more serious as a hydrocele. Only a physician can make the diagnosis. Therefore, any scrotal mass merits immediate medical attention. The treatment for hydrocele is surgical removal of the fluid. The condition can recur.

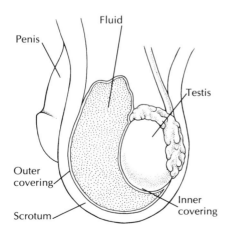

A hydrocele is an accumulation of fluid between the two layers covering a testis.

# Hydrocephalus

Hydrocephalus (sometimes inaccurately referred to as "water on the brain") is an abnormal accumulation of cerebrospinal fluid within the cavities (hollow spaces) of the brain.

Normally, cerebrospinal fluid is secreted in the cavities of the brain and absorbed by a membrane that lines the cavities. If the membrane does not absorb the fluid or if the fluid is blocked, it builds up in the cavities. The fluid buildup causes the head to become enlarged and the brain to become compressed. This condition can lead to paralysis, blindness, mental retardation, inability to speak, and convulsions.

Hydrocephalus is usually the result of a brain infection or a malformation in the fetus prior to birth. Although the baby's head may not appear abnormally large at birth, it expands rapidly from month to month; if untreated, the child usually dies by the end of the second year. If the blockage causing the fluid buildup is only partial, the child may live for a number of years or could possibly even live a normal life span.

Although hydrocephalus is usually a congenital (present at birth) condition, it can occur later as a result of an infection or tumor.

When hydrocephalus occurs in an infant, the loosely connected bony skull plates pull apart to accommodate the swelling. As a result, the head becomes greatly enlarged. In addition to having an oversized head, the child with hydrocephalus may have an abnormally enlarged forehead and swollen or enlarged blood vessels in the scalp.

Diagnosis is accomplished through the use of X rays and computed tomography. If infection is suspected, samples of the blood and cere-

Normal newborn skull

Fontanelles
(spaces
between bony
plates of the
skull)

Hydrocephalic newborn skull

When hydrocephalus—a buildup of fluid in the brain—occurs in a newborn infant, the loosely connected bony plates of the skull spread apart to accommodate the swelling.

brospinal fluid will be extracted for analysis.

Surgery can make it possible, in some cases, to bypass the blockage or obstruction, causing the fluid buildup to escape through other exits. Often, the insertion of a small tube connecting a brain cavity with the abdomen or a major blood vessel will allow the fluid to drain. As the child grows, the tube may become blocked, again allowing pressure to build in the brain. If this happens, the tube must be replaced or the blockage removed. When surgery is successful, the probability of mental retardation is greatly reduced, and the prospects of normal physical and intellectual development increase.

# Hyperemesis gravidarum

Hyperemesis gravidarum is a term that refers to excessive vomiting dur-ing pregnancy. This type of vomiting is more severe than that caused by ordinary morning sickness, which usually clears up on its own within a few months. In hyperemesis gravidarum, the vomiting leads to starvation, dehydration (excessive loss of water from the tissues), and a disruption of the chemical balance in the body.

Symptoms include loss of weight, dehydration, and, in very severe cases, jaundice (yellowing of the skin and the whites of the eyes). The condition is most often treated in the hospital through the use of antivomiting drugs and intravenous feeding to correct the possible malnutrition, dehydration, and chemical imbalance. A pregnant woman should not attempt to treat the vomiting with drugs without consulting her doctor.

# Hypertension

Hypertension, or high blood pressure, refers to persistently elevated pressure of blood within the arteries, which carry blood from the heart through the body. The exertion of excessive force on the artery walls may cause damage to the arteries themselves and thereby to the heart, kidneys, and brain, leading to heart attack, kidney failure, and stroke.

Although many people believe that hypertension is caused by extreme activity or tension, this theory has not been proved. When no underlying cause is discovered, the disease is called primary, or essential, hypertension. If another disease, such as kidney or heart disease, causes the elevated blood pressure, the condition is labeled secondary hypertension.

Contrary to popular belief, there is no typical hypertensive person. However, some people are more susceptible to developing high blood pressure than others. Heredity appears to play a role; persons whose parents are hypertensive are at greater risk of becoming hypertensive themselves. In the past, hypertension was attributed to aging, but current evidence indicates that age is not a primary factor. The incidence of hypertension in black persons, both children and adults, is about twice that in white persons.

Overweight, prolonged stress, smoking, drinking, and excessive sodium in the diet (which causes fluid retention) may increase blood pressure, especially in persons prone to hypertension. There are also indications that use of oral contraceptives may contribute to increased blood pressure; however, this is more likely to occur in women who are overweight, whose parents are hypertensive, or who have other hypertensive risk factors.

Hypertension has been called the "silent disease" because it often has no obvious symptoms. A person may have high blood pressure for years without noticing any symptoms. Symptoms may include headache, fatigue, dizziness, flushing of the face, ringing in the ears, thumping in the chest, and frequent nosebleeds. However, these symptoms may also result from other conditions.

To diagnose hypertension, a simple, risk-free, painless test using a stethoscope and a sphygmomanometer (a device for measuring the blood pressure) is used. Blood pressure is measured in a main artery of the arm by first shutting off and then releasing the flow of blood in the artery with the inflatable cuff of the sphygmomanometer while listening to the arterial pulse with the stethoscope.

The blood pressure measurements are given as the systolic pressure (the pressure at which the first beat of the pulse can be heard as gradual deflation of the cuff begins) over the diastolic pressure (the pressure at which

Using a sphygmomanometer—an inflatable arm cuff attached to a manometer—blood pressure is measured in a main artery of the arm by first shutting off and then releasing the flow of the blood in the artery with the cuff and listening to the artery pulse with a stethoscope.

steady flow through the artery can be heard as the cuff is deflated)—for example, 150/95. The systolic pressure essentially measures the pressure of the heart during a contraction. The diastolic pressure is that which exists when the heart is filling between beats. Although diastolic pressure is considerably lower than systolic, there is still pressure in the body when the heart is filling. Both values have diagnostic importance. An unusually high systolic pressure may mean that the heart is pumping too hard or the arteries are stiff; a high diastolic pressure means that the arteries have abnormally high muscular tone or resistance.

Normal blood pressure is about 80/46 at birth and climbs as age increases. The normal adult pressure is about 120/80.

Hypertension responds well to treatment, although female hypertensive patients seem to do better than male patients. When the condition is mild (a blood pressure of about 140/90) and there is no indication of other disease, a doctor may suggest lifestyle changes before prescribing medication. These changes may include weight loss, a regular exercise program, and strict limitation of sodium intake, which affects fluid balance and volume and therefore blood pressure. Controlling sodium in the diet requires restriction of table salt as well as careful scrutiny of all food and drug labels.

If medication is indicated, a physician may prescribe one or several drugs. There is no "cookbook" approach to treating hypertension. The choice of therapy is governed by multiple factors, including the patient's age, sex, and any coexisting illnesses, as well as by the severity of the hypertension.

While tension and stress do not directly cause hypertension, these factors do affect the condition. Persons with hypertension, therefore, are urged to avoid high-pressure situations and to learn to deal with stress. Biofeedback, self-hypnosis, and meditation have proved useful for reducing stress and may help someone with hypertension.

Blood pressure can be monitored at home with a special kit. If three separate elevated readings (above 140/90 in adults) are obtained, a trip to the doctor is in order. Furthermore, everyone should have his or her blood pressure measured by a healthcare professional at least once a year. Persons with a history of hypertension or with any of the risk factors for hypertension should carefully follow their physician's recommendations for periodic blood pressure checks. It is also recommended that children of hypertensive parents begin to receive regular blood pressure measurements early in life.

---

# Hyperthyroidism

Hyperthyroidism is a general term that encompasses several different disorders with the common feature of excessive production of thyroid hormone. The two most common forms of hyperthyroidism are Graves' disease and toxic multinodular goiter.

The production of thyroid hormone is normally regulated by the pituitary gland, which secretes thyroid-stimulating hormone (TSH) when a need for thyroid hormone is present and decreases secretion of TSH when it senses an adequate supply of the hormone. Generally speaking, some malfunction occurs in hyperthyroidism, and the thyroid is no longer sensitive to this regulatory mechanism. Graves' disease is probably due to the presence of an abnormal chemical stimulator of thyroid hormone production. In toxic multinodular goiter, nodules (lumplike clusters) of thyroid tissue form, for reasons that have yet to be determined, and secrete abnormally large amounts of thyroid hormone, independent of the amount of hormone in the body.

Because thyroid hormone is involved in so many vital processes throughout the body, including maintenance of body temperature, conversion of food to energy, and regulation of growth and fertility, the effects of an excess of that hormone are many and varied. The symptoms common to all forms of hyperthyroidism include rapid heartbeat, weight loss despite increased appetite and food intake, generalized hyperactivity, tremors (shakiness), increased sweating, severe nervousness and emotional instability, alterations of menstruation and fertility, and overall muscle weakness.

In addition to these symptoms, patients with Graves' disease often have bulging eyes. Their skin is characteristically warm, moist, and velvety, and there may be areas of raised, thickened, sometimes itchy skin with the texture of orange peel on the legs and feet. The thyroid gland is frequently enlarged, smooth, and soft. This disease occurs most frequently among those in their 30s and 40s. It is more common in women than in men.

In toxic multinodular goiter, the thyroid gland is lumpy but not uniformly enlarged. This condition occurs most often in the middle-aged and elderly.

The diagnosis of hyperthyroidism is made on the basis of the history and findings from a physical examination and various laboratory studies. Significant elevation of the level of thyroid hormone in the blood can be detected with special blood tests. The diagnosis can be further established through the use of nuclear medicine scans obtained after the injection of radioactive iodine, which becomes concentrated in the thyroid gland. The nuclear medicine study yields not only a picture of the gland, but also an estimate of the degree of hyperactivity.

Specific treatment of hyperthyroidism depends on which condition is present. However, treatment of the hyperthyroid state in general has several common elements. The drug propranolol, a beta blocker, is commonly used to block the effects of the hormonal overstimulation that greatly contributes to the tremors, increased heart rate, and sweating. This drug, although it diminishes symptoms, does not get at the root problem of too much thyroid hormone. To decrease the amount of thyroid hormone being produced, an antithyroid drug, such as propylthiouracil, is used. Antithyroid drugs actually interfere with the production of thyroid hormone. However, this is only a temporary solution; when the drug is stopped, the excess production usually resumes. The definitive therapy for hyperthyroidism is the destruction or removal of most or all of the gland using radioactive iodine or surgery.

Graves's disease is usually first treated by blocking hormonal overstimulation with the drug propranolol. Simultaneously, an antithyroid drug is started. This drug may be maintained for several years. If relapse occurs (which it frequently does) or if the level of thyroid hormone is not normalized, the question then is how to reduce the amount of thyroid tissue. Whether surgery or radioactive iodine is used depends on many complex factors. Both treatments frequently result in too little thyroid hormone in the blood, but this problem is easily remedied by supplementation with synthetic thyroid hormone.

The treatment of toxic multinodular goiter is less controversial. In addition to a beta-blocker and, frequently, an antithyroid drug, radioactive iodine is generally the therapy of choice.

See also Hypothyroidism.

# Hyperventilation

Hyperventilation is abnormally rapid and deep breathing, as a result of which large quantities of air are drawn into the lungs and abnormally large amounts of carbon dioxide are expelled.

Although hyperventilation can result from a physical disorder that interferes with the exchange of oxygen and carbon dioxide in the lungs, most often hyperventilation is a physical response to stress, anxiety, and emotional upset. It begins slowly and builds up to the point at which symptoms appear and the person panics. At this point, breathing often becomes even more rapid and difficult.

The diminished level of carbon dioxide in the blood can lead to buzzing in the ears; a tingling feeling in the fingers, toes, and lips; light-headedness; and fainting. It may also cause tightness in the chest and a feeling of suffocation. Episodes of hyperventilation may last longer than half an hour, and they may recur several times in a 24-hour period.

Symptoms of hyperventilation may be strikingly similar to those of heart disease and other serious illnesses. The individual experiencing these symptoms should, therefore, consult a doctor to rule out the existence of any of these conditions.

The symptoms of hyperventilation can often be relieved by having the person breathe into a paper bag. In this way, the needed carbon dioxide that has been exhaled into the bag can be inhaled again; as a result, the level of carbon dioxide in the blood can be restored to normal, and the breathing rate is slowed.

# Hypochondria

Hypochondria is persistent, exaggerated worry—usually based on self-diagnosis—about one's health, especially in the absence of any real illness. The condition reflects an often morbid concern over any unusual physical or mental sensation or feeling. For example, to the hypochondriac, a headache indicates a brain tumor; a cough has to mean tuberculosis; and a mole is sure to be cancerous. Despite normal test results and reassurances to the contrary, the individual is convinced that he or she either has a serious illness or will have one in the near future.

Frequently, the hypochondriac complains of pain or discomfort in the stomach, chest, head, or neck. Symptoms common among hypochondriacs include nausea, loss of appetite, vomiting, and belching. These symptoms become worse after the person has received expressions of sympathy and concern from family members and friends. It is not uncommon for a hypochondriac to make repeated visits to the doctor or consult several doctors at the same time, without their knowledge, in order to obtain prescriptions for a variety of drugs.

Hypochondria is very difficult to treat. It has been estimated that only a small percentage of persons afflicted with this disorder recover completely. Psychotherapy is sometimes useful in such situations; in many cases, however, a more helpful approach is to encourage the individual to divert the energy spent on worrying about his or her health to more productive interests and activities.

# Hypoglycemia

Hypoglycemia is the state of having an abnormally low blood glucose level. (Glucose is a sugar released into the blood as a result of digestion of carbohydrates.)

The two main forms of this condition are reactive hypoglycemia and fasting hypoglycemia. To understand how both forms of hypoglycemia occur, it is helpful to understand how glucose utilization is normally regulated.

During digestion, elevated blood glucose levels trigger the secretion of the hormone insulin from the pancreas. Insulin acts to reduce the sugar level in the blood by helping body cells absorb the glucose.

Reactive hypoglycemia is caused by oversecretion of insulin and consequent rapid lowering of blood glucose levels in response to ingestion of glucose. Reactive hypoglycemia is also known as postprandial (after meals) hypoglycemia because it occurs only in response to ingestion of food.

The specific causes of reactive hypoglycemia are unknown in most cases. However, certain persons—for example, those in the early stage of adult-onset diabetes mellitus and patients who have had part or most of the stomach removed surgically—are particularly susceptible to reactive hypoglycemia.

Fasting hypoglycemia is caused by insufficient production of glucose or overutilization of the glucose present in the blood. Often, these two factors combine to severely depress the blood glucose level. An insulin-producing tumor on the pancreas can also cause fasting hypoglycemia. Because alcohol disturbs the normal mechanisms of sugar storage and release within the liver, heavy drinkers are at greater risk of developing the disorder. Fasting hypoglycemia can also occur in anyone who has not eaten for an unusually long interval, but this is a temporary situation. Chronic (long-term) hypoglycemia is uncommon.

The symptoms of both types of hypoglycemia include fatigue, nervousness, perspiration, dizziness, headache, hunger pangs, visual impairment, and accelerated heartbeat. The condition may also cause anxiety, difficulty in concentrating, confusion, and blackouts. If sugar deprivation continues unchecked, severe hypoglycemia may produce convulsions (short-term loss of consciousness, accompanied by jerking muscle movements) or deep coma (prolonged loss of consciousness).

True hypoglycemia is an uncommon condition. Since many of the symptoms of anxiety and hypoglycemia are alike, the two conditions are often confused.

To diagnose hypoglycemia, a doctor analyzes a blood sample to detect abnormally low sugar levels. Blood drawn during an attack of the condition allows the most accurate assessment, since symptoms can then be correlated with actual blood glucose levels.

Treatment for hypoglycemia is often aimed at the underlying cause of the disease. For example, surgical removal of a pancreatic tumor or adjustment of a diabetic patient's insulin dosage may be necessary. In most cases of reactive hypoglycemia, however, there is no known cure for the tendency of the pancreas to overproduce insulin when it is not needed. The most effective treatment is to avoid all foods that generate attacks.

A good diet for a patient who is susceptible to episodes of hypoglycemia is one that is low enough in sugar and starches to moderate the reaction of the pancreas to sugar intake and rich enough in protein to help maintain gradual elevations of blood sugar. Eating several smaller meals a day, rather than three large meals, may help to keep blood sugar levels stable.

# Hypotension

Hypotension is low blood pressure. Unlike chronic high blood pressure, which can be a serious health problem, low blood pressure usually need not be a cause for concern or even treatment.

Blood pressures vary, depending on such factors as age, race, sex, and environment. On rare occasions, individuals may have medical problems that cause low blood pressure. Among such conditions are some types of heart disease, hormonal deficiencies, and malnutrition. In these cases, the hypotension will be corrected by the treatment of the medical problem.

Postural hypotension, or orthostatic hypotension, is a form of low blood pressure in which dizziness or faintness occurs when a person stands up abruptly from a sitting or reclining position. Normally, when an individual stands up, the blood vessels contract to maintain normal blood pressure in the new position. However, in persons with postural hypotension, this mechanism probably does not work properly, and on standing, a temporary reduction in the blood flow to the brain leads to feeling faint. Rising slowly from a sitting or reclining position will usually prevent the symptoms in this situation.

Sometimes postural hypotension results from taking a medication for high blood pressure; in these cases, the physician may reduce the dosage or change the medication.

Fluids, including blood, lost from the body may also cause postural hypotension, as may many diseases. Consequently, although postural hypotension is a benign condition in most individuals, it should be reported to a physician.

# Hypothermia

Hypothermia is a condition in which the body temperature falls well below the normal temperature of 98.6°F. The lowering of the temperature can occur accidentally, or it can be induced intentionally as part of a medical treatment plan.

When hypothermia happens accidentally, the person's condition can become serious if the symptoms or signs are ignored. Among the causes of accidental hypothermia are immersion in cold water, certain drugs, and long periods of being exposed to the cold without appropriate clothing. Hypothermia can easily occur in newborns and infants, because their heat-retaining mechanisms are not fully developed. Elderly persons are also at risk, because their heat-retaining mechanisms are easily overtaxed.

The signs and symptoms of hypothermia include an altered level of consciousness, slow breathing, low pulse rate, listlessness, and mental confusion. The hands, feet, and abdomen of the hypothermic person are cold to the touch.

Basic treatment for hypothermia is gradual rewarming of the body. The rewarming must be gradual to prevent the sudden enlargement of blood vessels at the surface of the body, which may divert too much blood from some of the body's vital internal organs. Medical help should always be obtained for a person with hypothermia. While waiting for help to arrive, the cold person should be covered with blankets and, if alert, should be offered a warm, nonalcoholic beverage. Alcoholic drinks do not help because they tend to reduce body heat. Also, briskly rubbing hands or feet to restore warmth is *not* recommended. Any other type of treatment depends on the underlying cause of the drop in body temperature. In severe cases in which body temperature is critically reduced, warm fluids may be given intravenously. Peritoneal dialysis (a process by which warm fluids are injected into and withdrawn from the abdominal cavity) is sometimes used to restore normal temperature, as is immersion in a specially designed tank filled with warm water.

# Hypothyroidism

Hypothyroidism is a disorder in which an underactive thyroid gland fails to produce enough thyroid hormone for the body.

Hypothyroidism can result from chronic (long-term) inflammation of the thyroid or a deficiency of thyroid-stimulating hormone, which is secreted by the pituitary gland. Autoimmune disorders (in which the immune system destroys the body's own tissues) are also a common cause of hypothyroidism. In addition, heredity may play a role in the development of the condition. Women seem more prone to thyroid disorders, and in some women, pregnancy triggers the hormonal imbalance. Hypothyroidism can also develop after suppression or partial removal of the thyroid gland as treatment for hyperthyroidism (a condition that results when an overactive thyroid gland produces too much thyroid hormone).

Because thyroid hormone influences every tissue in the body (for example, by participating in maintenance of body temperature, conversion of food to energy, and regulation of growth and fertility), the effects of having too little of the hormone are many and varied. People with hypothyroidism may be overweight, easily exhausted, and subject to recurrent infection. They may also experience menstrual disorders, be intolerant of cold, have dry skin and hair, exhibit puffiness of the hands and face, and suffer depression.

The diagnosis of hypothyroidism is based on laboratory tests of the blood. Determination of levels of thyroid and pituitary hormones is fundamental. Cardiac enzymes and cholesterol may also be measured. A special nuclear medicine study, which is an X ray taken after the injection of a radioactive isotope, may be performed.

Chronic hypothyroidism may cause signs of reduced general body functioning. Anemia (deficiency of red blood cells) may result from diminished function of the bone marrow, where red blood cells are formed. Heart rate may decrease, and reflexes may become sluggish. An electroencephalogram may reveal irregular patterns. Evaluation of growth patterns often provides the first clue to the diagnosis in children.

Since hypothyroidism develops from a shortage of thyroid hormone, the most effective treatment is generally thyroid hormone supplementation. Supplements are either natural hormones extracted from the thyroid glands of animals or synthetic hormones. Both types control the problem, but the newer, synthetic forms are much more efficient and their effects are more easily regulated. Although treatment provides the necessary hormone control, hypothyroidism often continues throughout life, and the patient may require lifelong follow-up to monitor treatment.

Contrary to popular belief, the correction of hypothyroidism will not cause an obese person to lose a significant amount of weight.

See also Hyperthyroidism.

# Hysterectomy

Hysterectomy is the surgical removal of the uterus, which causes the termination of menstruation and the inability to bear children.

A hysterectomy may be either total or partial. Total hysterectomy entails the removal of the entire uterus, including the cervix. Partial hysterectomy, which is rarely done today, involves removal of only the body of the uterus but not the cervix. Oophorectomy (removal of one or both ovaries) and salpingectomy (removal of one or both fallopian tubes) may be performed at the same time as hysterectomy.

Removal of the uterus may be done through an abdominal incision (cut) or through the vagina. In the latter procedure, the top of the vagina is stitched together after the uterus

A hysterectomy is the removal of the uterus. Oophorectomy (removal of the ovaries) is sometimes performed at the same time.

has been removed; this technique requires no external incision and leaves no external scar.

Hysterectomies are most commonly performed when the uterus is diseased. Symptomatic fibroid tumors, uterine prolapse (falling of the uterus out of its normal position), and cancer of the uterus are reasons for a hysterectomy.

Contrary to common belief, a hysterectomy, in and of itself, does not interfere with, or diminish the pleasure of, sexual intercourse, nor does it cause weight gain.

See also Fibroid tumors, Menopause, Ovarian cysts, and Prolapse of the uterus.

# I

# Ileitis

See Crohn's disease.

# Ileostomy

An ileostomy is the surgical creation of an opening, or stoma, through the abdomen into the ileum (the lower part of the small intestine). An ileostomy is performed if the large intestine and rectum must be removed because of disease or abnormality. The opening into the small intestine then becomes an artificial anus through which waste material is expelled, since waste matter can no longer travel through the ileum to the normal anus.

The waste matter that is discharged through the stoma is collected in a bag that the patient wears continuously. Because this waste matter does not pass through the large intestine,

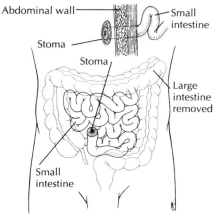

Abdominal wall — Small intestine

Stoma

Stoma

Large intestine removed

Small intestine

An ileostomy is the surgical creation of an opening through the abdomen into the ileum (lower part of the small intestine). Waste matter can then be expelled through that opening.

where water is absorbed from the waste matter, the material excreted through the stoma is watery.

Patients learn to care for their stomas in the hospital after the operation. Equipped with this knowledge, a patient can lead a normal life after an ileostomy.

See also Colostomy.

# Immunity

Immunity is the body's ability to defend itself against harmful organisms and substances. Essentially, it is a resistance to infection that may be inherited or acquired naturally or artificially.

Immunity develops when foreign organisms or substances, called antigens, enter the body, causing particular specialized cells to react either by attacking the antigen directly or by producing special proteins (microscopic molecules essential to living cells) that neutralize the foreign agents. The most common types of antigens are forms of bacteria (one-celled organisms that have the poten-

tial to attack body tissues or secrete poisonous substances called toxins) and viruses (the smallest infective agents, responsible for a variety of diseases).

See also Allergy, Anaphylactic shock, and Immunization.

# Immunization

Immunization is the means of producing immunity (resistance by the body) to a specific disease. There are two types of immunization—active and passive.

Active immunization is accomplished by injecting weakened or killed viruses or bacteria into the body. This stimulates the body's natural defense system. Certain specialized white blood cells produce substances known as antibodies, which are carried in the bloodstream and are tailor-made to fight invading organisms. These antibodies remain in the body for years—sometimes a lifetime—to protect it against that particular disease.

Passive immunization involves injecting ready-made antibodies into the body. These antibodies are usually extracted from the blood of humans who are immune to a certain disease or of animals that have been immunized solely for the purpose of producing antibodies to be used in passive immunization. Passive immunization is borrowed immunity and is only temporary, but it serves to protect a person who may already be infected until the body has time to create its own antibodies.

Immunization can protect against diphtheria, measles, mumps, pertussis (whooping cough), polio, rubella (German measles), tetanus, hepatitis B and certain kinds of meningitis.

Every child should receive injections of the combined diphtheria-tetanus-pertussis (DTP) vaccine at 2, 4, 6, and 18 months of age. The child should also receive a dose of the oral polio vaccine (OPV) at 2, 4, and 18 months of age. Every child should also receive injections of the vaccine against *Hemophilus influenzae* type B (HiB), the most common cause of bacterial meningitis in children. The recommended schedule for HiB vaccination depends upon the brand of vaccine used. For example, one brand of the vaccine should be given at 2, 4, and 12 months of age; another should be given at 2, 4, 6, and 15 months of age. The physician who performs the initial vaccination can tell you which schedule applies to your child. At 15 months, a child should receive the combined measles, mumps, and rubella (MMR) vaccine and a test for tuberculosis (TB). DTP and OPV boosters should be given around the time of school entry (when your child is four to five years old). A measles booster should be given when your child is 11 or 12 years of age, and anyone between 4 and 21 years of age should receive a measles booster during a measles outbreak. A diphtheria and tetanus toxoids (DT) booster shot should be given to teenagers between 14 and 16 years of age. And a tetanus booster should be given every ten years. A person with a high-risk wound, such as penetration into the foot by a rusty nail, should receive a tetanus booster if more than five years have elapsed since the last booster. Hepatitis B is given soon after birth, with two boosters administered during the first six months of life.

If the family does not have a physician, immunizations can usually be obtained through the local public health department. It usually has supplies of vaccines and may give shots free. If a child has an acute illness with fever, immunization should be delayed.

## Immunization and testing schedule

| | |
|---|---|
| Hepatitis B | Soon after birth; two boosters during first 6 months |
| DTP | 2, 4, 6, 18 months |
| OPV | 2, 4, 18 months |
| HiB | 2, 4, 6, 15, or 2, 4, 12 months |
| MMR | 15 months |
| TB test | 15 months |
| Measles booster | 11-12 years* |
| DT booster | 14-16 years |
| Tetanus booster | Every 10 years |

* If there is a measles outbreak, anyone between 4 years and 21 years of age should receive a booster.

Adults need a tetanus shot once every ten years. Otherwise, there are no routine immunizations necessary for adults in the United States, with the possible exception of influenza shots given annually (usually in the fall) to the aged and to patients with heart, lung, or other chronic diseases. A vaccine that would protect against 80 percent of serious cases of pneumonia is available. Immunization against the rabies virus is possible both before and after exposure. Vaccinations for hepatitis B are recommended for individuals at high risk, such as health-care workers or frequent travelers to areas in which the disease is endemic (in which the possibility of contracting disease is always present).

There are precautions to consider. Immunizations should not be given routinely to pregnant women, nor in general to anyone whose immune system has been weakened by leukemia, cancer, AIDS, or X-ray or corticosteroid treatment.

Most persons traveling abroad in developed countries need no additional vaccinations. In general, in the United States, Canada, Australia, New Zealand, Japan, and Europe, the traveler is safe without vaccinations.

Travel in Mexico and the less-developed countries of Africa, Asia, South America, Central America, the South Pacific, the Middle East, and the Far East may hold more risks, particularly in small villages and rural areas not usually visited by tourists.

In recent years, no vaccination has been necessary for direct travel from the United States to most countries or for return to the United States. However, some countries require proof of vaccination from travelers who have passed through infected areas, and it is best to get the shots before leaving home.

Any physician can give immunizations except for yellow-fever vaccinations, which must be given at an official "Yellow Fever Vaccination Center." Weeks before you plan to leave on your trip, call your local health department for the latest information about vaccination requirements and recommendations for all of the countries you plan to visit. The vaccinating physician must fill out and sign an "International Certificate of Vaccination," which must be validated by a health department or by an authorized physician.

Vaccinations against cholera, which is transmitted in contaminated food and water, and against yellow fever, which is transmitted by certain mosquitoes, are the shots most often required for foreign travel. Because no cholera vaccine is very effective and because the risk of acquiring cholera is small, the U.S. Public Health Service does not recommend vaccination against cholera unless the country to be visited requires it. However, yellow-fever vaccinations are strongly recommended, even if not required by law, for travel to infected areas (usually parts of Africa and South America) and for travel in countries in "yellow fever endemic zones" (areas in which the possibility of contracting the disease is always present).

In no case should anyone be immunized against smallpox. The World Health Organization has declared that smallpox has been eliminated from the world, and the vaccination itself is not without risk. Therefore, if you are traveling to a country that still requires proof of vaccination against smallpox, the U.S. Public Health Service suggests that you obtain a written statement from your physician recommending against smallpox vaccination for health reasons.

Anyone not already immune to measles and mumps should receive vaccinations before traveling abroad, as should children not immune to rubella. Travelers to developing countries need diphtheria, polio, and typhoid immunizations, unless they are already immune, and a tetanus booster shot if they have not had one in the previous ten years.

Vaccination cannot protect against malaria, a health threat in many developing countries. Travelers to infected areas should take along protective medications, sleep in well-screened areas, wear protective clothing, and use chemical repellents to ward off the long-legged *Anopheles* mosquito, which transmits the disease. Since antimalarial prophylaxis recommendations change, it is best to check with the U.S. Department of Health before travelling abroad.

# Impotence

Impotence is the inability to achieve and maintain an erection of the penis, which is necessary to penetrate the vagina during sexual intercourse. The corpora cavernosa of the penis normally fill with blood during sexual excitement, which causes the penis to become rigid and erect. Impotence is a partial or total impairment of this function.

There are two types of impotence: primary impotence, in which a man is never able to have an erection adequate for sexual intercourse; and secondary impotence, in which a man quite often fails to complete intercourse to the satisfaction of both partners. Secondary impotence is more common.

Many men experience temporary impotence at some point in their lives, but chronic (recurring) impotence can lower a man's self-esteem and put a strain on his marriage or social relationships.

Impotence can be caused by either physical or psychological problems. It may be brought on by job-related stress, fear of causing pregnancy, unresolved conflicts about sexuality, or fear of sex after a heart attack or major surgery. Drug and alcohol abuse are also among the leading causes of impotence.

Until recently, psychological problems were thought to be the only cause of impotence, but underlying physical factors are now also known to trigger the problem. These factors include the following: an imbalance in the hormonal system that causes a decrease in production of testosterone (the male hormone necessary for an erection); the use of certain drugs for the treatment of high blood pressure, particularly diuretics and beta-blockers; diseases of the nervous system, such as multiple sclerosis; structural abnormalities of the penis; injury to the penis; and malfunctioning of the circulatory system, which can interfere with the blood flow to the penis.

The major symptom of impotence is inability to attain or maintain erection of the penis for sexual intercourse. This may be accompanied by a lack of interest in sex, but not necessarily infertility (the inability to father a child).

Several tests can help to diagnose the cause of impotence. A blood test will show whether adequate levels of testosterone are present. With a blood pressure cuff specially designed to wrap around the penis and an ultrasound study (a technique that uses sound waves to create images of internal structures), blood vessel problems in the penis can often be detected. Another test registers the size of erections that naturally occur during sleep; if erections do not occur during sleep, a physical, rather than an emotional, cause is likely.

If impotence has a physical basis, a number of treatments are available. Injections of testosterone and other hormones may relieve some problems. Another nonsurgical option, external vacuum therapy, involves the use of a plastic cylinder and pump to enlarge the penis. In some cases, surgery may be necessary to repair the arteries and veins that carry blood to and from the penis.

The use of penile implants is a successful new treatment for impotence, with several varieties now in use. One is a silicone rod that is implanted in the corpora cavernosa, resulting in a permanent partial erection. Another is a flexible silver wire surrounded by silicone, which allows manipulation of the penis to an erect position for intercourse. A third model consists of balloon-like cylinders implanted in the corpora cavernosa and connected to a container of fluid; with the use of a hand pump, the cylinders may be filled with the fluid, in the same way that blood normally fills the penis during an erection.

Counseling by psychologists or trained sex therapists may be recommended for men whose impotence seems to stem from emotional problems. Counseling may also help those with physical disorders in learning to deal with their impotence.

Avoiding the abuse of alcohol and drugs, as well as eliminating or coping with stress, should help to prevent at least some episodes of secondary impotence.

# Incontinence

Urinary incontinence is the loss of voluntary bladder control. It occurs frequently in children and in older persons.

Most often, incontinence is caused by some underlying condition, such as obstruction, infection, or inflammation of any portion of the urinary tract. Successful treatment of the underlying cause clears up the problem of incontinence.

Stress incontinence is the leakage of urine on coughing, sneezing, straining, or laughing. This type of incontinence is common in women whose pelvic muscles have been weakened by childbirth.

Although the first step in treating incontinence is to detect and correct any underlying problem, it is important to remember that many children do not establish complete bladder control before they are four or five years old. Children of any age may have occasional accidents, especially if they become ill or extremely exhausted.

Persons who have problems with incontinence can help themselves by going to the bathroom often and regularly, by arranging sleeping and living quarters in close proximity to bathrooms, and by wearing clothes that can be removed quickly and easily. It may also help to keep a bedpan or urinal next to the bed and to drink only a small amount of water, if any, before going to bed.

Drugs are available to aid in controlling urination in certain conditions. Incontinence that is related to stress can usually be surgically corrected.

# Indigestion

Indigestion (also called dyspepsia) is the discomfort caused by difficulty in digesting food. It is an uncomfortable feeling of fullness, pressure, slight pain, or gassiness and is usually related to eating. (Constipation, diarrhea, heartburn, and nausea are not indigestion, although they may be related to the problem.)

Indigestion is usually caused by an eating problem, such as eating too fast or too much; chewing insufficiently; eating in an emotionally upsetting environment; eating particularly bothersome foods, such as spicy, fatty, or oily foods, or those that may cause an allergic reaction; or smoking, especially immediately before or after a meal. Indigestion can also be caused by serious disorders, such as cancer, ulcers, and diseases involving the organs associated with digestion (the esophagus, intestines, gallbladder, liver, stomach, and pancreas). In addition, heart attack, tumors, and emotional problems may be accompanied by symptoms that are similar to those of indigestion.

Any case of indigestion that lingers for some time or that cannot be controlled in any way should be reported to a doctor for diagnosis and appropriate treatment.

The cause of indigestion is diagnosed primarily by observing the symptoms and the conditions under which they occur. A doctor will want a description of the symptoms and of the patient's dietary habits; of the time, length, and location of the discomfort, as well as the circumstances surrounding it and the foods eaten preceding it; and of the emotional environment that usually exists during meals and snacks. X-ray studies of the gastrointestinal tract or analysis of stool (feces) may also be used to make a diagnosis of the cause of indigestion.

Antacids often relieve indigestion, but they should not be used without the advice of a physician. This is particularly true of people who have kidney disease.

The best treatment consists of preventing indigestion in the first place. Eating balanced meals in a relaxed setting, eliminating foods that can cause indigestion, and refraining from smoking, especially at mealtimes, should be beneficial in the prevention of indigestion.

# Infectious diseases

The human body is both surrounded and inhabited by billions of microorganisms (living organisms that are so small that they can be seen only with a microscope). Most microorganisms are harmless or even beneficial; for example, certain bacteria that normally live in the digestive system help digest food. Occasionally, however, a microorganism capable of causing a disease invades the body. Diseases caused by such microorganisms are called infectious diseases.

Infectious diseases are contagious; that is, they can be passed from one person to another. They can be transmitted by skin contact, through body fluids, in contaminated food or drink, or via airborne particles containing the microorganisms. Animal or insect bites are another means of transmission. (If an insect, for example, bites an infected person, the insect can carry the microorganism and pass the disease by biting another person.) The two most common types of infectious diseases are bacterial infections and viral infections.

Disease-causing, or pathogenic, bacteria either attack the body's tissues directly or cause damage by secreting poisonous substances called toxins. Fortunately, bacterial infections are frequently curable; certain bacteria can be killed by drugs. Other bacterial diseases can be prevented by vaccination.

Viruses are the smallest known microorganisms. They are responsible for diseases as relatively harmless as the common cold and as serious as meningitis. Viruses live and reproduce only within living cells, and only certain cells are susceptible to a specific virus. You can be host to many viruses without suffering any adverse effects, but if enough cells are attacked, you will become sick.

There is no effective medical treatment for most viral infections. Because a virus lives inside a cell, any treatment designed to kill the virus is also likely to harm the cell. In addition, there are thousands of different viruses—each with different properties—and an agent effective against one virus probably will not affect the others. Although there are vaccinations for some viral diseases, therapy for most viral diseases is limited to treating the symptoms.

Despite the prevalence of disease-causing microorganisms, the body is not defenseless against these invaders. The body fights infections in three ways: by preventing these organisms from entering the body, by attacking those that do manage to enter, and by inactivating those organisms it cannot kill. Sometimes, too, the body fights disease by developing defensive symptoms. Fever is an example. During an illness, the body's temperature regulator may respond to the illness by raising the body's temperature. Some researchers believe that this is an effective response because the microorganisms causing the disease may not be able to survive the higher body temperature.

The skin is the first barrier that guards the underlying tissues of the body. Where there are natural openings in the skin, there are also defenses. For example, tear glands in the eyes secrete and bathe the eyes with fluid that contains bacteria-fighting components. The salivary glands in the mouth and the tonsils in the throat help prevent microorganisms from attacking the mouth and throat. Many openings, as well as internal passages, in the body are lined with mucous membranes. These delicate layers produce mucus, a slippery secretion that moistens and protects by repelling or trapping microorganisms. Internally, certain body organs fight infection. For instance, the liver and the spleen (a large glandlike organ located in the abdomen) filter out harmful substances from the blood flowing through them. The lining of the stomach produces acids that attack germs in food that has been eaten. And the body's lymph system manufactures white blood cells, which attack and destroy invading organisms.

The lymph system is a network of vessels that carry lymph, a watery fluid containing white blood cells, throughout the body. Lymph drains from the blood vessels and body tissues, carrying away waste products. The waste products are filtered out of the lymph by small structures called lymph nodes (popularly known as lymph glands). Within the lymph nodes, harmful microorganisms are trapped, attacked, and destroyed by white blood cells. This is one of the body's primary and most efficient lines of defense.

Antibodies are manufactured in the lymph system. Antibodies are protective substances that the body produces in response to invasion by a hostile organism or the presence of a foreign substance. Antibodies counteract some invading bacteria and viruses by inactivating them so that they are powerless. Antibodies that neutralize toxins (poisons) produced by bacteria are called antitoxins.

The body's production of white blood cells and antibodies in response to an invading disease organism is called the immune reaction. Immunity is the body's ability to resist an invasion of disease-causing bacteria and viruses. Once antibodies have been made to fight a certain type of microorganism, that type usually no longer poses a threat to the body. That is why one attack of a disease often prevents the recurrence of that disease. The first attack causes antibodies to be produced, and these antibodies protect the system against subsequent attacks.

Immunity can be provided artificially by vaccination and other forms of immunization. A vaccine is a preparation containing the offending organism—usually in a weakened form that will not cause the actual disease. When introduced into the body, the vaccine stimulates the body to produce antibodies against the disease. These antibodies remain in the system for a long time, preparing the body to resist the actual disease.

A number of viral diseases can be prevented by immunization. There are vaccines for polio, measles, rubella (German measles), mumps, and some strains of influenza. Researchers are working on a vaccine against chicken pox and shingles; however, this vaccine is not yet available to the public. A vaccine against Hemophilus influenza type B is available to prevent the most common cause of bacterial meningitis in children. Hepatitis B vaccine is now available and recommended for all infants.

Besides vaccination, there are other measures that can be used to help the body's natural defenses fight off infectious diseases. Bacterial infections can often be conquered by medications called antibiotics. These are substances derived from living microorganisms that kill other microorganisms. Penicillin, for example, comes from a living mold called *Penicillium*. Penicillin is one of the most commonly used antibiotics, along with streptomycin, tetracycline, and erythromycin. Each of these is effective against specific diseases. Antibiotics work either by destroying bacteria or by preventing their reproduction.

Sulfonamides, or sulfa drugs, are synthetic antibiotic drugs that are also effective against infections. This type of drug is often prescribed for localized infections in the urinary tract.

Unfortunately, these medications do not attack viruses. Viruses, therefore, are responsible for many of the serious or fatal infectious illnesses today, since no generally effective cures have been developed. The virus that causes acquired immune deficiency syndrome (AIDS) is an example of a particularly lethal virus for which there is no cure.

Researchers are continually searching for new ways to help the body combat infectious diseases. Medical advances against these diseases have already been dramatic; not too many years ago infectious diseases were uncontrollable and thus a constant danger. The control of many infections has been one of medicine's greatest accomplishments.

# Infertility

Infertility is defined as a couple's failure to conceive a child after one year of regular sexual intercourse without birth control. In about 40 percent of all cases of infertility, the problem lies with the man; in 60 percent it lies with the woman or with both partners.

Infertility is not sterility. The term infertility implies that the condition can be treated and reversed—that it may be a temporary problem. The term sterility is applied to a permanent, irreversible inability to have children.

Recent research has shown that a woman's fertility drops off significantly between the ages of 31 and 35 and continues to decline thereafter until menopause, when it ceases. A man's fertility also declines after the age of 40, although men can remain fertile until old age.

One of the major causes of male infertility is a low sperm count. It is measured by the number of active sperm present in a milliliter (there are approximately five milliliters in one teaspoon) of semen (the fluid ejected from the penis during intercourse). An average sperm count is 90 million or more sperm per milliliter. A count of at least 40 to 60 million is thought to be necessary for fertilization; when the count is less than 20 million, it is less likely that the man can father a child (although, since only one sperm is needed to fertilize an egg, it is still possible).

A low sperm count can be caused by low levels of testosterone (the male sex hormone); by exposure to chemicals, pesticides, or radiation; by engaging in sexual intercourse too

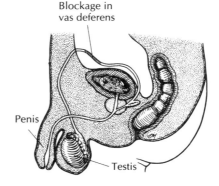

Blockage in
vas deferens

Penis

Testis

Male infertility can be caused by a blockage anywhere in the tubes that convey sperm from the testes to the penis.

frequently, which depletes the sperm supply too quickly; and by heat (which slows sperm production) generated by wearing tight underwear or pants, sitting for long periods in hot cars or trucks, or working near ovens and kilns. Infertility can also result if sperm cannot propel themselves through the female reproductive tract to reach the egg, or if sperm are irregularly shaped (only sperm with oval-shaped heads can fertilize an egg).

In addition to problems with the sperm themselves, male infertility can be caused by any obstruction in the tubes that convey the sperm from the testes (the male sex organs where sperm are produced) to the penis. Infertility may also be caused by varicose veins in the scrotum (the pouch containing the testes), perhaps because the increased blood flow in these swollen veins brings extra heat to the area, or by a local infection or injury; the infertility problem will probably reverse itself when the condition is corrected. In addition, surgical removal of part of the prostate gland (one of the organs in which most of the fluid in semen is produced), as well as the use of certain drugs for high blood pressure, can lead to retrograde ejaculation (a disorder in which the semen is passed backward into the bladder, to exit with the urine, rather than out through the penis).

Female infertility can be caused by an obstruction in a fallopian tube, through which the egg passes from the ovary to the uterus.

A woman may be infertile because of a variety of conditions. It may be that she is not ovulating (releasing an egg each month); this is true in about 25 percent of all cases of female infertility. The fallopian tubes (through which the eggs travel on their way from the ovaries to the uterus) may be obstructed, often as a result of pelvic inflammatory disease (PID), which irritates the tubes and causes scar tissue to form. PID can develop as a reaction to an IUD (intrauterine device used for birth control), a sexually transmitted disease, or an infection of the lower reproductive tract. Endometriosis (the displacement of tissue from the uterine lining to elsewhere in the body) may also cause the formation of scar tissue that blocks the fallopian tubes. An imbalance of the female hormones estrogen and progesterone or of other hormones secreted from the pituitary or thyroid glands can interfere with the reproductive cycle. A "hostile" cervix (one that creates an environment that in some way prevents sperm from surviving) may also be the cause of the infertility.

Diagnosis of the reason for the infertility problem will usually begin with physical examinations and complete medical and sexual histories of both partners.

A fresh sample of the man's semen will be examined under a microscope to determine the quantity and quality of the sperm. This will provide a sperm count and will also indicate whether the sperm are adequately mobile and whether the heads of the sperm are oval, both characteristics that are necessary for conception.

To determine whether ovulation is taking place in the female, the basal body temperature (the body temperature on awakening, before eating or drinking) will be taken every morning for several months. If the temperature rises by 0.6°F to 1.0°F for a few days in the middle of the menstrual cycle, ovulation is probably taking place. An endometrial biopsy, in which a sample of the lining of the uterus is obtained, can indicate whether ovulation is occurring and whether or not hormonal secretion is normal.

Obstruction of the fallopian tubes can be diagnosed by injecting a dye into the reproductive tract and then taking an X ray. Another test consists of injecting carbon dioxide gas into the fallopian tubes and waiting for the patient to feel pain in the upper part of the body, indicating that the gas is passing through the fallopian tubes and that there are no obstructions.

A hostile cervix can be identified by a microscopic examination of the mucus in the cervix shortly after sexual intercourse to determine the rate of sperm survival. Endometriosis is diagnosed by inserting into the abdomen a laparoscope (a small, lighted instrument), through which the doctor can actually see the uterus, fallopian tubes, ovaries, and any endometrial tissue that may be causing the infertility.

Hormonal imbalances in both men and women can be diagnosed with blood tests.

Treatment for a low sperm count caused by a testosterone deficiency is usually hormone therapy to increase testosterone levels. If the low sperm count is due to chemicals, radiation, or excess heat, exposure to these factors must be corrected or avoided. If the sperm count is low for some unknown reason, there is often little more that can be done.

If male infertility is caused by varicose veins, surgery may be necessary. If an obstruction exists somewhere in the tubes leading to and through the penis, microsurgery to open the blockage may correct the problem.

Failure to ovulate is often treated with a fertility drug called clomiphene, which stimulates production of the hormone that regulates ovulation. About 60 percent of the patients who receive clomiphene become pregnant; the chances of multiple births are very low. A stronger drug, which is a combination of certain pituitary gland hormones, may also be prescribed, but it carries with it a greater risk of multiple births.

Obstructed fallopian tubes may require microsurgery to open the blockage, or a new procedure in which an egg is removed and replaced beyond the point of the obstruction, where it may be fertilized normally. A hostile cervix can be treated with the female hormone estrogen, which stimulates the increased production of mucus, which is necessary to transport the sperm. Sometimes sperm can be placed directly into the uterus, bypassing the cervix completely. Endometriosis can be treated by the surgical removal of displaced tissue and the scar tissue that has formed around it. Hormonal imbalances can be corrected with hormone therapy.

Test-tube, or *in vitro*, fertilization is a relatively new technique in which an egg is removed from the woman's ovary and then placed in a test tube or special sterile dish containing the man's sperm. Once the egg has been fertilized, it is placed into the woman's uterus, where it will continue to grow. This technique is used primarily in women whose blocked fallopian tubes cannot be opened by surgery.

Another new technique used to treat infertility is called gamete intra fallopian transfer (GIFT). In this procedure, clomiphene or another fertility drug is given to the woman to stimulate ovulation. When an egg is produced by the ovary, it is removed via laparoscopy and immediately mixed with sperm from the man. This sperm-egg mixture is then transferred by laparoscopy into a fallopian tube, where fertilization may then take place normally. Fertilization occurs in the woman's body and not in a test tube. GIFT is a complicated and expensive procedure that should be used only by couples who have not been able to conceive using standard treatments for infertility.

Although recent advances in treating infertility have led to greater and greater success, about 15 percent of all female infertility problems and about ten percent of all male problems remain undiagnosed and therefore untreatable.

See also Birth control, Conception, Endometriosis, Menstruation, Ovulation, Pelvic inflammatory disease, Prostatitis, and Reproduction.

# Influenza

Influenza, more commonly called the flu, is a contagious disease that is accompanied by respiratory problems and fever. A bout of influenza is unpleasant, but it is usually not dangerous to otherwise healthy people.

Two types of viruses cause influenza: influenza A virus and influenza B virus. Each type encompasses several different strains, which are named for the place where they were first identified, such as Russian flu virus.

The unusual characteristic of the flu viruses is that once a strain has spread throughout a population, it changes in structure, becoming capable of causing a new form of influenza. The antibodies produced by the body to combat the virus are no longer effective because the virus has taken on different qualities. Scientists are generally able to predict what type of altered virus to expect each year, but about every ten years an entirely new strain appears.

Because influenza is thought to be transmitted by airborne particles from an infected person's respiratory tract, large numbers of people in a community or even in a country can easily contract the disease in a relatively short period of time. Overcrowded living conditions promote the transmission of the virus. Since flu spreads most easily when temperatures and humidity are low, most cases of influenza occur in the fall and winter months.

Flu symptoms usually develop one to three days after exposure to the virus. Some people experience symptoms in as short a time as 18 hours. Fever, chills, headache, muscle aches, and total exhaustion can occur suddenly. Fevers generally do not go above 104°F, but they may rise as high as 106°F.

Frequently, people experience a dry cough and a runny or congested nose as their initial symptoms begin to subside. These respiratory symptoms worsen and remain for three to four days. The cough and fatigue may persist for two weeks or more after the other symptoms have disappeared.

The most common complications are those that involve parts of the respiratory system—for example, pneumonia (infection of the lungs), which affects both adults and children, and croup (infection of the larynx), which affects young children. If the patient has extreme difficulty in breathing, blood in the coughed-up mucus, bluish skin, or a barklike cough, a physician should be consulted immediately.

One life-threatening complication of influenza that affects children and adolescents between the ages of 2 and 16 years is Reye's syndrome. It is a type of encephalitis (inflammation of the brain) that is accompanied by deterioration of the liver. Aspirin may place the child at higher risk for Reye's syndrome and should not be taken.

In most cases, influenza cannot be cured and is treated only by relieving symptoms. Amantadine, a drug used in the treatment of Parkinson's disease, can be used to prevent and treat some forms of influenza A infection. This drug can produce unpleasant side effects, however, so physicians usually prescribe it only when a patient is susceptible to additional complications.

Treatment for flu is generally the same as treatment for a bad cold or fever. Physicians recommend bed rest, extra fluids, and an aspirin substitute to reduce fever and muscle aches. Because an association has been established between aspirin use during a viral infection and Reye's syndrome in children, it is recommended that aspirin not be given to a child with influenza. Acetaminophen, however, has not been linked to Reye's syndrome and can be used. Nasal sprays or drops, when used sparingly so that nasal tissues are not damaged, and cough medicines can help relieve coldlike symptoms. Using a vaporizer in the patient's room to add moisture to the air will help to relieve congestion.

Each year, researchers prepare an influenza vaccine in an attempt to prevent spread of the virus. The vaccine is composed of inactivated organisms from several virus strains and provides protection against influenza caused by these strains. Unfortunately, protection is not necessarily afforded against new or different strains. Vaccines are typically between 67 percent and 92 percent effective. It is especially important for the elderly; people with lung disease, heart disease, or other chronic diseases; and those with immune system disorders to have this vaccine. Influenza can be devastating in these individuals.

Some people have reactions to the vaccine that range from inflammation at the injection site to mild flu symptoms. On very rare occasions, nervous system disorders result. Flu vaccines are commonly prepared using eggs. Therefore, individuals with known allergy to eggs should inform their physician before having the vaccine. Vaccination is not usually recommended for children unless they are in a high risk group, such as those with heart or lung conditions.

See also Reye's syndrome.

# Insect bite and sting

Insect bites and stings are minor inconveniences to most people, but to those who have an allergy to insect venom, the consequences can be serious.

Reactions to insect venom show themselves in various symptoms— shortness of breath, rapid heartbeat, coughing, wheezing, and light-headedness. The affected area swells and becomes tender or numb. In extreme cases, anaphylactic shock (a severe, potentially fatal reaction characterized by breathing problems, hives, collapse of blood vessels, and sometimes vomiting, diarrhea, and cramps) can occur.

Serious reactions to bites and stings are treated by slowing the spread of the venom throughout the body and getting emergency medical treatment as soon as possible. The progress of the venom can be slowed somewhat by applying an ice pack or a tourniquet (but not so tightly as to stop the blood flow) to the affected area. Emergency medical treatment will usually consist of an epinephrine injection and an injection of antihistamine. In some cases, a corticosteroid may be given as well. These serve to lessen existing symptoms and to halt progression of the reaction.

Prevention of recurrent allergic reactions to insect venom may be accomplished with a course of desensitization shots; starting with an initially weak solution of insect extract, doses are gradually increased with each shot. This allows the body to build up tolerance to the effects of the insect venom.

Persons with known sensitivity to insect bites should carry kits with injectable epinephrine, which are available by prescription.

See also Allergy and Anaphylactic shock.

# Insomnia

Insomnia is the inability to sleep during normal sleeping hours when there is no apparent reason for wakefulness. Insomnia may vary from simple restlessness, to wakefulness on and off throughout the night, to total sleeplessness.

Although the condition is most often associated with psychological or emotional problems, it can also be related to physical disorders or to conditions in the immediate environment.

Depression and anxiety are often the cause of insomnia. Among physical disorders that can lead to insomnia are urination problems, heart trouble, high blood pressure, infection, hardening of the arteries, spastic colon, and leg cramps. Less serious causes of insomnia can be found in the immediate environment—bright lights, noise, excessive heat or cold, or lack of ventilation. Insomnia may also be caused by having too many or too few bedclothes, by being constipated or hungry, or by having consumed too much coffee, tea, cola, or other beverage containing caffeine, which is a stimulant.

Strangely, drugs to promote sleep can cause insomnia. The careless or inappropriate use of tranquilizers and sedatives can disrupt sleep patterns. If high doses of tranquilizers or sedatives are taken, the waking-sleeping pattern can be reversed, and sleep can become irregular. The person may doze throughout the day and then be unable to sleep at night.

A person who has persistent insomnia should consult a physician so that the underlying cause—emotional or physical—can be diagnosed and treated.

Ways of preventing or coping with simple insomnia include taking a 10- or 15-minute walk before bedtime, taking a warm bath, drinking warm milk (milk contains a substance called tryptophan, which promotes drowsiness), reading, or watching television. Taking sleep-promoting medications should be discussed with a doctor.

# Intestinal and gastric bypass surgery

Intestinal bypass surgery and gastric bypass surgery are methods of treating massive obesity. Because of their potential dangers, such methods are usually limited to persons who are at least 100 pounds over their ideal weight and who have failed to lose weight by other means, such as diet and exercise. These persons are at serious risk for diabetes, high blood pressure, heart disease, arthritis, and other weight related disorders.

Various types of operations have been tried to detour digesting food around a long section of the small intestine, thus limiting the area of intestine that can absorb fats and carbohydrates from the food. One such operation is the jejunoileal bypass—named for the jejunum (the middle portion of the small intestine) and the ileum (the final portion of the small intestine). In this procedure, all but 18 inches of the 240 inches of the small intestine is bypassed (the unused portion remains in the body and drains into the colon). The method is very effective in reducing weight—from 80 to 150 pounds in most patients—but frequently produces persistent diarrhea, severe liver disease, imbalances in body salts, kidney stones, bladder stones, mental disturbances, and joint inflammations. Because the mortality rate associated with those complications may be as high as five percent, many physicians believe that the intestinal bypass method should no longer be used. This surgery is now seldom performed since there are other treatment methods that are safer.

Replacements for the intestinal bypass procedure, which are reported to have far fewer complications, are gastric bypass and gastric stapling. Both are designed to reduce the capacity of the stomach so that only a small amount of food can be eaten at one time. In the gastric bypass operation, the lower part of the stomach is cut off, and the remaining top part is connected to the upper portion of the small intestine. In the gastric stapling operation, stomach capacity is reduced by stapling off most of the fundus (the uppermost portion of the stomach).

Recently, a nonsurgical technique for reducing stomach capacity has been developed. A specially designed balloon is placed in the stomach and then inflated. Since the balloon takes up a significant portion of the volume of the stomach, there is less room for food. The patient feels full after eating a relatively small quantity of food. This technique has the advantage that it is readily reversible: the balloon can be removed relatively easily if problems arise or the patient reaches the desired weight.

The long-term results and side effects of gastric bypass, gastric stapling, and gastric balloon placement, when known, will determine whether these procedures are widely employed. Until then, it should be remembered that they are drastic measures that carry the risk of potentially serious complications. Currently, few of these procedures are performed.

# Irritable bowel syndrome

Irritable bowel syndrome, also called spastic colon or mucous colitis, is a collection of symptoms caused by irritability and irregularity in the movement of both the small and large intestines. The syndrome is usually influenced by emotions. Feelings of nervousness, anxiety, guilt, depression, or anger may bring on or aggravate this very common disorder. Coffee, raw fruits and vegetables, hormones, drugs, and overuse of laxatives can promote it, as can an inability of the body to digest the natural sugar found in milk.

Irritable bowel syndrome is not a disease, but a collection of symptoms that includes both constipation and diarrhea, often alternating and sometimes accompanied by abdominal cramps and straining during elimination. Stools may be loose or compacted and may include mucus, which is produced by the bowel lining in greater than usual amounts as a response to irritation. Gas, bloating, nausea, headache, and fatigue may accompany the other symptoms.

There are two main types of irritable bowel syndrome. The first type, spastic colon, is marked by cramps or a dull, aching pain in the abdomen, usually the lower part. The discomfort often begins at mealtime and may disappear after a bowel movement. The second type of irritable bowel syndrome is characterized by painless diarrhea, especially an urgent need for a bowel movement on awakening or during or right after a meal. Fecal incontinence (loss of voluntary bowel control) can occur.

If a patient appears to have irritable bowel syndrome, the doctor will first want to rule out diseases with similar symptoms. The patient may be asked to bring in a stool specimen to be examined for traces of blood and microorganisms. The colon may be x-rayed following a barium enema. The doctor may examine the lower portion of the colon with a proctosigmoidoscope (a lighted tubelike instrument inserted through the anus) to check for serious disorders, such as ulcerative colitis.

If no organic disease is found, the doctor will reassure the patient and discuss ways in which the symptoms can be relieved. There may be methods by which the patient can reduce the anxiety or depression that may be causing the syndrome. The doctor may prescribe a tranquilizer, sedative, antidepressant, or antispasmodic medication—but only on a short-term basis, so that the individual does not become dependent on the drug. Long walks, bike rides, or other exercise may help to relax the person while promoting better bowel action.

If constipation is a problem, the doctor will advise the patient to add bulk, such as whole bran, to the diet; to stop depending on laxatives; and to take pills that absorb water, add bulk, and help to stabilize the large intestine. If diarrhea is present, avoiding laxative foods, such as prunes, may help. Patients bothered by gas will be warned against foods such as cabbage and beans. Milk may be barred from the diet. Most people, with the general exception of those of northwestern European origin, lose

some or all of the ability to digest lactose, the natural sugar in milk, by the time they are 20 years old. A test for this is an oral dose of lactose. If it results in diarrhea and bloating, it is a tip-off that the symptoms could have been caused by drinking milk.

If irritable bowel syndrome continues despite treatment, it is important to remember that it is not dangerous. However, to be on the safe side, regular medical checkups should be scheduled, especially if the patient is over 40 years of age.

---

# Ischemia

Ischemia is a deficiency of blood in a specific part of the body caused by an obstruction of the blood vessels supplying that area. The obstruction may be due to narrowing, compression, or destruction of arteries caused by such conditions as blood clots and atherosclerosis (clogging of the arteries). The resultant oxygen deprivation, if prolonged, leads to tissue death in the affected area.

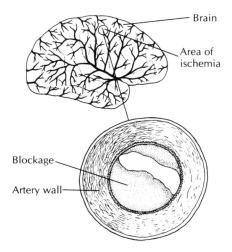

Ischemia is an inadequate flow of blood to a part of the body because of a blockage in the blood vessel nourishing that part of the body.

An ischemic attack in the brain occurs when the supply of blood to the brain is temporarily reduced. This type of attack resembles a stroke. If the brain is deprived of blood for more than several minutes, the result is irreversible brain damage and often death.

When the blood supply to the heart is reduced, angina pectoris (chest pain) results. When the blood supply to a region of the heart is completely cut off, a heart attack occurs. The lower the blood supply that gets through to the heart, the greater the severity of the attack. If a weakened heart is unable to pump an adequate supply of blood to the rest of the body, the efficiency of the other organs will also be impaired: They will not be able to work at their full capacity.

Ischemic attacks can be controlled by vasodilator medications, which have the effect of widening blood vessels. Angina pectoris is often managed in this way. In many cases, surgery to remove or to bypass the obstruction is recommended.

See also Angina pectoris, Coronary bypass surgery, Heart attack, Stroke, and Transient ischemic attack.

---

# Itching

Itching is an uncomfortable or irritating sensation on the surface of the skin, accompanied by an urge to scratch. It has been described as a pricking, stinging, burning, or crawling feeling.

The biological reactions that lead to itching are not clearly understood, but it is known that this stimulation of the nerve endings in the skin can be caused by both physical and psychological factors.

Itching can be caused by insect bites; small cuts or scrapes; hives and other allergic reactions; a fungal infection, and the rash that often accompanies infectious diseases, such as chicken pox. Dry skin, often stemming from bathing or showering too frequently or using harsh soaps; reactions to drugs; and psychological stress are other causes of itching.

Itching is characterized by a feeling of discomfort, the urge to scratch, and possibly redness, peeling, and other irritations of the skin as a result of scratching. Itching of just the scalp and forearms with no obvious cause may be triggered by psychological stress.

Treatment of itching depends on its cause. Itching from dry skin is usually treated by applying skin lotions or creams to small areas and using body lotions or bath oils for larger areas; reducing the frequency of showers and baths to only twice weekly (because water tends to dry the skin); and trying a new brand of soap or shampoo.

If itching seems to be a reaction to a drug, the doctor should be consulted before making any changes in medication. Generally, the doctor will either lower the dosage to relieve the itching or give advice on treatment of the itching while maintaining the original dosage.

If no outside substances seem to be triggering itching, psychological or emotional stress may be the cause. In these cases, treatment will center on removing the stress or learning how to deal with it.

If itching persists for more than a week after attempts at self-treatment, a doctor should be consulted because persistent itching with no visible cause may be a symptom of diabetes, thyroid disease, kidney failure, liver disease, or cancer.

Limiting bathing to twice weekly and using humidifiers to keep the air moist should help prevent the itching caused by dry skin.

# J

## Jaundice

Jaundice is a yellowish discoloration of the skin, the whites of the eyes, the mucous membranes, and other tissues of the body. The condition is caused by the abnormal accumulation of the bile pigment bilirubin in the blood.

Bilirubin consists primarily of the hemoglobin of used red blood cells and is found in bile, a bitter, yellow-green fluid that aids in digestion by breaking down fat. Bile is secreted by the liver, stored in the gallbladder, and discharged into the small intestine when it is needed for the process of digestion.

In many cases, jaundice occurs when bile is prevented from being discharged into the small intestine by an obstruction. The obstruction may be caused by gallstones, tumors, or parasites in the bile ducts. Jaundice may also be a sign of hepatitis, in which the inflamed or damaged liver cannot process the bilirubin it receives.

Occasionally, jaundice appears if red blood cells are destroyed too rapidly and the liver cannot accommodate the excess pigment. Jaundice is also associated with many other diseases in which the functioning of the liver is disrupted, including various forms of cancer and certain viral and parasitic infections. More than 50 percent of full-term newborn infants and 80 percent of premature newborn infants show signs of jaundice by the third day after birth. In most of these cases, the condition is nothing to worry about and disappears in a week or so.

Usually when jaundice occurs, the liver has become enlarged and is functioning less than optimally. Bowel movements may be clay-colored, and urine can vary in hue from light yellow to brownish green. Jaundiced skin ranges in color from lemon yellow to olive green.

Routine blood testing will determine the origin of some cases of jaundice, but usually it is necessary to examine the bile ducts using ultrasound, in which sound waves are used to create images of internal structures, and computed tomography, a special X-ray technique that provides cross-sectional pictures of an area.

Endoscopic retrograde cholangiopancreatography (ERCP) is a technique whereby the pancreas and bile ducts are examined after the direct injection of a contrast medium into a bile duct. This is accomplished by threading an endoscope (a flexible, lighted, tubelike instrument) through the mouth, down the esophagus, through the stomach, and into the duodenum. A small flexible tube is then inserted into the opening of the bile duct, and the contrast medium is infused. X rays are immediately taken. Bile samples for testing in the laboratory can also be obtained through this type of procedure. During this procedure, the patient is asleep but is not under general anesthesia. Usually the individual goes home the same day or the following day, depending on the underlying condition. Complications, such as perforation of an organ, pancreatitis (inflammation of the pancreas, an organ located behind the stomach), or infection, can occur but tend to be uncommon.

Surgery may be necessary if an obstruction is present. Otherwise, treatment depends on the underlying condition.

See also Gallstones and Hepatitis.

# K

## Keratitis

Keratitis is an inflammation of the cornea (the clear "window" in front of the iris and pupil of the eye), which commonly produces redness, tearing, tenderness, sensitivity to light, and blurred vision.

Interstitial keratitis is often caused by congenital (present at birth) syphilis in children or by tuberculosis. This type of keratitis produces deep deposits of scar tissue, which cause the cornea to become hazy and give it a ground-glass appearance. There is little that can be done for this condition, although the inflammation and redness usually diminish after a month or two. Vision may or may not be impaired thereafter.

A common type of keratitis is caused by the herpes simplex virus, the same virus that produces cold sores. Herpes simplex keratitis is usually not painful, although at first there is a sensation that foreign matter may be present. If the infection is left untreated, all feeling in the cornea will eventually be lost. Like a cold sore, the infection tends to come and go, but it should be taken care of when the first sign—a whitish lesion on the cornea—appears. Treatment usually consists of applying eyedrops or ointment, but some specialists prefer to scrape the cornea, after which they cover the affected eye temporarily.

Traumatic keratitis occurs when scar tissue remains after a corneal injury has healed. If a considerable amount of scar tissue covers the pupil, blindness may result. This condition can generally be cured by corrective surgery or corneal transplantation.

## Ketosis

Ketosis is an abnormal condition that occurs when the body burns fat instead of glucose (the form of sugar that is the body's chief source of energy) and, as a result, produces more of the chemical substances called ketones than is normal.

Ketones are the by-product of the chemical process that occurs in the cells when fat is broken down to produce energy. Under normal circumstances, ketones are broken down into carbon dioxide and water by the liver and other organs. In ketosis, the body is producing more ketones than it can process. The buildup of ketones disrupts the chemical balance of the body; if left unchecked, this condition can prove fatal.

Ketosis occurs most often in persons with insulin-dependent diabetes mellitus, a disorder in which the pancreas produces little or no insulin (a hormone secreted into the bloodstream to regulate glucose levels). This deficiency prevents the body from absorbing enough glucose and forces it to obtain its energy by burning fat. If ketosis is allowed to progress in a diabetic patient, diabetic ketoacidosis may occur. This is a life-threatening disorder that involves severe dehydration (excessive loss of body fluids) and coma (prolonged loss of consciousness).

Ketosis is also a consequence of starvation (and the self-induced starvation of excessive dieting), in which the body must rely on stores of fat for energy. Ketosis or ketoacidosis can also occur with heavy, long-term intake of alcohol.

The most common symptoms are a slightly sweet breath odor (similar to the smell of acetone or nail-polish remover), extreme dryness of the mucous membrane, weight loss, increased thirst and urination, weakness, abdominal pains, generalized aches, nausea and vomiting, and breathlessness.

Ketosis is diagnosed by testing the glucose and ketone levels in blood or urine. The urine test is less accurate than a blood test.

In insulin-dependent diabetics, administration of insulin corrects diabetic ketoacidosis. Diabetics are especially susceptible to ketosis before their condition is diagnosed, while they are fighting an infection, or when they neglect their diet or medication. Treatment of ketosis caused by starvation consists of feeding the patient substances that contain sugar or administering glucose solution intravenously. Alcoholic ketoacidosis is treated the same as that caused by starvation, usually with the addition of vitamin supplements.

See also Diabetes mellitus.

---

# Kidney failure

Kidney failure occurs when certain abnormalities within the kidneys prevent them from functioning normally, leading to chemical imbalances and the buildup of toxic (poisonous) substances and fluid within the body. This may eventually lead to organ damage and possibly death.

There are two forms of kidney failure. In the acute form, there is a sudden malfunction of the kidneys, leading to a rapid buildup of toxins and fluid within the body, often within several hours. In the chronic form of kidney failure, there is a slow, progressive deterioration of kidney function, leading to a buildup of toxins and fluid, often occurring over several months or years.

Numerous conditions can cause kidney failure. High blood pressure, kidney stones or other urinary tract blockage, adverse reactions to chemicals or drugs, serious injury, infectious disease, shock following surgery, heart attack, blood transfusion with incompatible blood, severe dehydration (excessive loss of body fluid), complications during pregnancy, immunologic disease, and congenital (existing from birth) kidney defects may all lead to kidney failure.

The most characteristic symptoms of kidney failure are a reduction in the volume of urine and edema (excessive accumulation of fluid in the tissues). As a result, the feet and hands and the area around the eyes may swell and become puffy. The urine may be bloody, wine-colored, or cloudy.

More generalized signs of kidney failure include drowsiness and fatigue, loss of appetite, diarrhea, nausea, dry skin, and difficulty in breathing. Delirium, coma, and death will eventually occur in untreated cases.

Analysis of blood and urine samples is used to diagnose kidney failure. Urine tests may show that white blood cells, sugars, or protein have slipped through the normally efficient filtering system of the kidneys. Similarly, when the kidneys are not filtering waste materials from the blood, blood analysis will detect waste products remaining in the blood. X-ray studies, ultrasound scans of the kidneys, or cystoscopy may identify structural abnormalities or blockage.

In the case of acute kidney failure, treatment begins with diagnosing and correcting the cause of the kidney damage and restoring normal kidney function as rapidly as possible. For example, shock may be treated with intravenous fluids, drugs, and, if necessary, blood transfusions; kidney stones may be removed.

Rest is essential as the kidneys recover. Limiting fluid intake, except in cases of unusual fluid loss from diarrhea or vomiting, may prevent congestive heart failure due to kidney overload. Physicians often recommend a low-protein diet due to the inability of the kidneys to process the waste products of protein metabolism.

Should these measures prove ineffective, the patient may be helped by dialysis. Dialysis is a process that cleans and filters toxic substances from the blood with an artificial kidney machine. Most dialysis patients receive treatment by traveling to the hospital three times a week. However, newer portable techniques allow considerably more freedom for dialysis patients.

In the case of chronic kidney failure, destruction of the kidney has progressed so much that treatment cannot bring kidney function back to normal. Treatment of these patients involves dialysis and a diet low in salt and protein. Dialysis will offer a chance to prolong life, but it is not a cure; only surgically replacing the damaged kidneys will cure the condition. In recent years, methods of matching kidney donors with recipients have improved, thereby limiting transplant rejection and serious complications. Today, kidney transplants are a highly successful treatment for chronic kidney failure.

See also Dialysis and Kidney stones.

---

# Kidney stones

Kidney stones are deposits of mineral or organic substances that form in the kidneys. When abnormally high levels of certain minerals, such as calcium, are in the urine, they may condense into hard masses, forming stones in the kidneys or urinary tract. The stones may be as small as a tiny pebble or as large as a walnut.

Increased levels of calcium in urine may come from drinking large quantities of milk. Eating foods rich in vitamin D, which helps the body absorb calcium, can also contribute to an overaccumulation of calcium. In addition, fractured bones can release extra calcium, which may later condense into stones in the kidneys.

Certain disorders encourage buildup of mineral deposits in the kidneys. Gout is a joint disease that results from high blood levels of uric acid (a waste product from the breakdown of protein), which may crystallize into stones in the urine. Urinary infections that impede bladder function can also cause retention of urine, which then harbors higher concentrations of elements that can solidify into stones. In addition, overactive parathyroid glands (endocrine glands that regulate calcium absorption) permit increased mineral absorption into the body.

Middle-aged men and persons with gout or chronic urinary tract infections are more susceptible to the development of kidney stones. However, in many cases, it is not possible to pinpoint the cause of the kidney stones.

Kidney stones may be present for years and never produce any symptoms. Problems arise when a stone obstructs or irritates a part of the kidney or causes problems as it passes out of the kidney. Symptoms include severe pain and tenderness over the affected kidney, frequent and painful urination, nausea, blood in the urine, fever, chills, and exhaustion.

A more serious condition can develop if a stone becomes lodged in a ureter. It produces excruciating pain across the back, abdomen, and reproductive organs. If blockage occurs in the urethra, urine output decreases. The trapped urine may back up, distending and injuring the urinary tract. An individual with this situation requires immediate medical treatment.

Kidney stones that are too small to be noticed may cause damage to delicate tissues in the urinary tract.

To determine the type of kidney stone formation, a physician analyzes blood and urine samples. Analysis of stone fragments or the actual stone is critical in determining the exact chemical imbalance. An ultrasound or X-ray study may reveal the location and nature of the stones.

Treatment is aimed at keeping the patient well hydrated and as comfortable as possible until the stone is passed.

For kidney stones too large to pass, surgical removal may be necessary. A new, nonsurgical method of treating kidney stones called extracorporeal shock-wave lithotripsy is becoming more widely available. With this technique, tiny shock waves are pulsed into a water bath in which the anesthetized patient is placed. The

shock waves are used to pulverize the stones so that they can pass out of the urinary tract. Removal of an impacted stone low in the urinary tract is frequently done through a cystoscope (a flexible, lighted, tubelike instrument). Once the cystoscope is in the bladder, a tiny guide wire attached to a basket is inserted into the ureter and withdrawn, hopefully with the stone inside.

To prevent recurrence of kidney stones, patients need to drink a great deal of fluid to dilute their urine. Drinking large amounts of fluids, particularly at night, reduces urine concentration so that stones cannot form. Surplus water can also flush the system of any small stones. For individuals with excess calcium and/or uric acid and other minerals in their urine, medication and dietary therapy can be helpful in preventing recurrences.

See also Cystitis and Gout.

# L

# Laryngitis

Laryngitis is an inflammation of the mucous membrane lining the larynx (voice box), which is located in the upper part of the respiratory tract. It causes hoarseness and possibly a temporary loss of speech.

Laryngitis may result from a bacterial or viral infection, such as a cold or the flu; from an irritation of the mucous membrane of the larynx, such as that caused by smoking; or from overuse of the voice.

Chronic or persistent laryngitis is most often caused by smoking, air pollution, dust, or smoke. It may also stem from tonsillitis, tuberculosis, the early stages of some forms of cancer, or paralysis of the vocal cords.

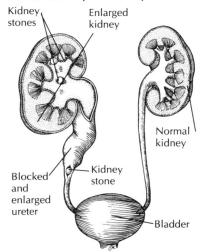

Kidney stones are formed in the kidney but may migrate to the ureter, creating an obstruction with swelling and damage above the blockage.

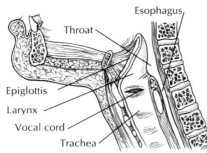

The larynx, or voice box, is located in the upper part of the respiratory tract.

Because laryngitis may be a symptom of a more serious condition, persons who consistently suffer from it should consult a physician.

Hoarseness, loss of the voice, dryness and scratchiness of the throat, coughing, and pain on speaking are common symptoms.

Laryngitis is best treated by totally resting the vocal cords. Pain may be eased with throat sprays, steam inhalations, and mild pain relievers, such as aspirin and acetaminophen.

# Legionnaires' disease

Legionnaires' disease is a severe bacterial infection of the respiratory tract. The first identifiable outbreak occurred in 1976 in Philadelphia. More than 180 people at the state convention of the American Legion became afflicted with the disease, and 29 of them died. Other outbreaks have since occurred in the United States and Europe. Studies have also shown that outbreaks of respiratory diseases that were later identified as Legionnaires' disease occurred as early as 1947.

Legionnaire's disease is caused by the *Legionella pneumophila* bacterium, which was not identified until the 1976 outbreak. The major environmental source of the infection is water from reservoirs and cooling units of air-conditioning systems. Lakes, creeks, and areas of excavation also may harbor the bacteria. Transmission is by breathing in droplets of contaminated water. Person-to-person transmission has not been documented.

Cigarette smokers, the elderly, and persons receiving drugs that depress the immune system are more likely to contract the disease than are other people. Individuals who have other medical complications such as heart trouble, cancer, respiratory illness, or kidney disease, are also believed to be particularly susceptible.

Legionnaires' disease has symptoms similar to those of many other respiratory diseases, making it difficult to differentiate and diagnose. Symptoms include dry coughing, high fever, chills, diarrhea, shortness of breath, chest pains, headaches, excessive sweating, nausea, vomiting, and abdominal pain. Occasionally, bloody sputum is produced. Lethargy and confusion may occur in progressive, serious cases.

Although Legionnaires' disease is uncommon, it should be considered in the case of anyone (particularly an elderly or chronically ill person) who has a respiratory tract infection that worsens over a period of about four days. The disease can initially be mild and appear to be an episode of the flu. The diagnosis is made from the history and physical examination, chest X rays, and special tests of the blood and sputum that determine the presence and changing numbers of antibodies (protective substances that fight off infection).

If an antibiotic (usually erythromycin) is given early in the course of the illness, the outlook for recovery is excellent.

There is as yet no preventive vaccine against Legionnaires' disease. If an outbreak is suspected, public health officials may search for and attempt to eliminate the source of infection.

# Leukemia

This is a disease that originates in the bone marrow, the site of blood cell production. The term *leukemia,* which is derived from Greek words that mean literally "white blood," refers to the fact that this disease is characterized by the presence of excessive numbers of white blood cells, especially immature and poorly functioning forms of these cells.

The symptoms of leukemia result from the impairment of normal blood cell functions.The primary role of white blood cells is fighting infection. Since many of the white blood cells present are immature, they function poorly and infections are common. Other blood cell types normally present in bone marrow (red blood cells, which carry oxygen throughout the body, and platelets, which are needed for blood clotting) may be crowded out by the cancerous leukemic cells. As a result, symptoms of deficiency of these cell types are often evident in leukemia patients. Symptoms include poor blood clotting ability (due to a shortage of platelets) and tiredness resulting from anemia (due to decreased numbers of red blood cells). Other symptoms are easy bruising, bleeding from the gums, blood in the stools, fever, and frequent infections. The spleen and lymph nodes are usually enlarged.

A diagnosis of leukemia should be made by a cancer specialist. The doctor will probably insert a needle into the hipbone to withdraw a sample of the bone marrow which will be tested for the presence of cancer.

Leukemia is often treated first with intensive chemotherapy to kill the cancer cells. The patient may appear

to become even more ill during treatment because of the side effects of the cancer-fighting drugs. After this initial treatment phase, radiation and additional drugs may be administered. Bone marrow transplants are now often used as a treatment.

Leukemia is the most common form of cancer in children. In recent years, the outlook has improved dramatically for children with this disease. Twenty years ago, nearly all children who suffered from leukemia died. Today, the life spans of many have increased; some live normal life spans.

See also Cancer.

# Leukoplakia

Leukoplakia is a tough, fibrous lesion that occurs on a mucous membrane. When it occurs in the mouth, it is often referred to as a smoker's patch or smoker's tongue. Although these oral lesions are generally not painful, they may cause difficulty and discomfort when the person talks or swallows.

The oral condition may be caused by badly fitted dentures, excessive smoking, overconsumption of alcohol, or a diet of highly spiced foods. Leukoplakia may also be a symptom of syphilis and may develop into a cancerous growth.

Leukoplakia most often appears in the form of a white patch on the lips, tongue, or gums or in other areas that are lined by mucous membranes, such as the female genital organs.

If a person notices the presence of these persistent white patches, a physician should be seen immediately. A biopsy specimen is often obtained because the presence of cancer cannot be determined by merely looking at the lesion.

One should never attempt to self-treat leukoplakia. After a physician has examined the lesion, he or she may advise having dentures refitted or cutting down on smoking and the consumption of alcohol and excessive amounts of spicy foods. These patches should be examined by a physician frequently, since cancer may develop in the future. In most cases, however, the physician will probably advise that the lesion be entirely removed surgically.

# Leukorrhea

Leukorrhea is an abnormal discharge from the vagina. All women have some normal discharge in the form of mucous secretions from the cervix and the vagina. This normal discharge helps to lubricate the vagina and, to some extent, prevent infection. This discharge is most noticeable at the time of ovulation (when an egg is released from the ovary), but it is generally present during the entire menstrual cycle.

Abnormal discharge is usually caused by an infection of the vagina by fungi, parasites, or bacteria. It may also be caused by an infection of the cervix, a tumor or other abnormal growth, the presence of foreign matter (such as a forgotten tampon) in the vagina, or an inflammation of the vagina caused by chemicals in douches or contraceptive creams or jellies.

An abnormal vaginal discharge usually is heavy, may be accompanied by itching of the genital organs and anal area, and may have a disagreeable odor.

To diagnose the cause of the discharge, the doctor will perform a pelvic examination and will often take a sample of the discharge for microscopic examination. Sometimes a culture of the discharge may also be performed so that the organism causing the problem can be grown in the laboratory and identified.

Once the cause of the abnormal discharge has been identified, specific steps are taken to treat it. If the discharge is caused by a bacterial infection, oral antibiotics or antibiotic vaginal creams may be prescribed. Specific oral drugs or vaginal preparations will be prescribed if the discharge is caused by a type of yeast or trichomonad (a single-celled parasite). In some cases, a biopsy of the cervix or vagina may be required if the doctor suspects that a tumor may be causing the discharge.

Douching with vinegar and water or other solutions available without a prescription generally will not cure the discharge, even though symptoms may improve for a few days. A woman with an abnormal vaginal discharge should consult her doctor rather than attempt to treat the condition on her own.

See also Vaginitis.

# Liver cancer

Liver cancer usually results from the spread of cancer cells from another site in the body. However, cancer that originates in the liver can sometimes be traced to environmental carcinogens. It is known that anyone who has worked with vinyl chloride, a chemical used in plastics manufacture, has a higher risk of this disease. It also appears that cirrhosis of the liver (a disease in which normal liver cells are replaced by fibrous tissue) may cause an individual to be more susceptible to cancer of the liver.

Symptoms of liver cancer are difficult to identify. They may resemble the signs of a peptic ulcer—aching or burning pain in the upper abdomen, nausea, and vomiting. A swollen or hardened liver often indicates to the doctor that there is need for further testing.

If this form of cancer is diagnosed early and is confined to the liver, it can be treated surgically. However, most often the prognosis for a patient with liver cancer is not good.

See also Cancer.

# Loss of appetite

Loss of appetite (also known as anorexia) is a lack of interest in or desire for food. Simple loss of appetite should not be confused with the illness called anorexia nervosa, which occurs most often in young women. Rather, loss of appetite is a common symptom that accompanies many illnesses.

Appetite is controlled by two areas of the brain, the "feeding" center and the "fullness" center, that work to regulate feelings of hunger depending on the body's need for food. In rare cases, appetite loss can be caused by damage to these areas of the brain. More commonly, it results from fatigue, the common cold, and psychological problems, such as anxiety and depression. Serious disorders that can lead to longer periods of appetite loss include certain types of cancers, as well as glandular and intestinal diseases.

Loss of appetite is indicated by a general lack of interest in food or eating, reduced food intake, and, in severe cases, weakness and a decrease in the body's natural resistance to disease.

A doctor's advice should be sought if appetite loss appears to be caused by emotional or psychological problems, if it lasts for long periods of time, or if it seems to have no obvious cause. Counseling may be beneficial if emotional problems are connected to loss of appetite.

See also Anorexia nervosa.

# Lung cancer

Cigarette smoking is generally accepted as the major cause of lung cancer. Lung cancer is the leading cause of cancer death in men, and in recent years the incidence of lung cancer in women has been growing, probably brought about because of the increase in the number of women who smoke. The incidence of lung cancer is also increasing among nonsmokers. This unfortunate change is possibly due to improved diagnostic techniques (many lung tumors were once diagnosed as tuberculosis) and to environmental pollution.

If you smoke and are over 45, or if you have a family history of lung cancer, you should be on the lookout for symptoms, since the early signs—a persistent cough or lingering respiratory discomfort—can be very mild. Later, coughing will increase, as will chest pain and shortness of breath, and blood may be found in the sputum (the material coughed up from the lungs).

A cancerous tumor in the lung is usually removed surgically. It is sometimes necessary to remove an entire lobe of the lung. Because lung cancers are usually not detected until they are well advanced, surgery alone may not be able to eliminate them, and radiation and chemotherapy may be used in combination with or in place of surgery.

In recent years, the deadliest form of lung cancer, which is referred to as small-cell carcinoma (also called oat-cell carcinoma), has yielded to a new drug therapy that has produced remission in many patients.

See also Cancer.

# Lumpectomy

See Mastectomy.

# Lungs

The respiratory system includes the nose, throat, larynx, trachea, bronchi, and lungs. The function of the respiratory system is to supply the blood with necessary oxygen and to relieve the blood of the waste product carbon dioxide. This exchange of oxygen and carbon dioxide occurs in the lungs. Air from the outside enters through the nose, where it is warmed, moistened, and filtered before it passes through the throat and past the larynx (voice box) into the trachea (windpipe). The trachea divides into two main bronchi (the airways connecting the windpipe and the lungs). Within each lung, the bronchi divide and subdivide, forming progressively smaller passageways called bronchioles. The smallest bronchioles end in small, cup-shaped sacs called alveoli. It is in the alveoli that the exchange of gas takes place. Each alveolus is served by numerous tiny blood vessels called capillaries. Oxygen in the alveolus crosses the thin alveolar and capillary walls to enter the blood, while carbon dioxide passes from the blood through the capillary walls into the alveolus. The oxygen is then carried by the blood to cells throughout the body, and the carbon dioxide is exhaled.

During inhalation and exhalation, the lungs are expanded and contracted by movements of the rib cage and the diaphragm (the large muscle separating the chest and abdominal cavities). During inhalation, the diaphragm contracts. The air pressure inside the chest cavity is then less than that of the air outside the body, and air from the outside rushes into the lungs. During exhalation, the diaphragm relaxes and moves upward, pushing air out of the lungs. The friction caused by expansion and contraction of the lungs is eased by the pleurae (membranes that cover the lungs and line the chest cavity), so that the surfaces of the lungs and chest cavity can move past each other smoothly.

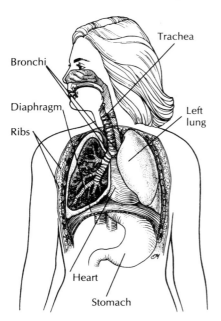

Bronchi

Trachea

Diaphragm

Left lung

Ribs

Heart

Stomach

The lungs are part of the respiratory system, the function of which is to supply the blood with oxygen and relieve the blood of carbon dioxide.

# Lupus erythematosus

Lupus erythematosus is a disorder that frequently affects the skin and the connective tissues (particularly the joints and muscles) but that can affect every tissue and organ in the body. The disorder occurs in two different forms—discoid lupus erythematosus and systemic lupus erythematosus.

**Discoid lupus erythematosus** Discoid lupus erythematosus is a chronic disease of the skin that is characterized by a red rash that appears on the cheeks and nose, as well as on other parts of the body. It often appears for the first time after the skin has been exposed to sunlight. Discoid lupus erythematosus is usually treated with drugs commonly used in the treatment of malaria (even though the two conditions are not at all related).

**Systemic lupus erythematosus** Systemic lupus erythematosus is a widespread autoimmune inflammatory disease of the blood vessels and connective tissues. The condition affects the joints, skin, and numerous other organs in the body, including the heart, lungs, liver, intestines, and kidneys. A red patch that resembles an open-winged butterfly may appear on the cheeks and nose. Symptoms may also include severe pain in the joints, intermittent fever, and unusual fatigue. The inflammation may cause severe and irreversible damage to the blood vessels and to the kidneys.

Cortisone and other steroids are used to control the inflammation in the joints and in other parts of the body; aspirin and other analgesics are used to control the pain. As with discoid lupus erythematosus, antimalarial drugs are used in the treatment of the rash.

This disease may be mild, or it may progress rapidly to seriously affect many organs. Death may result in severe cases.

See also Autoimmune diseases.

# Lymphocytes

Lymphocytes are a type of white blood cell. They are produced in the bone marrow and lymph nodes and stored in the thymus gland, spleen, and lymph nodes.

Lymphocytes play an important role in the body's immune system. Lymphocytes make their way through the lymph channels into the bloodstream, where they identify and "memorize" the characteristics of foreign elements called antigens. There are two types of lymphocytes—B cells and T cells. B cells manufacture antibodies (highly specialized proteins that destroy the antigens by combining with them). T cells, which make up 70 percent of the lymphocyte total, regulate antibody production and oversee immune responses.

Lymphocytes are the second most numerous type of white blood cell, normally constituting between 22 percent and 28 percent of the white blood cells in an adult's circulation. In cases of infection, especially those caused by viruses, the percentage of lymphocytes in the blood may increase to above 50 percent.

# Lymphoma

This cancer attacks the lymphatic system, particularly the lymph nodes and the spleen. These organs manufacture lymphocytes (cells that protect the body against infection).

The first symptom of lymphoma is usually a swollen spleen or swollen lymph nodes in the neck, armpit, or groin. Fever and sweating are later symptoms. If these symptoms persist, a doctor should be consulted. If the doctor suspects cancer, a biopsy of the enlarged organ will probably be ordered.

There are two major forms of lymphoma: Hodgkin's disease and non-Hodgkin's lymphoma. In recent years, there have been dramatic strides in the treatment of Hodgkin's disease. In the early stages, radiation alone can be very effective. Later in the course of the disease, more extensive radiation or a combination of radiation and chemotherapy may be required. Treatment of non-Hodgkin's lymphoma is much the same as that of Hodgkin's lymphoma. In the past, this form of lymphoma was usually discovered too late for treatment, but recent advances have made long periods of remission possible in many cases.

# M

# Macular degeneration

Macular degeneration is the deterioration of the macula (the yellowish depression in the central part of the retina of the eye). The macula is the part of the eye with the greatest density of visual receptor cells. As light enters the eye, the image that is focused on the macula is the one that is most clearly perceived in the brain. The function of the macula is to distinguish fine detail in the central visual field. Consequently, degeneration of the macula leads to blurring of central vision; peripheral (side) vision remains intact.

The exact cause of macular degeneration is unknown. In many cases, it may be a result of another disorder, atherosclerosis, which causes a narrowing of the blood vessels, including those that supply the macula with blood. In these cases, the macula "wastes away." This form is often referred to as the "dry" form. In another, less common, form of the disease, tiny blood vessels proliferate around the macula and leak blood or fluid, causing blurred or distorted cen-

tral vision. This is often called the "wet" form of macular degeneration.

Macular degeneration, in its dry form, usually develops slowly and painlessly. Therefore, the blurring of central vision is gradual. In the wet form of macular degeneration, blurring and loss of central vision may occur much more rapidly.

If both eyes are affected—as is almost always the case—activities requiring sharp vision, such as reading and driving, usually have to be curtailed. Eventually, all central vision disappears, although peripheral vision is unaffected.

There was no treatment for macular degeneration until recently. It has now been found that some individuals who have the wet form of macular degeneration may be helped by treatment with laser beams if the treatment is initiated early in the disease process, before significant damage to the eyesight has occurred. There is no treatment for the dry form of macular degeneration, although early in the course of the condition, vision may be improved by special powerful eyeglasses.

See also Eye.

# Mania

Mania is a term that refers to an abnormal elevation of mood, characterized by wild excitement, overactivity, and lack of concentration. It is also characterized by excessive irritability, hostility, and sometimes violence.

Mania is a component of the manic-depressive disorder, in which periods of mood elevation alternate with periods of depression, with periods of normalcy in between.

Persons in a manic state are likely to go on spending sprees; start, but not finish, new projects; become sexually promiscuous; exhibit restlessness and distractibility; and chatter rapidly and often incoherently. In addition, their judgment is often impaired. Because persons in the manic state think they are functioning at their very best, they tend to overextend themselves, becoming involved in many activities without considering the consequences.

Mania must always be diagnosed by a doctor because behavior that is apparently manic may actually have a physical basis. Certain disease states can cause similar symptoms. Mood elevation can also be a side effect of some medications. Both of these possibilities must be ruled out (and treated, if necessary) before assuming that a purely psychiatric disorder is present.

Mania and manic-depressive disorder are usually treated with medication and psychotherapy. The medication most commonly used is lithium carbonate. The chief value of lithium is in preventing manic episodes. However, it may take several weeks for the effects of the drug to become apparent. In the meantime, tests to monitor the level of lithium in the blood are essential, since excessive lithium can cause serious side effects. It is not known exactly how lithium works to combat mania, although it has been shown that lithium affects chemical transmitters in the central nervous system.

See also Depression.

---

# Marijuana

Marijuana, or cannabis, is the dried flower clusters, stems, and leaves of the Indian hemp plant (*Cannabis sativa*). It looks like coarse tobacco. It is also known as "weed," "pot," "grass," "tea," and "Mary Jane," as well as a number of other slang equivalents.

Marijuana has been smoked, drunk, eaten, and sniffed throughout recorded history. When marijuana is rolled into a cigarette, it is called a "joint" or a "reefer." The smoke has a very distinctive odor.

All of the effects of smoking or ingesting marijuana are not yet known because long-term studies are still under way. It is known that marijuana raises the heart rate by as much as 50 percent and lowers sex-hormone and fertility levels in both males and females.

Visible symptoms of marijuana use include reddened eyes, dilated pupils, and lack of physical coordination. Sometimes, users feel lethargic and nauseated. Reactions to marijuana differ: Some users feel happy, talkative, and silly; others may become withdrawn.

Marijuana relaxes the body and the mind. It gives a feeling of exhilaration and euphoria. In addition, marijuana alters perceptions—colors seem brighter, music more intense—and gives a sense of time being extended. However, these effects are often accompanied or followed by mood swings, panic, depression, hal-

Marijuana (cannabis) is obtained from the flowering tips and shoots of the *Cannabis sativa* plant, which grows wild or is cultivated all over the world.

lucinations, and fear of death, particularly if marijuana is being used in combination with other drugs.

Marijuana does not increase intellectual functioning or creative capacity, although it may produce that impression during use. Actually, marijuana affects the brain by interfering with the ability to think, to make judgments, and to solve problems. Marijuana also slows reaction time and hinders coordination and visual perception. For these reasons, driving a car while under the influence of marijuana is dangerous.

It is believed that use of marijuana may cause long-term physical effects, including damage to the brain, heart, lungs, and reproductive system.

Users of marijuana often experience a decrease in motivation and become psychologically dependent on the drug because it represents a way to avoid facing the problems and stresses of life. Marijuana users do not, however, appear to become physically addicted to it and generally do not suffer serious physical withdrawal reactions when they abstain from its use. Most users of marijuana do not progress to the use of hard drugs, such as heroin or cocaine, although that risk does exist.

Occasional use of marijuana does not appear to pose highly dangerous long-term effects. Nevertheless, there are several reasons for concern about the use of this substance. First, much of the marijuana used is smoked by young people in their formative years; they tend to use the drug more regularly than adults. Second, improved methods of cultivation have resulted in harvests of the plant that are increasingly more potent. Third, unlike alcohol, the mind-altering chemical in marijuana can remain in the body for a week or more. Fourth, because the substance is illegal, there are no quality controls over its content; large quantities of marijuana have been found to be contaminated with pesticides or laced with more dangerous or addictive narcotics. Fifth, because marijuana cigarettes do not have filters, their smoke irritates lung tissue much more than the smoke of regular filtered cigarettes. Marijuana cigarettes also contain more tar and benzopyrene (a cancer-causing agent) than do tobacco cigarettes.

# Mastectomy

Mastectomy is the surgical removal of a breast or part of a breast, usually as a treatment for cancer.

There are several types of mastectomy, each characterized by which muscles, glands, and other tissues are removed.

- Lumpectomy—removal of the tumor along with some of the surrounding breast tissue
- Partial mastectomy—removal of the tumor along with as much as one half of the breast
- Simple mastectomy—removal of the entire breast
- Modified radical mastectomy—removal of the entire breast plus the armpit lymph nodes on the affected side
- Radical mastectomy—removal of the entire breast, the armpit lymph nodes, and the muscles below the breast
- Extended radical mastectomy—removal of the entire breast plus additional tissue in the chest, as well as the armpit lymph nodes and chest muscles
- Super-radical mastectomy—removal of the same tissues and muscles as in the extended radical mastectomy, as well as some tissues and lymph nodes in the neck

The type of mastectomy to be performed is determined by a multitude

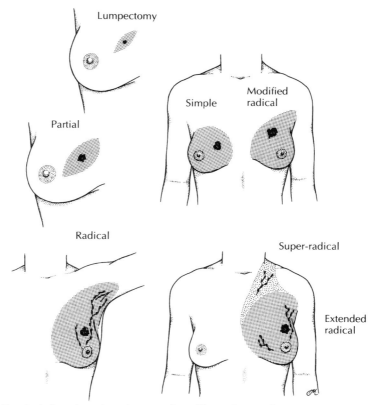

The shaded portions show the area affected by each type of mastectomy.

of factors, including the location, size, and type of tumor. The age and general health of the patient are also extremely important. A biopsy (removal of a small tissue sample for microscopic examination) will be performed prior to mastectomy. In addition, other tests may be done to determine if the cancer has spread to other areas of the body.

There is some question about how extensive the surgery should be. In recent years, the modified radical mastectomy has become the most frequently chosen procedure. However, there are differences of opinion about surgical choices in medical circles, and a woman facing a mastectomy should thoroughly discuss all of the procedures and available options with her doctor.

The operation is performed while the patient is under general anesthesia. Afterward the patient remains hospitalized for about a week and may begin radiation therapy or chemotherapy. Checkups every 6 to 12 months are recommended.

One of the best measures a woman can take is establishing the habit of examining her breasts monthly. With this simple routine, a woman can often detect a cancerous lump before cancer cells can spread beyond the breast. The effectiveness of breast self-examination (BSE) is shown by the high percentage of tumors that are discovered by patients themselves during a monthly BSE.

Many experts recommend annual mammography (X-ray examination of the breasts) for women over the age of 50 and for younger women who are considered to be at high risk of developing breast cancer (those who have had breast cancer in the past or who have a mother or sister who has had the disease). For women between 40 and 50 years of age, semiannual exams are recommended, and all women are urged to have a mammogram at the age of 35 to provide a baseline for later comparison.

See also Cancer.

# Mastitis

Mastitis is an inflammation of the breast, most often caused by bacterial invasion and infection.

This condition occurs most frequently in nursing mothers and is caused by bacteria normally found on the skin and nipples. The bacteria enter the breast through the nipple and infect the milk glands and ducts. In many cases, the condition occurs on the third to fifth day after the birth of the baby because of the development of cracked nipples, through which the bacteria may enter the breast.

Symptoms of mastitis include pain, swelling, redness, high fever, and a tender lump in the breast. Sometimes the lymph nodes in the armpit next to the affected breast may be tender and swollen. In cases of severe infection, there may be pus in the breast.

The diagnosis is generally made on the basis of the physical examination and the medical history. If there is a severe infection, signaled by the appearance of pus coming from the nipple, a specimen of the pus may be examined to identify the causative organism.

The treatment for mastitis is antibiotic medication to combat the infection. A breast-feeding mother can continue nursing from the unaffected breast, but her physician may recommend that she discontinue nursing from the infected breast and expel the milk by hand to prevent painful swelling of the breast. Even though most antibiotics will enter the breast milk in small quantities, this will not harm the baby. When the infection clears up, nursing from the previously infected breast can be resumed. If there is a great deal of pus, the pus may have to be drained.

A woman who is breast-feeding a baby can reduce the risk of developing mastitis by keeping her nipples clean and dry between feedings and by wearing clothing that does not irritate the nipples.

See also Fibrocystic disease of the breast.

# Mastoiditis

Mastoiditis is a bacterial infection of the mastoid air cells (small, air-filled cavities located in the mastoid process, which is the bulge in the skull behind the ear). Mastoiditis is most often a complication of a middle ear infection.

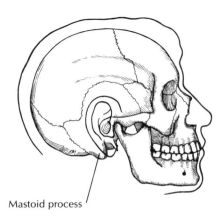

Mastoid process

Mastoiditis is an infection of the air-filled cavities in the mastoid process.

Mastoiditis is characterized by ringing in the ear, a discharge of pus from the ear canal, and fever. Other indications include swelling and tenderness over the mastoid process.

In severe cases, an abscess may develop in the mastoid process. This is a serious complication because it carries the risk that infection will spread to the interior of the skull and cause meningitis (inflammation of the membranes covering the brain and spinal cord).

Because antibiotics are so effective against ear infections and mastoid infections, mastoiditis is fortunately now a rare occurrence. Sometimes, however, surgery is required to remove the infected cells if antibiotic treatment is started too late or is not effective.

# Measles

Measles (also called rubeola) is a contagious disease that mainly affects the respiratory system, skin, and eyes. It was once considered one of the more dangerous childhood diseases because the threat of serious complications was so great. Fortunately, development of a vaccine to prevent measles has drastically reduced its occurrence.

Measles is caused by a virus. The virus is transmitted via droplets of moisture from the respiratory tract of an infected person that travel through the air. Some researchers contend that the virus enters the body through the eyes.

The incubation period (the time between being exposed to the infectious organism and actually showing symptoms) for measles is 8 to 12 days. An infected person is contagious for up to four days before symptoms appear and for up to six days after the rash develops.

Measles usually begins much like a cold, with a runny nose, nasal congestion, sneezing, a dry cough, and a fever of 102°F to 104°F. After three or four days, the eyes may become sensitive to bright light as they grow red and swollen. Then the fever drops, and red spots with tiny white centers (called Koplik's spots after the physician who first identified them) appear in the cheek pouches of the mouth.

By the fourth or fifth day, the fever increases again, and a rash appears. The rash usually starts on the face and neck and behind the ears, and then spreads to the rest of the body. As the

The measles rash—dark red spots that blend together as they spread—usually begins on the face, neck, and behind the ears and then spreads to the rest of the body.

spots multiply, they grow larger, become raised, and sometimes blend together. They turn dark red and then brown before the skin begins to peel in small flakes. This process takes about one week after the rash first emerges, although skin discoloration can last as long as two weeks. Other symptoms usually disappear within seven to ten days after the appearance of the first symptoms.

Breathing problems, increased coughing, earache, or extreme drowsiness may indicate complications that warrant consulting a doctor immediately. The more serious complications are pneumonia (inflammation of the lungs) and encephalitis (inflammation of the brain). Subacute sclerosing panencephalitis, a rare but often fatal disease of the brain, has also been linked to measles. Severe ear infections can occur, particularly in young children. In addition, bronchitis, laryngitis, and swelling of the lymph nodes in the neck can prolong the course of the illness or make it appear to return.

Generally, physicians diagnose measles by the initial symptoms. To confirm diagnosis, nasal discharge, blood, or urine can be tested for signs of the virus.

Since measles is caused by a virus, it does not respond to antibiotics, and treatment must focus on relieving the patient's discomfort. A vaporizer in the patient's room will ease coldlike symptoms by adding moisture to the air. If the eyes are irritated, warm compresses may relieve the inflammation. Also, dim lights are easier on the eyes. Soaps that may irritate the skin should not be used. The doctor may suggest adding baking soda to bath water or applying a soothing lotion, such as calamine lotion, to the rash to relieve itching.

An association has been established between aspirin use during or immediately after a viral infection and Reye's syndrome (inflammation of the brain accompanied by deterioration of the liver). It is recommended that aspirin not be given to a child with measles. A doctor can suggest an aspirin substitute, such as acetaminophen, if needed for relief of discomfort or fever.

Until recently, measles had been almost eliminated through childhood immunization. Unfortunately, over the last few years, the number of measles cases in the United States has increased dramatically due to low rates of immunization. This new epidemic has occurred in young children and older adolescents. The newest recommendation is that children receive the initial measles vaccine by injection at 15 months of age; a measles booster vaccine should be given at 11 or 12 years of age. If a measles outbreak occurs, anyone between 4 years and 21 years of age should receive a measles booster. If measles or vaccine history is unknown in an adult, it is best to check with your doctor. Blood tests that can show immunity to the disease are available. The vaccine, which is prepared from measles virus, stimulates production of antibodies (protective substances) in the body. Because the vaccine effectiveness rate is very low in young infants, babies are not vaccinated before 15 months of age unless measles cases have been reported in the area. The infants of women who are immune to measles (either because they have had measles or have been immunized against it) acquire temporary natural immunity that lasts for about the first six months of life. If a baby is exposed to measles, however, a doctor should be consulted. Measles is dangerous for anyone under three years of age and for anyone with a chronic (long-term) illness.

# Ménière's disease

Ménière's disease is the result of an increase in pressure in the inner ear because of a buildup of fluid in the semicircular canals of the inner ear, which control balance and equilibrium. This buildup of pressure distorts and sometimes ruptures the lining of the walls of the canals.

The cause of Ménière's disease is unknown, although it is thought that the pressure changes may be brought on by an infection, a small hemorrhage in the ear, or an allergic response. It occurs most commonly in men aged 40 to 60.

The symptoms of Ménière's disease include recurring and violent attacks of vertigo or dizziness, ringing in the ears, muffling or distortion of noises, and nausea that is sometimes accompanied by vomiting. Deafness in one or both ears may eventually develop.

Mild attacks of Ménière's disease may last from a half hour to several days before fading away naturally. They may recur regularly at intervals of weeks, months, or years. Severe attacks may last for several weeks, requiring the person to be confined to bed. In such cases, almost any movement of the head will result in bizarre and disturbing sensations that the floor and the furniture in the room are spinning around. Severe cases may also be accompanied by anxiety attacks and migraine headaches.

The use of certain drugs, such as diuretics, tranquilizers, and antihistamines, may help to relieve severe and recurrent attacks. In severe cases, surgery may be necessary.

See also Dizziness.

# Meningitis

Meningitis occurs when bacteria or viruses enter the spinal fluid and

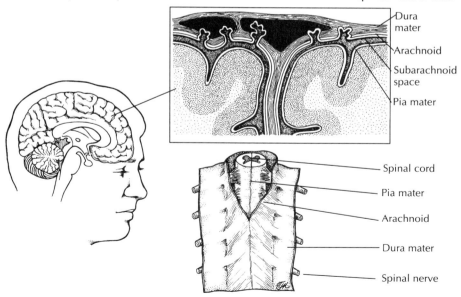

The meninges are the three membranes that cover the brain and spinal cord: the dura mater (outer layer), the arachnoid (middle layer), and the pia mater (inner layer). Between the pia mater and the arachnoid is the subarachnoid space, which is filled with cerebrospinal fluid to the meninges.

infect the meninges, the three layers of membrane that surround the brain and spinal cord. Meningitis can be fatal, although this is becoming less common because of the increased use of effective medications.

Meningitis seems to strike males more often than females and is most commonly seen in children up to the age of four years and in adults over the age of 60. Swelling of the brain, as well as epilepsy, blindness, amnesia, and deafness, can result when meningitis is not properly and promptly treated.

The three layers of meninges are the dura mater (the outermost layer), the arachnoid (the middle layer), and the pia mater (the innermost layer). The space between the inner two layers, called the subarachnoid space, is filled with clear cerebrospinal fluid, which is produced in the brain. When bacteria or viruses invade this fluid and form pus, the surrounding membranes soon become infected, resulting in meningitis.

Meningitis is caused by an infection that enters the system through a serious head wound or through the bloodstream from a source of infection in another part of the body. The bacteria may also reach the meninges from an abscess (localized infection) of the brain itself, but this is quite rare.

A deficiency in the immune system, which can be either inherited or acquired over time, may lead to a greater chance of contracting this disease. Also, newborns may be at a greater risk if the mother had a genital infection, such as herpes, during the last week of pregnancy, if the membranes of the uterus ruptured prematurely, or if labor was prolonged.

The symptoms of meningitis are a "bursting" headache, high fever, rising pulse rate, irregular breathing, vomiting, and sensitivity to light. Pain extends down the neck, into the back and lower limbs; the neck may be stiff, and it will be difficult for the patient to bend forward. As the disease progresses, convulsions or coma may occur.

Unless increased pressure in the brain is suspected, meningitis is diagnosed with a test called a lumbar puncture, or spinal tap, in which a sample of the cerebrospinal fluid is withdrawn and examined to see if it is clear (normal) or cloudy (pus-filled) and to identify the bacteria causing the infection. A physical examination, blood cultures, and cultures from the secretions of the respiratory tract may also be useful in determining the type of bacteria present. A viral infection is much harder to diagnose; it may not show up on any tests.

Because immediate treatment is so important, medication may be prescribed before the specific infecting agent has been identified. Once the cause has been determined, a more appropriate medication, most often an antibiotic, can then be administered. The patient will be admitted to the hospital, where measures can be taken to reduce fever and control brain swelling.

Viral infections are much more difficult to treat. Fortunately, most cases run their course without causing serious consequences. Treatment is generally limited to hospitalization, so that supportive therapy can be administered.

Prevention of meningitis caused by certain strains of bacteria may be possible with some vaccines that are now available. Research continues on vaccines against other bacterial strains.

Rifampin, an antituberculosis drug, is used for prevention of meningococcal meningitis (a bacteria known as meningococcus is the causative agent). The drug is given orally to individuals who have been in close contact with a person who has a documented case of meningococcal meningitis.

---

# Menopause

Menopause is the normal, natural stage in a woman's life when her menstruation and ovulation cycles stop, ending her reproductive years. Also called the climacteric, or the change of life, it occurs around age 50 but can start anywhere between the ages of 40 and 60.

Scientists do not fully understand what causes menopause. They believe it is triggered when the ovaries stop responding to the sex hormones that are secreted by the pituitary gland to control normal functioning of the ovaries. The subsequent decline in the production of the female hormone estrogen by the ovaries sets off the bodily changes.

During the years immediately preceding the onset of menopause, menstrual periods may become irregular and menstrual flow scanty.

Other physical symptoms may include hot flashes (a warm and flushed feeling over the face, neck, and chest that lasts a few minutes and recurs throughout the day), excessive perspiration, dryness in the vagina (which can lead to painful or difficult sexual intercourse), pounding heartbeat, joint pains, headaches, itching skin, increased facial hair, and decreased armpit and pubic hair.

Nonphysical symptoms may include depression, anxiety, irritability, apprehension, decreased ability to concentrate, lack of confidence, and insomnia.

The duration of symptoms may range from a few weeks to more than five years. Not every woman experiences the same changes, other than an end to menstruation; about 25 percent notice no other changes, 50 percent discern some physical or psychological symptoms, and the other 25 percent are troubled by very uncomfortable or distressing symptoms.

It is important not to attribute all physical changes to menopause to the point of overlooking the symptoms of some disease. This is a good time to schedule an examination and discuss the bodily changes with a doctor. A woman should see a doctor immediately if she starts to bleed in between menstrual periods, bleeds excessively, or has another period six months or more after they had apparently stopped.

The primary treatment for the physical symptoms of menopause is replacement of the female sex hormones (commonly estrogen or a combination of estrogen and progesterone in the form of an oral tablet). Estrogen in the form of a vaginal cream may be prescribed specifically to treat vaginal dryness. The lowest effective dose is administered (because of possible side effects). Any treatment merely lessens the discomfort of menopause, however; it cannot stop or slow down the process. Because of the many beneficial effects of hormone replacement therapy, most physicians now believe that it should continue for the remainder of the patient's life.

Estrogen is not usually given to women with severe circulatory or liver disorders and is carefully controlled when prescribed to those with diabetes, epilepsy, or heart or kidney disease. Progesterone is not prescribed for women with liver disease and is carefully controlled in those with asthma, epilepsy, or heart or kidney disease. The benefits and hazards should be discussed with a doctor; other medication is available to treat certain menopausal symptoms in women who cannot take hormones for some reason.

Treatment for the psychological or emotional symptoms may include tranquilizers, antidepressants, sleeping pills, or psychotherapy. During this time, it may also be difficult for a woman to face the aging process and its physical ramifications—the end of the childbearing years and a sense of uselessness because of a possible decrease in family responsibilities. Counseling may be helpful.

Fertility and the need to practice birth control at this stage depend upon a woman's age at the time of her last period. In general, a woman under the age of 50 may still be able to conceive for up to 24 months after the date of her last period; over 50, conception may be possible for up to one year.

After menopause, a woman is more liable to suffer osteoporosis (a disease that makes bones porous and brittle). This can often be prevented or controlled with estrogen therapy and calcium supplementation under medical supervision. The risk of heart attack also increases after menopause, and it is currently believed that estrogen therapy helps to substantially decrease that risk.

See also Hypertension and Osteoporosis.

# Menorrhagia

Menorrhagia is a term referring to an abnormally long (more than seven days) or heavy menstrual flow, frequently accompanied by the passing of large blood clots.

The condition, which is especially common in women in their late 30s and 40s, seldom indicates the existence of a serious disorder. However, it may result in iron deficiency anemia because of excessive blood loss.

Menorrhagia is a common problem, often caused by a disturbance in the hormones controlling the menstrual cycle. It can also be caused by fibroid tumors in the uterus, inflammation of the pelvic region, and hypothyroidism (underactivity of the thyroid gland).

If abnormal menstrual flow continues or recurs or if there is any chance of pregnancy, a physician should be consulted. The physician may perform a number of tests (including a Pap test) to determine whether there is a serious underlying cause. Biopsy (removal of a small tissue sample for laboratory examination) of the cervix or the uterine lining may be performed to check for cancer or other abnormalities. The physician may also do a blood test to check for iron deficiency anemia.

It is suggested that women who experience this disorder reduce the level of their activities during menstruation. They should also be sure to get enough iron so that they will not become anemic.

Hormones (estrogen and progesterone) may also be used to control heavy bleeding if the underlying problem is a hormonal disturbance. Hysterectomy may be necessary in severe cases that do not respond to estrogen therapy and in cases of extensive fibroid tumors.

# Menstruation

Menstruation is the monthly breakdown and discharge of portions of the endometrial tissue that lines the uterus.

Endometrial tissue thickens during each menstrual cycle to prepare the uterus for possible pregnancy. Approximately midway through the cycle, ovulation occurs. Ovulation is the process by which an ovary produces and releases an egg. The fingerlike projections at the end of the

Stages of menstrual cycle

In the first stage, while the egg is still inside the ovary, the endometrium (lining of the uterus) is fairly thin.

When the egg is released and begins to move into the fallopian tube, the endometrium begins to thicken in preparation for a possible pregnancy.

The egg moves through the tube toward the uterus. This is the point at which conception may occur. The egg is met by the male sperm cell in the fallopian tube, and the fertilized egg moves on to the uterus. During this time the endometrium continues to grow.

If conception does not occur, the endometrium ceases to grow and thicken. At this stage, the endometrium breaks down and is discharged, along with the unfertilized egg, from the uterus. This is menstruation. (In this drawing, the egg has been enlarged for the sake of illustration; normally the egg is only visible under a microscope.)

nearby fallopian tube sweep the egg into the tube, where it begins inching toward the uterus. If the egg is fertilized by a sperm, the fertilized egg moves to the uterus and becomes implanted in the rich uterine lining, where it grows for the next nine months. If the egg does not become fertilized, the thickened endometrial tissue breaks down and passes, along with the unfertilized egg, out of the body as the menstrual discharge. This monthly cycle is controlled by the female hormones estrogen and progesterone, which are secreted by the ovaries.

Young women start menstruating and ovulating at puberty, which usu-ally occurs between the ages of 9 and 14. Thereafter, they normally menstruate and ovulate once every month (except while pregnant) until they reach menopause.

Menstruation may be accompanied by complications of varying degrees of seriousness. Most women will experience at least one such problem at some point in their reproductive lives. The most common problems are dysmenorrhea (painful menstruation), amenorrhea (the absence of one or more menstrual periods), and premenstrual syndrome (a complex of physical and emotional symptoms that appear in the days before the period begins).

For many years, the symptoms of these disorders have been attributed to emotional factors. Research has shown, however, that most are caused by very real physical changes, and many new methods of treatment for various menstrual complications have been developed.

Although the disorders themselves are generally not dangerous, they can be physically and emotionally incapacitating. Furthermore, they may be symptoms of disease in the reproductive organs. Therefore, to be on the safe side, medical treatment for annoying symptoms accompanying menstruation should always be sought.

See also Amenorrhea, Conception, Dysmenorrea, Ovulation, and Premenstrual syndrome.

# Middle ear infections

The ear can become infected in any one of its three parts—the inner ear, the middle ear, or the outer ear. However, ear infections most commonly settle in the middle ear. The medical term for middle ear infection is otitis media.

Ear infections are much more likely to affect children than adults; children are most susceptible between the ages of six months and six years. Children who contract ear infections in their first year are more likely to have chronic (long-term) ear infections later in life. By the age of eight, almost every child has had at least one ear infection.

Middle ear infections develop when viruses or bacteria in the nose or throat travel to the ear through the eustachian tube, which connects the middle ear to the nose and throat. The middle ear also can become infected when infection spreads from a severe outer ear infection or injury.

Middle ear infections can be recognized by severe throbbing pain in the ear, fever as high as 105°F (102°F in adults), hearing loss, and possibly dizziness, nausea, vomiting, or sore throat. The eardrums may bulge out or may even burst, oozing blood and pus into the outer ear and relieving the pain. Symptoms may worsen over a period of hours or days. A child too young to talk may seem ill or feverish or may pull on an ear.

Ear infections are diagnosed by an inspection of the eardrum. If it is red and swollen or bulging, middle ear infection can usually be confirmed.

Middle ear infections are usually quickly eliminated by treatment with an antibiotic, often a form of penicillin. Decongestants may also be used. If a viral infection is present, however, antibiotics are not used, since viruses do not respond to antibiotics. If the eardrum is bulging and the pain is severe, the doctor may make a small cut in the eardrum (called a myringotomy) to relieve the pressure. If the eardrum bursts, the outer ear must be kept clean to prevent infection from spreading.

The development of more effective antibiotics has lessened the need for surgery. In rare cases, however, the infected tissue may have to be surgically removed.

Middle ear infections usually clear up quickly, but the more severe or persistent infections can lead to a variety of serious complications, including temporary or permanent hearing loss, infection of the semicircular canals in the inner ear, facial paralysis, brain abscess, meningitis (inflammation of the membranes covering the brain and spinal cord), and infection of the mastoid process (the bulge in the skull behind the ear).

# Migraine

See Headaches.

# Minerals

Minerals are natural, nonorganic substances with a specific chemical composition and characteristic crystalline structure. Minerals are essential for health and growth. They are important components of the bones and soft tissues, and they play a vital role in regulating the cardiovascular system, the internal pressure of body fluids, nerve responses, and oxygen conduction.

The body requires some minerals in relatively large amounts; these "macrominerals" are calcium, chloride, magnesium, phosphorus, potassium, sodium, and sulfur. Others are called trace minerals (or micronutrients) because they are needed only in minute quantities; these include iron, manganese, copper, iodine, zinc, chromium, cobalt, fluoride, and selenium. Large amounts of these minerals taken for nonmedical reasons can cause serious health problems. Still other minerals, such as lead, mercury, and cadmium, are toxic even in small amounts.

Although minerals are essential, they can be harmful if taken in excess. Those who use mineral supplements should take care not to surpass the daily requirement. An overload can upset the balance of other minerals and block their performance, can result in decreased physical capabilities, and can contribute to such conditions as anemia, bone demineralization (mineral depletion) and brittleness, nervous system disease, and fetal abnormalities. With certain minerals, even consuming twice the

daily requirement or taking one day's requirement all in one dose can lead to severe illness. Taking minerals in excessive quantities is especially risky for children, pregnant or nursing women, and the elderly.

**Calcium**  Calcium is the most prevalent mineral in the body; in fact, the bones and teeth together contain an average of two to three pounds of calcium. In addition to its role in the structure of bones and teeth, calcium regulates certain body processes— normal nerve function, muscle tone, and blood clotting. Major sources of calcium are milk and milk products.

**Phosphorus**  Phosphorus coexists with calcium in the bones and teeth but is also present in most body tissues. Phosphorus is present in so many foods that a deficiency is rare; it is most abundant in meat, poultry, fish, eggs, and whole-grain products.

**Sodium chloride**  Sodium and chlorine combine to form sodium chloride (table salt), yet each element functions separately. Sodium maintains regular water balance both inside and outside the cells, and is found in blood plasma and fluids outside the cells. Foods rich in sodium include meat, fish, poultry, eggs, milk, and such processed foods as bacon, ham, bread, and crackers. Chloride is a constituent of hydrochloric acid, which is concentrated in gastric (stomach) juices and is necessary for the functioning of the digestive system. People who perspire heavily may have to add salt to their diet, but most people eat too much salt because of their high consumption of processed foods and added table salt. Surplus salt increases water retention and, in predisposed individuals, has been associated with edema (excess fluid retention in the tissues) and high blood pressure.

**Potassium**  Potassium, mainly present in the fluid in cells, regulates the balance and volume of body fluids in tandem with sodium. Because most foods (both plant and animal) are rich in potassium, a nutritional deficiency is very rare, although it may occur in conjunction with prolonged diarrhea, use of diuretics (medications that remove water from the body), or a diet that lacks protein. Use of potassium supplements without medical supervision is very dangerous.

**Magnesium** Magnesium is contained mostly in bones, although it is present in all body tissues. It is vital to the enzymes that help convert food into energy. Magnesium deficiencies usually occur only in postsurgical patients, alcoholics, and others who do not eat a well-balanced diet. Magnesium-rich foods include wholegrain cereals, dried peas and beans, cocoa, nuts, seafood, and dark-green vegetables.

**Sulfur** Sulfur, found in all tissues, is a part of several important amino acids and of the vitamins thiamin and biotin. It is not fully understood how sulfur works in the body.

**Iron** Iron is found throughout the body, chiefly in the blood, liver, spleen, and bone marrow. It is an integral part of the compounds that are necessary to transport oxygen to the cells and to regulate its use there. Foods that provide significant amounts of iron include liver, seafood, meats, egg yolks, fish, and green vegetables, as well as dried peas and beans.

An inadequate supply of iron in the diet causes iron deficiency anemia, which most often affects women in their reproductive years (especially pregnant women), infants, and teenagers (particularly during the adolescent growth spurt).

**Manganese** Manganese is fundamental for the normal building of tendons and bones and is part of some enzymes. Foods rich in this mineral include whole-grain breads and cereals, coffee, tea, nuts, peas, and beans.

Manganese deficiency in humans is virtually unknown.

**Copper** Copper, an element involved in the storage and release of iron to form the oxygen-carrying hemoglobin in red blood cells, is most vital in the early months of life. If a pregnant woman's intake is sufficient, her baby will be born with enough copper. It is most available in processed foods, organ meats, shellfish, nuts, and dried peas and beans.

**Iodine** Iodine is indispensable to the normal working of the thyroid gland. A shortage can result in goiter (thyroid enlargement). Before the introduction of iodized salt in the United States in 1924, iodine-deficiency goiter was common in inland areas. Foods obtained from the sea are rich in iodine.

**Zinc** Zinc is a fundamental part of the enzymes that move carbon dioxide in the red blood cells from the tissues to the lungs for exhalation. A deficiency of zinc may show up as a loss of the sense of taste or delayed healing of wounds. Associated with protein, zinc is found in meats (especially liver), cheese, dried beans and peas, seafood, egg yolks, and milk. Although it is available in whole-grain cereal, it is not likely to be absorbed because of the presence of other substances.

**Cobalt** Cobalt is not needed in the body by itself, but is part of the nutrient cyanocobalamin (vitamin $B_{12}$), which is available in meat, eggs, fish, and dairy products.

**Chromium** Chromium acts with insulin in the use of glucose (a form of sugar). A shortage produces a condition that is similar to diabetes. Chromium is present in dried brewer's yeast, whole-grain cereals, and liver.

**Selenium** Selenium appears to work in conjunction with vitamin E. Not much is known about selenium, except that it is important in the body and that it is found in animals and plants where it is accessible in the earth. A deficiency may cause muscle pain and impairment of heart function.

**Fluoride** Fluoride is important in the formation of teeth and resistance to dental caries (cavities), especially in children, and may help maintain calcium in the bones of the elderly. It is available in fluoridated water, seafood, and meats.

See also Fluorides and Vitamins.

# Miscarriage

A miscarriage (in medical terms, a spontaneous abortion) is the ending of a pregnancy due to the premature delivery of the fetus before the beginning of the twentieth week of pregnancy. At that point, the fetus is not developed enough to survive outside the uterus on its own. (After the twentieth week of pregnancy, a spontaneous abortion is considered a premature delivery or, if the fetus is dead at delivery, a stillbirth. A pregnancy that is ended artificially is commonly known as an abortion, although the medical term is termination of pregnancy.) Most miscarriages occur within the first 14 weeks of pregnancy.

It is impossible to know the number of miscarriages that occur during the first month of pregnancy before a woman realizes that she is pregnant; the only indication is a slightly late menstrual period with a heavier than normal flow. However, about 12 percent of known pregnancies end in miscarriage.

There are several different types of miscarriages. A *threatened miscarriage* is experienced by about one of every five pregnant women when vaginal bleeding occurs during the first three months. Although such bleeding may indicate a spontaneous abortion, it is rarely more than a threat, and the pregnancy will continue normally. An *inevitable miscarriage* refers to a situation in which bleeding occurs, the cervix begins to dilate (open), but the uterine contents are not yet expelled. A *missed miscarriage* occurs when the fetus dies in the uterus but is not naturally expelled, and the woman has no bleeding or pain to signify that the pregnancy is not progressing; the physician usually diagnoses the condition when he or she observes that the uterus stops enlarging.

The reason that a miscarriage occurs is not always understood, but it is believed that a fetus is usually aborted because it is not developing normally. Several factors can contribute to a miscarriage, including abnormalities in the father's sperm; abnormalities in the egg; disease in the mother (for example, an infection, a glandular disorder, high blood pressure, kidney or heart disease, or diabetes); uterine abnormalities; the mother's poor nutrition or use of cigarettes, alcohol, or drugs; and exposure to environmental pollutants. Because the fetus is so well protected within the uterus, a fall or other trauma suffered by the mother is rarely, if ever, the cause of miscarriage.

The expulsion of the fetus resulting from an abnormality is thought to be a chance event, not due to a problem or defect in either parent. Of women who miscarry once, most (about 80 percent) have a successful subsequent pregnancy.

The symptoms of miscarriage are vaginal bleeding (from a few drops to a heavy flow) and cramps (either dull and constant or sharp and intermittent) in the lower abdomen or back. The bleeding can start suddenly or follow a brownish discharge. A solid clot of material or tissue may pass from the vagina. If possible, this should be saved for the doctor, who may be able to examine it and determine a reason for the expulsion. A miscarriage can be complete (the uterus expels all the tissue) or incomplete (tissue remains inside the uterus).

A pregnant woman who starts bleeding or experiences pain should contact her physician immediately.

Depending on the type of miscarriage, diagnosis may be made on the basis of the medical history, physical examination, analysis of any discharge, blood and urine tests (to detect the presence of infection or anemia caused by hemorrhage), or ultrasound studies (to establish the absence of a fetus or the presence of an abnormal fetus or parts of a fetus).

There is no medical treatment to stop or avert an inevitable miscarriage. (The drug diethylstilbestrol, or DES, used to be prescribed to deter miscarriages until it was discovered that it had little effect and could cause fetal abnormalities.) The physician generally directs the woman with symptoms to rest in bed and abstain from sexual intercourse.

After an inevitable, incomplete, or missed miscarriage, any remaining fetal or placental tissue must be removed by a surgical procedure known as dilatation and curettage (D&C), in which the physician expands the cervix and gently scrapes out residual material from inside the uterus. Without this precaution, a woman is more susceptible to infections and heavy bleeding.

It is normal for a woman to feel depressed by the loss of the expected child, but it is usually safe for her to attempt to conceive soon afterward (six to eight weeks later) on the advice of her physician.

More and more information is becoming available about the effect of drugs and nutritional and environmental factors on pregnancy. It is advisable for a woman, at the beginning of her pregnancy, to obtain adequate prenatal care and the most up-to-date information on the substances and practices that may contribute to a miscarriage.

See also DES and Dilatation and curettage.

# Mole

A mole is a cluster of cells, usually pigmented (colored), that appears on the skin. Moles are sometimes present at birth, but more often they appear during childhood, adolescence, or pregnancy. Although moles, which are commonplace, can become cancerous, they seldom do.

Moles vary in size, shape, and color. They may be large or small, flat or raised, smooth or warty. They may be the same color as the skin, or their color may vary from yellow-brown to black. Some moles have one or more hairs in them.

The most common type of mole is the intradermal nevus, which forms in the lower layer of skin. It is a raised cluster of cells that ranges in color from skin-tone to black. Other types of moles include the lentigo nevus (a flat, uniformly pigmented brown or black spot), the junctional nevus (a flat or slightly raised blemish that ranges in color from light brown to nearly black), the compound nevus (a raised mole that is usually dark in color), and the halo nevus (a pigmented mole in the middle of a ring of skin from which the pigment has been lost).

Moles are often removed for cosmetic reasons. However, any mole that enlarges suddenly, becomes darker, begins to bleed, or changes in any other unexplained way should be removed by a physician and examined microscopically.

# Mononucleosis

Infectious mononucleosis, or "mono," is a contagious viral illness that initially attacks the lymph nodes in the neck and the throat. When these tissues become less effective in fighting infection, sore throat, swelling of the lymph nodes, and fever result.

Mono is caused by the Epstein-Barr virus, which is named after the scientists who first identified it in the mid-1960s. The virus enters the lymph nodes and attacks the lymphocytes (the white blood cells manufactured there). As the white blood cells come into contact with the virus, they change shape and multiply. At first there are no symptoms, because it takes several weeks before enough of the altered cells can accumulate to generate a reaction. Gradually, however, symptoms appear. First, there is a mild sore throat, sluggishness, and fever. The symptoms worsen as the body tries to fight the infection by creating more white blood cells. The symptoms usually diminish and disappear about six to eight weeks later.

Mono spreads by contact with moisture from the mouth and throat of an infected person. Kissing, sharing drinking glasses and toothbrushes, or touching anything that has been near the mouth of an infected person may result in transmission of the disease.

Teenagers and young adults seem most susceptible to mono. However, even children less than one year old can develop mono. The disease is uncommon in persons over the age of 35.

In all cases, the infection develops so slowly with such mild symptoms that it may be initially indistinguishable from a cold or the flu. However, a sore throat that lasts two weeks or more; swollen lymph nodes in the neck, throat, armpits, and groin; a persistent fever (usually about 102°F); and tiredness and malaise (a vague feeling of discomfort) may indicate mono. Mono symptoms can be mild or so severe that throat pain impedes swallowing and fever reaches 105°F. Some people also experience a rash, eye pain, and photophobia (discomfort in bright light).

Most cases of mono run an uncomplicated course. Occasionally, however, the infection spreads to other parts of the body besides the throat and lymph nodes. For example, mono may lead to monohepatitis (an inflammation of the liver that is not the same as hepatitis A, B, or non-A, non-B). Jaundice, a symptom of this complication, appears as a yellow discoloration of the skin and whites of the eyes. A much more serious problem is pain or tenderness in the abdomen. This discomfort may mean a swollen spleen (an organ in the lymph system), which could burst. Any of the above symptoms should be reported to a physician for immediate attention. Anyone whose spleen is swollen should avoid contact sports and any type of trauma to the abdomen.

To diagnose infectious mononucleosis, blood samples are analyzed to detect the presence of antibodies to the Epstein-Barr virus and to determine overall blood cell count. Inflammation of the liver can also be detected and followed up with blood tests.

As long as there are no complications, the best treatment is to rest, drink plenty of liquids until the temperature returns to normal, and then gradually resume normal activities as strength returns. If the patient feels well enough, complete bed rest is probably not necessary or beneficial.

Antibiotics are ineffective against mono, since it is a viral infection and viruses do not respond to antibiotics. However, mono can be accompanied by a streptococcal infection of the throat, in which case an antibiotic will be prescribed to treat that condition. In severe cases, corticosteroid drugs that reduce swelling are prescribed. If the spleen is swollen, the doctor may recommend avoiding strenuous activities, such as lifting and pushing, which may cause sudden rupture of the spleen. Hospitalization is necessary if there is a serious complication, such as rupture of the spleen.

Most people recover in six to eight weeks, but some cases take as long as six months for complete recovery. A tired feeling, which may include depression, is the last symptom to disappear. Mono may return in a milder form within a few months. Fortunately, mono almost never reappears in its full-blown form after a year.

In a related condition, chronic Epstein-Barr virus infection, symptoms of mono recur periodically over a period of years. This illness, among others, is often referred to as "chronic fatigue syndrome." Symptoms are similar to acute mono in that the individual notices severe fatigue, aches and pains in the muscles and joints, and low-grade fevers (less than 100°F). These symptoms generally tend to flare and subside chronically. There is no specific treatment for this illness, but analgesics, low doses of antidepressants, and rest during acute flare-ups are often helpful. It is important that these symptoms be differentiated from other diseases, such as malignancies of the lymph system. There is no specific diagnostic test for "chronic mono," but persistent high blood levels of antibody to the E-B virus can be found with a simple blood test and is helpful in establishing the diagnosis. Other than feeling miserable at times and perhaps los-

ing work days, there are generally no serious complications of this condition.

# Mucous colitis

See Irritable bowel syndrome.

# Multiple sclerosis

Multiple sclerosis is a chronic disease of the central nervous system (the brain and spinal cord) in which the protective myelin sheath (the insulating covering) of the nerve fibers degenerates. When this protection disappears, body functions may become impaired. In some cases, the patient ultimately becomes wheelchair-bound or even dies. In other cases, the disease may flare up only once in a lifetime and leave the individual with no or only minimal disabilities.

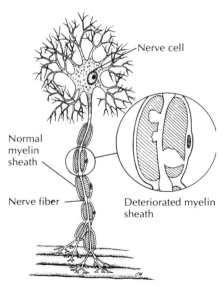

Multiple sclerosis results when the myelin sheath, the substance that insulates the nerve fibers, deteriorates.

Researchers have not yet determined the exact cause of multiple sclerosis. Some studies indicate that the disease follows exposure to a virus that may lie dormant (inactive) until some factor, such as stress or a second exposure to the virus, triggers the disease.

Another theory suggests that multiple sclerosis affects people who have some defect in their immune system (the body system responsible for protection from foreign substances or infective agents). It is thought that following viral exposure, the immune system mistakenly identifies the myelin covering of the nerves as foreign tissue and tries to destroy it. The symptoms of multiple sclerosis may be the consequence of this destructive process.

Initial attacks of multiple sclerosis are most common in people in their late 20s and early 30s. The disease begins with one or more of the following symptoms: tingling and numbness in the arms and legs, muscle spasms, partial loss of vision, difficulty in walking, and impaired bladder control. After the first attack, there is usually a period of remission (a time without symptoms) for as long as two to three years.

Subsequent attacks occur at irregular intervals and cause gradually increasing disability. Frequent episodes cause weakness, general incoordination, impaired speech, and burning sensations. Sexual function deteriorates, and mood swings are common.

More extensive nerve damage may result in loss of muscle control and may necessitate the use of a wheelchair. Usually, the earlier the onset of disease, the more slowly it progresses. Ten years after onset, fewer than half of patients with multiple sclerosis can continue regular daily activity. After 20 years, fewer than one fourth are able to function normally. Often, however, an individual may suffer one attack and never have further symptoms.

Physicians diagnose multiple sclerosis through physical examination and observation of symptoms. Often, diagnosis remains unconfirmed until a second attack occurs. Analysis of the spinal fluid in conjunction with magnetic resonance imaging (MRI) studies is very useful in establishing the diagnosis.

Since there is no cure for multiple sclerosis, treatment concentrates on relieving the symptoms. Muscle relaxants may ease muscle spasms and corticosteroid drugs may shorten attacks by reducing nerve tissue inflammation. Newer drugs that act on the immune system are showing promise. Many patients are more comfortable if they are well rested; afternoon naps and adequate sleep at night are advised. Cold temperatures sometimes relieve symptoms, whereas heat makes them worse.

# Mumps

Mumps is a contagious viral disease that is usually contracted during childhood. More than 85 percent of the cases occur before the age of 15, especially between the ages of six and ten years.

Mumps is caused by a virus that attacks cells of the parotid salivary glands. This invasion results in painful swelling of the face beneath the ear along the jawline. Mumps virus spreads by contact with airborne moisture from an infected person's nose or throat. Sometimes, the infection comes from someone who has the disease without symptoms or who is not yet aware of the symptoms. The disease occurs most often during the spring months, although it can happen at any time of the year.

Symptoms can be so mild that they are almost nonexistent, or they can be very severe. Fever (101°F to 103°F), headache, and loss of appetite usually develop first, followed by earache; then the characteristic swelling of the salivary glands appears. Swelling may start on one side of the face and then appear on the other side within a few days. Sometimes, however, only one side swells. The inflammation may cause soreness and difficulty in eating or swallowing.

The sex glands may become swollen as well. Orchitis (inflammation of one or both testes) can cause considerable pain. Affected testes may shrink somewhat, but contrary to popular belief, it is not common for mumps to lead to sterility in males. Girls may have swelling in the ovaries, but there is seldom any severe discomfort. In addition, swelling may occur in other glands and organs, including the breasts, other salivary glands, the liver, and the brain.

Although mumps can be unpleasant, it rarely has long-term complications. Encephalitis (inflammation of the brain) is the most dangerous complication of mumps because it carries the risk of death. Another possible consequence of mumps encephalitis is hearing loss or even deafness. Hearing may return to normal after several months, however. A milder complication is meningoencephalitis (inflammation of the brain and its covering, the meninges). This disease causes a stiff neck, headache, high fever, drowsiness, sensitivity to bright light, and sometimes delirium; these symptoms usually disappear without damage to the brain.

Pancreatitis (inflammation of the pancreas) can also result from mumps. Symptoms of pancreatitis include stomach pain, vomiting, chills, fever, and extreme weakness. Although these signs usually vanish and leave no damage, diabetes can result in rare cases. Other complications of mumps include nerve inflammation, heart problems, and nervous system disorders—all usually temporary. An adult male with mumps can develop inflammation of the testes, which may possibly lead to sterility. Symptoms of any of these conditions should be brought to the attention of a doctor.

A doctor diagnoses mumps on the basis of the characteristic form and texture of the swollen parotid glands. Boys may have swelling and tenderness in the testes. Exposure to the disease is also a clue. The incubation time (the time between exposure to

Parotid gland

Outline of jaw bone

Mumps is caused by a virus that infects the salivary glands, especially the parotid gland. The infection causes a painful swelling of the face in front of the ear.

the virus and the appearance of signs and symptoms) is 14 to 21 days. If mumps is suspected, secretions from the salivary glands can be tested for mumps virus.

Treatment for mumps involves relieving the discomfort of the symptoms, since there is no cure for the disease. Bed rest is usually not necessary. Soft foods and liquids may be easier to swallow. However, fruit juices with a high acid content, like orange and grapefruit juice, may sting the mouth.

If the glands are severely swollen, a physician may prescribe painkilling drugs. Steroid drugs may be recommended for men or boys with extremely swollen testes, but these drugs may prove ineffective. Warm or cold compresses or an ice pack may relieve some pain. Most mumps symptoms disappear within about ten days.

There is a vaccine that is 95 percent effective in preventing mumps. The vaccine stimulates the production of antibodies to resist the disease. Mumps vaccine is usually combined with measles and rubella (German measles) vaccines and given to children by injection when they are 15 months of age. There are usually no side effects from the mumps vaccine.

# Muscles

There are three types of muscle: striated, smooth, and cardiac.

Striated, or striped, muscle consists of layers of tissue divided into bundles of interwoven fibers that run parallel to one another. These layers are attached to the skeleton, and they aid the body in voluntary movement.

Smooth, or organic, muscle is present in several of the internal organs, including the intestines and the bladder, and in the larger blood vessels.

This type of muscle functions under involuntary control by the autonomic nervous system. Among its functions, smooth muscle helps circulate blood and glandular secretions throughout the body, move material through the digestive tract, and regulate breathing. Smooth muscle contains elongated, spindly cells arranged parallel to one another that are often grouped into bundles.

Cardiac muscle is the muscle of the heart, and its job is to pump blood within and from the heart. The unique characteristic of this muscle is that although it is striated (like the muscles of the skeleton), it is controlled by the autonomic nervous system (like the muscles of the internal organs).

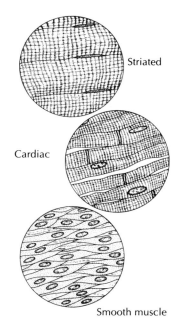

Striated

Cardiac

Smooth muscle

Muscles are connective tissues that have the ability to contract. There are three types of muscles: striated, that aid in voluntary movement; smooth, that assist functions under involuntary control; and cardiac, that is the muscle of the heart.

# Muscular dystrophy

Muscular dystrophy is the general term for a group of rare diseases in which the body's muscles weaken and waste away. Muscular dystrophy almost always strikes in childhood and is usually inherited. Duchenne muscular dystrophy, which is usually inherited through the mother, is the most common form of the disease.

The disease is progressive (it becomes gradually worse once it takes hold). In severe forms the child must use a wheelchair by the age of 11 or 12. Scoliosis (curvature of the spine) may also result from the disease. Severe cases may be fatal, often when the patient is a young adult. Pneumonia is sometimes a fatal complication because of weakening of the muscles involved in breathing.

Muscular dystrophy is sometimes confused with multiple sclerosis, which is a disease of the nervous system that can ultimately result in spasticity and paralysis. There is no deterioration of the nervous system in muscular dystrophy.

Symptoms of muscular dystrophy vary. Muscles usually begin to weaken first in the hips, legs, and shoulders. A child of four or five who waddles from side to side, who has difficulty standing up properly, or who falls frequently should be examined by a physician. The child may also have difficulty in standing up straight or raising an arm high above the head.

Parents should not be overly concerned about the natural awkwardness that occasionally overtakes the older toddler. However, a child near five years of age who consistently has problems with muscular coordination should be checked.

The diagnosis of Duchenne muscular dystrophy is rarely made before the age of three. It is most commonly seen in boys; girls are rarely affected.

The physician may want to obtain a muscle biopsy specimen (a small tissue sample) to confirm a diagnosis of muscular dystrophy. The biopsy may be done on an outpatient basis in a hospital or in a physician's office.

There is no treatment for the disease, but an exercise program designed by a physical therapist may be helpful. The patient's diet should be regulated so that he or she does not become overweight; excess weight taxes the child's weakening muscles and hastens the course of the disease.

Because muscular dystrophy is an inherited disease, women in the family of an affected child should be tested to see if they are carriers (they can pass on the disease to their children). Such women should receive genetic counseling regarding any pregnancy.

# Myasthenia gravis

Myasthenia gravis is an uncommon disease of the nerves and muscles, characterized by great fatigue and weakness in the muscular system, most notably in the face and throat. Although the muscles do not atrophy (wither or waste away), there is slow and progressive paralysis. The disease is most likely to strike adults, especially women between the ages of 18 and 25 and men older than 40, but it can affect persons of any age.

Myasthenia gravis is sometimes associated with thyroid disease, excessive growth of the thymus (a gland in the chest that is an essential part of the immune system), or tumors in the thymus.

The condition is a neuromuscular disorder; the muscles fail to receive messages from the nerves because of a lack of the important neurotransmitting chemical acetylcholine. Experts believe that the disorder originates in the immune system and causes the body to destroy or block the sites responsible for receiving acetylcholine.

The muscular weakness first shows up in the face: the eyelids droop, often causing squinting and double vision; there is an inability to move the mouth and lips, with subsequent difficulty in talking, chewing, and swallowing; and the cheeks generally droop or sag. Sometimes the arms and legs are afflicted, affecting basic motor movements, like walking and standing, and the performance of simple tasks, like lifting a cup. The progressive muscular weakness can also impair breathing. The degree of paralysis or weakness varies from hour to hour and day to day, although it tends to be least severe in the morning and worst at night. Blood tests and chest X rays aid in the diagnosis.

Myasthenia gravis is usually not curable, but drugs are available that restore nerve transmission to the muscles. The drugs neostigmine and pyridostigmine help to reestablish muscle strength and enable the patient with myasthenia gravis to live a more normal life. If a disorder of the thymus gland is found to be the underlying problem, the gland can be surgically removed. Corticosteroids are used to help regulate the immune system in myasthenia gravis patients.

# Myopia

Myopia, or nearsightedness, is a common optical defect in which close objects can be seen clearly but faraway objects look blurred. About one in every five persons is myopic. The condition tends to be hereditary, developing around age 12 and getting progressively worse to about age 20.

The defect occurs if the eyeball is too long from front to back. Normally, the cornea and the lens (the disk-shaped structure just behind the front of the eye) refract (bend) light coming from a viewed distant object so that the image is focused on the retina (the layer of specialized, light-sensitive cells that line the back of the eyeball). In myopia, the focused image falls short of the retina because of the greater length of the eyeball, resulting in a fuzzy image.

There are several kinds of myopia. *Curvature myopia* occurs when there is an excessive curve of the refractive (light-bending) surfaces of the eye, which causes light to enter the eye in an abnormal path. The curvature is in the front surface of either the

Normal

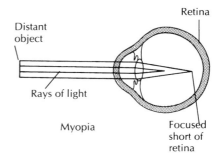

Myopia

Myopia is a vision defect in which close objects can be clearly seen, but distant objects appear blurred. This defect occurs if the eyeball is too long from front to back, which causes incoming light from distant objects to fall short of the retina.

cornea or the lens. In *index myopia*, there is an increase in the light-refracting properties of the lens. This is sometimes associated with future development of cataracts or iritis (inflammation of the iris). *Progressive myopia* is an uncommon form in which the eyeball continues to elongate throughout a person's life, eventually leading to degeneration or detachment of the retina.

Blurred or fuzzy vision should be evaluated by an ophthalmologist (a physician who specializes in eye disorders), who will look inside the eyes with a special instrument called an ophthalmoscope, diagnose any disorders, and test the acuity (sharpness) of vision.

Nearsightedness is easily corrected with a concave (inwardly curved) lens that pushes the images back toward the retina and focuses them clearly.

A surgical procedure known as radial keratotomy has been used to correct myopia. It involves cutting numerous "spokes" into the corneal surface, coming out from the center; the cornea flattens as it heals, which counteracts the problem. This procedure, however, is considered controversial by many ophthalmologists.

Myopia rarely progresses after age 30. In fact, the onset of middle age sometimes lessens the severity of the condition.

# N

# Narcolepsy

Narcolepsy is a disorder in which a person is recurrently subject to an irresistible, uncontrollable desire to sleep.

Narcolepsy is not necessarily related to any other abnormal condition, although it may be the result of an abnormality in the hypothalamus that causes a disorder in the endocrine system.

The most obvious symptom is the pattern of uncontrollable lapses into deep sleep during waking hours, often at inopportune times. These episodes of sleep last only a few minutes; the person wakes up feeling refreshed but is likely to fall asleep again a few hours later. The condition may be associated with cataplexy, a disorder in which stress or an unexpected emotional reaction causes collapse due to a sudden attack of muscle weakness.

The diagnosis is confirmed by observation in a sleep laboratory or by special electroencephalographic (EEG) studies.

Central nervous system stimulants are often prescribed.

# Nasal congestion

Nasal congestion occurs when the blood vessels in the nose enlarge. These enlarged blood vessels leak fluid into the surrounding tissues, which fills the nasal cavity and impairs breathing.

Nasal congestion is not a serious problem in itself, although it may be bothersome enough to interfere with daily activities and sleep. Persistent cases should be reported to a doctor, as nasal congestion may be a symptom of mild infections or more serious disorders.

The common cold, influenza, allergy, and bronchitis are the most frequent causes of nasal congestion. Persistent cases may be caused by structural abnormalities in the nose or by the daily use of certain drugs, particularly those often prescribed for high blood pressure, which act to enlarge all blood vessels, including those in the nose.

Occasional nasal congestion is often treated with over-the-counter (nonprescription) decongestants, such as nasal sprays, nose drops, and nasal inhalers, all of which act to shrink swollen blood vessels in the nose and stop fluid secretion. However, they can also shrink blood vessels elsewhere in the body, resulting in increased blood pressure and heart rate, as well as nervousness and insomnia. For this reason, over-the-counter decongestants should not be used without the advice of a physician by those with high blood pressure, heart disease, diabetes, or thyroid disorders.

Those who do use nasal decongestants should use them only for brief periods, perhaps three days at the most. Since they act to constrict the blood vessels, their overuse tends to tire the blood vessels, relaxing them completely and making the nose more congested than it was before decongestants were used. This is called rebound congestion.

In addition, specific medicine that is inserted in the nose may be prescribed by a doctor. Also, the use of vaporizers or humidifiers is often beneficial in relieving some of the discomfort of nasal congestion.

# Nausea and vomiting

Nausea is an extremely uncomfortable or queasy feeling in the stomach area, often accompanied by an urge to vomit. Vomiting is the forceful ejection of the contents of the stomach through the mouth.

Both nausea and vomiting can be symptoms of relatively mild upsets in the body, such as motion sickness, or of more serious disorders, such as peptic ulcer.

The sensation of nausea and the urge to vomit originate in an area of the brain called the vomiting center. In response to certain messages from nerves in the digestive system or the inner ear (part of which controls balance) or to direct stimulation by certain drugs, the vomiting center can trigger the muscular actions that result in vomiting.

Nausea and vomiting are usually temporary conditions and may be beneficial if they result in the expulsion of something potentially harmful to the body. However, persistent or recurring vomiting can lead to a dangerous loss of fluids and salts (called dehydration) and of nutrients, and can also damage the esophagus (the passageway from the mouth to the stomach) and the upper portion of the stomach.

Several relatively mild conditions and disorders may cause nausea and vomiting, including motion sickness, the "morning sickness" that can accompany pregnancy, excessive alcohol intake, emotional upset, and drug side effects. Eating too much, eating especially bothersome foods (such as oily or greasy foods), and eating spoiled food may also be responsible for episodes of vomiting. More serious conditions that may be accompanied by nausea and vomiting are severe injury or pain, serious disorders of the digestive system (such as peptic ulcer or gastritis), heart disease, and certain glandular disorders. Vomiting without a preceding feeling of nausea may be a symptom of brain injury or brain tumor.

The symptoms that accompany nausea include a "sour" or queasy stomach, chills, perspiration, drowsiness, headache, rapid heartbeat and breathing, and excessive production of saliva.

In most cases, nausea and vomiting require little or no treatment—they will subside when the cause is removed or corrected. However, if vomiting occurs regularly or frequently without an obvious cause, or if blood or red or dark brown spots appear in the vomitus (the material discharged during vomiting), medical treatment should be sought immediately. (The physician may want to examine a sample of the vomitus.)

Home remedies will often help to relieve the discomfort of occasional bouts of nausea and vomiting. Drinking tea, noncola beverages (especially ginger ale), and soup or broth is often suggested to replace the fluids lost due to vomiting. Solid food usually is not recommended during episodes of vomiting, but when vomiting subsides, toast may be tried before returning to a normal diet.

Several medications can successfully control the urge to vomit, but they must be prescribed by a doctor and should be used only with caution. Any woman who is pregnant or thinks she may be pregnant should consult her doctor before taking this (or any other) type of medication.

See also Dehydration and Hyperemesis gravidarum.

# Nephrotic syndrome

Nephrotic syndrome is a kidney disorder in which the glomeruli (tiny clumps of blood vessels, which filter the blood to produce urine) do not work properly. The defective glomeruli allow proteins, most notably albumin, to escape from the bloodstream and seep into the urine, while letting fluid that should be eliminated as waste accumulate within the tissues.

Nephrotic syndrome most often affects children, particularly those between the ages of one and six years. Boys are more likely than girls to be affected.

Nephrotic syndrome is caused by other diseases that affect the kidneys. The syndrome in turn creates vulnerability in the body to other infections, including peritonitis (inflammation of the lining of the abdominal cavity).

As a result of fluid accumulation, the body gradually swells (a condition called edema), becoming especially bloated around the face, abdomen, and ankles. The child may urinate very little (approximately one-fifth the normal amount).

To prevent complications, a doctor should be consulted as soon as either less frequent urination or unusual swelling in the face, abdomen, or ankles is noted.

If initial blood and urine tests point to nephrotic syndrome, the doctor will order more tests and possibly a kidney biopsy (removal of a tissue sample for microscopic examination).

The condition can be controlled with proper medical care, usually in a hospital, where medication (diuretics to eliminate excess fluid and steroids to control inflammation) and diet can be carefully supervised. Symptoms are likely to clear up after a few weeks, and the patient can finish recuperating at home, sometimes with no aftereffects.

# Nervous system

The nervous system is a complex network of specialized tissues that regulates thoughts, emotions, actions, sensations, and basic body functions.

The basic element of the nervous system is the nerve cell, or neuron. In combination, neurons form nerves, which transmit impulses throughout

Brain

Spinal cord

The nervous system has two major divisions: the central nervous system (brain and spinal cord) and the peripheral nervous system (nerves that branch out from brain and spinal cord).

rotransmitters from their sacs. The neurotransmitters travel across the synapse (the junction between the neighboring neurons) and stimulate the production of an electrical charge, which carries the nerve impulse forward. This process is repeated over and over again until a muscle is moved or relaxed or a sensory impression is noted by the brain. These electrochemical events can be considered the "language" of the nervous system, by which information is transmitted from one part of the body to another.

There are two major divisions of the nervous system: the central nervous system and the peripheral nervous system. The central nervous system consists of the brain and the spinal cord. The brain lies within the skull (the bony framework of the head). It governs body functions by sending and receiving messages through the spinal cord. Protecting the brain and spinal cord are bones, layers of tissue, and cerebrospinal fluid.

Once messages leave the central nervous system, they are carried by the peripheral nervous system. The peripheral system includes the cranial nerves (nerves branching from the brain) and the spinal nerves (nerves branching from the spinal cord). These nerves convey sensory messages from receptor cells in the body to the central nervous system. They also transport motor impulses from the central system out to the body, where muscles and glands can respond to the impulses.

The autonomic nervous system, which is part of the peripheral nervous system, regulates all activity that is involuntary but necessary for life, including activity of the internal organs and glands.

Working together, these divisions coordinate adjustment and reaction of the body to internal and external environmental conditions.

See also Brain.

the body. A protective covering of myelin, a fatty substance, insulates parts of those fibers.

The action of nerve cells is both electrical and chemical. At the ends of each nerve cell there are specialized regions called synaptic terminals, which contain large numbers of tiny membranous sacs that hold neurotransmitter chemicals. These chemicals transmit nerve impulses from one nerve cell to another. After an electrical nerve impulse has traveled along a neuron, it reaches the terminal and stimulates the release of neu-

# Neuralgia

Neuralgia is pain that runs along the course of a damaged nerve. The condition ranges from mild and temporary to severe and chronic. The pain itself is sharp and extreme, lasting only a few seconds but tending to recur. There are various types of neuralgia. These include carpal tunnel syndrome, sciatica, and the three types listed below.

**Peripheral neuropathy** In peripheral neuropathy, impairment of the peripheral nerves (those outside the brain and spinal cord) occurs as a complication of another disorder, such as diabetes mellitus, alcoholism, certain vitamin deficiencies, anemia, or a tumor, or as a result of overexposure to particular chemicals or drugs (the typical cause for farm and industrial workers). The first symptom is frequently a tingling sensation in the hands and feet, which slowly spreads up the limbs to the trunk; numbness follows in the same pattern, the skin becomes sensitive, and neuralgic pain ensues. Numbness in the hands leads to a loss of dexterity and susceptibility to accidents. A special risk is that a numbed part of the body can sustain an injury without the patient's being aware of what has happened until it becomes infected or ulcerated. The muscles gradually atrophy (wither away), and paralysis may set in.

**Shingles** Shingles, or herpes zoster, is a viral infection characterized by intense pain and skin rash along the course of a nerve. Red blisters appear in a band, usually along one side of the chest, trunk, or abdomen. Shingles occurs almost exclusively in persons who have already had chicken pox (which is caused by the same virus) and appears during times of stress or after a subsequent exposure to the chicken pox virus. Shingles can often be diagnosed by sight.

**Trigeminal neuralgia** Trigeminal neuralgia, or tic douloureux, primarily affects elderly persons (most commonly, those over age 70), although it may also occur in younger persons with multiple sclerosis. The pain arises from the trigeminal nerve, which controls sensation in the face, teeth, mouth, and nasal cavity and movement of the jaw. The pain, usually excruciating, covers one side of the face and can be set off by eating, by washing, or even by being exposed to a gust of air. With time, the stabbing pains occur more and more frequently, until they become constant. The cause is unknown. Although the condition is not life-threatening, it can become very disabling.

Treatment for the various types of neuralgia depends on the location of the damaged nerves, the severity of the pain, and the reason behind the impairment. Therapy may vary from cold or hot packs and aspirin to stronger prescription painkillers. For shingles, ointments may soothe and dry up blisters, and the antiviral drug acyclovir may shorten the course of the illness. A physician may refer a patient to a neurologist (a specialist in problems of the nervous system). In rare instances, neurosurgery to sever a damaged nerve is necessary to eliminate the pain.

There is virtually no way to prevent neuralgia, except to treat underlying diseases that may precipitate nerve damage and to avoid overexposure to chemicals and drugs.

See also Carpal tunnel syndrome, Sciatica, and Shingles.

# Night blindness

Night blindness, or nyctalopia, is a condition in which a person can see well in good light but not in dim or fading light.

The retina contains a layer of photoreceptors (specialized, light-sensitive cells) that lines the interior of the eyeball. These photoreceptors make the adjustments that are responsible for adaptation to varying degrees of light. There are two types of photoreceptors—cones and rods. Cones, concentrated in the center of the retina (the region called the macula), distinguish fine detail and color, while rods, which predominate around the edges of the retina, are sensitive to the intensity of light and do most of the work of seeing in dim light. Rods contain the pigment rhodopsin, or visual purple, which becomes temporarily bleached by bright light. The speed at which rhodopsin adjusts to darkness depends on a sufficient supply of vitamin A in the body.

Night blindness is caused either by a severe deficiency of vitamin A or by retinitis pigmentosa, an inherited degenerative disorder of the retina. In cases of extreme vitamin A shortage, the cornea may soften or start to dissolve (a condition called keratomalacia), or the eyes may become excessively dry (a condition called xerophthalmia).

A vitamin A deficiency can be treated with doses of the vitamin. However, consuming large doses of vitamin A without a doctor's recommendation and without documentation of a deficiency can be extremely dangerous.

The only preventive measure is to obtain enough vitamin A in the diet (for example, from liver, egg yolks, yellow and dark green vegetables, butter, and cream).

See also Retinitis.

# Nose

See Ear, nose, and throat.

# Nosebleeds

A nosebleed occurs when there is a break in the blood vessels in the inner lining of the nose, causing bleeding from the nose. Nosebleeds seldom require medical attention, but it is possible for nosebleeds to be a symptom of serious illness such as an underlying blood disorder.

Nosebleeds can be caused by an injury to the nose, breathing dry air for prolonged periods, repeated blowing or picking of the nose, tumors in the nose, high blood pressure, and certain blood diseases.

Very persistent or frequently recurring nosebleeds will require the attention of a doctor, who may cauterize (use heat or the chemical silver nitrate to seal off) the blood vessels in the back of the nose.

However, occasional nosebleeds can be treated simply by sitting up and leaning forward, so as not to swallow the blood, and pinching the entire soft portion of the nose between the thumb and forefinger for

An occasional nosebleed can be treated by sitting up, leaning forward, and pinching the entire soft portion of the nose between the thumb and forefinger for ten minutes.

ten minutes. If the bleeding does not stop, cold packs can be applied to the bridge of the nose for 15 to 20 minutes. If bleeding still persists, a doctor should be notified.

Frequent nosebleeds from breathing dry air may be relieved by the use of a humidifier. Also, those who have frequent nosebleeds should not blow the nose too harshly or blow through one nostril.

When nosebleeds occur along with colds or other respiratory infections, a nasal decongestant may help to temporarily shrink the blood vessels in the nose. However, these decongestants should not be used by anyone with high blood pressure, heart disease, diabetes, or thyroid disorders, because decongestants also shrink blood vessels in parts of the body other than the nose, which can lead to complications for these patients.

# Nystagmus

Nystagmus is the involuntary, rhythmic, and rapid movement of the eyeballs in a horizontal, vertical, or rotary direction. The eye movements of a person who sits in a moving vehicle and watches the scenery flashing by are an example of normal nystagmus.

Abnormal nystagmus is brought on by one of three problems: defective vision, such that the eye does not receive enough stimulation to concentrate on one object; disturbances in the elaborate mechanisms in the inner ear responsible for balance; and diseases of the nervous system, especially those affecting the parts of the brain responsible for eye movement and coordination. Generally, the only symptoms of abnormal nystagmus are double vision, vertigo, and dizziness. Treatment depends on the underlying cause.

# O

# Obesity

Obesity is a term commonly applied to the condition in which the body weight is 20 percent or more above normal. It has been linked statistically to high blood pressure, diabetes, cardiovascular disease, and chronic back and joint pains, among other ailments. It is a potentially serious condition that shortens the life span.

The risk of disease and death among the obese is greater for men than for women, but for both it increases in direct proportion to the degree of overweight. For example, it has been estimated that among those who are 20 percent overweight, there are 25 percent more deaths for men and 21 percent more for women than among those of normal weight in a given age group; for those who

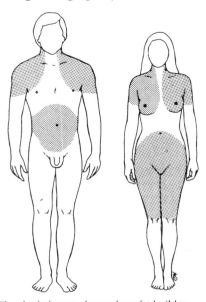

The shaded areas show where fat buildup most commonly occurs in men and women.

are 30 percent overweight, there are 42 percent more deaths for men and 30 percent more for women.

Obesity tends to occur more frequently in some families than in others. This may indicate a hereditary tendency, or it may be due to shared food consumption patterns and attitudes toward food. Women tend to gain weight after menopause, and men gain in middle age. Overweight children often grow up to be overweight adults. This is particularly true when food is used as a reward for a child or is withheld as a punishment. Food may then come to represent security and love—an attitude toward food that often continues into adult life.

Obesity is most often the direct result of taking in more food than is "burned off" in activity. Certain glandular (endocrine) disturbances can affect the appetite or the distribution of fat in the body, but these conditions are uncommon. It is said that only one percent of all obesity is due to factors other than diet. The appetite for food is influenced by habit as well as by emotional factors, and it is not always prompted by hunger. The appetite control center, or feeding center, is thought to be located in the area of the brain called the hypothalamus. The term appestat (suggested by the word thermostat) has been coined to describe the mechanism of appetite control.

The connection between smoking, appetite, and weight gain is unclear. Because smoking has been said to decrease appetite, giving up smoking is often thought to be followed by increased appetite and weight gain. The gain in weight that may follow when smoking is stopped has also been attributed to the dependence of some smokers on oral satisfaction; when they stop smoking, they may be compelled to substitute the oral satisfaction of eating for that of smok-

ing. Many smokers, however, gain no weight whatsoever after quitting.

The treatment for obesity is twofold: eat less and exercise more. A low-calorie diet that is nutritionally well balanced and that can form the basis of permanent eating habits is the first step. Combined with a regular exercise program, such a diet can eliminate obesity. Anyone embarking on such a program, however, should consult a physician for a medical checkup and for guidance.

Appetite-decreasing drugs can be harmful and should be taken only under medical supervision. Even physicians who prescribe them in selected cases recognize that these drugs are, at best, only a temporary prop, not a long-term answer to the problem of obesity.

Crash diets and fad diets can lead to nutritional deficiencies; if they are effective at all, it is basically only because they furnish fewer calories. The quick weight loss that many such diets promise is often merely a loss of fluid from body tissues; weight lost will quickly be regained as fluid is replaced. Other complications, such as gallbladder disease, may be associated with these diets as well.

Massage is not effective in removing or redistributing local fat deposits. Hot baths and sweating serve only to remove water from the tissues—water that will soon be replaced.

In extreme cases, surgery is sometimes performed to remove excessive layers of fatty tissue. However, the expense of the operation and the inherent dangers of any surgery make this a treatment to be used only in very select cases. The same caution should be exercised with stomach-stapling surgery or intestinal bypass surgery.

Although there are a variety of medical and surgical treatments for obesity, these are mostly reserved for those individuals who are severely obese and have had no success with more conventional diets. In the vast majority of cases, a diet and exercise program prescribed and supervised by a qualified medical professional is all that is necessary.

It is particularly important for parents to teach their children good eating habits and to control any tendency toward obesity before it becomes a serious problem. The old notions that children should have food urged on them and that a fat child is a healthy child should be recognized as not only false but harmful.

Older people, too, need to take special care to avoid obesity. They tend to be less active than they were in their younger days yet may continue to follow their established eating patterns. Reduced activity may make it necessary for the elderly to seek out a form of regular exercise—whether it be calisthenics or sports, such as swimming, bicycling, or hiking—that is suited to their capacities and tastes.

One safeguard for those of all ages is to control weight strictly, at an early stage, by weighing themselves frequently and embarking on a program of diet and exercise as soon as the weight is three to five pounds above the norm for the individual's height and body type. It is far easier to take off a few pounds than to wait until massive obesity requires a protracted and difficult struggle. Increased life span and improved health and vigor—not to mention improved appearance—will be a satisfying reward.

# Occult blood

Occult blood is blood that is present in an amount so small that it is detectable only with a chemical test or microscopic examination. This term is generally used to refer to blood in the stools that indicates bleeding along the gastrointestinal tract.

Often, the only symptom of occult bleeding is fatigue due to loss of oxygen-carrying red blood cells. A significant amount of blood can be passed in one stool with no visible indication that it is present.

Occult bleeding is not always constant, so tests are typically performed on stool samples obtained on three separate occasions if a problem is suspected. The patient must not eat red meat for three days before the samples are obtained because even cooked blood from meat that has been eaten can cause a positive test result. Aspirin can also cause minute amounts of blood to appear in the stools and should not be taken for at least several days before starting to test for occult blood in the stools. Tests for occult blood are commonly done as a screening examination for colon cancer and polyps. These tests are highly effective in early diagnosis of these conditions.

# Onychogryphosis

Onychogryphosis (or onychogryposis) is unusual growth of the fingernails or toenails, to the extent that they begin to resemble claws or horns.

Injuries due to going barefoot or wearing tight shoes are the usual cause of onychogryphosis, but the condition can be hereditary. It may also be related to congestive heart failure, in which there may be a shortage of blood circulation to the feet; peripheral neuritis, which affects nerves in the legs, causing decreased sensation in the feet and thereby increasing the chance that the foot will be injured; dry, scaly skin; hormonal disorders; syphilis; and stroke.

The nail becomes thick, long, raised, and green or black in color with an opaque surface. This condition occurs most often in toenails, especially on the big toes.

Properly fitting shoes, hot baths, massage with warm oil or hydrogen peroxide, or treatment of underlying disease may clear up the condition. Trimming or removal of an abnormal nail should be done only by a physician or podiatrist; serious complications can arise if this is done improperly.

# Onychomycosis

The most common of inflammatory nail disorders, onychomycosis is a fungal infection of the nails that is prevalent among persons with a low resistance to infection (diabetics and patients taking corticosteroid or other hormonal drugs), those who work with their hands in water and are prone to paronychia (inflammation of the skin around the nail), and those with ingrown toenails. Onychomycosis is caused by a number of fungi and is often associated with paronychia.

The condition is chronic but painless. The affected nails look dull, opaque, and brittle; are marked with grooves or ridges; and appear flaky. The surrounding cuticle may become red, tender, and swollen and may ooze pus if a bacterial infection accompanies the disorder. The fungi can be identified by examining nail scrapings in the laboratory.

The condition is sometimes treated with griseofulvin, an antifungal drug that can be taken orally or applied topically. However, it may take months to cure. Furthermore, the condition may never clear up at all, especially if the toenails are affected. Shortening or removing the nail can help the healing process.

To prevent onychomycosis, fingernails and toenails should be dried thoroughly after bathing, because fungi thrive in a moist environment. Footwear should be changed often if the feet tend to perspire.

# Oophorectomy

Oophorectomy is the surgical removal of an ovary. An oophorectomy is a major operation, usually performed through either a vertical or a horizontal incision in the abdominal area, but occasionally the procedure is performed through an incision in the vagina.

Removal of one ovary is called a unilateral oophorectomy. A salpingectomy (removal of all or part of the nearby fallopian tube) is usually performed at the same time. Removal of both ovaries is called a bilateral oophorectomy. A bilateral oophorectomy ends a woman's ability to conceive children and brings on menopause (if it has not already occurred). A hysterectomy (removal of the uterus) is generally performed in conjunction with a bilateral oophorectomy because the uterus has no purpose without both ovaries and, if left, can later harbor tumors.

Oophorectomy is used to correct a number of conditions in which the ovaries are the site of the trouble, including ovarian ectopic pregnancy (in which the embryo begins to develop in the ovary, rather than in the uterus) and benign (noncancerous) and malignant (cancerous) ovarian cysts and tumors. In women with recurrent cancer or endometriosis (the displacement of tissue from the uterine lining to areas elsewhere in the body), oophorectomy is performed to stop the production of hormones, which tend to aggravate the problem. Breast cancer, as well, may be dependent on hormones to grow; about one third of women with breast cancer show a decrease in breast cancer growth after removal of their ovaries.

Some physicians recommend a bilateral oophorectomy when a hysterectomy must be performed. There are pros and cons when it comes to removing healthy ovaries. Arguments for their removal are that it reduces the risk of ovarian cancer; that a small number of women will develop painful cystic ovaries, which would necessitate a second operation; and that for a woman in her 40s, the ovaries will naturally stop functioning within a few years anyway. Arguments against routine oophorectomy are that it causes the premature onset of menopause, which brings with it a greater risk of osteoporosis (loss of bone mass) and heart attack; that the abrupt end of hormone production is less natural than the gradual tapering off of natural menopause, provoking severe menopausal symptoms, such as hot flashes and vaginal shrinkage; and that estrogen, the hormone usually prescribed for a woman after oophorectomy, may increase the risk of cancer of the reproductive system.

If a woman is in her childbearing years, her doctor will make every effort to save healthy ovarian tissue. Because the ovaries are fed by an excellent blood supply, they heal quickly and even a small bit of preserved ovarian tissue will function, secrete hormones, and release eggs. The woman remains fertile and avoids early menopause.

In women past menopause, for whom fertility is no longer an issue and in whom the ovaries are no longer producing estrogen anyway, both the ovaries and the uterus are commonly removed even if only one ovary is abnormal.

See also Hysterectomy and Ovarian cysts.

# Osteitis deformans

See Paget's disease.

# Osteoarthritis

See Arthritis.

# Osteomyelitis

Osteomyelitis is inflammation of the bone and bone marrow. It is usually caused by a bacterial infection. Osteomyelitis is considered a childhood disease, due to the fact that it occurs most often in boys between the ages of 5 and 14 years, but it also occurs in adults. Since the introduction of antibiotics, osteomyelitis is rarely encountered in the United States, but it is still common in countries lacking good medical care and proper nutrition.

Along with essential oxygen and nutrients, blood may also carry bacteria and other organisms, which tend to settle in the capillaries (tiny blood vessels) of the long bones of the arms and legs. Infectious agents can also reach the bones directly from adjacent infected tissue or through an open wound or through a fracture. Osteomyelitis usually affects only one area of the bone or bone marrow, but it can attack more than one bone at a time.

Symptoms include pain and excruciating tenderness near a joint or at the affected area, fever in the range of 102°F to 104°F, redness, and swelling.

Although it is often possible for a physician to diagnose osteomyelitis from the symptoms, X rays and blood tests help to confirm the presence of the disease.

The child with osteomyelitis may be hospitalized and given antibiotics in liquid, tablet, or intravenous form. It may be necessary to drain any pus and clean the area in a minor surgical procedure and then immobilize the limb in a splint. The child is released from the hospital once the healing begins, but may have to undertake a course of antibiotics for six more weeks.

Possible complications of osteomyelitis include septicemia (blood poisoning); destruction of the bone; spread of the infection to a nearby joint, possibly resulting in a permanent deformity; transference of the infection to the surface of the skin, where it erupts as an abscess. Damage to the cartilage adjacent to the bone, which may retard bone growth, and suppurative (infectious) arthritis are additional complications.

Chronic (long-term) osteomyelitis may be a delayed complication of acute (sudden-onset) osteomyelitis, especially if it results from a fracture or the presence of a foreign body in the wound, such as a bullet or a piece of metallic debris. The major sign of chronic osteomyelitis is a flare-up or reopening of an abscessed wound, with periodic pain and discharge of pus. X rays show irregular bone and pieces of dead bone. Treatment for chronic osteomyelitis may require several operations to remove all the dead bone and other tissue, completely drain the abscess, and repair the bone structure when possible. Large doses of antibiotics may also be necessary in order to cure the problem.

To prevent osteomyelitis, clean and disinfect all wounds thoroughly and, especially in children, apply a bandage to keep the area clean until it has healed. Chronic osteomyelitis can be prevented by immediate antibiotic treatment of acute osteomyelitis.

# Osteoporosis

Osteoporosis is a relatively common disorder characterized by a decrease in the calcium content of the bones, which leaves them thin and susceptible to fracture.

The causes of osteoporosis are largely unknown. However, chances of acquiring the condition seem to increase dramatically with age, especially for women. One prevailing theory maintains that osteoporosis results from a loss of the female hormone estrogen, which affects the calcium content of the bones. Menopause (cessation of menstruation) may lead to osteoporosis because the body's production of estrogen is reduced at that time. Almost one third of all women over 60 years of age have the condition to some extent.

For reasons not entirely known, osteoporosis is more likely to affect white and Oriental women than black women. In addition, slender women, especially those with fair skin, run a higher risk than stouter, darker-skinned women.

Osteoporosis can also occur as a result of other conditions. Surgical removal of both ovaries (the female sex glands, which produce estrogen) and chronic arthritis (inflammation of the joints) may lead to osteoporosis. People who are inactive, either by choice or due to confinement because of illness, seem more susceptible to the disorder. A diet deficient in nutrients, especially calcium (which promotes bone development), may also contribute to osteoporosis.

Depending on the strength of the bones, osteoporosis may initially cause either no symptoms or extreme pain. If there is pain, it is most commonly in the lower back. The disease is not life-threatening, but it may lead to fractures, which, for the elderly,

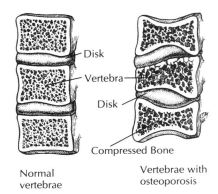

Disk

Vertebra

Disk

Compressed Bone

Normal
vertebrae

Vertebrae with
osteoporosis

Osteoporosis, a condition in which the
bones weaken and break easily, may lead to
compression of the vertebrae (bones of the
spine).

can result in serious complications. Initially, sudden back pain may follow fracture of the vertebrae (the bones of the spine). Pain from the fracture itself may subside but discomfort from osteoporosis may continue. This pain may lead to further inactivity, which may weaken additional vertebrae. Hence, a vicious cycle develops whereby pain leading to inactivity encourages osteoporosis, which in turn increases bone fragility and the cycle repeats itself.

As the disease progresses, the spinal column may decrease in length, causing a height loss of as much as several inches, or may become curved, producing the characteristic "dowager's hump." These changes are the result of successive fractures due to the pressure of body weight on the deteriorating vertebrae.

Often, osteoporosis progresses undetected until a bone is fractured and an X ray is taken. At that time, a physician may notice that bone thinning has become a generalized condition throughout the body.

Physicians urge patients with osteoporosis to follow an exercise program that will strengthen the muscles supporting weakened bones. To

protect bones in the spinal column, however, lifting heavy objects should be avoided. For advanced cases, a back brace may be necessary to help support body weight while sitting or standing. Crutches, walkers, or a cane may assist walking.

Physicians often prescribe estrogen or estrogen-progesterone combinations to women who are no longer menstruating in order to prevent osteoporosis. Women taking this medication need careful supervision because the hormone may cause adverse side effects. Anyone receiving estrogen therapy should have frequent physical and gynecologic examinations. Linkage between the use of estrogen and increased incidence of breast and/or gynecologic cancer is controversial. Women at high risk of breast cancer or with a history of gynecologic cancer should consult with an expert prior to undertaking hormonal therapy. Calcitonin, a hormone that promotes addition of calcium to bone, and fluoride may be given to treat osteoporosis in special cases. Men may be given the male hormone testosterone, which stimulates growth of body tissues, to treat osteoporosis if their own hormone production is inadequate.

For people prone to injury from osteoporosis, a balanced diet is an important factor in preventing or controlling the disease. Foods rich in vitamins and minerals, particularly calcium and vitamin D, encourage bone formation. When the diet is deficient in these nutrients, vitamin and mineral supplements may be prescribed by a doctor.

# Otitis media

See Middle ear infections.

# Otosclerosis

Otosclerosis is a condition in which an abnormal spongy overgrowth of bone in the middle ear leads to totally or partially muffled hearing or deafness. The excess bone grows at the entrance to the middle ear, where it immobilizes the base of the stirrup, or stapes (one of the three tiny, interconnected bones that transmit sound waves to the inner ear). As a result, sound-conducting vibrations are diminished, and hearing is impaired. In most cases, both ears are eventually affected. The cause of otosclerosis is unknown, but the condition tends to be hereditary.

Hearing loss generally begins in the late teens or early 20s; the rate of deafness may accelerate and stabilize several times, but ordinarily the loss is complete within 10 to 15 years of onset—sooner if the disease began in childhood. In some cases, the hearing loss stops just short of deafness, and the affected person can still hear loud sounds. Otosclerosis usually affects one ear before the other and is preceded by tinnitus (ringing in the ear). Special hearing tests aid in diagnosis.

The only way to halt or reverse otosclerosis is surgery, which is successful about 70 percent of the time. Although a hearing aid can help, most doctors prefer to operate. In a procedure called a stapedectomy, a surgeon folds back the eardrum, removes the affected stirrup, and replaces it with a synthetic or wire substitute that restores the conductive vibrations of the middle ear. Because the bones involved are the tiniest in the body, the surgery is very delicate and entails a risk of failure. In most cases, the operation is done on only one ear at a time, thereby reducing the risk.

After surgery, the hearing of most patients is greatly improved within two to three weeks. In some cases, a residual blood clot at the site of the surgery temporarily blocks hearing until it dissolves. Patients with advanced otosclerosis in both ears are usually advised to undergo stapedectomy as soon as possible.

See also Deafness.

# Ovarian cancer

This is the most dangerous form of cancer of the female reproductive organs, because it is so difficult to diagnose in its early stages. Women over 50 have a higher incidence of the disease, as do childless women and those with a family history of ovarian cancer.

Symptoms may include pelvic discomfort, constipation, abdominal swelling, and irregular menstruation. Diagnosis is often not possible without an exploratory operation known as a laparotomy, in which a surgical incision is made in the abdominal wall. Laparoscopy, during which a lighted tubelike instrument is inserted through a small incision in the abdominal wall for direct examination of the female organs and occasional treatment, has become a very useful tool in detecting ovarian cancer. Sometimes, removing only one ovary is sufficient, but usually it is necessary to remove both ovaries and the uterus. Radiation therapy and chemotherapy may then be administered, if necessary.

See also Cancer.

# Ovarian cysts

An ovarian cyst is an abnormal swelling or saclike growth on an ovary.

Ovarian cysts may be filled with liquid or may contain a semifluid substance. Most cysts are small, but they can vary in size from less than an inch in diameter to as large as 15 to 20 inches in diameter. Depending on their size, type, and location, they can cause severe pain and complications or no symptoms at all. They are common among women between the ages of 20 and 50 and can grow alone or in groups, on one ovary or both. Approximately 85 percent are benign (noncancerous).

The origin of most ovarian cysts is unknown. In some instances, they develop from an abnormal egg. Others originate as eggs in polycystic ovaries (ovaries in which the eggs are not released after they mature). Still others are related to abnormalities in the ovary. Women with endometriosis (the displacement of tissue from the uterine lining to elsewhere in the body) tend to develop growths on the ovaries. Dermoid cysts, which are most often found in women under the age of 30, arise from the ovarian cells that produce the eggs, and may contain fragments of hair, teeth, bone, and sweat and oil glands.

Cysts can rupture during sexual intercourse, a fall, childbirth, or surgery, or for no apparent reason. The resulting effect depends on how irritating the cystic fluid is to the surrounding tissues. The situation can be dangerous if the fluid is infected, cancerous, or extremely irritating. Also, in response to the injury caused by cystic fluid, surrounding tissues may produce adhesions (fibrous, scarlike material), which can further complicate the situation.

Symptoms of ovarian cysts vary with the type of growth. Some cause no symptoms and are discovered during a routine pelvic examination. Others cause firm, painless swelling in the lower abdomen; pain during sexual intercourse; frequent urination (if they press against the bladder); irregular vaginal bleeding; or pain, nausea, and fever (if the cysts rupture or grow on stalks that become twisted). Excessive and abnormal body hair growth and the development of acne may result from hormonal imbalances caused by polycystic ovaries.

Ovarian cysts are diagnosed by pelvic examination, ultrasound (a technique that uses sound waves to create an image of internal structures), or laparoscopy (a surgical procedure in which a tubelike instrument is inserted through the abdominal wall to view the pelvic organs). The condition may be difficult to diagnose accurately because the symptoms can resemble those of acute appendicitis or other abdominal problems. In addition, it can be hard to determine if a cyst is malignant and if it is actually on the ovary rather than some other pelvic organ. Ovarian cysts that develop during pregnancy are also difficult to diagnose.

Cysts that are small, are not creating any problems, or are likely to disappear on their own require no treatment. If treatment is necessary, cysts may be removed surgically. Removal of the cyst involves either taking out the entire ovary (oophorectomy) or taking out only the cyst (cystectomy).

Surgery for both oophorectomy and cystectomy can be performed in one of two ways. The first involves making a four- to five-inch incision in the abdomen. The surgeon then manually removes the cyst or ovary. This is the traditional method. The second method is a newer technique that involves removing a cyst or ovary using a laparoscopic procedure. In this technique, three small incisions are made into the abdomen; each incision is about a half inch to one inch in length. Through one incision, the surgeon inserts the laparoscope (a small, lighted, tubelike instrument).

Through the other two incisions, fine operating instruments may be inserted into the abdomen. By looking through the laparoscope and by manipulating the instruments, the surgeon is able to remove the cyst or diseased ovary. The advantage to the laparoscopic procedure is that it involves a very short recovery time and often can be performed in an outpatient surgical center. While traditional surgery can involve a hospital stay of two to three days and a recuperation time of two to four weeks, the patient who has a laparoscopic procedure may be able to go home two to four hours after surgery.

If the ovarian cyst is found to be cancerous, it is necessary to remove both ovaries, both fallopian tubes, and the uterus, since the cancer may have spread from the ovarian cyst to these other structures. This procedure is also performed if an ovarian cyst is found after menopause because these cysts are cancerous.

See also Cyst, Hysterectomy, and Oophorectomy.

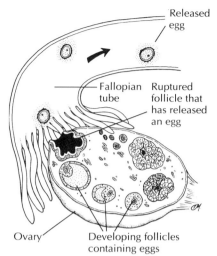

During ovulation the ovary releases the ripe egg (shown greatly enlarged) which moves up the fallopian tube toward the uterus.

# Ovulation

Ovulation is the process by which an ovary produces and releases an egg into the uterus.

The egg develops within the ovary in a small, fluid-filled sac called a follicle. When the egg is mature, this sac ruptures, releasing the egg from the ovary. The fingerlike projections on the nearby fallopian tube sweep the egg into the tube, where it begins to inch toward the uterus. If the egg is fertilized by a sperm, the fertilized egg moves along the tube to the uterus and becomes implanted in the rich uterine lining, where it grows for the next nine months. If the egg does not become fertilized, the uterine lining breaks down and passes, along with the unfertilized egg, out of the cervix, through the vagina, and out of the body as the menstrual discharge.

Ovulation is regulated by a complex system of hormonal and chemical secretions from the ovaries, the hypothalamus (part of the brain), and the pituitary gland (the master gland, which controls most hormonal secretions). Ovulation and menstruation begin during puberty, which usually occurs between the ages of 9 and 14, and normally continue every month (except during pregnancy) until menopause occurs (around age 50).

One way to recognize when ovulation is happening is to take the body temperature with a basal thermometer (a special thermometer that will show even slight changes in body temperature) before rising in the morning. In most women, the body temperature rises slightly soon after ovulation occurs each month and does not return to normal until the menstrual flow begins. Another way is to count 14 days forward from the first day of the last menstrual period in an average 28-day cycle (count 15 days for a cycle that is normally 29 days long, 16 days for a cycle that is normally 30 days long, and so on). However, this method is less accurate than the thermometer method because the length of the menstrual cycle can vary from month to month. Some women feel cramps in the lower abdomen during ovulation.

A sperm that has been released into the vagina as long as two days before the release of a ripe egg can still fertilize it; and an egg, once released, is capable of being fertilized for about two days. Because of this variability, there is a period of four to ten days in each menstrual cycle during which a woman can become pregnant.

See also Birth control, Conception, and Reproduction.

---

# P

---

# Paget's disease

Paget's disease (known medically as osteitis deformans) is a disorder in which the normal process of breakdown and replacement of bone tissue is greatly accelerated. The disease develops in three stages. In the first, or destructive, stage, bone tissue breaks down and is replaced with blood vessels and dense fibrous tissue, making the bones very vascular (having a greater-than-normal number of blood vessels). During the second, or mixed, stage, new bone formation takes place at a rate geared to the breakdown process. In the third, or sclerotic, stage, the breakdown process slows, allowing the hardening of new bone, which becomes quite dense.

Although any bone can be affected, Paget's disease most commonly invades the pelvis, skull, thighbones, shinbones, vertebrae (the bones of the spine), collarbones, and ribs.

The condition affects one percent to three percent of the adult population. Men are more commonly afflicted than women. The incidence of the condition is higher in some European countries than in others; it is rare in Asia, Africa, and South America. The cause is unknown.

Bone pain is one of the most prevalent symptoms. Complications sometimes develop. The thickened, enlarged bones are susceptible to fracture, particularly during the destructive phase of the disease. When the disease attacks the skull bones, the auditory nerve, which relays signals from the ear to the brain, is often compressed, causing deafness. Heart failure can result from the stress of the increased blood flow through the bones. Malignant bone tumors are another complication, but fortunately they are uncommon. The disease can affect appearance if it enlarges the head, bends the back, or bows the legs. In some severe cases, particularly if the person is immobile, calcium levels in the blood and urine increase and may lead to formation of kidney stones.

A history and physical examination, blood tests, and particularly X-ray studies are used to confirm the diagnosis.

Although there is no cure, analgesics (painkillers) like aspirin offer some relief. Severe pain and other complications are sometimes managed with drug therapy. Injections of calcitonin (a hormone normally produced in the thyroid gland, which promotes calcification of bone) may help block excessive breakdown of bone. Oral drug therapy is now also available. In most cases, however, medication (oral or injectable) is not necessary.

# Pain

Pain is an unpleasant or uncomfortable sensation that can range from mild irritation to excruciating agony. It is probably the most commonly reported symptom and may be associated with innumerable disorders and diseases.

Pain occurs when specialized nerve endings are stimulated; within a fraction of a second this pain "signal" travels through a network of nerves to the brain. Pain can be a warning sign, indicating impending damage to the body, or it can be a protective mechanism, causing a person to remove the cause of the pain or to reflexively draw away from the source. Most healthy people have occasional, brief twinges of pain that have no specific cause and are usually harmless. However, bothersome, recurring, or persistent pain can be caused by thousands of factors. Most commonly, pain is a symptom of disease, injury, or abnormal changes in the body.

There are many types of pain. Pain can be dull and constant, sharp and sudden, crushing, burning, piercing, or aching. When it is felt in areas other than the location of the disorder (for example, when the pain of heart attack is felt in the arm), it is called referred pain.

Unexplainable pain should be reported promptly to a doctor for investigation and possible treatment. It is best to observe any accompanying symptoms and to be prepared to answer two questions that the doctor will almost certainly ask in trying to identify the cause of the pain: "What brings on the pain?" and "What brings relief?"

The ideal treatment for pain consists of finding and correcting its source. In some cases, however, such as in widespread cancer, this would be impossible, so the pain itself needs to be treated, most commonly with analgesic drugs (painkilling medications). Aspirin and acetaminophen are probably the most common painkillers that can be obtained without a prescription. More potent painkillers, such as narcotics, must be prescribed by a doctor. Other drugs, both prescription and nonprescription, are designed to treat and relieve the pain of a specific disorder (for example, antacids treat the discomfort of heartburn or ulcers).

If the pain comes from the muscles (such as that from overexertion or from a bruising injury to the soft tissues), adequate rest of the affected area may bring relief. Surface treatment of this type of pain is often very beneficial; this consists of massage or application of heat or cold (depending on the injury and the time elapsed since incurring it) to the painful area.

# Pancreatitis

The pancreas has many functions. The endocrine portion of the pancreas secretes hormones directly into the bloodstream, such as the hormones insulin and glucagon, which are critical to the processing of glucose (the form of sugar used by the body for energy). The exocrine portion of the pancreas secretes digestive enzymes (proteins that promote chemical reactions), such as amylase, which aids in the breakdown of starches, and lipase, which aids in the breakdown of fats. Pancreatitis is an inflammation of the pancreas.

Pancreatitis commonly results from an obstruction of the pancreatic ducts, which convey enzymes to the small intestine. Why these blockages occur is often hard to determine; however, most cases of pancreatitis are related to gallbladder disease or alcoholism. Acute attacks are frequently associated with gallstones or alcoholic binges. If hereditary factors are involved, the disease may begin in childhood, as early as eight or ten years of age. Direct blows to the abdomen or injury during an operation may also lead to pancreatitis, sometimes a year or more after the event. Mumps and other viral infections; use of certain drugs, including steroids, thiazide diuretics, and oral contraceptives; and tumors have all been associated with pancreatitis.

The disease is characterized by the sudden onset of steady, severe, piercing, upper abdominal pain (frequently radiating to the middle portion of the back) accompanied by nausea and persistent vomiting. Eating—or even the sight of food—may bring on the pain or make it worse. Vomiting provides no relief, a feature that distinguishes pancreatitis from some stomach or intestinal disorders. Fever, shock (circulatory collapse), jaundice (yellowish discoloration of the skin and whites of the eyes), dehydration (excessive fluid loss), bleeding, and infection may occur in severe attacks.

The existence and degree of inflammation in the pancreas may be hard to determine, not only because of the hidden position and dual purpose of the gland, but also because the symptoms are easily confused with those of other abdominal disorders. Blood and urine tests, as well as microscopic tissue examination, may be inconclusive, but these tests can at least be helpful in excluding other abdominal disorders.

A special X-ray study, endoscopic retrograde cholangiopancreatography (ERCP), may be used to inspect the pancreatic ducts. The technique is performed by inserting a endoscope (a flexible, lighted, tubelike instrument) through the mouth and stomach into the duodenum. In the duodenum is the opening to the common bile and main pancreatic ducts. A special device is inserted through this opening, and X-ray contrast material is injected. Obstructions, tumors, and characteristic ductal patterns associated with chronic pancreatitis can be seen on the X-ray films obtained.

The patient is usually hospitalized for 3 to 14 days for a mild to severe acute attack. Correction of an underlying problem (for example, removal of stones) improves the chances for complete recovery.

Initial treatment is aimed at relieving the pain and reducing stomach secretions, which can stimulate the pancreas. To allow the pancreas to rest, eating and drinking are replaced by intravenous feeding, and stomach acids are suctioned out through a tube inserted through the nose. Antacids and antibodies are also frequently given.

During convalescence, a low-fat, high-protein diet should be followed, and antacids may be prescribed. If the disease is chronic, it may be necessary to use pancreatic extracts to supplement the insufficient quantities of enzymes secreted by the diseased pancreas. This helps to normalize digestion and thereby maintain adequate nutritional status.

After an acute episode of pancreatitis, tissue debris, blood, and pancreatic enzymes may form a pseudocyst (an internal space filled with a collection of material but not within a sac). Rupture or enlargement of a pseudocyst can be a very serious or even fatal event. If a pseudocyst does not clear up spontaneously, surgery is necessary to drain it.

Chronic pancreatitis is an indication of continued degenerative tissue damage, which may impair pancreatic function. In some cases of recurrence, surgical exploration might be considered to locate a previously unidentified blockage or to remove diseased tissue; however, surgery is unlikely to help the patient who continues to drink excessive amounts of alcohol. Recently, procedures to remove stones or otherwise relieve obstruction have been successfully performed through a gastroscope, eliminating the need for surgery.

# Paralysis

Paralysis is the loss of the ability to move a part of the body, usually brought on by damage to either the muscles or to the nervous system. The condition can vary in severity and degree from paralysis of one small muscle to paralysis of almost the entire body. Irreversible and permanent paralysis results when a nerve is completely severed and destroyed, whereas paralysis caused by some diseases that cause inflammation without actual destruction of nerve tissue may diminish as the condition is treated and the body recuperates.

There are numerous causes of paralysis. Brain damage resulting from disease or a stroke can lead to partial or total paralysis of various parts of the body. Such damage interferes with the transmission of nerve impulses from the brain to the muscles. Certain other diseases (for example, poliomyelitis, a viral infection of the central nervous system, and myasthenia gravis, a severe muscular disorder of the neurochemical transmission system) and poisons (such as nerve gas and the toxin that causes botulism) also prevent nerve impulses from making contact with muscles, but do not necessarily cause complete loss of movement.

Damage to the spinal cord at the level of the middle or lower back can cause paralysis of the legs and the structures in the lower part of the body, including the bladder and rec-tum; this condition is called paraplegia. Injury to the spinal cord at the level of the neck affects both arms and both legs; this is known as quadriplegia.

Diabetes, cancer, alcoholism, vitamin deficiency, and drug reactions, among other conditions, can injure peripheral nerves (those outside the brain and spinal cord), occasionally weakening or totally immobilizing the muscles they control, as well as causing loss of sensation in the areas they serve.

Well-being and survival depend on the cause and extent of the paralysis. Obviously, paralysis that affects the muscles involved in breathing is life-threatening, and the job of breathing must be taken over by machines (called ventilators or respirators) until the paralysis improves or disappears.

Patients whose paralysis does not require artificial measures for survival may benefit from physical or occupational therapy. These patients can learn to reuse a muscle or to develop other muscles to compensate for a disabled muscle. All patients with disabled muscles require special attention to prevent muscle atrophy (withering away) and ulcers (pressure sores or bed sores).

# Paranoia

Paranoia is a personality disorder characterized by delusions of grandeur and/or suspicions of persecution.

An internal conflict between the need for recognition and the compulsion to guard certain aspects of emotional life may be the root of paranoia. Unconscious sexual conflicts often play a role.

Paranoid persons display unreasonable distrust and constant unfounded suspicion that others are out to do them harm; interpret innocent comments as personal attacks; develop grandiose or exaggerated estimations of their own worth, yet feel that others do not recognize their value; believe they are the center of attention because everyone else openly criticizes them; and strenuously defend their fears with reason and logic. Paranoia differs from paranoid schizophrenia, a much more serious problem in which the individual not only has delusions of grandeur and a persecution complex, but also demonstrates deranged thought processes, hallucinations, and other signs of disturbed personality.

Almost everyone exhibits short-lived symptoms that suggest paranoia at some time, usually from excessive worry over an embarrassment or from disappointment. It is only when paranoid behavior persists or worsens and impairs the person's ability to function that concern is warranted. Like the symptoms of many other mental disorders, paranoid symptoms can have an underlying physical cause, such as a brain disease or a drug side effect. Diagnosis should always be made by a physician, who will first rule out (and treat) purely physical causes and then recommend appropriate therapy.

Paranoid persons can often be helped with psychotherapy and medication.

# Parkinson's disease

Parkinson's disease is a progressive disorder characterized primarily by uncontrollable tremors in the limbs, a shuffling gait, and generalized muscular rigidity. It most often strikes people over the age of 60.

Parkinson's disease is usually not fatal, but it leads to changes in the entire body, making the patient more

"Cogwheel rigidity" is noted in a patient with Parkinson's disease when the arm moves in a jerky fashion (as if controlled by a ratchet in a cogwheel) after being pulled straight from a flexed position.

susceptible to other diseases. It can be present in a mild form for 20 or 30 years, but a severe form can lead to serious disability within five to ten years.

The cause of Parkinson's disease is unknown. No inherited, physiological, or environmental factors have been identified as causes of the disease. It is known, however, that Parkinson's disease is a reflection of a chemical imbalance in the brain. Those with the disease have been shown to have low levels of a neurotransmitter called dopamine. (Neurotransmitters are chemicals in the brain that transmit impulses across junctions between neurons; the delicate balance of neurotransmitters in the brain is responsible for brain function and muscular control.) To date, no cause for this chemical deficiency has been found.

The symptoms of Parkinson's disease are uncontrollable shaking of the limbs, stiff muscles, drooling, reduced blinking, an expressionless face, stooping posture, and a shuffling walk. Tremors may worsen during rest periods and times of increased anxiety. Interestingly, the tremors may decrease when the patient makes a conscious effort to perform some action.

As the disease progresses, speech slurs and sentences trail off into unintelligible muttering. Small muscle movements become increasingly difficult—reducing the ability to write, eat, chew, and swallow—and all movements seem overly stiff and slow. The term "cogwheel rigidity" is often used to describe the typical arm motion these patients display; when the arm is pulled straight from a flexed position, it seems to jerk up and down as if controlled by a ratchet in a cogwheel.

Excitement and tension can cause these symptoms to worsen, as can depression. Depression is common among Parkinson's disease victims, who are upset by their loss of muscle control.

Diagnostic evaluation involves a history, physical examination, and observation of the symptoms. If tremors are the only symptom displayed, tests may be done to rule out the possibility that other disorders are causing the tremors, such as liver disease, multiple sclerosis (a debilitating nervous disorder), chronic alcoholism, or overactivity of the thyroid gland.

Treatment of Parkinson's disease consists of correcting the dopamine deficiency. Dopamine itself cannot be absorbed directly into the brain from the bloodstream, so a substance called levodopa is prescribed to help the brain manuacture more of its own dopamine.

Levodopa has several undesirable side effects, among them nausea (which is decreased if the drug is taken with meals), an uneven "on-off" effect (causing symptoms to disappear and then reappear), and a loss of effectiveness over time. Levodopa preparations are often given in combination with anticholinergic drugs, which decrease nerve-to-muscle transmission, thereby reducing tremor and rigidity, and also decrease drooling. Levodopa is most often prescribed in combination with carbidopa, a substance that prevents destruction of levodopa in the body

before it reaches the brain, thus allowing the use of smaller amounts of levodopa. Bromocriptine, a drug that enhances the effects of dopamine, has also been successful, as have other drugs.

Surgery to halt the tremor of Parkinson's has been helpful in select groups of patients. Physical therapy and exercise are also important in a treatment program for patients with Parkinson's disease. In addition, emotional support and understanding are critical.

# Patent ductus arteriosus

Patent ductus arteriosus is a congenital (present at birth) heart disorder in which the ductus arteriosus, an extra blood vessel present in the fetus that allows the blood to pass from the pulmonary artery (which conveys blood from the heart to the lungs) to the aorta (the main blood vessel that conveys blood from the heart to the rest of the body) fails to close after birth. This condition is most commonly encountered among babies born prematurely.

During the nine months of growth and development in the uterus, the fetus is immersed in amniotic fluid, and the lungs are not used. The blood bypasses the lungs through the ductus arteriosus, and the fetus receives its supply of oxygen directly from the placenta.

If the ductus arteriosus remains open after birth, some blood is rerouted from the aorta back through the lungs. As a result, less oxygen-rich blood can be supplied to the tissues throughout the body, and the workload of the left side of the heart (which pumps blood from the heart to the rest of the body) is increased.

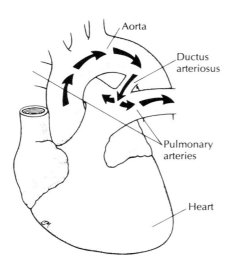

If the ductus arteriosus fails to close after birth, incorrect flow of blood will put a strain on the baby's heart.

In most babies, the duct begins to close before birth and is completely closed by the age of three months. The reasons for this normal closure (and for failure to close) are poorly understood.

Although obvious symptoms are rare, the affected infant may display shortness of breath or develop congestive heart failure.

Patent ductus arteriosus can be treated with medication if diagnosed very early. Various prenatal (before birth) tests have become available in recent years for diagnosis if the condition is suspected. After birth, the condition can easily be corrected by tying off the duct in a relatively simple surgical procedure.

# Pellagra

Pellagra is a disorder caused by a deficiency of niacin (also known as nicotinic acid), a vitamin found in many foods. Niacin is vital to many of the important chemical reactions by which energy is generated in the body, as well as to maintenance of healthy skin and normal functioning of the nervous system. Since niacin is abundant in many foods, only those who seriously neglect their diets, such as alcoholics, are likely to lack the daily requirement of between 9 and 20 milligrams of niacin. Pellagra was once widespread in the United States, especially in the South, but today it occurs far less frequently.

Physical symptoms of pellagra include weakness; loss of appetite; sore, red, cracked skin with symmetrical spots that turn scaly and brownish; a painful scarlet mouth, tongue, and gums; a burning sensation throughout the digestive tract; diarrhea; and headaches. Psychological symptoms are anxiety, forgetfulness, insomnia (inability to sleep), irritability, and dementia (loss of intellectual abilities).

The deficiency can be reversed by eating a balanced diet and taking niacin supplements.

# Pelvic inflammatory disease

Pelvic inflammatory disease (PID), or salpingitis, is an inflammation of one or both of the fallopian tubes. Although the term is widely used to refer to infections of other organs in the pelvic cavity, PID properly refers only to an inflammation of the fallopian tubes.

Pelvic inflammatory disease is usually caused by certain bacteria transmitted during sexual intercourse, the presence of an intrauterine device (IUD) that has become a source of infection, or certain vaginal infections.

Pelvic inflammatory disease is an inflammation of the fallopian tubes (salpingitis) that can lead to an abscessed ovary, an inflammation of the abdominal lining, and perhaps blocked fallopian tubes.

Two of the most common causes of PID are gonorrhea and chlamydia, both sexually transmitted diseases.

Under normal circumstances, the cervix prevents bacteria in the vagina from entering the uterus. However, a woman becomes more vulnerable to PID if the opening of her cervix has been dilated (enlarged) by recent surgery, childbirth, or miscarriage.

Symptoms include severe pain and tenderness in the lower abdomen, fever, a foul-smelling vaginal discharge, menstrual irregularities, pain during sexual intercourse, nausea, vomiting, fatigue, and pain during urination or defecation.

It is important to seek medical attention as soon as symptoms occur, so that the infection can be treated before it worsens and spreads. The physician will perform a physical examination and take a sample of fluid from the cervix to identify the infecting organism.

If PID is not diagnosed and treated early, the infection can cause abscesses (pus-filled cavities) to form in the fallopian tubes or around the ovaries. The inflammation can also damage and irreversibly scar pelvic tissues. If the fallopian tubes are blocked, conception can become impossible. The infection can also result in septicemia (in which bacteria enter the bloodstream and are spread to other parts of the body) and in peritonitis (inflammation of the membrane lining the pelvic and abdominal cavities).

The doctor will prescribe antibiotics to fight the infection and aspirin or other painkillers for pain relief. The woman may be advised to rest in bed, abstain from sexual intercourse, and apply heat to the lower abdominal area. In some cases, the woman may have to enter the hospital to receive antibiotics intravenously. Laparoscopy (examination of the internal organs through a special tubelike instrument) or surgery to drain blocked tubes or abscessed tissue may be performed. Sometimes, however, the damage is too extensive, and the fallopian tubes, the uterus, and the ovaries have to be removed surgically.

When the cervix is dilated for any reason, a woman is more susceptible to PID for several weeks. Since the cervix is dilated in childbirth, abortion, miscarriage, and the surgical procedure called dilatation and curettage (D&C), a woman can minimize her chances of contracting PID by taking special precautions after any of those events. Such precautions include avoiding sexual intercourse, tub baths, and the use of douches and tampons. She should check with her doctor before resuming any of these activities. Also, if a woman suspects that she may have gonorrhea or chlamydia, she should seek treatment immediately. The use of condoms during sexual intercourse will help prevent these infections.

# Peptic Ulcer

See Ulcer.

# Pericarditis

Pericarditis is an inflammation of the pericardium (the membranous sac surrounding the heart). The inflammation is often accompanied by development of an effusion (a collection of fluid) between the membrane and the heart, which may lead to complications.

The inflammation commonly stems from an infection, such as bacterial pneumonia, tuberculosis, or a viral infection. Pericarditis can also occur in noninfectious diseases, such as connective tissue disorders and chronic kidney failure. Pericarditis sometimes follows a heart attack or chest injury.

Occasionally, long-term pericarditis arises from a chronic condition, most notably tuberculosis. The chronic inflammation causes thickening and contraction of the pericardium to the point that it restricts the heartbeat. Called constrictive pericarditis, this condition is no longer common because of the decrease in the incidence of tuberculosis, but it is a severe condition calling for immediate attention.

Pain in the center of the chest (and possibly the shoulders, neck, and upper arms) that worsens with coughing, lying flat, or breathing and is relieved by leaning forward may signify pericarditis. Since this type of pain is a symptom of a number of serious illnesses, a doctor should be consulted about any severe chest pain.

Constrictive pericarditis is signaled by difficulty in breathing, swelling of the veins in the neck, and edema (fluid retention) in the legs and abdomen.

A chest X ray, electrocardiogram, and blood tests, along with the medical history and physical examination, are used to diagnose pericarditis. If an effusion is present, a sample of the fluid may be obtained to identify any infectious agent.

When a large effusion exists, the motion of the heart may be restricted, thereby preventing it from filling and pumping effectively. This life-threatening condition must be corrected as soon as possible. The fluid may be drained by inserting a needle through the chest and into the pericardial sac.

Once the underlying cause of pericarditis has been identified, the doctor can treat it (for example, by using dialysis in kidney failure or antibiotics for bacterial infection).

Constrictive pericarditis cannot be corrected without a surgical procedure, called pericardiectomy, to remove scarred tissue.

# Periodontal disease

Periodontal disease (also known as periodontitis or, less accurately, as pyorrhea) is a progressive deterioration of the gums, bones, and other tissues around the teeth.

One theory is that the condition begins with an accumulation of bacteria and food particles within tissues surrounding the teeth. These bacteria emit toxins (poisons) that cause gum tissues to swell, bleed, and deteriorate.

Gingivitis (inflammation of the gums) is the first stage of periodontitis. The second stage results when the soft tissues become separated from the bone and teeth, leading to "pocket" formation. Pockets of bacteria and pus accumulate around the teeth, leading to weakening of the tissues holding the teeth in their sockets, as well as to destruction of the bone supporting the teeth. As the disease advances, teeth become loose and fall out. They may also move out of alignment with one another, causing problems with chewing.

In the early stage of periodontal disease, gums become sore, red, and slightly swollen. They may be sensitive to the touch and may bleed when brushed or flossed. The presence of pus in the gums around the teeth signals the beginning of the second stage. If pus remains in the gum tissue without draining, extreme pain and swelling can result.

The diagnosis of periodontal disease is based on the presence of swollen gums and deposits of plaque around the teeth.

Once periodontal disease has been detected, continued care of the mouth at home can help prevent extension of disease and can reduce gum problems.

Oral hygiene to prevent gum disease is the same as treatment to prevent tooth decay. Ideally, the mouth should be cleaned after every meal. At the least, a thorough cleansing at bedtime is necessary to reduce the risk of gum disease. Dentists suggest brushing with a soft-bristled toothbrush. Gentle movements within the crevices dislodge decay-causing material, and firm strokes over the teeth remove plaque. Flossing is recommended to clear plaque from between teeth. After brushing and flossing, vigorously rinsing the mouth with mouthwash containing an antimicrobial agent (a substance that kills bacteria) can also help eliminate bacterial growth, but using mouthwash alone cannot completely prevent plaque formation.

For self-checking, a dental mirror provides a view of the teeth and gums in the back of the mouth. Disclosing wafers, which discolor plaque when chewed, reveal any invisible film that needs to be removed.

In advanced cases, a dentist may scrape the affected tissue pockets and apply antiseptics (germ-killers) every few months in an effort to kill the bacteria. Should this procedure fail to check the spread of the disease, surgery by a periodontist (gum specialist) may be needed to remove deep pockets in the gums. Once the bacteria have been eliminated, good oral hygiene should control the disease.

See Tooth decay.

# Peritonitis

Peritonitis is a term used to describe an inflammation and/or infection of the peritoneum, the thin, double-layered membrane that lines the abdominal cavity and covers the abdominal organs.

The condition occurs when the peritoneum is invaded by bacteria or irritated by toxins (poisons), bile (a substance produced by the liver and stored in the gallbladder), blood, or urine. Because the peritoneum is well sealed, it can be infiltrated only when one of the hollow organs of the abdomen ruptures; when a solid

Plaque buildup

Pocket of bacteria

Receding gum tissue

Bone deterioration

The left side shows plaque buildup and deterioration of bone and gums from periodontal disease; the right side shows healthy tooth, bone, and gums.

organ is somehow damaged, causing it to leak; or when there is a penetrating injury from the outside. If the colon is perforated, feces, which contain bacteria and toxins, are discharged, causing bacterial peritonitis. Immediate treatment is necessary for this condition.

A main symptom of peritonitis is severe pain that intensifies with any movement and often forces the person to lie very still with the legs drawn up. The abdominal area becomes very tender and rigid; commonly there is vomiting, fever, and dehydration (excessive loss of body fluids). When the peritoneum is inflamed, fluid begins to leak out of the blood vessels into the peritoneum. If this condition is not corrected, it may lead to shock (failure of the circulatory system). Swelling of the abdomen is a sign that the intestines have become paralyzed and bloated with air and/or a large amount of fluid is accumulating.

These symptoms of peritonitis call for immediate medical care, including intravenous administration of antibiotics to fight infection. Intravenous fluids are also given to replace lost fluids. In addition, a tube is usually inserted through the nose and into the stomach to relieve bloating and remove pooled fluids. After the patient's condition has been stabilized, surgery is performed to remove or repair the cause of peritonitis. Chances for recovery are usually excellent.

# Phenylketonuria

Phenylketonuria (PKU) is a congenital (present at birth) disorder characterized by the presence of increased amounts of certain amino acids in the blood and urine. (Amino acids are the chemical building blocks of protein.)

The condition is caused by the inability to convert phenylalanine (an amino acid essential for optimal growth in infants and for maintenance of nitrogen balance in adults) into tyrosine (another amino acid). Excess phenylalanine is normally eliminated from the body by conversion to tyrosine. In PKU, this mechanism does not work, permitting an accumulation of phenylalanine. If untreated, the result is mental retardation in infants or young children.

Phenylketonuria is hereditary and is found in most population groups, although it is very rare in Jewish and black children. The incidence in the United States is about one in every 16,000 live births.

Early diagnosis of phenylketonuria is essential because symptoms are usually not obvious in a newborn infant. Therefore, screening tests are now mandatory for all babies born in the United States and Canada. Sometimes, infants with PKU will have nervous system disorders, very light coloring of the skin and hair, eczema (a skin disorder), and a musty odor. Older children may be extremely hyperactive. The light coloring is often an early clue to the disease; the infant's skin, hair, and even eyes will be lighter than those of other members of the family.

Treatment of this disorder within the first few days after birth is essential if mental retardation is to be prevented. Treatment consists of limiting the child's phenylalanine intake so that the essential amino acid requirement is satisfied without any excess. This can be done by feeding the infant special formulas with little or no phenylalanine. Milk is a protein food rich in phenylalanine, so it must be avoided. When it is time to introduce solid foods into the infant's diet, low-protein natural foods, such as fruits, vegetables, and certain cereals, are permitted.

If PKU is not diagnosed in the first few days of life, extreme hyperactivity, seizures, and mental retardation usually occur. Some physicians think that treatment and special diet must be continued throughout the child's life; others believe it can be ended when brain development is virtually complete (which occurs at about five years of age).

It is important to remember that, although untreated PKU can lead to retardation and other problems, early diagnosis and treatment can enable the child to develop normally and to lead a normal life.

# Phimosis

Phimosis is a constriction of the foreskin (the skin fold over the head of the penis), which prevents the foreskin from being drawn back over the glans (the head of the penis).

Phimosis is either congenital (present at birth) or acquired. The acquired form is usually due to an infection involving the penis that leaves adhesions (growths of tissue that adhere both to the inner aspect of the fore-

Tight foreskin

Glans penis

Phimosis occurs when the foreskin cannot be pulled back over the penis.

skin and to the glans itself). Phimosis also allows debris (dirt, dead cells, and normal fluid secretions) to accumulate between the foreskin and the glans, providing a breeding ground for bacteria to grow.

If infection becomes established, ulcers (open sores) may appear on the glans, and swelling of the lymph nodes in the groin may occur.

The condition will be apparent on physical examination of the child. If infection is present, cultures may be performed.

The definitive treatment for this condition is circumcision (the surgical removal of the foreskin). If, for some reason, circumcision must be delayed, there must be careful attention to keeping the area clean and dry and free from infection until the procedure can be performed.

See also Circumcision.

# Phobia

A phobia is a psychological disorder characterized by persistent, abnormal, excessive, or unfounded dread of something that is often not inherently dangerous or considered threatening by most people. A phobic reaction resembles acute or chronic anxiety, but rather than being a generalized response, it is linked to specific environmental stimuli, such as being alone or in an open space, seeing a spider, or hearing thunder.

Phobias affect fewer than one percent of the total population. They seem to occur more often in some families and more often in women than in men.

Anxiety is a fearful reaction to the emergence of forbidden or unconscious drives. In most cases, the psychological mechanisms called projection and displacement focus anxiety on specific external objects, persons, or situations, which then come to represent the original cause of the anxiety. In shifting attention to a secondary symbol, a patient learns to use avoidance of the object or situation (spiders, heights, open places, and so on) to prevent rearousal of the painful anxiety. The "choice" of the phobic object is often at random; it may be the first object, location, or situation at hand when the original anxiety first appeared.

Phobias usually begin in early adulthood and follow a long course of alternate improvement and worsening of symptoms. The longer a patient has phobic symptoms, the less likely he or she is to achieve a complete recovery.

The symptoms of a phobia depend on the phobic object. Often, the very thought or mention of the object induces anxiety in the patient. The more inescapable the exposure or contact becomes, the more anxiety mounts toward panic. As a result, the patient spends more and more time avoiding the phobic stimulus, and this avoidance often begins to restrict his or her daily activities (for example, he or she becomes unable to travel because of fear of flying).

Agoraphobia (a fear of open, public places, such as stores, malls, parks, theaters, and stadiums, or of crowds and crowded situations) is the most common phobia, accounting for about 60 percent of all cases. This abnormal fear of being in open places greatly restricts the life of the victim, who in extreme cases will not leave home, except perhaps if accompanied by a close friend or relative. The first sign of the condition may be a panic attack when out in public, with feelings of anxiety and a sense of approaching doom, restlessness, breathlessness, and rapid or irregular heartbeat. Thereafter, the person may stay at home to avoid another panic attack. Often, the agoraphobic per-

son experiences the phobia selectively—the phobic situation can be faced fairly well in the company of someone close.

Another common phobia, claustrophobia, is an intense and unrealistic fear of being confined in an enclosed space, such as an elevator or a small room. Commonly, the claustrophobic person becomes anxious at even the thought of being "trapped" in a small room or passageway. If the person unexpectedly has to face the phobia, as when caught in a stuck elevator, real panic may result. Unlike some phobias, such as a fear of mice, snakes, or spiders, which the average person seldom sees, claustrophobia can cripple one's vocational and social life, since enclosed spaces are part of the everyday environment.

Some childhood phobias, such as fear of the dark or of animals, disappear with age. But adults, too, experience phobias of specific objects or situations, such as arachnophobia (fear of spiders), ophidiophobia (fear of snakes), acrophobia (fear of heights), and monophobia (fear of being alone). If the objects are easily avoided, like spiders and snakes, there is usually no great problem. However, fear of flying due to acrophobia may cause great inconvenience for a person whose work or social life involves frequent air travel, and monophobia may handicap a worker whose job requires long periods of isolation to complete a project.

The phobias of function, or social phobias, are those in which the presence of others causes the anxiety. Among them are erythrophobia (fear of blushing), haphephobia (fear of being touched), and phagophobia (fear of being seen eating, which makes the victim incapable of eating in the presence of others).

A type of psychotherapy called insight therapy may be helpful in less severe cases; patients learn to recognize the real, underlying object of anxiety and come to see the phobic object as merely symbolic of that other fear. More extreme cases often respond better to behavioral therapy, in which the patient is deconditioned to the phobic stimulus by being required to confront it. At the same time, the patient is encouraged to try various relaxation techniques to combat anxiety. In the most severe cases, a psychiatrist may use a technique called flooding, by which the patient is forced to experience prolonged phobic anxiety with a constant exposure to the dreaded object or situation.

Although drug therapy generally is less effective when used alone than when it is combined with psychotherapy, mild tranquilizers and antidepressants can often delay the onset of panic attacks or reduce their severity.

# Photosensitivity

Photosensitivity is an abnormally increased sensitivity of the skin to the rays of the sun.

The causes of this condition are not fully understood, although it is known that certain substances, when combined with ultraviolet light, produce the reaction. Among those substances are contraceptive pills, hexachlorophene (a skin antiseptic), sandalwood oil, coal tar, certain perfumes and soaps, certain sunscreen agents, and a variety of orally administered drugs, including chlorothiazides, phenothiazines, sulfonamides, and tetracyclines.

The symptoms of photosensitivity include burning reactions similar to those ordinarily suffered after prolonged exposure to the sun, rashes, scaling, welts (raised areas) on the skin, dizziness, nausea, and vomiting. The most common symptom is a rash.

The most effective treatment is to discover the basic cause of the heightened sensitivity and to eliminate it. If, for example, photosensitivity is a reaction to a contraceptive pill, a different kind of pill or form of contraception could be prescribed. Treatment of photosensitivity symptoms is similar to that used for sunburn: ointments, topical anesthetics, and creams. It should be remembered that these treatments are standard topical therapy for the skin but do not eliminate the causes of photosensitivity.

If it is impossible to isolate the cause of photosensitivity, the next best step is to avoid exposure to sunlight by wearing light-colored clothing, white gloves, and broad-brimmed hats. Commercial sunscreen products are also helpful. Contact with the substances already listed should be avoided.

# Pica

Pica is an abnormal craving to eat substances not ordinarily considered to be foods.

The causes of pica are not completely understood. In the case of a pregnant woman who eats laundry starch, pica may be an almost instinctive effort to make up for deficiencies in the diet. In the case of a child who eats chips of lead-based paint (a common cause of lead poisoning in children), the cause is less clear: it could be a teething impulse, or it could be the result of unconscious drives that are not fully understood.

Although lead poisoning is the most serious pica problem with children, the effects of pica are as varied as the substances that are consumed. The substances most commonly eaten as a result of pica are those that are used as ingredients in the manufacture of such products as paints, matches, soaps, cleaners, and pesticides. Some doctors also include consumption of a variety of growing plants, such as mushrooms, century plants, and toxic (poisonous) plants (for example, poison ivy), as pica.

Some pica sufferers (especially children) eat nonfoods indiscriminately; others exhibit pica as a compulsion to consume only one or several specific inedible substances.

The treatment for pica is not simple, since medical science has not yet pinned down the root of the compulsion. Obviously, if the craving is induced by a deficiency of an element such as iron, the treatment is to remedy the deficiency. Medical treatment for the effects of ingested nonfoods depends on the nature of the substance consumed. If a child is the pica sufferer, the first line of defense is to remove the material from his reach and to search the immediate area for other such substances.

# Pinworms

Pinworms (any of a variety of worms called oxyurids) are parasites that may infect the gastrointestinal tract and occasionally other sites, such as the female reproductive tract. These worms are tiny (about one-eighth to one-half inch in length).

The usual cause of the infection is eating food contaminated with fertilized oxyurid eggs. Contamination results from contact with infected feces. Eggs can also survive on clothes and bedding for two or three weeks.

After being ingested (taken into the body), the eggs hatch and release their larvae (an immature form of the worm) into the upper portion of the small intestine. The larvae mature as they pass through the first part of the large intestine. After mating, the adult male worms die and the females migrate down the large intestine and lay their eggs around the anus. The eggs are transferred by the child's hands from the anus to the mouth, and the cycle continues. Pinworms can be transmitted to other children and adults in the same manner. Also, the hatched larvae can migrate back through the anus and into the bowel.

Many children who have pinworms do not have obvious symptoms. Symptoms that may occur are itching and inflammation around the anus. Worms can also cause irritation, inflammation, and obstruction in the appendix. In girls and women, pinworms can work their way into the vagina and urethra (the passageway connecting the bladder to the outside) and cause an inflammation or infection in the reproductive system and in the bladder.

Aside from noting the symptom of itching, diagnosis is made by identifying the eggs or worms through a microscope. The physician will usually place a piece of clear adhesive tape against the child's anus. The eggs will adhere to the tape, which is placed under a microscope for examination.

Treatment of pinworms is not difficult. Usually one dose of the drug pyrantel pamoate is sufficient. Other medications are also available. In addition, all members of a family should be treated simultaneously, and their bedclothes, towels, and underwear should be laundered at the same time. Also, the eggs around the anus should be removed by cleaning the anal area thoroughly at the time of treatment. Reinfection is common, and when symptoms develop, another course of treatment is necessary.

It is important to teach children clean eating habits, to encourage them to wash their hands frequently, and to be alert to other children who may be infected (as evidenced by scratching around the anus).

# Pituitary disorders

Because of the vital role of the pituitary gland in regulating many body functions, disorders of this gland (often due to tumors) can result in disastrous abnormalities in growth and body maintenance.

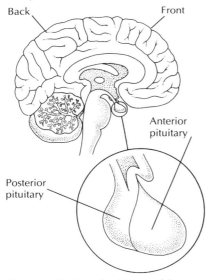

Back                          Front

Anterior
pituitary

Posterior
pituitary

The small pituitary gland is one of the most important glands in the body.

Persons who have excessive secretion of growth hormone by the anterior lobe during the years in which the skeleton is growing become giants; those who have deficient secretion at that time become dwarfs. If oversecretion occurs after a person has become an adult, a condition called acromegaly results, in which the victim's hands, feet, jaws, and facial bones grow disproportionately large.

A condition known as diabetes insipidus (which is related only symptomatically to the more common diabetes mellitus) is due to a malfunction of the posterior lobe. In this disorder, a deficiency of the pituitary hormone vasopressin results in abnormally high urinary output of water. Control can be regained with the use of synthetic vasopressin.

See also Endocrine system.

# Placenta previa

Placenta previa is an abnormal condition in which the fertilized egg, or zygote, travels to the lower portion of the uterus and attaches itself to a part of the uterine wall near or even over the uterine opening. As a result, the placenta (a temporary organ in the uterus, which develops during pregnancy to conduct nourishment and oxygen from the mother to the fetus) forms in such a way as to cover all or part of the uterine opening and thus interfere with normal delivery.

There are three types of placenta previa: partial, in which only a portion of the cervix is covered; complete, in which the cervix is completely covered; and low-lying (or marginal), in which the placenta does not cover the cervix, but is close enough to it to potentially interfere with normal delivery.

Placenta previa occurs in one of every 100 to 500 pregnancies. It is more prevalent among women who have had two or more children than those in their first pregnancy.

The cause of placenta previa is unknown. Some authorities believe that placental implantation cannot take place on the same part of the uterine wall more than once. If a woman has had several pregnancies, the lower part of the uterus may be the only place left on which the placenta can implant.

The major symptom of placenta previa is painless vaginal bleeding.

Profuse bleeding may begin as early as the twenty-fourth week of pregnancy, with no apparent cause. The blood will be bright red, indicating that it is fresh. Bleeding occurs as the placenta separates from the wall of the uterus near the uterine opening. This bleeding occurs without any injury (from a fall, for example). In some cases, there is only spotting (light blood flow).

Any vaginal bleeding during pregnancy is abnormal and should, therefore, be reported to the doctor immediately. An ultrasound scan of the woman's abdomen will then be performed. If placenta previa is present, it will be seen on an ultrasound scan.

There are two types of treatment: delayed and active. The purpose of delayed treatment is to give the fetus sufficient time to mature. In the case of active treatment, the fetus is delivered by cesarean section as soon as possible.

The degree of vaginal bleeding will usually dictate the type of treatment. If vaginal bleeding is slight, delayed treatment is generally chosen. If vaginal bleeding is heavy, a cesarean section will be performed immediately.

Bleeding from placenta previa may be extremely heavy, leading to severe blood loss by the mother. This bleeding stops only after the fetus and placenta have been delivered by cesarean section. Unless treatment is rapid, death of both the mother and fetus may occur.

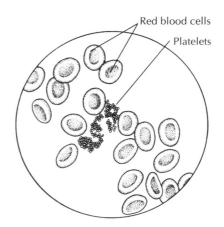

Compared with red blood cells, platelets are tiny, yet they play a vital role in blood clotting.

# Platelets

Platelets (also called thrombocytes) are tiny, disk-shaped, cell-like structures that play a critical role in the process of blood coagulation (clotting). They are manufactured in the bone marrow and usually survive for about ten days.

Blood coagulation is a complex process requiring the presence of many substances in the blood besides platelets. However, without platelets, coagulation would be impossible. Platelets initiate the coagulation process by aggregating (clumping together). Adequate coagulation usually takes five minutes or less.

The number of platelets per unit volume of blood plays an important role in proper platelet function. The normal number ranges between 200,000 and 500,000 platelets per cubic millimeter of blood.

A low platelet count may be seen with many different diseases, including certain liver diseases, uncommon forms of anemia caused by vitamin deficiencies, and certain cancers (such as leukemia) of the blood-forming organs. Use of certain drugs also may cause a low platelet count.

The most common cause of a low platelet count is destruction of platelets by the body's immune system. For some unknown reason, the immune system mistakenly identifies the platelets as foreign and forms antibodies to destroy them.

When a lack of platelets prolongs bleeding time, several types of treatment may be attempted, depending on the cause of the low platelet count. The usual method of immediately increasing the number of platelets in the blood is by transfusion (this procedure is generally reserved for patients with severe platelet deficiencies). Care must be taken to avoid increasing the platelet count too much, however, because emboli (clots that obstruct blood vessels) may develop.

Care should be taken by any patient whose platelet count is low, since bleeding will be prolonged and coagulation will not occur within normal time limits. For this reason, many physicians recommend that until normal platelet counts are attained, patients should not take aspirin and should avoid doing anything that may cause bleeding, such as vigorous toothbrushing, eating abrasive foods, and having enemas. They should also avoid contact sports and use caution regarding any activity that might lead to personal injury.

# Pleurisy

Pleurisy, or pleuritis, is an inflammation of the pleurae (thin, moist membranes that cover the lungs and line the chest cavity). The pleurae normally reduce the friction between the chest structures as the lungs expand and contract. Inflammation of the pleurae causes breathing to become painful and less effective.

There are two types of pleurisy: dry pleurisy and wet pleurisy. In dry pleurisy, the more common condition, the inflamed pleurae rub directly against each other. In wet pleurisy, fluid oozes from the inflamed tissue into the space between the lungs and the chest wall. This fluid may compress the lungs, making breathing difficult.

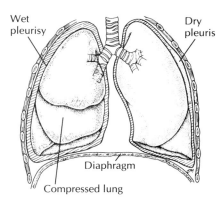

Pleurisy is an inflammation of the pleurae (the membranes that cover the lungs and line the chest cavity). In dry pleurisy, the inflamed plurae rub directly against each other, causing painful breathing. In wet pleurisy, fluid oozes from the inflamed tissue into the space between the lungs and the chest wall, compressing the lung.

Both types of pleurisy often occur as complications of respiratory tract infections, such as pneumonia, viral infections, and tuberculosis, and are more likely to develop in persons who are highly susceptible to such infections. They can also be caused by a tumor or an injury. Some cases are due to certain gastrointestinal tract diseases, particularly of the liver and pancreas, which can inflame the diaphragm (the large muscle separating the chest and abdominal cavities) and the portions of the pleurae that cover the diaphragm.

The major symptom of dry pleurisy is a sharp, stabbing pain toward the side and lower part of the chest. The pain may also be felt along the shoulders, neck, and abdomen. Any movement involving the chest, such as breathing or coughing, will aggravate the pain, which may be accompanied by shortness of breath, a dry cough, and fever. Wet pleurisy is characterized by similar symptoms, but there may also be difficulty in breathing.

A diagnosis of pleurisy usually begins with a physical examination, during which the doctor listens to the chest with a stethoscope for the low-pitched, grating sound that occurs with each breath in a case of dry pleurisy. If fluid in the lungs is suspected, the physician may percuss, or tap on, the chest wall (usually on the back) to determine the level or amount. The skin near the affected area is often found to be tender. If wet pleurisy is suspected, a sample of the fluid oozing from the pleurae will usually be obtained (by inserting a needle directly into the pleura) and analyzed. A tuberculin skin test may be done to learn whether tuberculosis is a factor. An X-ray study is very helpful in detecting the presence of pleural fluid.

To treat pleurisy, the doctor will first need to treat the underlying infection or disease, often with antibiotics. The symptoms of pleurisy can be relieved somewhat by resting. Strapping the chest firmly with a non-adhesive elastic bandage is sometimes recommended; however, it may prevent deep breathing and coughing up of mucus, both of which are necessary to clear the respiratory tract. Painkillers may help to relieve chest discomfort at least enough so that the patient will not need to stifle the painful coughing that is necessary to loosen the mucus. Anti-inflammatory medications and even cortisone drugs are very effective in relieving the inflammation and pain, particularly in dry pleurisy.

# Pneumonia

Pneumonia is an infection of the lungs in which the alveoli in one or more sections of the lungs become inflamed and filled with fluid and white blood cells, which try to fight off the infection. Pneumonia can be fatal, especially in the very young and the very old.

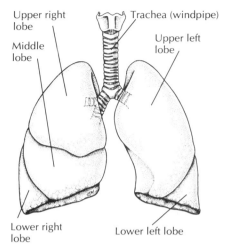

Upper right lobe — Trachea (windpipe) — Upper left lobe — Middle lobe — Lower right lobe — Lower left lobe

The lungs consist of five sections, called lobes.

There are several types of pneumonia, distinguished by the location, causative agent, and extent of infection. Lobar pneumonia is an infection in only one lobe (section) of the lungs. Double pneumonia is an infection in all or parts of both lungs. Bronchial pneumonia is an infection in the areas of the lungs near the bronchi (the main airways connecting the windpipe and the lungs). Walking pneumonia is a general term often used to describe a form of pneumonia that an individual may have for a week or more with no symptoms other than cough. When seen by a physician, a chest X ray reveals pneumonia. This type of pneumonia is often caused by an organism known as *mycoplasma pneumoniae.* Although often mild, it can be quite serious if left unrecognized.

Pneumonia most often strikes the person whose resistance is lowered, frequently by an upper respiratory tract infection or a systemic (affecting the body generally) disease. It is commonly a secondary disease stemming from inadequate defense mechanisms, from a cold or the flu, or from long-term diseases, such as chronic bronchitis, emphysema, asthma, diabetes, cancer, or sickle cell anemia. In the elderly, pneumonia is a much-feared consequence of being bedridden for long periods.

Viruses, bacteria, fungi, and other microorganisms may cause pneumonia. It may also develop if a person inhales certain chemicals or if food, vomit, or a foreign object passes through the trachea (the windpipe) instead of the esophagus (food tube) and settles in a lung ("aspiration pneumonia"). Smoking, excessive drinking, a prolonged period of being bedridden, anesthesia, and use of sedatives and drugs that suppress the immune system may make an individual more susceptible to pneumonia if he or she is exposed to an infectious organism. Pneumonia is most common during flu and cold epidemics and during the winter months, when people are more likely to be indoors, where bacteria and viruses are easily spread.

Pneumonia is generally characterized by four major symptoms: chest pain, a sudden rise in temperature, coughing, and difficulty in breathing. Viral pneumonia is signaled by coughing and other cold symptoms, as well as by general fatigue. Bacterial pneumonia generally comes on suddenly with shaking chills; a rapid, steep rise in temperature; shallow breathing; and a cough that brings up bloody, dark yellow, or rust-colored sputum. An oxygen shortage that is sometimes a result of fluid and debris blocking small airways in the lungs will be indicated by other symptoms, such as headache, nausea, vomiting, and bluish discoloration of the lips and fingertips.

Pneumonia is diagnosed by listening to the chest with a stethoscope to detect the presence of fluid in the lungs. An analysis of the sputum and an X-ray examination are also done to identify the type and location of the infection.

Viral pneumonia is generally treated by staying in bed, drinking lots of fluids, maintaining a light diet, and using pain-killers to combat discomfort. Hospitalization is not usually necessary. Viral pneumonia, however, can be quite serious and even fatal, particularly in those with underlying diseases affecting the immune system and in premature newborns. Newer antiviral drugs, which are available in both intravenous and aerosol form, have been extremely helpful in select cases.

Bacterial pneumonia is treated with antibiotics, such as penicillin. Patients also need to rest or, in severe cases, to enter the hospital for care, supervision, and intravenous drug therapy. If breathing is difficult, oxygen may be administered.

There are vaccines that may help in preventing some types of pneumonia. Pneumonia caused by certain bacteria may be prevented with a vaccine, which is especially recommended for the elderly or for those with chronic diseases that may weaken the respiratory system. Pneumonia caused by one type of influenza virus may also be prevented with a vaccination.

The very young, the very old, and the chronically ill are the most likely to contract pneumonia, so care must be taken to protect them from respiratory infections.

# Polycythemia vera

Polycythemia vera is a relatively rare chronic disorder characterized by an increase in red blood cell mass and in the concentration of hemoglobin (the substance in red blood cells that carries oxygen). Polycythemia literally means "many blood cells."

The immediate cause of polycythemia is excessive production of red blood cells by the bone marrow, but the underlying cause remains unknown. The condition is most often seen in the elderly and in persons of Jewish descent.

The initial symptoms include fatigue, difficulty in concentration, headache, drowsiness, forgetfulness, and dizziness. About half of the patients with polycythemia vera complain of itching, especially after a hot bath. Reddish skin color, or flushing, may be observed; however, patients may have completely normal skin color, with redness only of the mucous membranes, especially the inner lids of the eyes. Patients may complain of blurred vision, ringing in the ears, and circulatory disturbances.

Diagnosis can usually be made on the basis of a physical examination, medical history, and analysis of the blood.

Phlebotomy (withdrawal of blood from a vein) to counterbalance the overproduction of red blood cells is probably the safest treatment since it does not interfere with the functioning of the bone marrow. Radiation therapy to suppress bone marrow activity may also be useful.

# Pregnancy

Pregnancy is the condition that exists in a woman between the time one of her eggs is fertilized by a sperm and the time her child is born. This period is usually nine months in duration.

During normal pregnancy, many changes take place in a woman's body. The abdomen expands, and the breasts enlarge, grow sensitive, and prepare to produce milk for the baby. Blood volume increases by up to 30 percent. Breathing proceeds more from the chest and less from the abdomen. The bladder is pushed higher into the abdomen because of the increased abdominal space taken up by the growing fetus. The amount of blood flowing through the kidneys increases by 25 percent to 40 percent because wastes must be eliminated from both the mother and fetus. There is a slight increase in the acidity of the saliva (this may be one of the causes of the nausea and vomiting that are so common). The nipples and external genitalia may darken, and brown spots or splotches may appear on the skin. A hormone called relaxin causes the ligaments (connective tissues that link bones together at joints) to begin to loosen during the tenth or twelfth week of pregnancy; this will be particularly important in the pelvic area because it will allow greater flexibility at the time of delivery. Many of the glands increase in size.

Usually the first symptom noticed by a pregnant woman is a missed menstrual period. Nausea and vomiting (commonly called "morning sickness") are frequently encountered symptoms of pregnancy.

The nine months of pregnancy are usually thought of medically as three three-month periods, or trimesters. During the first trimester, the woman may experience nausea and vomiting, her breasts and nipples will become enlarged, and her waistline may expand. In the second trimester, the uterus expands, abdominal enlargement becomes more apparent, and the woman can feel the fetus move. Many women feel their best during this trimester. During the last three months, pregnancy tends to become a more cumbersome condition, and the woman may feel tired much of the time. The fetus often "drops" lower in the uterus in the last month.

Many women wait until they have missed a second period before consulting their doctor. Once the doctor has confirmed the pregnancy, a program of prenatal (before birth) care

One month    Three months    Six months    Nine months

As the unborn fetus grows within the uterus, the mother's body changes both internally and externally.

will be prescribed for the mother-to-be. Prenatal care consists chiefly of making sure that nothing goes wrong with this completely normal and natural process—in other words, that there are no complications.

Good nutrition is especially important during pregnancy. The body's requirements for calcium and phosphorus, two essential minerals in food, almost double, and there is an increase in the demand for iron and many other elements. Gradual caloric increases are not only allowed but advisable, provided that the additional food does not consist of empty calories, such as excess starches and sugars. Fresh fruits and vegetables and appropriate amounts of high-protein, low-fat foods are good choices. Generally, if the woman was consuming 2,000 calories before pregnancy with no weight gain, she should raise her intake to 2,200 to 2,400 calories in early pregnancy; she may be advised to increase that figure to 2,600 calories by the later stages.

If the baby's weight is included, most women should gain approximately 23 to 26 extra pounds by the ninth month. This additional weight puts more stress on the back and on the legs, sometimes resulting in such problems as swayback and varicose veins (swollen veins close to the skin surface) in the legs. These conditions can be eased by getting proper rest and exercise and by wearing special hosiery.

Once the initial period of nausea and vomiting is over (usually after two or three months), many women increase their caloric intake too much, sometimes in a mistaken attempt to "make up for what the baby is taking." As a consequence, they experience a drastic gain in weight. At the other extreme are those mothers who cannot eat normally because nausea persists throughout pregnancy. In each of these cases, both the mother and the fetus may suffer. If any sudden weight gain or loss is experienced, the physician should be informed.

Due to either rapid weight gain or inadequate kidney function, some women will experience significant swelling in the ankles and lower legs and, to a lesser extent, in the hands and fingers. Under no circumstances should nonprescription diuretics (drugs that increase urinary output) be taken for this condition. The doctor should be consulted.

Proper rest and exercise are important throughout pregnancy. In general, a woman can participate in most, if not all, of the activities and sports she was taking part in before her pregnancy. Her doctor can advise her about any limitations.

Many substances and organisms have been found to affect the development and survival of the fetus. It is estimated that 20 percent of all birth defects are directly related to environmental factors such as drugs, viruses, and vitamin deficiencies. Another 60 percent are caused by the interaction of an environmental factor and an inherited predisposition. So it is important for every woman who is contemplating pregnancy or is already pregnant to beware of the possible hazards to which her baby may be vulnerable.

One of the most important aspects of prenatal care is safety in the use of medications and the ingestion of nonfood substances. A pregnant woman (or one who even suspects she is pregnant) should never take a medication without her doctor's recommendation or approval. This caution includes over-the-counter preparations and medications—even aspirin —as well as prescription drugs. In addition, a woman should not smoke during pregnancy, and she should limit, if not eliminate, consumption of alcoholic beverages. Smoking has been linked to miscarriage (the expulsion of the fetus before it is capable of surviving on its own), low birth weight, and prematurity. Alcohol, too, has been linked to miscarriage, and studies have shown that alcohol can affect the brain of the fetus. Products containing caffeine should probably also be limited. The best guideline to remember is that no drug or nonfood substance can be assumed to be harmless during pregnancy.

The fetus is also susceptible to infections that affect the mother-to-be, especially rubella (German measles) and certain sexually transmitted diseases, such as herpes. A pregnant woman should avoid immunizations with live viruses and postpone travel to foreign countries where infectious diseases are prevalent. Toxoplasmosis, an infection spread by eating or preparing uncooked meat or handling a cat's litter box, presents another risk. The parasite that causes toxoplasmosis is harbored in the bodies of some food animals (pigs, sheep, and cattle) and in the intestinal tracts of cats. A pregnant woman need not forgo meat or get rid of her cat. She should, however, be certain to cook meat thoroughly and to avoid emptying or cleaning the cat's litter box.

A woman's doctor will also advise against unnecessary X rays during pregnancy.

As the medical profession has learned more about inherited diseases, it has been able to offer genetic counseling to couples concerned about the possibility of having a child with an inherited disease or abnormality. A genetic counselor or specialist in genetic disorders can estimate the likelihood that a couple's offspring will be afflicted with a problem due to an inherited trait or to the age of the parents. For some genetic disorders, tests can determine whether one or both parents are carriers or can detect whether a defect is present in a fetus. However, genetic counseling cannot guarantee the health of a child; it can only be a source of advice.

A normal pregnancy that has run its full course is called a "full-term pregnancy"—the baby is born after a full gestational (developmental) period of about 40 weeks. If the birth occurs earlier than the thirty-seventh week, it is considered premature.

There are three stages of normal labor and vaginal childbirth. During the first stage, contractions of the uterus open the cervix (the neck of the uterus). The plug of mucus that has been sealing off the uterus from the vagina for nine months is expelled. This is often followed by either a slow trickle or a sudden gush of amniotic fluid as the amniotic sac, in which the baby has been growing, breaks. At this point, the woman should notify her physician and go to the hospital.

The second stage begins when the cervix is completely dilated (opened). The contractions become much stronger, accompanied by an urge to bear down and push the baby along the birth canal. A doctor or midwife will instruct the woman to push down only during a contraction so that she conserves her energy and strength. After the baby has emerged, the umbilical cord, which connects the baby to the placenta, is tied and cut.

The baby, who usually gasps and cries on delivery, is immediately checked by the obstetrician or pediatrician. After being cleaned off, the baby may be given to the mother to hold at the doctor's discretion.

Five or ten minutes later, the placenta, or afterbirth, is pushed out by more contractions of the uterus. After this third stage has been completed, the physician will stitch any tears or incisions that were made in the vagina and give the woman medication to stop any excessive bleeding from the uterus.

The entire birthing process can last anywhere from 5 to 24 hours; the average is about 12 hours. Childbirth usually takes longer if it is the woman's first delivery.

In about one out of six pregnancies, vaginal delivery is not possible or desirable, and a cesarean section must be performed. The baby is delivered through an incision in the mother's abdominal wall.

More and more expectant fathers are taking active roles in the birthing process by attending prenatal classes and participating in the delivery. Most hospitals now welcome fathers into the delivery room so that they can witness the miracle of childbirth and can comfort and support the mother while she goes through labor.

Although once the norm, general anesthesia is now rarely used during vaginal childbirth because, among other reasons, it slows uterine contractions and causes sluggishness and the possibility of respiratory problems in the baby. Other forms of anesthesia that are used during childbirth include pudendal block; paracervical block; and spinal, epidural, and caudal anesthesia.

In pudendal block, local anesthetic is injected through the wall of the vagina or through the skin of the buttock to reach the pudendal nerve. Blocking this nerve eliminates pain and feeling from the lower part of the vagina, the rear portion of the vulva (the external genitals), and the surrounding skin. It is often used when delivery is going well and the mother wants to push. Sometimes this type of anesthesia is used following a paracervical block, in which a local anesthetic is injected around the opening of the uterus.

Various types of spinal anesthesia are used in childbirth. In one method, a solution containing local anesthetic is injected between the fourth and fifth vertebrae of the lower back into the fluid-filled sac surrounding the spinal cord. The heavy solution mixes with the spinal fluid and settles downward, blocking off pain messages from below the waist for about an hour.

Epidural anesthesia has an effect similar to that of spinal anesthesia. The anesthetic is injected at the same place, but instead of being introduced into the spinal fluid in a single injection, it can be administered over a period of hours through a fine plastic tube with its tip resting against the tough dural membrane covering the spinal cord (the prefix *epi* means upon, hence the term epidural). The nerves are blocked where they enter the spinal cord, producing a numbing effect. Because the dural membrane is not punctured, the chance of complications, such as headache and infection, is reduced. Caudal anesthesia, which is seldom used today, is the same as epidural except that the tube is introduced at the very tip of the spine (caudal comes from the Latin word meaning tail). Because both epidural and caudal anesthesia can slow labor if administered too soon, they are not given until the woman is in active labor.

See also Cesarean section, Conception, and Ovulation.

---

# Premenstrual syndrome (PMS)

Premenstrual syndrome (PMS) is a term used to encompass the varying complex of physical and emotional symptoms experienced by some women during the week before their menstrual period begins. In the past, this and other menstrual problems were thought to be caused by emotional instability or hysteria, but current research, while not yet offering conclusive findings, indicates that there may be physical reasons for such disorders.

Many researchers believe that PMS is caused by fluctuations in the production of female hormones during the course of the menstrual cycle. Hormonal changes influence the amounts of salt and fluid retained in the body, especially during the week before the period begins. Neither the exact cause for this fluid and salt retention nor the reason for its effect on certain women is fully understood.

The symptoms of PMS appear from 5 to 14 days before menstruation and usually disappear as soon as the menstrual flow begins. In addition to nervousness and irritability, a bloated or puffy feeling that results from edema (fluid retention) often characterizes this disorder. Other possible symptoms include depression, headache, fatigue, tenderness in the breasts, and acne.

The diagnosis of premenstrual syndrome is based on a physical examination and the menstrual history. The occurrence of any of the symptoms with some regularity before each menstrual period and their disappearance soon after menstrual flow begins are the key diagnostic clues.

At present, there is no single or sure remedy for PMS. Depending on the symptoms present, various medications may be helpful. The edema is often treated by reducing salt intake or by taking diuretics, medications that help to eliminate excess fluid from the tissues by increasing the production of urine. The avoidance of methylxanthines (chemicals contained in coffee, tea, cola, chocolate, and certain medications) will often help reduce headache and irritability. Tranquilizers and psychological counseling may be recommended for patients in whom PMS causes emotional distress. A balanced diet, moderate exercise, and adequate rest may also be beneficial in treating the condition. The use of hormones (for example, progesterone in the form of a suppository inserted into the vagina) is controversial but has significantly reduced PMS symptoms in some women.

A reduction of salt intake may help to prevent the initial edema that often accompanies PMS. Self-treatment with diuretics without the advice of a physician is not recommended.

# Prolapse of the uterus

Prolapse refers to a collapse, descent, or other change in the position of an organ in relation to surrounding structures. Prolapse of the uterus may be one of three types, depending on severity:

Normal

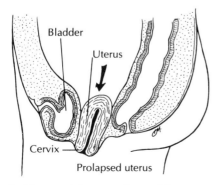

In this second degree prolapse of the uterus, the organ has fallen to a point where the cervix is outside the vagina.

- First-degree prolapse, in which the uterus sags downward so that the cervix is flush with the entrance to the vagina
- Second-degree prolapse, in which the cervix is outside the vagina
- Third-degree prolapse, in which the entire uterus is outside the vagina

Prolapse of the uterus occurs when the muscles and ligaments that normally hold the uterus in place become stretched or slack. This is most often due to a long or difficult childbirth or multiple childbirths. There may be a feeling of heaviness in the vagina, backache, or inability to control urination. Prolapse of the uterus is apparent during a pelvic examination.

It is especially important to treat prolapse of the uterus because it can make childbirth difficult and may damage other organs. In mild cases, exercises for the muscles of the pelvic floor may be helpful. If the prolapse is the result of injury or stress, surgical repair may be indicated, in which the uterus is returned to its proper place and sewn or stapled into position. If the prolapse is due to disease or swelling, the underlying disorder must first be controlled or eliminated before the uterus can be returned to its original position and secured there. In some cases, a pessary (a plastic ring or donut) may be inserted into the vagina to hold the uterus in its proper position. If childbearing is no longer desired, a hysterectomy may be performed.

# Prostate cancer

After lung cancer, this is the most common cancer among men. Black Americans have a higher incidence of prostate cancer than any other group in the world. In general, it is more common in men over 55. Cancer of the prostate (the male sex gland that lies at the base of the bladder) can develop very slowly, often producing no symptoms until the disease is far advanced. Sometimes a routine examination discloses a lump in the prostate, which proves to be cancerous in about 50 percent of cases. Prostate examinations should be incorporated into regular medical checkups performed on all men over the age of 40.

Newer diagnostic blood tests for prostate cancer such as PSA (prostatic specific antigen) may be helpful in early detection. It is important to note, however, that a positive blood test in itself does not necessarily mean that a patient definitely has cancer, nor does a negative test mean he does not.

When symptoms occur, they are usually the result of enlargement of the prostate, which causes difficult urination or blood in the urine. Prostate cancer often spreads to the bone, and patients may complain of bone pain before they show any other symptoms.

In cases in which prostate cancer is discovered before it has begun to spread, the cancer can frequently be cured by means of surgery or by treatment with radiation. When the disease has spread, usually only its symptoms are treated as they occur. Often a patient can live a long time with this form of treatment.

See also Cancer.

---

# Prostatitis

Prostatitis is an infection or inflammation of the male sex gland called the prostate. It predominantly affects older men, usually in the form of chronic (recurring) flare-ups. Though not generally a serious disorder, prostatitis can be irritating and uncomfortable because it disrupts normal urination; in advanced stages, it can cause bladder or kidney damage.

Located just below the bladder, the prostate is a small, doughnut-shaped gland that surrounds the neck of the bladder and the urethra. As men get older, the prostate often becomes enlarged, which may constrict the urethra. This will eventually develop into a condition called prostatism, which causes disruption of normal urination, marked by prolonged effort or repeated attempts to start the flow, decreased force, and dribbling toward the end of the flow. Some urine is almost always left in the bladder, providing a fertile breeding ground for bacteria. Bladder infection is a common consequence of prostatism, which may in turn cause prostatitis. Advanced cases of prostatitis may cause a sudden, total blockage of urine flow, requiring emergency treatment before the backup of urine can cause bladder and kidney damage.

Sexually transmitted diseases and urinary tract infections are the most common underlying causes of prostatitis.

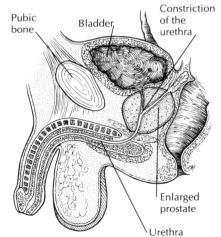

Enlargement of the prostate gland due to inflammation may constrict the urethra, thereby interfering with urination.

The most common symptoms are trouble in starting the urine flow, reduced force in urination, dribbling at the end of urination, and increased frequency of urination. Prostatitis may be signaled by discomfort in the lower back and genital area, a burning sensation while urinating, fever, and chills.

Prostatitis is diagnosed by an examination of the prostate to check its size, shape, and firmness. A physician does this by inserting a finger into the rectum. An infected prostate will be tender to the touch; when it is massaged by the doctor, pus cells will be forced out and will then appear in the urine. A culture of the urine specimen will be examined for bacteria, although very often no bacteria are identified in a case of chronic prostatitis. Nevertheless, a urinalysis may show some evidence of infection, and if a trace of blood is present, the urine may be additionally tested for the presence of malignant cells.

Enlargement of the prostate is frequently diagnosed by a digital examination. Ultrasound and intravenous pyelogram are also helpful. The definitive test is a cystoscopy (the examination of the urinary bladder by means of a tubelike instrument that is lighted).

Most prostate infections can be treated quite successfully with antibiotics. Chronic nonbacterial prostatitis, however, is not treated with antibiotics. Instead, drinking large quantities of water and taking hot baths are often recommended.

Enlargement of the prostate gland that causes symptoms is normally treated by surgical removal of the excess tissue through one of two procedures: transurethral surgery, in which the center of the prostate gland is scraped out by an instrument that has been inserted into the penis; or prostatectomy, a more complicated procedure requiring an incision. There is danger of impotence and incontinence resulting from either of these surgical procedures. The prostatectomy rarely causes such problems, but it may lead to retrograde ejaculation, a condition in which the semen is passed back into the bladder to be expelled with the urine, rather than being released during intercourse (although this condition presents no health risk, it is a cause of male infertility).

# Proteinuria

Excessive proteinuria (protein in the urine) is a symptom of some types of kidney problems.

Proteinuria can be caused by, among other conditions, kidney malfunction, heart disease, the consumption of certain foods, pregnancy, and overexertion from certain sports, such as jogging and marathon running.

Most cases of proteinuria in adults are discovered unexpectedly in a routine physical examination. Usually, the person will have experienced no symptoms and will be essentially healthy, with no evidence of kidney disease.

Treatment of proteinuria depends on its cause and severity. In about half of the diagnosed cases, proteinuria ceases spontaneously within a year to several years. However, there are instances in which the patient continues to lose greater and greater amounts of protein in the urine. Eventually, high blood pressure and kidney failure may develop.

When proteinuria is constant, measurements of protein excretion should be made on a regular basis. Alteration in the protein level should be followed up along with other appropriate testing of kidney function.

# Psittacosis

Psittacosis is a rare form of pneumonia caused by a microorganism called *Chlamydia psittaci*, which may be transmitted to humans by certain birds. It is often called parrot fever because it was first found to be transmitted by members of the parrot family, including parakeets and lovebirds. It may also be transmitted by other birds, such as sea gulls, pigeons, canaries, and poultry, in which case it is called ornithosis.

Infection usually takes place when a person inhales dust from the feathers or droppings of infected birds. It can also be transmitted directly to a person by a bite from an infected bird. Person-to-person transmission is rare. Eating poultry has not been reported as a source of infection.

The incubation period (the time between exposure to the illness and the appearance of symptoms), is one to two weeks. The disease usually begins with fever, chills, headache, muscle aches, and loss of appetite. Nausea, vomiting, and enlargement of the spleen may also be present. The patient's temperature continues to rise, and a dry cough develops. Coughing brings up mucus and pus in the later stages. Chest X rays made during the first week of noticeable symptoms often show inflammation of the lungs. During the second week, the typical symptoms of pneumonia develop. The patient's temperature will remain above normal for at least two weeks and then will begin to fall slowly. A steady increase in the pulse and breathing rate may be serious. About 30 percent of untreated cases end in death. Recovery of those people who receive treatment may be gradual.

The drug most commonly used to treat psittacosis is oral tetracycline, an antibiotic. Complete bed rest is necessary in most cases. Cough preparations with codeine are also advised. In severe cases, tetracycline may be given intravenously.

Flocks of infected pigeons or other birds, dust from feathers, bird-cage contents, and sick domestic birds or fowl should be avoided. Specially treated feed is often used to prevent the spread of infection among imported parrots, parakeets, and lovebirds and among turkeys raised for market.

# Psoriasis

Psoriasis is a persistent skin disease characterized by thick, red eruptions, often covered by silvery scales, either in small patches or over large areas of the body. Psoriasis is fairly common, affecting one to two percent of the population. The condition often first appears between the ages of 15 and 30 years and usually requires lifelong treatment.

Psoriasis is not contagious. The cause of psoriasis is unknown, but researchers believe that the condition is related to a malfunction in the process of skin growth and regeneration (cell replacement). With normal skin, old cells are continuously being shed from the epidermis and replaced by new cells formed in the deeper layers. Cells live for about one month before they die and flake off. With psoriasis, the rate of cell growth accelerates. Skin cells may move to the surface and die in as short a time as four or five days. Increased cell growth causes buildup that can be extremely dry and irritating. The normal shedding process is usually unnoticeable, but psoriasis can produce very obvious blemishes.

Psoriasis seems to involve a strong hereditary factor, although only one third of its victims can recall having

Psoriasis is characterized by reddened, raised patches of skin with silvery scales called plaques. These clearly defined plaques appear most commonly on the elbows, knees, trunk, and scalp, although the underarm and genital areas may also be involved. Patches on the scalp shed large, silver-white scales at the hairline that resemble severe dandruff. Those patches found in moist areas, such as the underarms, are usually less scaly and less red. All patches may itch. If fingernails are involved, they may be pitted, frayed, thickened, or discolored; in more advanced cases, the nails may be separated from the nail beds.

Psoriasis that has spread to the fingernails may cause fraying, pitting, thickening, and discoloration of the nails.

Psoriasis of the knee has reddened, raised patches of skin with silvery scales called plaques.

Usually, psoriasis produces no general health problems. Sometimes, however, the disease becomes so severe that chills, painful reddening of the skin, cracking of the skin around the joints, and shedding of large areas of scaled skin result. This condition, called exfoliative psoriasis, may necessitate hospitalization for intensive therapy.

As yet, there is no known cure for psoriasis, and treatment offers only temporary relief from symptoms. Normal cleaning of the skin around the affected areas is important to prevent infection. Over-the-counter lotions and creams can cleanse irritated skin and reduce itching as well. These preparations often contain small amounts of coal tar and other ingredients designed to remove scales. If the skin becomes sensitive after application, use of these preparations should be discontinued. Many patients find regular and controlled exposure to sunlight helpful. Where sunlight is scarce, a special sunlamp may be used, but only under a doctor's supervision.

a relative with the disease. There seems to be some relationship between the condition and a certain type of arthritis as well.

Once psoriasis develops, outbreaks of the disorder can be triggered in several ways. Injury to the skin, such as a cut or burn, may provoke a flare-up, usually 8 to 18 days after the trauma. Seasonal changes may also affect psoriasis, with the disease worsening during winter months. Many patients have greater problems during periods of physical and emotional stress. Infections, particularly upper respiratory tract infections, may aggravate psoriasis.

Various drugs have recently been shown to be effective in relieving the symptoms of psoriasis. Cortisone and newer steroids (hormonally based medications) can clear plaques in about 50 percent of the cases when applied directly to the affected skin. Many physicians recommend covering the treated areas with a thin plastic wrapping in addition to the cream. This is called occlusive therapy.

Some drugs slow the growth rate of cells. The most commonly used of these drugs, methotrexate, reduces symptoms in severe cases. Because its side effects may be severe, however, the drug is prescribed for use only under the close supervision of a physician.

Another form of treatment is called PUVA therapy, which combines medication and ultraviolet light treatments. The benefits of this form of therapy should be carefully weighed against the premature skin aging and skin cancer that it may cause.

# Psychosomatic illness

Psychosomatic illnesses are a broad category of disorders in which psychological or emotional factors cause or contribute to physical symptoms. Psychosomatic illnesses are often considered to be imaginary. This is unjustified, since the patient is not pretending to be ill, and his or her symptoms are no less real than if there were a purely physical basis for the complaint. (There is a psychiatric disorder called Munchausen's syndrome, in which a person knowingly pretends to be ill or intentionally injures himself or herself in order to become ill; however, this rare condition is quite different from psychosomatic illness).

It is known that psychological factors can contribute directly or indirectly to some physical disorders. For example, having a Type A personali-

ty (characterized by aggressiveness, competitiveness, preoccupation with deadlines and time constraints, and chronic impatience) has been associated with an increased risk of heart disease. In addition, there is new evidence that stress can change the response and ability of the body's immune system to disease.

Emotional stress may also be reflected in the appearance of physical symptoms, especially if a person has a hard time expressing emotions. In some families, having pain due to physical illness is accepted and elicits a caring response, whereas expressing unhappiness and anger is not tolerated. For someone in such a family, a physical symptom may be an unconscious expression of his or her emotional state.

It is also quite common for someone who is unhappy at home or at work to become preoccupied with everyday aches and pains. For that person, a genuine—albeit minor—illness may take on unwarranted importance because of the emotional state.

Almost any type of symptom may be psychosomatic. In fact, it has been estimated that one third of all complaints reported by patients to their doctors are at least partially psychosomatic. The most typical psychosomatic symptom is pain—for example, facial pain, headaches, generalized abdominal pain, and backache.

It is important not to dismiss a person's seemingly psychosomatic illness as being "all in his head." A physician should always give serious consideration to a patient's complaints, even when it may seem obvious that they are psychosomatic. There have been cases in which symptoms with a purely physical basis have been disregarded because of a suspicion that they were psychosomatic. It should also be remembered that psychosomatic factors can set the stage for a serious physical disorder, and that psychosomatic symptoms, although they may be exaggerated, may reflect a physical illness.

A physician who takes the time to learn about the patient's life circumstances can often discover the stresses that may be contributing to an illness, even though the patient may be overlooking or denying the underlying emotional factors.

If, after a thorough examination, no physical cause can be discovered for a disorder, the best treatment the doctor can offer may be to listen sympathetically and to show concern. Some patients may demand more dramatic treatment methods and may go from doctor to doctor until they find someone who will prescribe the treatment they want. It is important to avoid risky or expensive procedures and testing, as well as unnecessary medication. Helping the patient to recognize that certain symptoms are caused or worsened by stress and to learn how to deal effectively with that stress can often be helpful.

# Pulmonary embolism

Pulmonary embolism is a serious and potentially fatal condition that occurs when an embolus (a clump of matter originating elsewhere in the body and traveling via the bloodstream) blocks a blood vessel in the lungs.

Emboli (the plural of *embolus*) may be solid (detached blood clots, clumps of tumor cells, or bits of foreign objects); liquid (globules of fat); or gaseous (air). Pulmonary emboli are venous thrombi (blood clots that form in the veins) that have originated most often in the lower extremities and pelvis, usually as the result of injury, surgery, or blood vessel dis-

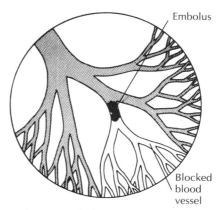

Pulmonary embolism occurs when a blood vessel in a lung is blocked by an embolism (clump of matter), cutting off the blood supply in the area beyond the blockage.

eases. Such thrombi are common in persons on prolonged bed rest, particularly after surgery, due to the lack of movement of blood in the legs.

The presence of a pulmonary embolus is indicated by the sudden development of wheezing, dyspnea (labored or difficult breathing), chest pains, and hemoptysis (spitting up of blood).

Diagnostic procedures for detection of pulmonary embolism may include an electrocardiogram and analysis of arterial blood obtained from the wrist, arm, or groin. Radioisotope scanning is very helpful. The definitive diagnostic procedure is pulmonary angiography, which is an X-ray scan of the lungs done after the introduction of a special dye into the pulmonary circulation (via a catheter inserted into the groin and floated up to the right side of the heart).

Initial treatment may include administration of oxygen, pain relievers, and medication to maintain cardiovascular functions. An anticoagulant (usually intravenous heparin or oral warfarin) is given to prevent the development of additional emboli.

If it is determined that the embolism was caused by a venous thrombus, and there is some reason why anticoagulants should not be used, the inferior vena cava (the main vein draining blood from the lower limbs and the pelvis) may be deliberately blocked with an "umbrella filter" or a clip to keep other venous thrombi from traveling to the lungs. Surgical removal of the embolus is done only in rare cases for large clots that can be removed immediately after detection. Clot dissolvers have been helpful in occasional cases.

The best prevention of pulmonary embolism is prevention of venous thrombosis. Persons predisposed to embolism may be given injections of heparin or low doses of oral warfarin to prevent the formation of thrombi. Recently, "compression boots," soft plastic bags or sacks wrapped around the legs and rapidly inflated and deflated, have been shown to prevent clot formation in postoperative and bedridden individuals. However, early ambulation—walking—after surgery is probably the best preventive measure.

See also Embolism.

# Purpura

The term purpura refers to a group of bleeding disorders that are all characterized by purplish or brownish-red discolorations, easily visible through the skin's outer layer, that are caused by hemorrhaging (internal bleeding) into the tissues.

Common purpura (also called simple purpura or senile purpura) is the most widespread of such disorders and is marked by easy bruising and increased blood vessel fragility. It is an inherited condition that occurs mostly in women, particularly following menopause. The condition often affects thigh tissue and produces large bruises rather than hemorrhages. The bleeding is usually under the skin and may be intensified by surgery or injury.

Henoch-Schonlein purpura (also known as allergic purpura and anaphylactoid purpura) most often affects children. The condition could possibly be associated with arthritis, gastrointestinal disorders, kidney failure, and erythema (redness of the skin).

Purpura fulminans is most often seen in children, mainly after an infectious disease. It is marked by fever, shock (dangerous, sudden lowering of blood pressure), anemia, and rapidly spreading symmetrical skin hemorrhages in the lower limbs, as well as by intravascular thrombosis (blockage of a blood vessel by a solid mass) and gangrene.

Thrombocytopenic purpura is a disorder in which the number of platelets (the tiny elements in the blood that are vital to clotting) is decreased, whether because of a primary disease or as a consequence of another blood disorder. This form of purpura is characterized by anemia, side effects in the nervous system, and blood clots in tiny blood vessels.

Causes vary with the type of purpura. Common purpura in postmenopausal women appears to result from decreased estrogen (female hormone) levels and thinning of the deep layers of the skin. Henoch-Schonlein purpura may result from the development of sensitivities following an infection or allergic reaction. Purpura in the elderly is often due to the fragility of their skin. There are also temporary forms of purpura in which vascular bleeding occurs as a result of fever, hypothyroidism (low output of thyroid hormone), generalized illness, defects in the small blood vessels, or a drug reaction to certain medications, such as aspirin. Purpura can sometimes stem from wearing overly tight clothing or from sustaining an injury, such as a black eye.

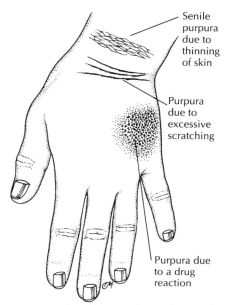

Senile purpura due to thinning of skin

Purpura due to excessive scratching

Purpura due to a drug reaction

In purpura, bleeding from the smaller blood vessels beneath the skin surface may have many causes.

Laboratory testing is essential in all cases of possible purpura in order to exclude other causes. Perhaps the most difficult of the forms of purpura to diagnose is Henoch-Schonlein purpura. Joint pain and bouts of abdominal pain in this disorder may mimic acute abdominal conditions or. forms of arthritis. Later, kidney involvement during the course of this form of purpura may cause a misdiagnosis of kidney disease.

In the case of allergic purpura, it is advisable to eliminate the possible allergic cause. Corticosteroid medications (artificial hormones) are often prescribed, but may produce disappointing results. Immunosuppressive therapy (suppression of the immune system by means of drugs) is sometimes useful. If the purpura is thrombocytopenic, the spleen (an abdominal organ that is a component of the circulatory system) may be removed if it is hoarding too many platelets. Milder cases of purpura often improve spontaneously.

Estrogen therapy has proved helpful in preventing or relieving common purpura in post-menopausal women. Other than preventive measures to avoid infections or allergic reactions, there is little that can be done to prevent purpura.

# Pyelonephritis

Pyelonephritis is an inflammation of both the kidney tissue and the renal pelvis (the funnel-shaped expansion of the upper end of the ureter where it joins the kidney).

There are two types of pyelonephritis, descending and ascending. In the descending type, the bacteria reach the kidney through the bloodstream, infecting first the kidney tissues themselves and then moving downward to infect the renal pelvis of the kidney. In the more common ascending type, the bladder is infected first, and the infection then spreads upward to the kidney.

Most cases of pyelonephritis are caused by bacterial infection. Conditions that increase the likelihood of such an infection include scars from previous infections, urinary tract infections, abnormal growth of the prostate gland, kidney stones, tumors, stagnation of urine due to backflow from the bladder, diabetes mellitus (a condition characterized by the presence of an excessive amount of sugar in the bloodstream), and pregnancy.

Symptoms of acute pyelonephritis include fever, back pain, difficulty in urinating, a burning sensation on urination, mental confusion, nausea, vomiting, and, in extreme cases, loss of consciousness. Although some cases of chronic pyelonephritis can be traced to an initial attack, many patients will have no evidence of past or current infections.

Acute pyelonephritis is treated with antibiotics given orally or intravenously. Recurrent episodes should be treated with an appropriate antibiotic. Chronic pyelonephritis requires careful management and frequent reevaluation. Patients are generally treated with an antibiotic even during periods when they feel no symptoms and usually receive long-term therapy after that.

# Pyloric stenosis

Pyloric stenosis is a constriction (narrowing) of the passage between the stomach and the small intestine. The stomach has two openings—one at the top, where it joins with the esophagus (food tube), and one at the bottom, where it joins with the small intestine. The lower opening is called the pylorus.

Pyloric stenosis can be caused by many conditions, including cancer,

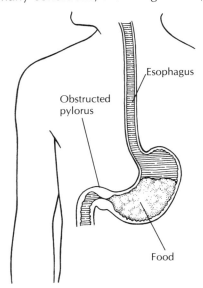

Obstructed pylorus

Esophagus

Food

When pyloric stenosis occurs, food has no way of entering into the intestines from the stomach.

spasm, a nearby ulcer in the part of the intestine directly below the pyloric opening, gastritis (inflammation of the stomach), and enlargement of the pyloric sphincter (the muscle that rings the pyloric opening and controls the opening's movement).

In the case of congenital (present at birth) pyloric stenosis, ten days to three weeks after birth the infant will experience regurgitation ("spitting up"), projectile vomiting (vomiting with great force), weight loss, and dehydration (excessive loss of body fluids) without appetite loss. Adult subjects with pyloric stenosis will experience discomfort in the upper and middle portions of the abdomen, pain, bloating of the abdominal area, nausea, vomiting, and weight loss.

In mild cases of temporary pyloric stenosis, such as that due to an ulcer, the condition can be treated by offering only small meals or intravenous feeding, restoring normal fluid levels, and administering antacid drugs (drugs that block the production of stomach acid).

In severe cases, a pyloromyotomy (a lengthwise incision into the pyloric muscle) may be indicated. A portion of the pyloric sphincter may also be removed.

# Pyorrhea

See Periodontal disease.

# R

# Rabies

Rabies (formerly known as hydrophobia) is an acute infectious viral disease of mammals, especially carnivores (meat eaters), which is characterized by central nervous system irritation followed by paralysis and, in some cases, death. Human infection usually follows the bite of a rabid animal (dogs, skunks, cats, raccoons, bats, foxes, and coyotes are among those that may be affected). In the later stages of the disease, it is marked by paralysis of the swallowing muscles and by throat spasms, which are set off by drinking or even the sight of liquids (hence the name hydrophobia, meaning fear of water). Convulsions, tetanus (a condition characterized by severe muscular contractions), and paralysis of the respiratory (breathing) muscles are other symptoms of the last stages. Fortunately, because of animal immunization programs, only a handful of rabies cases are reported in the United States each year.

Rabies is caused by a virus that is present in the saliva and respiratory secretions of rabid animals. Rabid animals transmit the infection by biting other animals or human beings. Rabies can be acquired by exposure of a mucous membrane or an open skin wound to infected animal saliva or by inhalation of the virus.

The rabies virus travels from the site of entry to the spinal cord and brain, where it multiplies. It then spreads to the salivary glands and into the saliva itself. In human beings, the incubation period (the time between exposure to the virus and development of symptoms) may extend from ten days to one year, but the average incubation period is 30 to 50 days. The incubation period is shortest in persons who have been bitten on the head or trunk and in those who have multiple bites.

The first symptom is a short period of mental depression, restlessness, and fever. In the next stage of the disease, the restlessness increases to uncontrollable excitement and hyper-activity. There is excessive salivation ("foaming at the mouth") and painful spasms of the throat muscles. The spasms can be easily initiated—by a breath of air, a slight breeze, an attempt to drink water. Generally, the patient experiences overwhelming thirst but cannot drink. In untreated cases, death occurs within three to ten days. However, patients often survive the disease if diagnosis and treatment are prompt.

In human patients, rabies is usually suspected if there has been a report of an animal bite or exposure to the saliva of a rabid animal. The diagnosis is confirmed by testing for the virus once the symptoms appear. A domestic animal with no symptoms that suddenly bites a human should be confined and observed by a veterinarian for ten days. If the animal still shows no symptoms, it was most likely not infectious at the time of the bite and is usually released. However, if the animal is apparently rabid or is a wild animal, it should be captured. The police or local health department should be notified so that they can capture and examine the animal. Only an experienced professional should attempt to capture an animal suspected of being rabid.

As soon as possible after the bite or exposure of an open wound to animal saliva occurs, the contaminated area should be cleansed thoroughly with soap and water or an antiseptic solution.

The next step is administration of antirabies serum or human rabies immune globulin for passive immunization. This is followed immediately by vaccine for active immunization. A new active immunization, called HDCV, is said to have only mild side effects for most people. Subsequent HDCV injections are given on days 3, 7, 14, and 28 after exposure. The World Health Organization recommends that a sixth injection be given 90 days after the first injection.

The best preventive measure for rabies is to minimize contact with animals that may be rabid. In many cases, persons with a high occupational risk of animal bites receive pre-exposure injections. This is especially helpful for zoo personnel and persons whose work or hobbies take them into areas where they might encounter rabid animals.

As for domestic animals, restraining dogs and cats from contact with wild animals and impounding stray animals are important preventive measures. Immunizing 70 percent or more of the dog population of major cities has helped to restrict the transmission of rabies, even in areas where wild animals carry the disease.

Controlling rabies in wildlife areas is more difficult, although rabies as a disease is self-limiting, because it tends to kill off susceptible hosts in an area. Expensive control efforts are generally limited to areas where humans are apt to be exposed to wildlife—in campgrounds, parks, wildlife preserves, and so on.

# Rash

A rash is an eruption on the surface of the skin, covering either small areas of the body or extensive areas, in the form of red spots, patches, or blisters. A rash often causes itching, but this is not always the case. A rash is usually a temporary condition, appearing and disappearing within a few days, if not sooner. If so, there is little need for worry; however, a rash can also be a symptom of infectious diseases or other disorders.

Allergic rashes may be caused by exposure to the sun, heat, cold, the chemicals in household cleansers or detergents, fabrics, or certain foods.

A rash may also appear as a symptom of disease, such as measles, rubella (German measles), chicken pox, and shingles.

Rashes that appear regularly with no other symptoms may indicate the presence of an allergy. On the other hand, if a rash is accompanied by other symptoms, such as fever, it is more likely that the cause is an infectious disease.

Any rash that lasts for more than a few days should be examined by a doctor. A rash will usually disappear when its cause is treated. In the case of an allergy, the only treatment may be something to relieve itching and irritation, but allergy testing may indicate which irritant to avoid in the future.

# Raynaud's disease

Raynaud's disease involves spasm of the arterioles (small artery branches), especially in the fingers and hands and occasionally in other parts of the body, such as the nose and tongue. It is often accompanied by intermittent paleness or cyanosis (bluish discoloration) of the skin.

Attacks of Raynaud's disease are most often precipitated by exposure to cold temperatures or by emotional stress. When the symptoms are caused by another condition, such as scleroderma (a connective tissue disorder), a nerve disorder, a drug reaction, or pulmonary hypertension, the condition is called Raynaud's phenomenon. Raynaud's disease is most commonly encountered among young women.

The color changes that come about in the skin in the classic form of the disease manifest themselves in three stages—pallor (extreme paleness), cyanosis, and then extreme redness, called reactive hyperemia.

Sometimes the color changes may go through only two stages, cyanosis and then redness. Normal color and sensation are restored when the hands are warmed. Color changes in the hands do not affect the joints and seldom affect the thumb. Pain is usually not present, but numbness, tingling, and burning are common complaints. Ulcers (open sores) may appear on the tips of the fingers. Raynaud's disease differs from Raynaud's phenomenon in that both sides of the body are involved.

A wide range of other symptoms may be associated with Raynaud's phenomenon. Individual symptoms depend on the underlying disease process.

Mild cases of Raynaud's disease can be relieved substantially by protecting the body and extremities from exposure to cold. This is extremely important because prolonged spasm of the small arteries leads to severe tissue injury. Mild sedatives, taken orally, can sometimes be of help. The patient is strongly advised to stop smoking, since nicotine acts as a constrictor of blood vessels. Drugs known as calcium-channel blockers, such as nifedipine, verapamil, and diltiazem, are of great benefit in relieving symptoms but do not cure the condition.

A more extreme measure, which is not often used, is regional sympathectomy (an interruption of certain portions of the nerve pathways). This operation is reserved for patients with progressive disability; while it abolishes the symptoms, the relief may last only for a year or two. Results of the surgical procedure are usually better in patients with Raynaud's disease than in those with Raynaud's phenomenon.

Therapy for Raynaud's phenomenon depends chiefly on correctly diagnosing and then treating the underlying disorder.

# Rectocele

Rectocele is a condition in which a part of the rectum (the terminal portion of the large intestine) protrudes into the vagina.

The usual cause of this condition is a weakening of the back wall of the vagina due to the stretching caused by childbirth.

A minimal protrusion may produce no symptoms or only a mild pressure sensation during bowel movements. More severe protrusion of the rectum may lead to chronic constipation and painful bowel movements.

A rectocele is easily identified by the doctor during a pelvic examination. On straining or coughing, the rectum may be found to bulge into the vagina.

Rectocele is not a dangerous condition and generally requires no treatment. If severe constipation or painful bowel movements develop, surgical repair is often curative. Mild symptoms may be relieved by avoiding straining and heavy lifting and by ensuring soft bowel movements with use of drugs and careful selection of diet.

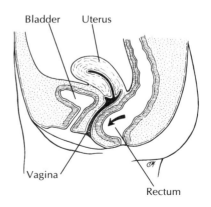

Rectocele occurs when the rectum protrudes onto the back wall of the vagina.

# Reiter's syndrome

Reiter's syndrome is characterized by the occurrence of urethritis (inflammation of the urethra, which is the tube from the bladder to the outside of the body), conjunctivitis (inflammation of the membrane that covers the front of the eyeball and the insides of the eyelids), and arthritis (joint inflammation). It affects males more often than females.

It is thought that Reiter's syndrome is caused by a bacterial infection that is often sexually transmitted.

Reiter's syndrome exhibits multiple symptoms, any one of which might be mistaken for a sign of another disease. The conjunctivas become inflamed, with corresponding discomfort around the eyes. Urethritis causes discomfort during urination. Arthritic symptoms appear, with joint swelling and pain. Furthermore, many victims have a fever; diarrhea; sores on the palms of the hands, the soles of the feet, the trunk, the mouth, and the penis; and inflammation of the iris (the part of the eye that gives it color).

Treatment for Reiter's syndrome is similar to that for rheumatoid arthritis—aspirin or, if aspirin is ineffective, another nonsteroidal anti-inflammatory drug, such as ibuprofen, indomethacin, or naproxen. The antibiotic tetracycline may help control the urethritis. Conjunctivitis can be treated with eye drops.

# Reproduction

The reproductive system includes those organs in the male and female body that function to create a new life and, in the female, to nourish it during the developmental stage until birth. Some doctors include breasts

as reproductive parts, because they may nourish the new life after birth.

**The Female Reproductive System**
The female reproductive system consists of those structures within the female body that are designed to create and nourish new life. The system includes the ovaries, fallopian tubes, uterus, cervix, and vagina.

Although the breasts, or mammary glands, are actually a type of sweat gland, their function (supporting new life) is closely related to that of the reproductive system.

The reproductive process begins in the ovaries. The ovaries are small, egg-shaped glands located in the lower abdomen. These glands control the cyclic functions of the reproductive system—ovulation and menstruation. Ovulation is the monthly production and release of a mature egg (occasionally two or more eggs). This process and other reproductive functions are regulated by two hormones, estrogen and progesterone, which are secreted by the ovaries. Estrogen regulates the secondary sex traits of body hair growth, breast development, ovulation, and menstruation. Progesterone is responsible for preparing the uterus for pregnancy, as well as contributing to enlargement of the breasts during pregnancy and milk production after childbirth. The two hormones coordinate to control the menstrual cycle.

Once an egg has been released, it travels through the fallopian tubes, which extend from each ovary into the uterus. Their reproductive function is to contain the egg until fertilization (union of an egg and a sperm, or male sex cell) takes place and to provide a passageway leading the sperm to the egg and the fertilized egg to the uterus.

The uterus is a pear-shaped, hollow organ that is normally about the size of a lemon. Its muscular walls are lined with rich, soft tissue called

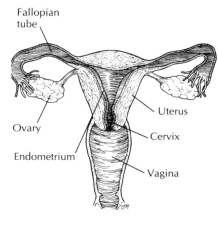

A side view of the female reproductive organs.

A front view of the female reproductive organs.

the endometrium. Each month, the lining adds layers in anticipation of receiving a fertilized egg. Should fertilization occur, the lining nourishes the fertilized egg in the uterus until birth. However, if the egg remains unfertilized, the uterus sheds the endometrium and the egg, which leave the body as menstrual discharge.

The cervix is a narrow structure with an inch-long canal connecting the lower end of the uterus to the upper portion of the vagina. This canal is the conduit for sperm on their way to fertilize an egg and for menstrual discharge and babies leaving the uterus.

The vagina, or birth canal, is a passageway leading from the cervix to the outside of the body. In the average adult woman, it measures four to five inches in length. Although the vaginal walls are normally close together, they separate to accommodate the infant during childbirth and the erect penis during sexual intercourse. The vagina continually pro-

duces secretions that lubricate and cleanse it.

**The Male Reproductive System** The male reproductive system consists of those structures in the male body designed to create life. The system includes the two testes, a network of ducts, the seminal vesicles, the prostate gland, and the penis.

The testes are two oval glands located in the scrotum. They produce the male sex hormone testosterone and sperm (male reproductive cells). Sex hormones control the secondary male sex characteristics (such as growth of the penis and of body hair, voice change, and increased muscle mass), which begin to appear at puberty.

The testes discharge sperm into the epididymis, the first structure in the duct system. Other passageways include the two vasa deferentia (the plural of vas deferens), the ejaculatory duct, and the urethra (the tube that connects the bladder to the outside of the body).

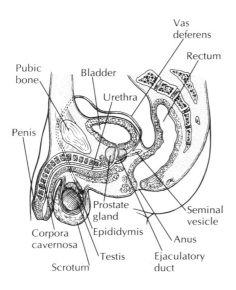

A side view of the male reproductive organs.

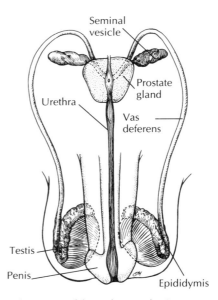

A front view of the male reproductive organs.

The epididymis runs along the top and side of each testis. Inside the epididymis are several ducts that conduct sperm from the testis into the vas deferens. The vas deferens loops up into the body before descending into a duct in the seminal vesicle. This duct joins the ejaculatory duct, which extends through the prostate gland and enters the upper segment of the urethra. At different times, the urethra functions as a passageway for urine and for sperm.

As sperm travel through the duct system, they combine with fluids from the seminal vesicles, the prostate gland, and the urethra to form semen. The two seminal vesicles, which lie near the underside of the urinary bladder, discharge a thick, sticky fluid. The prostate gland is a small, doughnut-shaped organ that completely surrounds the urethra. The prostate gland secretes an alkaline substance that makes up the major portion of seminal fluid. The sperm are protected from acid (present both in the male urethra and in the vagina) by the alkalinity of the prostatic secretions. Sperm are also capable of the greatest mobility when in a slightly alkaline medium. Proper prostate secretion is thus essential to effective sperm action.

The penis is the external organ that propels sperm into the female during sexual intercourse. During sexual excitement, the corpora cavernosa (large internal spaces within the penis) become filled with blood, making the penis rigid enough to enter the vagina (the entryway to the female reproductive tract). The semen, which is formed in the urethra, then travels out of the penis during ejaculation (sudden discharge of fluid).

See also Conception.

# Respiratory system

The respiratory system includes the nose, throat, larynx, trachea, bronchi, and lungs. The function of the respiratory system is to supply the blood with necessary oxygen and to relieve the blood of the waste product carbon dioxide. This exchange of oxygen and carbon dioxide occurs in the lungs. The first step in the process begins when air from the outside enters through the nose, where it is warmed, moistened, and filtered before it passes through the throat and past the larynx (voice box) into the trachea (windpipe). The trachea divides into two main bronchi (the airways connecting the windpipe and the lungs). Within each lung, the bronchi divide and subdivide, forming progressively smaller passageways called bronchioles. The smallest bronchioles end in small, cup-shaped sacs called alveoli. It is in the alveoli that the exchange of gas takes place. Each alveolus is served by numerous tiny blood vessels called capillaries. Oxygen in the alveolus crosses the thin alveolar and capillary walls to enter the blood, while carbon dioxide passes from the blood through the capillary walls into the alveolus. The oxygen is then carried by the blood to cells throughout the body. Meanwhile, the carbon dioxide is removed from the system by exhalation.

During inhalation and exhalation, the lungs are expanded and contracted by movements of the rib cage and the diaphragm (the large muscle separating the chest and abdominal cavities). During inhalation, the diaphragm contracts. This causes the diaphragm to descend and the chest cavity to expand. At this point, the air pressure inside the chest cavity is less than that of the air outside the body; consequently, air from the outside rushes into the lungs. During exhalation, the diaphragm relaxes and moves upward, reducing the chest capacity and pushing air out of the lungs. The friction caused by expansion and contraction of the lungs is eased by the pleurae (thin, moist membranes that cover the lungs and line the chest cavity), so that the sur-faces of the lungs and chest cavity can move past each other smoothly.

# Restless legs syndrome

Restless legs syndrome (also called Ekbom syndrome, "jimmy legs," and "jitter legs") is a feeling of uneasiness, shakiness, twitching, and restlessness that affects the legs after a patient has gone to bed for the night. Insomnia is almost always a result of the syndrome.

The precise cause of the syndrome is not known, although some authorities consider it to be brought about, or intensified, by poor blood circulation. Some physicians believe that it is more common in hyperactive patients; others say that it can be brought about by intense activity, especially physical activity, just before bedtime.

The patient often has difficulty falling asleep in the evening because of an uncomfortable feeling or a jerking sensation within the legs, usually in the thighs and calves. The discomfort is often relieved by moving about, but as a result, normal sleep is largely prevented. Consequently, the person may be excessively tired the next day. The condition most commonly affects middle-aged women.

The diagnosis can generally be made on the basis of the patient's medical history and report of symptoms. The physician will perform a physical examination to rule out more serious disorders.

Since the syndrome has been connected with circulatory disorders, drugs that increase the circulation to the lower extremities may prove helpful. A mild sedative at bedtime may also be useful.

# Retinitis

Retinitis is an inflammation of the retina, the light-sensitive innermost lining of the eye.

There are several types of retinitis. *Toxoplasmic retinitis*, which may be either acquired or congenital (present at birth), is caused by a microorganism. If the condition is congenital, the microorganism was passed to the fetus through the placenta (the temporary organ in the uterus that nourishes the fetus during development). A similar type of retinitis is caused by a blood-borne infection that settles in the eye. *Exudative retinitis* stems from unknown causes, but may result in detachment of the retina from the internal surface of the eyeball. *Retinitis pigmentosa* is an inherited disorder in which excessive amounts of a substance called phytanic acid accumulate and cause extensive damage to the retina. This form of retinitis also usually accompanies the rare inherited disorder of fat metabolism called Refsum's syndrome.

The symptoms of retinitis pigmentosa are night blindness, inflammation of the retina, marked limitation of the field of vision (tunnel vision), loss of kinesthetic sense (sense of body movement), shrinkage of the retina, clumping of retinal pigment, and dislodging of the blood vessels of the retina. Many of the same symptoms are found in the other forms of retinitis. They are sometimes accompanied by cloudiness of the vitreous humor (liquid filling the eyeball). This can be detected by a physician examining the interior of the eye with a special lighted instrument called an ophthalmoscope.

In the case of retinitis pigmentosa, there is little that can be done. If the retina is detached (a condition often caused when a hole in the retina allows fluid to seep into the eye and create a pocket), surgery is usually the treatment. The pocket is eliminated either by freezing or by heat, sometimes with a laser. If retinitis is the result of blood-borne infection, that condition must be treated first.

Other than genetic counseling for persons with a family history of retinitis pigmentosa, there are no clear-cut preventive measures that can be taken against retinitis.

See also Detached retina.

# Retinopathy

Retinopathy is a condition in which deterioration of the retina is caused by damage to or overproduction of the blood vessels in that structure.

The vast majority of cases of retinopathy are due to diabetes. Although fewer than five percent of all diabetics completely lose their sight because of retinopathy, diabetes is one of the leading causes of irreversible blindness today. Other conditions that increase susceptibility to retinopathy include high blood pres-

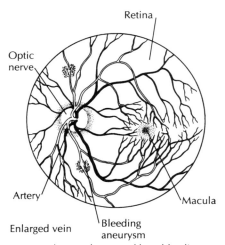

Retinopathy may be caused by a bleeding aneurysm (saclike bulging) in one of the arteries that supply the retina.

sure; hemorrhaging due to sudden vessel blockage by a blood clot, fat globule, or cholesterol plaque; and chronic kidney failure.

If a sudden hemorrhage is triggered, total blindness in the eye can strike swiftly; immediate medical attention is necessary. In cases of retinopathy due to hypertension (high blood pressure) or diabetes, vision usually worsens over time.

Hypertensive retinopathy is primarily treated by strict control of the blood pressure through diet and, in many cases, medication (depending on the severity of the condition). Diabetic retinopathy is also treated through diet and medication; if diabetic patients continually allow their glucose levels to exceed normal bounds, retinal damage can be extensive and may require laser treatments to seal off leaking blood vessels.

# Reye's syndrome

Reye's syndrome is a relatively rare condition in which encephalitis (inflammation of the brain) is associated with liver damage due to the collection of fatty deposits in that organ. It strikes children and adolescents (most commonly, children between the ages of 5 and 11 years), often while they are recovering from a viral infection, such as influenza or chicken pox. For some unknown reason, it occurs most often between December and March.

Reye's syndrome is a serious disease that requires *immediate* treatment. Brain damage, coma, or death can result if it is not diagnosed and treated quickly. It is fatal in about 25 percent of cases.

The exact cause of Reye's syndrome is not known, but since it almost always follows a viral infection, scientists suspect that the virus combines with an unknown substance in the body to produce a toxin (poison). There is some evidence that use of aspirin during a viral illness increases the risk of Reye's syndrome. Thus, physicians caution parents not to give aspirin products to their children during chicken pox or influenza infections.

The symptoms of Reye's syndrome are sudden vomiting, abnormal sleepiness or hyperactivity, and confusion. Convulsions and coma may possibly occur as the disease progresses.

Early diagnosis is crucial. Reye's syndrome is diagnosed by careful observation of the symptoms, testing of a sample of cerebrospinal fluid (the clear fluid of the central nervous system, which is produced in the brain), blood tests to determine the presence of liver damage, and tests of the blood sugar level, which is often low in young children with this disease.

There is no known cure for Reye's syndrome. Treatment consists in helping the child to weather the first few days of the illness, maintaining normal blood sugar levels and reducing pressure on the swollen brain. Usually, if the child survives for three or four days, the symptoms will subside and recovery will follow.

Sponge baths can be used instead of aspirin to reduce fever in children with viral illnesses, especially chicken pox and influenza.

If the blood sugar level is low, a normal concentration is restored with the intravenous administration of glucose (a form of sugar). Increased pressure on the brain from the swelling is also reduced with medication.

An association has been established between aspirin use during and immediately after viral infections (particularly chicken pox and influenza) and Reye's syndrome. It is therefore strongly recommended that aspirin not be given to a child or adolescent with such an infection. A doctor can suggest an aspirin substitute, such as acetaminophen, if needed for discomfort or fever. Sponge baths may also be helpful in reducing fever.

# Rheumatic fever

Rheumatic fever is the result of a bacterial disease characterized by inflammation, swelling, and soreness of the joints—especially the ankles, knees, and wrists—and inflammation of the heart. Occurring most commonly in children and adolescents, it is a serious illness that can result in permanent damage to the heart. The attacks of fever may recur over a period of years and last from a few weeks to several months.

The disease is considered to be a late stage of a streptococcal infection, such as strep throat; however, not all species of *Streptococcus* bacteria cause rheumatic fever. In some cases, the earlier infection may have been so minor that it cannot be recalled. Some researchers believe that rheumatic fever is an autoimmune disorder, in which the immune system forms antibodies to attack the body's own healthy tissues, such as those of the joints and the heart. The disease is more prevalent in some families than in others, but whether this indicates a hereditary factor or is due simply to sharing the same environment and living habits is not clear. Because only one percent of all cases of streptococcal infection in children and adolescents are followed by rheumatic fever, it is believed that a special susceptibility may be involved.

Rheumatic fever should be immediately suspected when a child or teenager develops an unexplained fever with joint inflammation a few weeks after a throat infection or tonsillitis, even if that preceding condition was very mild. The joints then become inflamed one after another. A peculiar skin rash of large, reddened, nonitchy areas with irregular borders develops, lasting a day or two. Nodules may emerge over the elbows, kneecaps, and other bony prominences; they may also form within the heart. Chorea (involuntary movement of the limbs and facial features) may occur if the infection spreads to involve the brain. Fortunately, chorea leaves no lasting brain damage and passes after some time, even without specific treatment.

The acute stage of joint involvement leaves no permanent deformity or crippling, but damage to the heart is permanent when it involves destruction of heart valve tissue. Scar tissue is then eventually formed on the valves, so that they cannot open and close properly. The heart, unable to efficiently carry out its function of pumping blood through the circulatory system, must work harder and becomes enlarged. Blood clots may form on its inner lining and may be carried in the blood throughout the body, often lodging in a blood vessel and blocking it.

Joint inflammation, heart abnormalities, chorea, and the appearance of the rash and the nodules are the most common manifestations of rheumatic fever, but these signs may appear alone or in a number of different combinations. Because no single laboratory finding or symptom is common to all cases of rheumatic fever, the diagnosis is made presumptively on the basis of the total clinical picture.

The chief treatment for rheumatic fever is the use of antibiotics for an extended period of time to eliminate any remaining *Streptococcus* bacteria. Aspirin is commonly used to bring down fever and relieve inflammation and pain. Corticosteroid drugs are sometimes given if there are signs of heart involvement, and sedatives may be prescribed if chorea becomes severe. The long periods of immobilization in bed that were once recommended are now believed to be unnecessary, although bed rest during acute attacks may be prescribed. Seriously damaged heart valves can often be repaired surgically or replaced by prosthetic (artificial) valves.

The only preventive measure is prompt diagnosis and adequate treatment of all streptococcal infections, especially those involving the throat and ears. Since dental procedures can sometimes be a source of bacterial infection, special precautions (such as the administration of antibiotics) may be recommended for persons whose heart valves have been injured.

See also Rheumatic heart disease.

# Rheumatic heart disease

Rheumatic heart disease consists of a variety of abnormal cardiac conditions, including heart valve scarring and endocarditis (inflammation of the lining of the heart).

This disease is a potential aftermath of rheumatic fever, once one of the prime killers of children. Rheumatic fever may cause inflammation of the heart valves and scarring of the valve leaflets. This scarring can result in valve leakage, allowing blood to flow backward, or severe narrowing of the valve, restricting blood flow out of the heart.

The most common symptom is a heart murmur, caused by abnormal blood flow across a scarred valve. There may be hemorrhaging (excessive bleeding) and impairment of vision if microscopic blood clots that have formed in the heart block tiny blood vessels in the eye. Kidney function may deteriorate in middle or later life. Muscle shrinkage due to inactivity may be accompanied by lack of muscular and cardiovascular endurance. Irregular pulse, shortness of breath, and fainting spells are also common symptoms.

Many persons who have suffered rheumatic heart disease have gone on to live extremely active lives, despite heart murmurs, heart enlargement, and damaged valves. Although rheumatic heart disease is a serious matter, regular exercise, a sensible diet, and determination can mean the difference between a sedentary and an active life.

Supervision by a physician is a necessity for anyone who suffers from rheumatic heart disease and wants to embark on a regular exercise program. In some cases, however, it may be impossible for a patient to participate in vigorous physical activity, especially if the heart damage is advanced or severe. For some of these individuals, surgery to implant an artificial valve can offer relief.

Persons with rheumatic heart disease must consult their physicians about antibiotic treatment before undergoing any dental or surgical procedures.

See also Rheumatic fever.

# Rheumatoid arthritis

See Arthritis.

# Rh factor

Rh factor refers to a specific antigen present in the blood. ("Rh" is derived from the name of the rhesus monkey, in which the factor was discovered.) An antigen is a substance that can induce the production of antibodies, which are crucial to the functioning of the body's immune system. Rh-positive blood has the antigen on its red cells; Rh-negative blood does not. An estimated 85 percent of the population has Rh-positive blood; that is to say, they possess Rh antigens.

Blood normally has no anti-Rh antibodies. Anti-Rh antibodies can develop in Rh-negative blood, however, if Rh-positive blood is introduced into the bloodstream. This can come about in two ways: if a person with Rh-negative blood receives a transfusion of Rh-positive blood or if a woman with Rh-negative blood conceives a child with Rh-positive blood (inherited from the father) and some of the Rh-positive cells from the fetus find their way into the bloodstream of the mother. In either case, the Rh-positive red blood cells will stimulate the person's body to form anti-Rh antibodies. If this happens, the blood will form clumps, and a potentially lethal situation will develop—the clumps may block the blood vessels, leading to death.

If difficulties do not appear with the formation of these antibodies during the first transfusion or the first pregnancy, they will surely appear if Rh-positive blood is ever again intro-duced into the person's bloodstream. The antibodies are already present, and the introduction of additional Rh-positive blood will result in a mobilization of existing antibodies and the production of even more. In addition to clumping of blood, other problems will arise. For example, hemolysis (the breakdown of red blood cells and release of their hemoglobin) will make it impossible for those cells to carry oxygen, resulting in anemia.

There are potential dangers to the fetus if the mother's blood contains anti-Rh antibodies. If the fetus has Rh-positive cells, anti-Rh antibodies may pass through the placenta from the mother's bloodstream to cause hemolysis of the child's blood cells. Once born, the baby may need to have massive, possibly even total, transfusions of Rh-negative blood to prevent clumping of the red blood cells and hemolytic anemia. This situation is now relatively rare because injections of gammaglobulin are routinely given to an Rh-negative mother after every pregnancy. These injections inhibit the formation of the potentially dangerous antibodies.

# Ringworm

Ringworm is a skin infection caused by a fungus, not a worm. The name originated because the infection is often characterized by round patches that enlarge as healing proceeds from the center, leaving red rings that persist on the skin for a few months.

There are several different types of ringworm, each caused by a different type of fungus. Ringworm of the scalp, or *tinea capitis*, appears as scaly patches with stubs of broken-off hairs or as bald areas. Ringworm of the body, or *tinea corporis*, appears as round or oval, scaly, red patches on the torso. Ringworm of the groin, or *tinea cruris* (popularly referred to as "jock itch"), is characterized by a scaly, red or brown rash in the crotch and genital area. Ringworm of the feet, or *tinea pedis*, is more commonly called athlete's foot.

Ringworm spreads by direct contact with an infected person or pet or by contact with contaminated objects, such as combs, pillows, towels, and clothing. Tight-fitting clothing, obesity, and heavy perspiration may be contributing factors in the development of ringworm of the body and the groin.

Ringworm infections are generally unsightly rather than threatening to general health. However, several other skin infections resemble ringworm, so it is important that a physician make the diagnosis. The doctor may want to examine the rash under ultraviolet light and obtain a skin scraping to be examined microscopically.

An antifungal ointment to be applied to the skin may be prescribed for ringworm of the body or the groin. Special medicated shampoos are available to treat ringworm of the scalp. In some especially resistant cases, an oral medication called griseofulvin may be necessary as well.

To prevent spread of the infection, personal articles that have been in contact with infected areas, such as hats, combs, and bed linen, should be discarded or laundered in very hot water.

# Rubella

Rubella, or German measles, is a relatively mild viral infection with cold-like symptoms and a short-lived rash. The disease is contagious; however, rubella outbreaks have become infrequent since the development of a vaccine to prevent the illness. Rubella is usually not dangerous, unless it occurs during pregnancy. In that circumstance, it can cause birth defects that are serious.

Rubella is caused by a virus. The virus spreads from one person to another via airborne droplets from an infected person's respiratory system. The incubation period (the time between exposure to the infection and appearance of symptoms) is usually 14 to 21 days. An infected person can spread the virus as early as one week before the rash appears and as late as five days after the rash has faded. A child with congenital (existing at or before the time of birth) rubella syndrome can transmit the virus until he or she reaches about 12 to 18 months. Second infections have been reported, but they are rare.

Although rubella is generally a mild infection, some complications can arise. Encephalitis (inflammation of the brain) occurs in one in 5,000 cases. Thrombocytopenic purpura, a blood disease characterized by a lowered platelet count, can prove fatal when it accompanies rubella. High or prolonged fever and extreme fatigue should be reported to a physician in order to prevent further complications.

Congenital rubella syndrome occurs when the disease is transmitted to the fetus during pregnancy. Rubella virus may cause one or more serious organic and growth disorders of the fetus, particularly if contracted during the first three months of pregnancy. The most common problems include congenital heart defects, hearing and vision problems, and blood disorders. Mental retardation and other brain disorders are additional common problems encountered in congenital rubella syndrome.

The first symptoms of rubella are a runny nose, swollen lymph nodes in the neck, and a low-grade fever (up to 101°F). About two days later, a rash of very small red or pink spots appears on the face and neck. The spots are flat initially. They then become slightly raised and fade within a day or two. As the first spots fade, more spots develop until the rash has spread over most of the body. The rash lasts only two to three days, but swelling of the lymph nodes may persist for as long as a week. All other symptoms usually will have disappeared by that time. When joint pain is in evidence, as is common with older women, discomfort may last another week.

Under normal circumstances, rubella is difficult to diagnose because the symptoms are so mild and variable. Sometimes there is no rash, and the disease resembles a cold. Other cases may be so severe that the infection may be confused with measles. A doctor can identify the virus by testing a blood sample. Tracing a history of exposure to the disease also helps in the effort to properly establish the diagnosis.

Most patients require little or no treatment for rubella because the symptoms are so mild. An aspirin substitute may afford relief from joint pain. Otherwise, drugs are not needed. Some patients may want bed rest, but most people feel well enough to be somewhat active.

Rubella rarely occurs now because children routinely receive rubella vaccine at about 15 months of age. The vaccine is usually combined with measles and mumps vaccines in one injection, but it can be given alone. The rubella vaccine can cause some mild muscle or joint aches, but they are rarely significant. The rubella vaccine also goes to work in the body to stimulate the production of antibodies (protective substances manufactured by the body) that counteract or fight off the disease.

Women who want to become pregnant should have a blood test to

The light pink rubella rash first appears on the face and the neck and then gradually spreads over most of the body. The rash is in evidence for only two or three days, but the swollen lymph nodes may last for a week.

determine whether they are already immune to rubella; if not, they can be vaccinated. Vaccination is not recommended during pregnancy because of the possible risk to the fetus. Doctors also caution women to wait at least three months after rubella vaccination before trying to become pregnant.

# S

# Scarlet fever

Scarlet fever (also known as scarlatina) is a highly contagious illness caused by *Streptococcus* bacteria and is almost always accompanied by a strep throat.

The symptoms of scarlet fever include fever; sore throat; widespread scarlet rash beginning in the armpits and groin and spreading to the neck, chest, back, extremities, and even the tongue; and peeling and scaling of the skin, even on the palms of the hands and the soles of the feet. The incubation period (the time between exposure to the disease and the appearance of symptoms) is two to four days.

In the past, scarlet fever was often fatal, but today it is easily treated with penicillin, and complications are rare. Bed rest and a nourishing diet with plenty of fluids help speed recuperation.

# Schizophrenia

Schizophrenia is not a single mental disorder, but rather a group of mental disorders that are characterized by disturbances of thought processes, emotional response, and behavior. Among the characteristics common to most types of schizophrenia are extreme mental confusion, withdrawal from reality, delusions, hallucinations, extreme mood changes, and bizarre behavior.

Most cases of schizophrenia are due to a combination of inherited and environmental factors. A genetic predisposition appears to be an impor-

tant factor in schizophrenia. It has been estimated that approximately ten percent of relatives of schizophrenics are schizophrenic themselves. Schizophrenia is not inherited, however. Even if the genetic predisposition is present, the occurrence of the illness is often related to stressful life events and the individual's ways of coping with them.

Schizophrenia affects persons of all ages, although it commonly begins in late adolescence or early adult life. There is no specific personality type that can be singled out as predisposing to development of schizophrenia, but many schizophrenics show such traits as extreme sensitivity, shyness, lack of emotion, antisocial behavior, and paranoid attitudes early in life.

The onset of schizophrenia may be sudden or gradual. Some or possibly all of the following symptoms will be present:

- Mental disturbances—progressive confusion of thought and speech; disruption of logical reasoning
- Emotional disorders—absent or inappropriate emotional responses; extremes of depression, excitability, anxiety, and elation
- Hallucinations—distorted or imaginary perceptions involving any of the senses, such as hearing voices or seeing things that are not there
- Delusions—mistaken notions that one is being persecuted, that one is more powerful or important than one is (called delusions of grandeur), or that one's thoughts are being broadcast to others or are being controlled by some outside agency
- Movement disorders—extreme hyperactivity; immobility and stupor; adoption of strange positions, facial expressions, mannerisms, and abnormal activity patterns, like rocking and pacing
- Violent behavior—such as threats of violence and assassination

attempts against authority figures and persons in the public eye
• Withdrawal from reality and social contact

As with other mental disorders, the physician will obtain a personal and medical history from (or about) the patient and will conduct a physical examination to rule out the possibility that some medical condition or drug reaction may be causing the symptoms of schizophrenia.

The chief treatment measures for schizophrenia include drug therapy, psychotherapy, counseling, social support, and rehabilitation. For a first illness or acute relapse, hospitalization is usually indicated in order to stabilize the patient's condition. However, hospitalization for more than a few months may be inadvisable; if the patient is able to function outside an institution, leading some semblance of a normal life may be therapeutic.

Schizophrenia is not necessarily a chronic condition. In fact, about 30 percent of patients recover completely, and most of the remainder show marked improvement with appropriate treatment, although impaired emotional response and motivation may persist.

See also Depression, Electroconvulsive therapy, and Paranoia.

# Sciatica

Sciatica is a condition characterized by pain that extends along the entire length of the sciatic nerve (which runs down the lower back and outer side of the thigh, leg, and foot), radiating across the back of the pelvis through the buttocks and into the leg.

Sciatica is commonly associated with injury to or rupture of a lumbar disk, one of the cartilaginous disks located between the lumbar (lower

back) vertebrae. When the injured disk exerts pressure against the sciatic nerve, pain radiates down the nerve.

The symptoms of sciatica vary in intensity, depending on the extent to which the injured disk presses on the sciatic nerve and according to the individual's susceptibility to pain. In mild cases, the pain may be a slight discomfort in the lower back and along the leg. In severe cases, the pain is excruciating and often completely immobilizes the victim. Since the cause is frequently a ruptured ("slipped") disk, it is difficult to know when an attack will begin. A sudden cough may cause the disk to move and press on the sciatic nerve, resulting in the pain that such pressure causes. It is commonplace for sciatica patients to be free from pain one moment and in agony the next.

Area of lumbar vertebrae

Path of sciatic nerve

Sciatica occurs when pressure on the sciatic nerve in the area of the lumbar vertebrae causes pain to radiate along the path of the sciatic nerve.

Repeated problems with a ruptured lumbar disk can cause general inflammation of the sciatic nerve. In these cases, it is not a matter of pain that comes and goes. Instead, it is a matter of having somewhat less pain at one time than at another.

The primary treatment of sciatica is rest, to allow the inflammation of the nerve to subside. In an effort to alleviate the pain, various medications, such as analgesics and muscle relaxants, may be prescribed or anesthetic agents may be injected into the area around the spinal cord. In cases that do not respond to such conservative measures, surgery may be necessary. Recently, new surgical techniques, such as microsurgery and percutaneous (through the skin without cutting, as with a needle) removal of disc fragments, have been developed. These techniques have considerably decreased hospital stays and loss of work time. So far, success at relieving pain and neurologic symptoms has been good. Not all individuals with disk problems, however, are suitable for this surgery.

Physical therapy (under a doctor's supervision or according to a doctor's prescription) is often used to relieve the pain of sciatica. This treatment includes hydrotherapy, in which a stream of water is directed at the affected area. Many therapists advise their patients to overcome the effects of a ruptured disk by developing the core muscles (the four muscle groups that form the waist) in order to provide a supportive column of muscle that will help keep the disk in place.

See also Neuralagia and Slipped disk.

---

# Scoliosis

Scoliosis is curvature of the spine. There is usually a main curve in one direction and an upper curve or lower curve, or both, to compensate for it in the opposite direction.

Before the age of three years, boys are more likely to be affected, developing an upper curve to the left and a lower curve to the right. Between the ages of four and ten years, boys and girls are affected in equal numbers, and the direction of curvature varies. Most prevalent is the adolescent form, usually affecting girls between the age of ten and the time their skeletons mature. Most often, the upper spinal area (behind the chest) curves to the right, with compensating curves to the left in the lower neck area and in the small of the back.

Severe, untreated scoliosis can cause diminished lung capacity, back pain, spinal arthritis, and disease of the cartilage disks between the vertebrae.

Scoliosis can result from unequal leg lengths, or it may be due to defective development of the vertebrae (the bones of the spine) while the fetus was growing in the uterus. Paralysis of the trunk muscles on one side of

Severe scoliosis can be seen when viewing a child from the back, and even mild scoliosis can be noticed when the child bends at the waist. Bending forward rotates the chest, making one side of the back more prominent.

the body caused by polio, cerebral palsy, or muscular dystrophy; tilting of the pelvis due to hip disease; or deformities of the spine caused by rickets or rheumatism can also lead to scoliosis. Idiopathic scoliosis, the most common kind, has no known cause.

Parents should be alert for the signs of scoliosis. At first the child may appear to have an uneven hemline, unequal pant legs, or one hip higher than the other. To make a preliminary assessment, ask your child to stand up straight with his or her shirt off while you observe from the rear. Notice if one shoulder is higher than the other or if one shoulder blade sticks out. When the child's arms hang loosely at the sides, notice if one arm hangs farther away from the body than does the other. See if one hip appears higher or more prominent than the other. See if the child seems to tilt to one side. Finally, ask your child to bend forward, arms hanging in front and palms together at the level of the knees. A hump on the back at the ribs or near the waist may also be a sign of scoliosis.

If you have any suspicions, report them to your child's doctor, who will give the child a similar checkup and, if necessary, take X rays or refer you to an orthopedic surgeon (bone specialist) to confirm the diagnosis.

Treatment of scoliosis may involve only exercises if the curvature is mild. Sit-ups, exercises to stretch the spine, and breathing exercises may strengthen the muscles of the trunk enough to correct the situation. Frequent X rays and physical examinations may be needed to determine if the exercises are working.

More severe scoliosis may require the wearing of a special leather brace or a plastic pelvic girdle with one vertical brace in front and two in back, connected to a ring around the neck. In many cases, this must be worn 24 hours a day, except when the patient is bathing or exercising, until the child's skeleton has matured. It is adjustable for growth.

The use of specially designed electrical stimulation devices has met with some success.

The most severe scoliosis requires spinal-fusion surgery, in which certain vertebrae are fused together, with stabilization provided by metal rods, cable, or staples. Frequent checkups are needed after surgery to make sure that the correction is being maintained.

# Scurvy

Scurvy is a disease caused by vitamin C deficiency. It is characterized by anemia (deficiency of red blood cells), spongy gums, a tendency to bleed, and abnormal bone and tooth formation. The disease may be either acute (short-term) or chronic (long-term).

Vitamin C is essential for the formation and maintenance of connective tissue, bone tissue, and teeth. It is also essential for the healing of wounds and burns.

There are two forms of scurvy, infantile and adult. Vitamin C deficiency in infants is due simply to lack of sufficient quantities of vitamin C. In adults, scurvy is usually due to improper diet. Adult scurvy may also result from being on an "ulcer diet" for gastrointestinal disorders that limits citrus fruits and juices because of their acid content. Pregnancy and breast-feeding increase the vitamin C requirement; pregnant women and nursing mothers must be sure to include adequate vitamin C in the diet. In addition, diarrhea, inflammatory disease, burns, surgery, and exposure to intense cold all increase the vitamin C requirement.

Infantile scurvy usually appears between the ages of six months and one year. The earliest symptoms include irritability, loss of appetite, and failure to gain weight. Often the child screams or cries whenever he is moved and may hold his legs motionless because of the pain caused by internal bleeding of the bone surface. There may be abnormal enlargement or hardening of the joints or long bones (especially in the thighs) and a tendency toward gum hemorrhage as the teeth erupt. Fever, anemia, and increased pulse and respiration rates are also common signs.

Adult scurvy usually takes a long time to develop. Early symptoms include extreme fatigue, weakness, irritability, weight loss, loss of appetite, multiple splinter hemorrhages at the nails, failure of wounds to heal, loosening of teeth, and swollen, purplish, and spongy gums. Secondary infections, gangrene (death and decay of tissue, frequently due to inadequate blood supply), breaks in old scars, spontaneous hemorrhaging, muscle pain, pain in the joints, and small hemorrhagic spots on the skin of the legs are all symptoms of a more advanced stage of the disorder. In some cases there is edema (fluid retention) in the lower extremities and a form of arthritis that resembles rheumatoid arthritis. There may even be bleeding in the conjunctiva (the membrane that covers the front of the eye and lines the inside eyelids).

In a case of infantile scurvy, an X-ray study of the ends of the long bones of the legs will show areas of crosswise thickening and increased density, the so-called white lines. If the diagnosis is doubtful, a therapeutic dose of vitamin C given orally will stop the pain of infantile scurvy almost immediately and reduce the swelling and bleeding of the gums within 72 hours.

In adults, scurvy can mimic arthritis, hemorrhagic disease, and gingivitis (inflammation of the gums). The blood level of vitamin C is usually low, but this is not always an accurate diagnostic indication. The level of vitamin C in the urine will be low, and there may be anemia not caused by blood loss.

Fortunately, scurvy is easy to treat. Vitamin C given orally for one week, supplemented with orange and tomato juice, is the remedy for infantile scurvy. If diarrhea or vomiting is present, half the recommended oral dose can be given intravenously (in a vein).

For adult scurvy, vitamin C is taken orally until symptoms have disappeared; the patient can then receive maintenance doses. Vitamin C is given for several months for chronic scurvy that appears in connection with gingivitis, hemorrhaging, or joint symptoms.

A balanced diet with plenty of vitamin C is the best preventive measure for scurvy. Fortunately, natural sources of vitamin C are plentiful: Besides citrus fruits and tomatoes, many green vegetables, such as green peppers, are rich in vitamin C. In the case of patients on bland diets or ulcer diets, a physician should be consulted about how to prevent vitamin C deficiency.

See also Vitamins.

# Senility

Senility is the medical term applied to the gradual process of mental and physical deterioration that is sometimes associated with old age.

The causes of senility are many—arteriosclerosis (hardening of the arteries), other blood vessel diseases, heart diseases, and lung diseases (all of which may decrease the amount of oxygen available to the brain and other body tissues) and diseases of the liver, the kidneys, and other organs. Senility is not linked to a single disease, nor is it inevitable. However, the years take their toll, and chronic disorders hasten senility. Lifelong harmful habits are also a cause of early senility; alcohol, tobacco, and drug abuse are among the worst offenders.

Gradual loss of physical and mental vigor is the most common symptom of oncoming senility. A lack of interest in the surroundings or in activities once enjoyed is another symptom. Victims experience a loss of complex skills, such as the ability to do puzzles, math problems, or logic problems, or even to balance their checkbooks. If the onset of senility is relatively sudden, as it is with a condition called Alzheimer's disease, the victim will often be in a panic, as he or she feels the mental powers waning. Short-term memory is one of the first faculties to go, and many victims are painfully aware of their condition.

Physical senility is gradual, unless a chronic illness accelerates the process. The skin becomes dry and loses its resilience, the muscles lose their tone and become weak, the bones become brittle, and the organs gradually fail.

Do not assume that a relative is suffering from senility simply on the basis of confusion and apparent loss of mental skills. Depression and a number of physical conditions can cause similar symptoms. Such symptoms may also be related to the use of certain medications (or combinations of medications). Always consult a physician so that such conditions can be ruled out (or, in some cases, treated).

Although there is no way to stop the clock, there are many ways that one can continue leading a vigorous, active life. Getting regular exercise; avoiding toxic substances, such as tobacco, alcohol, drugs, and pollutants; and eating a balanced diet, with adequate amounts of vitamins and minerals, seem to have a positive effect at any age. Protection from debilitating disease and avoidance of injuries (such as broken bones) can also add years of activity to the lives of the elderly.

Mental senility can often be avoided simply by not "turning off" the mind on retirement. The mind begins to deteriorate quickly if it is not used, in much the same way that muscles shrink when they are not used.

See also Alzheimer's disease, Atherosclerosis, and Osteoporosis.

# Septicemia

Septicemia, often called blood poisoning, is a form of bacteremia (invasion of the blood circulation by bacteria).

The cause of septicemia is sometimes traceable to a surgical procedure, to the use of intravenous devices or catheters, or to childbirth injury complicated by infection. Septicemia is also a common effect of intravenous drug injections, particularly in drug abusers. Other diseases and disorders associated with septicemia include endocarditis (inflammation of the lining of the heart), genitourinary tract infections, and diseases of the skin, bones, and joints. However, relatively minor problems such as untreated cuts that become infected or untreated sinus infections can lead to septicemia.

Because few symptoms are unique to septicemia, it is often confused with other illnesses. Fever is generally present, although it may be variable and intermittent. Chills may occur at the onset of the disease. Skin eruptions are common and may be petechial (small red dots or splotches) or purpuric (purple and bruiselike) or may take any of several other forms. Septicemia often begins abruptly with chills, fever, nausea, vomiting, and diarrhea, leading to collapse.

Complications may include secondary infections of the organs and bones.

The diagnosis of septicemia is established by testing cultures of blood and other tissues for various kinds of bacteria. Normally, there should be no bacteria in the blood. A single negative culture does not exclude septicemia, particularly in some patients who have had antibiotic therapy.

Septicemia is treated by intravenous administration of antibiotics. Therapy should continue until the patient has been free of symptoms for at least one week.

# Sexually transmitted diseases

See Aids, Genital warts, Chlamydia, Gonorrhea, Herpes, Nongonococcal urethritis, and Syphillis.

# Shingles

Shingles, or herpes zoster, is a painful viral infection of one or more nerves. The infection produces a blistery, itchy skin rash on the area of skin supplied by the affected nerve. Shingles rash looks identical to the rash of chicken pox, which should not be surprising because shingles and chicken pox are both caused by the varicella zoster virus.

Shingles usually occurs only in persons who have already had chicken pox. Some scientists believe that after a case of chicken pox has run its course, the varicella zoster virus lies dormant in a nerve root but can be reactivated by injury to the affected area or even after emotional or physical upset among other causes. Others believe that the number and strength of antibodies produced by the body to fight the varicella zoster virus diminish with time, making the person susceptible to another attack of the virus; because some antibodies endure, the person gets shingles rather than chicken pox. If an adult who has not had chicken pox is exposed to the virus, he will get chicken pox, not shingles.

The incidence of shingles increases with age. It rarely occurs in people under the age of 15. More than 50 percent of those who get shingles are over 45 years of age.

Shingles begins with prickling or tenderness in the skin over the affected nerve. Burning or shooting pain in the same area is also an early symptom. Within two to four days, a rash of small, red spots appears over the affected part of the body. As the spots enlarge, they blister and sometimes blend together. Eventually they fill with pus, burst, and crust over, much the same as with chicken pox rash. With shingles, however, the process takes longer and is confined to the skin area above the affected nerve.

The shingles rash is very itchy. Pain increases as the area beneath the rash becomes redder and more swollen. Shingles most often attacks nerves of the chest, back, neck, arms, and legs; however, facial nerves are frequently involved. The rash appears in a band or strip following the distribution of the nerve, usually on one side of the body. The rash persists for two to three weeks before clearing; the pain continues for about three or four weeks. In persons over age 60, pain may persist for months to years

Shingles is an infection of a nerve characterized by a blistering skin rash following the path of the affected underlying nerve. The rash itself is identical to that of chicken pox, since both diseases are caused by the same virus.

(a disorder that temporarily paralyzes one side of the face) can result. Shingles in other parts of the body can cause similar temporary paralysis of the area in close proximity to the affected nerve.

Since there is no known cure for shingles, treatment focuses on reducing pain. An analgesic (pain-killing drug) may relieve the burning sensation. Some physicians prescribe steroid drugs to reduce nerve inflammation in older patients. To be effective, steroids must be taken soon after shingles begins. Steroid treatment is usually not recommended for persons with underlying disease because steroids can interfere with resistance to infection. Acyclovir, an antiviral drug given in ointment, oral, and intravenous forms, has been shown to shorten the course and decrease the severity of the illness in many cases.

Preventing infection is also important. Baths in warm (not hot) water soothe and clean the skin. If itching is severe, patients should cut their fingernails and wear gloves when asleep to control unconscious scratching.

See also Bells palsy.

after the rash has disappeared; this condition is called postherpetic neuralgia. This condition is difficult to treat. Antidepressants, antiseizure medications, electrical stimulation of the affected areas, and analgesics have been helpful in reducing the pain related to shingles.

Occasionally, the shingles rash spreads over the entire body. This develops most often in people who have some underlying disease, such as Hodgkin's disease (cancer of the lymph system) or leukemia (cancer of the blood). When these serious disorders already exist, shingles can cause death, but this is very unusual. An indication that other illness may be present is recurrence of shingles, since the condition seldom occurs more than once.

The most common complication of shingles is bacterial infection of the rash. This can prolong the rash and cause scarring of the skin.

Less common complications may follow a shingles attack on facial nerves. Eye disorders and Bell's palsy

# Sickle cell anemia

Sickle cell anemia is an inherited blood disorder, occurring almost exclusively in black persons, in which the normally round, red blood cells are transformed into crescentic, or sickle-shaped, cells that are less able to transport needed oxygen. The disease is chronic, marked by fatigue, breathing difficulty on exertion, swollen joints, attacks of extreme illness, complications from other diseases, and shortened life. In the past, half of all victims died by the age of 20 and few survived past 40. With new technology and forms of treat-

Normal red blood cells

Sickle-shaped red blood cells

Sickle cell anemia is a blood disorder in which the normally round red blood cells are transformed into crescentic, or sickle-shaped, cells. The sickle-shaped cells tangle together and interfere with blood circulation.

ment, the outlook is much better, but sickle cell anemia remains a chronic debilitating disease.

The deformation of the red blood cells occurs because of the presence of defective hemoglobin (the iron-protein compound in the red blood cells that carries oxygen). It occurs when part or all of the body is not getting enough oxygen. Because of their hooked shapes, the blood cells tend to tangle together and pile up, temporarily clogging tiny blood vessels and slowing circulation. Tissue formerly nourished by the clogged blood vessels becomes starved for oxygen and may die. The anemia (deficien-

cy of red blood cells) that results from the accelerated breakdown of defective red blood cells not only weakens the body, but increases oxygen deficiency, which results in more "sickling" of the cells.

The disease occurs in about one of every 330 black persons in the United States. About one in ten black persons in America is a carrier of the defective gene for sickle cell anemia but has no symptoms and is not affected by the disease. However, if two carriers conceive a child together, the risk that their child will be afflicted by the disease is one in four. The risk that the child will also be a carrier is one in two. Both the carrier state and the active state of the disease can be established by a simple blood test.

In half the victims, symptoms of sickle cell anemia begin between the ages of six months and two years.

Among the first signs is unusual swelling of the fingers and toes. The bones of the hands and feet thicken, and clumping of sickle cells may affect the bone marrow, where new blood cells are produced. Youngsters are especially subject to "sickle cell crises," marked by severe pain in the abdomen, joints, bones, and muscles due to lack of oxygen. These crises may last from four days to several weeks, and commonly occur eight to ten times a year before the age of ten. They occur much less often in later years. Signs of a sickle cell crisis include paleness of the lips, tongue, and palms; lack of energy; sleepiness and difficulty in awakening; irritability; pain; and a temperature of 104°F (or one over 100°F that lasts for at least two days).

Thickening of the heart muscle; enlargement of the heart, liver, and spleen in children; heart murmurs; and gallstones are common. The heartbeat is usually rapid. Children with the disease are usually small for their age. Those who survive to adult-hood may have narrow shoulders and hips, a barrel chest, a curved spine, long arms and legs, and an elongated skull.

At present, there is no cure for the disease. Treatment includes giving painkillers, making the patient as comfortable as possible, and treating problems as they occur. These problems include severe anemia, which may require a blood transfusion, and frequent infections, which occur because of impairment of the immune system.

Avoiding cold, fatigue, and other stress may help to reduce the number of sickle cell crises.

Screening programs are available for those who wish to know whether they carry the gene for sickle cell anemia. Those who have the gene can obtain genetic counseling. There is no risk of disease in offspring if only one parent is a carrier, but each child will have a one in two chance of being a carrier.

# Sinusitis

Sinusitis is an infection (usually bacterial) of one or more of the sinuses. It occurs more commonly in adults than in children.

The sinuses are air-filled cavities located within the facial bone structure and connected to the nose. There are four major groups of sinuses: frontal, ethmoidal, sphenoidal, and maxillary sinuses.

The sinuses are lined with mucous membrane and are normally kept clear when mucus drains through them into the nasal passages. If they are obstructed for any reason, such as from the congestion present during a cold, normal drainage cannot occur, and infection of the sinuses can result.

It is rare but possible for long-lasting sinusitis to lead to more serious disorders. A persistent infection may travel to the brain, causing meningitis (inflammation of the membranes covering the brain and spinal cord), or to the bone, resulting in osteomyelitis (inflammation of a bone and its marrow).

A sinus infection may be triggered by anything that prevents the mucus in the sinuses from draining properly into the nasal passages. Possible causes include swimming and diving, injuries, abnormal structure of the facial bones, congestion from the flu or a cold, allergies, or an abscess (inflamed pocket of pus) in a tooth, which may penetrate the sinuses and allow bacteria to enter them. Many different types of bacteria can cause sinusitis, including some of the same strains that lead to pneumonia, laryngitis, and middle ear infections.

Sinusitis is characterized by pain and tenderness above the infected sinus, which is felt in the face and

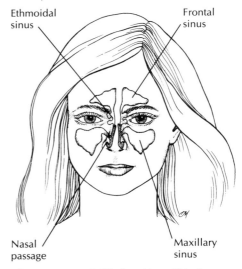

Ethmoidal sinus

Frontal sinus

Nasal passage

Maxillary sinus

The sinuses are air-filled cavities within the facial bone structure that are connected to the nasal passages. The four major groups are the frontal, ethmoidal, sphenoidal, and maxillary. The sphenoidal sinuses are located behind the ethmoidal.

forehead, behind the eyes, in the eyes, near the upper part of the nose, and even in the upper teeth (but not in a single tooth). This facial pain may be accompanied by headache, slight fever, chills, sore throat, nasal obstruction, and a discharge of pus from the nose.

Sinusitis usually lasts about two weeks, with the pain often subsiding in the morning and worsening as the day goes on, or fluctuating as the patient moves about and changes positions.

The sinuses cannot be seen directly by a doctor, so diagnostic evaluation may include an X-ray examination to check for the presence of fluid or abnormalities in the sinuses and to determine which sinuses are infected. Computed tomography is an excellent tool for evaluating serious sinus problems.

Sinusitis is treated by encouraging drainage of the sinuses. Nasal decongestants and moist heat work to aid sinus drainage. The doctor will usually prescribe an antibiotic that will kill the bacteria that most commonly trigger sinusitis.

If these treatments bring no relief, the doctor may perform a sinus puncture to determine exactly which bacteria are present. In this procedure, a needle is inserted into the sinus, and a sample of the fluid is removed. (This is necessary because the nasal discharge may contain bacteria different from those in the sinuses.) On the basis of analysis of the fluid sample, a more specific antibiotic may be prescribed.

In severe cases, codeine may be prescribed to dull the pain, and the doctor may clear the sinuses by injecting a solution through the nose to flush out the sinus cavities.

In some cases, surgery may be necessary to remove a nasal polyp (a mass of swollen tissue), repair abnormal bone structures, or remove infected sinus tissue.

There is some evidence that smokers are more likely to suffer from sinusitis than are nonsmokers. Those who frequently have colds are also more susceptible to sinusitis. Avoiding smoking and limiting exposure to persons with colds may help to prevent sinusitis.

# Skin

The skin is the largest organ of the body, covering 18 square feet and weighing about seven pounds in an average adult. This waterproof barrier affords protection from invasion by dirt, bacteria, and other harmful substances and helps to regulate body temperature.

The skin is composed of three layers—the epidermis, the dermis, and the subcutaneous layer.

The outermost layer of skin is referred to as the epidermis. The epidermis contains pigment cells that determine an individual's skin color and shield the skin against damaging sun rays. Specialized cells are located within this layer that manufacture keratin, a tough substance that is part of the composition of hair and nails.

Epidermal cells are continuously being worn away and replaced. This reconstruction process is usually invisible, except when skin becomes irritated, as in psoriasis, a disease that appears as scaly red patches. Since the outer skin layer repairs itself quickly, any injury to the epidermis rarely causes injury to the body as a whole.

The dermis contains blood vessels, nerve endings, hair follicles, sweat glands, and sebaceous (oil) glands. Damage at this level can send infection both into the bloodstream and throughout the body.

Within the dermis, blood vessels and sweat glands help the body reg-

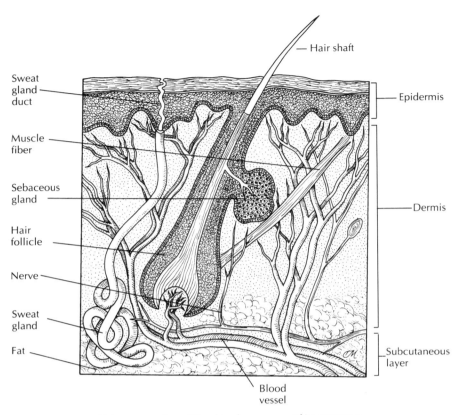

Hair shaft

Sweat gland duct

Epidermis

Muscle fiber

Sebaceous gland

Dermis

Hair follicle

Nerve

Sweat gland

Fat

Subcutaneous layer

Blood vessel

This cross section of the skin shows many of its structures.

ulate heat. If the temperature of blood rises, the brain stimulates secretion by the sweat glands. Sweat then flows to the surface of the skin through ducts and cools the skin by evaporating. The sebaceous glands prevent excessive evaporation by coating the surface of the skin with an oily substance called sebum.

Beneath the dermis is the subcutaneous layer, in which the sweat glands originate and fat is stored. This layer also supports the blood vessels and nerves that supply the outer layers of the skin.

Because the dermis and the subcutaneous layer are rich with nerve endings, the skin is also a sensory organ. Nerves throughout these layers transmit tactile perceptions to the brain.

# Skin cancer

About 300,000 cases of skin cancer are discovered every year. Its incidence increases every year, particularly among women, perhaps because people currently are getting more exposure to sunlight. The ultraviolet rays of the sun are a major cause of skin cancer. Fair-skinned people have less melanin (a protective substance in the skin) than dark-skinned people do and are therefore more susceptible to the effects of these rays. Skin cancer can also result from prolonged exposure to certain chemicals, such as arsenic compounds. Burn scars and skin diseases sometimes develop into cancer.

Symptoms of skin cancer include a change in the surface of the skin, a wound that does not heal, and a sudden major change in a wart, mole, or birthmark. All such suspicious signs should be examined by a doctor.

Most skin cancers are highly treatable. Some can be removed in a doctor's office or an outpatient clinic. But since some forms of skin cancer can spread throughout the body, it is important that they be treated early. The most dangerous skin cancer, malignant melanoma, can metastasize through the lymph and vascular (blood vessel) systems. Melanomas can develop from moles.

Skin cancer is an unusual form of cancer in that it can be prevented easily. Fair-skinned people and anyone with a family history of skin cancer should avoid exposure to the sun. Additionally, everyone who spends time in the sun should apply a protective sunscreen to exposed portions of the body. It is important that children, whose skin is more sensitive, be protected against the sun. The use of certain drugs, such as barbiturates, antibiotics, and birth control pills, can increase the sensitivity of the skin.

See also Cancer.

# Slipped disk

A slipped disk is a back problem involving the disks of soft elastic tissue located between the vertebrae (bones of the spinal column). The vertebrae are loosely strung together by bands of tissue called ligaments, which allow body movement and flexibility. The main function of each disk is to prevent friction and trauma between adjacent vertebrae as the body moves.

When this intricate spinal structure experiences strain and overexertion, the rim of a disk may weaken and tear, causing part of the gelatinous center of the disk to be forced out of position ("slip" or "herniate"). In its new location, the protruding material often presses against an adjacent spinal nerve, which causes pain along the path of the affected nerve.

Often, a slipped disk occurs when there is strain or injury to the spinal structure resulting from bending and straightening the back to lift heavy objects. Damage to the disk may not be realized for many months. More often, low back pain radiating into the buttock(s) and/or thigh(s) occurs soon after the injury.

Disks also seem to deteriorate with age. They lose some fluidity and become more compressed. This form of degeneration usually results in only mild pain and intermittent backache and stiffness.

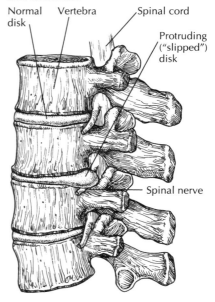

Cushioning disks of cartilage lie between the vertebrae (bones of the spine). If the rim of a disk weakens or tears, part of the jellylike center becomes pushed out. This protruding "slipped" disk presses on a nearby spinal nerve, causing pain along the path of the nerve.

Symptoms may vary with the location of the disk. The most common site for a slipped disk is the lowest movable disk in the small of the back. Injury to this disk causes pain along the sciatic nerve, a condition called sciatica. Mild or disabling pain and tenderness may result. Any straining, such as coughing or moving, can aggravate the discomfort. Weakness, tingling, or numbness in parts of the arms, legs, or feet may also result from damage to a particular disk in the neck or back.

To determine the source of back pain, a physician obtains a medical history; observes the patient sitting, walking, and bending; and explores for sensitive areas by maneuvering the patient's legs in different positions, checking ankle and knee reflexes, and testing muscle strength. Structural changes in bones, joints, or disk spaces (but not the disks themselves) can be seen on an ordinary X-ray study.

To locate a particularly problematic disk or to prepare for a surgical procedure, special tests are necessary. A myelogram is an X-ray study obtained after the injection of dye directly into the space surrounding the spinal cord and nerve roots. Discography gives much the same information as myelography; before this X-ray study, dye is injected directly into the disks. Computed tomography and magnetic resonance imaging are also highly accurate in the diagnosis of disk problems. However, prior to surgery, most orthopedists and neurosurgeons prefer to do a myelogram to best visualize the area.

The first course of treatment for a slipped disk involves bed rest on a firm mattress. Rest relieves pressure exerted by the disk on the nerve. Some form of back support may improve comfort when moving about. Under no circumstances should a patient lift heavy objects.

For severe pain, a physician may prescribe an analgesic or anti-inflammatory drug. Frequently, direct injection of a steroid (cortisone) drug and local anesthetic into the area around the spinal cord (epidural space) will break the cycle of pain and nerve-root swelling and provide long-lasting relief. Several injections may be needed, however, before significant relief is obtained. After the pain has completely subsided, an exercise program may be recommended to gradually strengthen muscles in the region.

Partial or complete relief from the pain of a slipped disk can usually be obtained without surgery. However, in some cases, surgery provides the only remedy. Newer microscopic techniques as well as percutaneous (through the skin without cutting) disk removal have greatly shortened recovery time and reduced surgical complications.

See also Sciatica.

---

# Smoking

Smoking usually begins as a social behavior and results in significant physical consequences to the body. Cigarette smoke is much more hazardous in this regard than pipe or cigar smoke. Cigarette smoking is habit-forming, and the accumulated effects increase the risks for development of life-threatening disease.

The chemical makeup of cigarette smoke is complicated and still under scientific investigation. Nevertheless, it is clear that one of the chemicals in tobacco is tar, a powerful carcinogen (cancer-causing agent). Another chemical, nicotine, produces harmful effects on the nervous system. Various chemicals in tobacco interfere with other biochemical processes and body functions.

Smoking cigarettes, pipes, and cigars and chewing smokeless tobacco have been linked to oral cancers. Oral cancers include those of the mouth, lips, salivary glands, tongue, and throat. Symptoms of oral cancers include a persistent sore, which may bleed; a thickened area; discoloration; difficulty in chewing or swallowing; and persistent sore throat. Such symptoms should be called to a physician's attention immediately.

Cigarette smoking has also been implicated in lung cancer. Initially, cigarette smoke may destroy the tiny hairs that normally function in clearing away mucus in the respiratory tract. The bronchial lining may then undergo changes that result in cancer-cell production. Early symptoms of lung cancer may include coughing, wheezing, and chest pain. Anyone with a history of smoking should be alert to these symptoms. If you have not smoked cigarettes, your chances of developing lung cancer are very greatly reduced. If you do smoke, stopping will decrease your risk of developing lung cancer.

Emphysema and chronic bronchitis are most often caused by smoking. Both of these diseases are considered chronic obstructive pulmonary diseases, in which airways are blocked. Emphysema and chronic bronchitis frequently coexist. In emphysema, abnormally large amounts of air accumulate in the air sacs of the lungs, making exhalation especially difficult. In chronic bronchitis, the bronchi (large airways) undergo changes that impede the flow of air into the lungs.

The initial symptom of emphysema is shortness of breath. This may be accompanied by a persistent cough. Progression of the disease, usually occurring over a course of years, results in severe breathing difficulty and restriction of activity. In chronic bronchitis, a persistent cough develops initially and is usually accompanied by excessive production of mucus. If you experience shortness of breath or develop a persistent cough, consult your physician. Stopping smoking will generally provide the best means of slowing the course of these diseases in smokers. Fortunately, emphysema and chronic bronchitis can usually be prevented by avoiding cigarette smoking.

Stopping smoking can also significantly reduce the incidence of arteriosclerosis, in which the walls of the arteries thicken and lose elasticity. This condition is associated with heart attacks and strokes.

Smoking can also produce indirect adverse reactions in the body. Chemicals in smoke can interfere with the action of some medications by altering the absorption rate and duration of effect. Always mention your smoking habits to the physician when drugs are being prescribed. The physician will then be able to make the proper adjustments in dosage.

Nonsmokers who continuously breathe the cigarette smoke of others are known as passive smokers. Research indicates that passive smokers suffer ill effects from exposure to cigarette smoke, including increased heart rates and blood pressure levels in addition to constriction of the airways in the lungs. Children are especially vulnerable to the respiratory effects of breathing "second-hand" smoke.

Stopping smoking is beneficial to yourself and to those around you, even if there are not yet any signs of disease. (Never starting is even better.) Unfortunately, despite the proven medical risks of tobacco use, many smokers who want to quit seem unable to break the habit. For those who cannot do it on their own, help is available from many sources, such as the American Cancer Society.

Nicotine in the form of gum has been on the market for several years.

Since nicotine is a dangerous drug, the gum is available only by physician's prescription. The gum can ease the physical symptoms of withdrawal from nicotine while the individual removes cigarettes from his or her routine. However, certain people with medical conditions such as heart or blood pressure problems may not be able to use the preparation. Furthermore, it must be remembered that nicotine is a drug. Therefore, directions for use of nicotine gum must be strictly adhered to.

Many over-the-counter preparations are also available as nicotine substitutes. It is best to check with your doctor prior to using one of these. The purpose of such preparations is to make quitting smoking less unpleasant, not to substitute one habit for another.

If you want to try quitting by yourself, it may help first to figure out why you smoke and then to substitute other activities or substances when you feel the urge to light up. The motivation for smoking may be addiction, habit, a response to anxiety, a need to have something to do with the mouth and hands, or a desire for stimulation or relaxation.

There is no single method for quitting smoking that is right for everyone. Ex-smokers have quit in a variety of ways. If one plan fails, try another; if you don't succeed the first time, keep trying. Remember, smoking is a learned behavior that can be changed.

See also Atherosclerosis, Bronchitis, Cancer, Emphysema, and Lung Cancer.

# Sore throat

A sore throat is a painful irritation in the throat, often a symptom of the common cold. A sore throat can range from mild scratchiness to severe pain and difficulty in swallowing.

A sore throat is most frequently seen as a symptom of the common cold, when the nasal passages are congested and the person is forced to breath through the mouth, leaving the throat dry and irritated. Coughing may also irritate the throat, as will the secretions that drain into the throat from the back of the nose during a cold.

Irritating environmental substances, such as smoke, pollen, pollution, and dust, can cause a sore throat when inhaled; also, soreness of the throat may result when hot liquids or foods are swallowed.

A severe sore throat may be caused by a bacterial (frequently streptococcal) infection of the throat, middle ear, nose, or sinuses. Left untreated, a certain type of strep throat can lead to rheumatic fever (a disease that can affect the heart valves) or to glomerulonephritis (a disease of the kidneys).

A sore throat is characterized by dryness and scratchiness in the throat and pain when swallowing. A doctor should be notified if a sore throat lasts more than several days, if it occurs without a cold, or if no obvious irritant can be found; these circumstances may indicate a serious disease, a blood disorder, or a severe infection. If a sore throat is accompanied by fever, achiness, and fatigue, or if the throat and mouth are very red or covered with yellow or white spots, a bacterial infection may be present, and appropriate cultures should be obtained. A recently developed screening test allows the physician to diagnose a streptococcal infection (strep throat) within minutes of testing.

A simple sore throat accompanying a cold is treated by relieving the other cold symptoms. A nasal decongestant may be used if the nose is congested. A cough suppressant may be used if coughing is irritating the throat; cough suppressants are not always recommended, however, because they allow mucus to accumulate and thus may trigger further complications. Sour, hard candy can stimulate saliva production, which will moisten the throat. Frequent gargling with warm salt water soothes the irritated tissues of the throat by reducing swelling.

If a strep infection is the cause of the sore throat, antibiotics are prescribed to prevent rheumatic fever and to fight the infection and aspirin or an aspirin substitute, such as acetaminophen, is prescribed to relieve pain and fever.

See also Rheumatic fever.

# Spastic colon

See Irritable bowel syndrome.

# Spina bifida

Spina bifida is a congenital (present at birth) defect of development, marked by defective closure of some of the vertebrae (the bones of the spine) that normally encase the spinal cord. If the meninges (the membranes that cover the brain and spinal cord) protrude as a sac through the gap in the spine, the condition is known as spina bifida cystica; if not, it is called spina bifida occulta. The severity of the defect can range all the way from a form with few visible symptoms to a completely open spine.

The cause of spina bifida is unknown.

Spina bifida commonly affects the chest and lower back regions of the spine and extends for three to six segments of the spinal column. If there is a sac, it may collapse while the

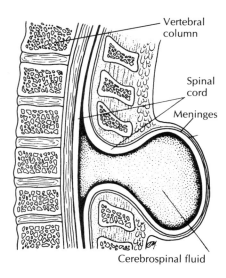

Vertebral column

Spinal cord

Meninges

Cerebrospinal fluid

Spina bifida cystica is a defect of development in which there is defective closure of the bony encasement of the spinal cord, allowing the meninges (membranes surrounding the brain and spinal cord) to protrude as a sac through the opening.

child is still in the uterus, but it fills with cerebrospinal fluid soon after birth. If the sac is not covered with skin, it can rupture, perhaps leading to meningitis (inflammation of the meninges).

Spina bifida can be accompanied by varying degrees of paralysis, depending on the extent of involvement of the spinal cord and its nerve roots. The paralysis can lead to orthopedic problems, such as clubfoot and dislocated hip, and may also affect the sphincters (closure muscles) of the bladder and rectum, resulting in genitourinary disorders. Abnormal curvature of the spine can hinder surgical closure. Hydrocephalus (accumulation of cerebrospinal fluid within the skull) also accompanies many cases of spina bifida.

Diagnostic evaluation of the condition begins with X rays of the spine, skull, hips, and lower extremities. Urine tests are also necessary. The need for further tests depends on the extent of the defect. Such tests may include a computed tomography scan and an evaluation of the cerebrospinal fluid.

Treatment requires an extensive evaluation of the child's condition by neurosurgeons, urologists, orthopedists, and pediatricians. In some cases, social service workers and psychiatrists will work with the parents. Closure of the defect ensures a better outcome. Long-term survival and quality of life depend on the type and extent of the spinal defect, other defects present, the infant's general health, and treatment resources. In addition to surgical closure of the spine, the infant may need other surgery to correct accompanying problems. The most common complications are loss of kidney function, clubfoot, dislocation of the hip joints, scoliosis (curvature of the spine), pressure sores, and muscle weakness and spasm.

There is no known preventive for spina bifida. Prenatal (before birth) diagnosis through amniocentesis is growing progressively more accurate.

See also Hydrocephalus.

# Stomach cancer

The incidence of stomach cancer has decreased by 50 percent in the last 25 years. A change in diet may account for this. Stomach cancer is more common in men than in women and usually occurs between the ages of 50 and 70. The high-risk group includes those with a history of pernicious anemia or alcoholism and those who choose a diet rich in smoked, pickled, or salted foods.

The symptoms of stomach cancer are similar to those of peptic ulcer (heartburn and abdominal discomfort), which makes diagnosis more difficult. It may not be until the disease

is well advanced that the identifying symptoms of bloody stools or vomit appear. A special X-ray study may be obtained after the patient swallows barium (a contrast substance that coats the lining of the stomach), which allows visualization of irregularities in the stomach (such as the presence of a tumor) on X-ray films. If a tumor is identified, a flexible, lighted, tubelike instrument called an endoscope may be inserted down the throat into the stomach to examine the tumor more closely and perhaps obtain a biopsy specimen of it.

Surgery is the most effective treatment of this disease, but only about ten percent of victims survive more than five years after diagnosis. Surgery is most useful when the tumor has not begun to spread. It is sometimes necessary to remove all or part of the stomach. After such surgery, the patient will be required to follow a modified diet.

See also Cancer.

# Strabismus

Strabismus is commonly referred to as "squint-eye" or "cross-eye." Technically, the term refers to a deviation of one eye from being parallel with the other.

In most cases, strabismus is congenital (present at birth), although it can result from later injury to one eye or impaired vision because of disease. The cause of congenital strabismus is unknown, but the effect is generally paralysis or malfunction of the tiny muscles that control the movement of the eyes.

Symptoms include obviously crossed, wandering, or squinting eyes, although in some cases lack of parallelism of the eyes is so subtle that it can be detected only by special testing.

The eyes shown above are properly aligned, while the eyes below exhibit strabismus and are not parallel. When a light is shined into the eyes, the highlight should normally be on the same spot in each eye.

Complete evaluation of the eyes is essential to rule out more serious eye or nervous disorders and to determine how best to correct the strabismus. Such a test is usually done by an ophthalmologist (a physician who specializes in eye disorders).

If muscle imbalance alone is responsible, the strabismus can usually be treated easily with corrective glasses or contact lenses. Eye exercises are effective in many less severe cases. Surgical restoration of the muscle balance can be done in more extreme cases. Permanent visual loss can result if strabismus is not treated by the time the child is four to six years old.

See also Amblyopia.

# Stroke

Stroke is a nervous-system disorder of abrupt onset caused by interruption of the blood supply to an area of the brain, resulting in malfunction or loss of function in those parts of the body that the damaged area controls. Generally speaking, each side of the brain controls the motor and sensory functions of the opposite side of the body (for example, damage to cells on the left side of the brain will impair function on the right side of the body). Stroke can have a wide range of consequences, among them temporary or permanent loss of memory and difficulty in speaking, walking, and controlling emotions.

Stroke can be caused by several conditions. One is called cerebrovascular embolism, which occurs when a blood clot formed elsewhere in the body (usually in the heart or in one of the carotid arteries in the neck) lodges itself in an artery in the brain or leading to the brain. Interruption of blood flow also occurs when a clot is formed in the arteries that supply blood to the brain, usually due to atherosclerosis (clogging of the arteries).

Stroke can also be caused by cerebral hemorrhage, in which a diseased artery in the brain bursts, depriving the cells that are normally nourished by that artery and flooding the surrounding tissue with blood. This accumulation of blood forms a clot, which displaces and compresses brain tissue and thus interferes with brain function. This type of stroke often afflicts people who have both hypertension (high blood pressure) and atherosclerosis.

A third condition that can lead to stroke is rupture of an aneurysm (a bulge in an artery because of a defect in its wall), which interrupts blood flow to an area of the brain and floods the area with blood. The formation of aneurysms is sometimes associated with hypertension. Congenital (present at birth) aneurysms are often the cause of cerebral hemorrhage in young people.

People who have both hypertension and atherosclerosis are the most likely to suffer a stroke, since both diseases weaken and damage the arteries. Hypertension probably also encourages hemorrhage. Heredity may play a role in stroke, since the

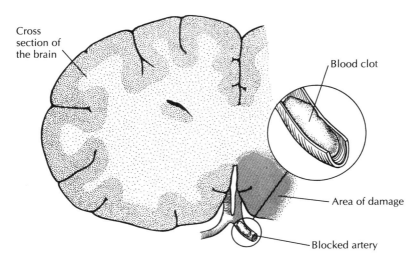

A stroke is caused by an interruption in the blood supply to an area of the brain.

tendencies to develop both hypertension and atherosclerosis appear to be inherited. Black persons are more susceptible to stroke because high blood pressure is about twice as common in the black population as in the white population.

Smoking, diabetes, and high blood cholesterol levels may also contribute to stroke. Stroke is more likely to occur if there is a history of mild strokelike episodes called transient ischemic attacks (TIAs), which are like mild strokes that clear up within 24 hours, leaving no residual effects.

A stroke can present itself in many ways, but some of the more common symptoms are sudden weakness or numbness in the face, arm, and leg on one side of the body; loss or slurring of speech or difficulty in understanding others; unexplained unsteadiness; and persistent falling to one side. It is possible to suffer a mild stroke and experience minor degrees of these symptoms.

Stroke is diagnosed mostly from the history and physical examination. Sophisticated X-ray techniques are also employed. For example, angiog-

raphy will show damage or clots in the arteries in the brain or leading to the brain. In this procedure, a thin catheter is inserted into an artery in the arm or leg and advanced to the site to be studied; a special dye is then injected through the catheter to outline the area so that X rays may be taken. Computed tomography will provide cross-sectional images that may indicate whether the stroke was caused by a hemorrhage or by blockage of blood flow. Tumors, which can cause symptoms identical to those of stroke, are also frequently diagnosed by these means.

Treatment of stroke begins with immediate hospitalization. Blood pressure is normalized, and drug therapy to prevent further damage, as well as to reduce swelling of the brain tissue, is often begun. Anticoagulants (drugs that inhibit the normal clotting of blood) are sometimes administered in the hope of limiting the progress of the stroke or preventing additional strokes. After the acute period, rehabilitation is begun by speech, physical, and occupational therapists. For those who have experienced TIAs or other warning signs of stroke, precautions can be taken to prevent an actual stroke. After a TIA, some form of angiography (also called arteriography) is usually performed to locate obstructions or ulcerated areas of the arteries supplying blood to the head. Depending on the results of the angiogram, the general condition of the patient, and many other factors, surgery to "clean out" the arteries or treatment with anticoagulants or other medications may be elected.

Prevention of stroke mainly involves control of high blood pressure and other risk factors, such as smoking and high cholesterol intake.

See also Aneurysm, Atherosclerosis, and Transient ischemic attack.

---

# Sty

A sty is an inflamed or infected swelling of the sebaceous (oil-producing) glands in the eyelid.

The infection is commonly caused by *Staphylococcus* bacteria. An external sty appears on the surface of the skin at the edge of the eyelid. An internal sty is due to inflammation, infection, or obstruction of a sebaceous gland on the inner surface of the eyelid. This type of sty is often seen as a protrusion or lump on the eyelid without visible pus or redness.

Initially, a sty feels like a foreign object in the eye. Tearing, redness, swelling, and tenderness in or around a particular area of the eye soon follow. The eye may be sensitive to light and touch. In addition, pustules (small, yellow bumps filled with pus) may develop. These pustules often burst, release the pus, and begin to heal. Once the pressure has been released, the pain usually subsides.

Treatment for a sty often involves antibiotic eyedrops or ointments. Applying warm, moist compresses to the eye for about ten minutes three or four times a day may encourage the sty to burst. In some cases, particularly if there is an internal sty, surgical opening may be needed to cure the condition. One should never attempt to open a sty on his or her own, because the risks of spreading and worsening the infection are quite high.

A sty is an inflamed or infected swelling of the sebaceous (oil-producing) glands of the eyelid. An external sty appears on the surface of the skin at the edge of the eyelid.

---

# Sudden infant death syndrome (SIDS)

Sudden infant death syndrome (also called crib death) is the unexplained and sudden death of a baby—often, the baby is perfectly well when put to bed but dies silently during sleep. In the United States, SIDS is second only to accidents as a cause of death in infants from two weeks to one year of age, causing 8,000 to 10,000 deaths per year. Most deaths from SIDS occur in the third or fourth month of life, with higher death rates for boys, children of teenage mothers, infants from poor families, and babies who were premature. Cigarette smoking by the mother during pregnancy appears to be one of the biggest risk factors for SIDS, and the use of drugs such as cocaine or heroin during pregnancy also places the child at increased risk. More deaths from SIDS occur in the winter than in the summer.

It once was thought that SIDS is caused by smothering in the bedding, but this is untrue. It is also not attributable to clogging of the airways by vomited food, to bottle feeding, or to any other cause that parents could prevent. Some investigators believe that a combination of conditions is necessary to trigger SIDS, including a narrowed and inflamed airway, temporary airway obstruction, chronic oxygen deficiency, and irregular breathing, leading to a spasm of the trachea (windpipe) and death. Research continues.

Parents who lose a child to SIDS are totally unprepared for the death and usually have overwhelming guilt feelings—that something they did or did not do caused the death of their child. An autopsy will usually prove that the death was not the parents' fault. Doctors and nurses who take the time to discuss the death fully with the parents can be very helpful. So can another parent who has lost a child to SIDS. There are now many local chapters of the National Sudden Infant Death Syndrome Foundation and the International Council for Infant Survival, both of which can be valuable sources of counseling and information.

# Sunburn

Sunburn is an inflammation of the cells of the skin caused by overexposure to the ultraviolet radiation of the sun or a sunlamp. Damage to the skin can be either insignificant or serious, depending on the intensity of the light source, the length of exposure, and the sensitivity of the individual to ultraviolet radiation.

Sunburn is caused by overexposure to ultraviolet radiation. Certain substances (such as deodorants, soaps, perfumes, cosmetics, and certain medications) may produce heightened sensitivity to ultraviolet radiation, with a corresponding increase in the severity of the burn. While light-skinned people usually burn more easily than dark-skinned people, skin color is not always a dependable guide to individual susceptibility.

Irritation of the skin and a prickling sensation mark the onset of sunburn; the skin also feels hot to the touch. Capillaries (tiny blood vessels) in the skin become congested because of the release of certain inflammatory agents, thus producing the characteristic redness. Oral contraceptive users may develop irregularly shaped dark splotches, and some sensitive individuals may have allergic reactions in the form of rashes or welts.

As the burn progresses in severity, the skin will feel tight, swollen, and dry or brittle and may become hypersensitive to touch. Overheating and loss of fluids through the damaged skin may also produce dizziness, nausea, vomiting, hyperventilation (rapid breathing, which causes excessive loss of carbon dioxide from the blood), impaired vision and hearing, irregular heartbeat, and loss of consciousness.

The aftermath of severe sunburn often includes blistering and peeling, as well as permanent freckling, splotching, or scarring of the skin. Long-term effects may include premature skin aging, marked by chronic dryness, wrinkling, leathery texture, and loss of elasticity. In some cases, melanoma (a form of skin cancer) may be induced by chronic overexposure to sunlight.

Minor sunburn can be effectively treated by a wide variety of nonprescription ointments, oils, powders, creams, and sprays that restore fluids and prevent further drying, relieve discomfort, and promote healing. Many over-the-counter medications contain mild anesthetics to relieve stinging and suppress the desire to scratch itching areas. One of the most common complications is the infection of blistered and peeling areas of the skin. This condition should be treated by a physician.

In the case of severe sunburn, overheating and dehydration (loss of too much fluid) must be avoided. The victim should be taken out of the sun immediately and placed in a cool, shaded area until medical attention can be obtained. Cool (but not cold), wet cloths can be applied to the arms, the head, and the legs. Chills should be avoided. Ice water and other cold drinks may trigger unwanted responses. If the victim is perspiring profusely, a fan may help evaporate the water on the skin's surface, thus aiding a natural cooling process.

The best prevention of sunburn is simply to avoid prolonged exposure to the direct rays of the sun or a sunlamp. When this is not possible (because of one's occuption, for example) the first line of defense is to cover the skin completely, preferably with loose-fitting, light-colored clothes made of loose-weave fabrics. Wearing a wide-brimmed hat will also help.

The second line of defense is a sunscreen, available as an oil, cream, paste, or liquid. Most sunscreens are intended to block ultraviolet rays. Many contain para-aminobenzoic acid (PABA). This compound may affect some individuals adversely, particularly those with photosensitivity (abnormal sensitivity of the skin to light) who are taking certain drugs. For these people, opaque (light-blocking) creams, pastes, and lotions are available, as well as other chemical sunscreens known as benzophenones. Anyone who is uncertain about a possible interaction between sunlight and a medication that has been prescribed should contact his or her doctor before exposure to sunlight.

# Syphilis

Syphilis is a serious, highly contagious disease spread primarily by direct sexual contact. Syphilis is caused by spiral-shaped bacteria called spirochetes.

Over time, syphilis can affect all parts of the body—the brain, bones, spinal cord, and heart, as well as the reproductive organs. If left untreated, blindness, brain damage, heart disease, and even death can result. Syphilis can also be passed from a mother to her unborn baby, causing congenital syphilis in the child, which may eventually result in blindness and deafness, among other serious consequences. Syphilis in a pregnant woman must be treated prior to the eighteenth week of the pregnancy in order to prevent passage of the disease to the fetus.

Syphilis is a progressive disorder that passes through three stages: primary, secondary, and tertiary.

Primary syphilis is characterized by the appearance of a painless, open sore (called a chancre) 10 to 90 days after exposure to the disease. As a rule, there is usually only one sore, appearing most commonly on the genital organs, but also at times on the rectum, cervix, lips, tongue, fingers, or anywhere that direct contact was made. The chancre first appears as a red bump, sometimes surround-

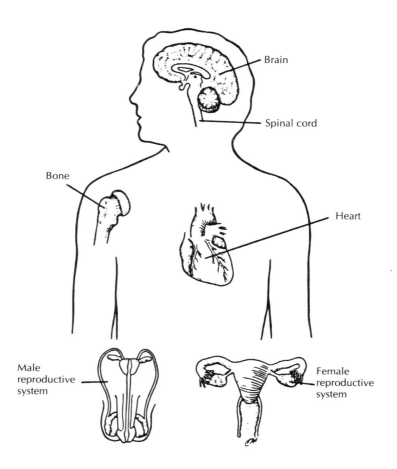

In its final stages, syphilis can seriously damage the brain, spinal cord, bones, heart, and reproductive organs.

ed by a red ring that oozes clear fluid; it soon turns into a painless ulcer and disappears within several weeks without treatment. Although the chancre is gone, the disease is still active in the body.

Secondary syphilis usually appears within six weeks to six months of initial contact. Symptoms resembling those of the flu (fever, sore throat, headache, fatigue, aching joints, and enlarged lymph nodes) are common. Secondary syphilis is also characterized by extremely contagious, red or reddish-brown erosions that can be seen on the lining of the mouth, the penis, the external female sex organs,

the anus, and warm, moist areas, such as the underarms. Other symptoms of secondary syphilis include growths resembling warts in the genital area (not to be confused with the more common nonsyphilitic genital warts) and a rash on the palms of the hands or the soles of the feet in the form of round, reddish spots that occur in patches and do not itch. These sores, growths, and rashes heal within three to six weeks without treatment, and the disease enters the third stage.

At the beginning of the third stage, all symptoms disappear and the disease becomes latent (present but not showing symptoms) for a time. The patient appears to be healthy, and the disease is probably no longer contagious (except in the case of pregnant women, who can still pass it on to their offspring). This latent stage of syphilis can last indefinitely, but in about one third of patients the disease will most likely progress, and the entire body may come under siege. The brain, bones, spinal cord, and heart may be affected, with the result that blindness, brain damage, heart disease, or even death could occur.

Syphilis is diagnosed on the basis of the patient's medical and sexual history and findings from the physical examination, blood tests, and microscopic examination of a sample taken from the sores or rash areas. Several blood tests may be necessary because evidence of infection may not show up on blood tests during the first one to two weeks after exposure to the infection.

Treatment of syphilis is accomplished with the administration of penicillin (or another antibiotic, if the patient happens to be allergic to penicillin). Some cases of late syphilis are so advanced, however, that they cannot be treated.

A person who has syphilis or any other sexually transmitted disease should abstain from sexual activity until all tests have confirmed that the disease is no longer contagious. Every sexual partner of the infected person needs to be tested and, if necessary, treated.

Syphilis can be prevented by avoiding sexual contact with someone who has the disease. Because the chances of contracting this or any other sexually transmitted disease increase with the number of sexual partners a person has, limiting the number of partners is the first step toward prevention. Using condoms also helps to reduce the risk of contracting syphilis.

# T

# Tay-Sachs disease

Tay-Sachs disease is a hereditary metabolic disorder that chiefly afflicts infants of eastern European Jewish descent. This disease is fatal, usually by the age of four years. It is marked by retarded development, loss of vision, and paralysis.

The disease is caused by a deficiency of a certain digestive enzyme. This deficiency results in the accumulation of fatty acids in the brain.

The symptoms of Tay-Sachs disease in an infant are most often noted after four to six months of normal development. A previously well infant begins to lose motor coordination skills that had been attained and to exhibit loss of interest in his or her surroundings. As the condition becomes more advanced, seizures occur, and the head becomes considerably enlarged.

The physician may notice poor muscle tone and an exaggerated startle response to sound. A distinctive cherry-red spot may be seen in the retina of the eye. The diagnosis is confirmed with special blood tests.

Diagnosis of the disorder may be made before birth by amniocentesis, a procedure in which a small amount of amniotic fluid is removed.

There is no known treatment for Tay-Sachs disease, other than supportive care.

There is a blood test available that will help identify carriers of the defective gene. (A carrier has the defective gene but does not have the disease.) This test is especially recommended for all Jews of reproductive age. If two carriers have children, each child conceived has a one in four chance of having the disease. It is, therefore, a good idea for carriers to seek genetic counseling before starting their families.

# Tendinitis

Tendinitis is an inflammation of a tendon (a band of fibrous tissue connecting muscle to bone). The condition appears most often as a result of physical activity. It also can be a symptom of a more generalized inflammatory disease, such as rheumatoid arthritis.

Improper activity, lack of conditioning, and poor athletic equipment encourage the development of tendinitis. Nonathletes who suddenly begin long-distance jogging or another athletic activity and athletes who resume strenuous sports after a period of inactivity are especially susceptible. In addition, people who wear shoes with run-down heels put needless tension on the Achilles tendon, which joins the two major muscles on the back of the leg to the back of the heel bone. Similarly, women who wear high-heel shoes may have problems with inflamed Achilles tendons because the extreme stress created by the shoes considerably strains the tendons.

Tendinitis causes pain in the affected tendon, which is worsened by activity. The tendon may grow thicker than normal and be tender to the touch or very painful. When minor injuries are continually placed under stress, an already inflamed tendon can rupture and become a greater problem.

Physicians diagnose tendinitis problems by first acquiring an exercise history to determine the patient's normal activity and to identify any changes in routine. Muscle lengths in

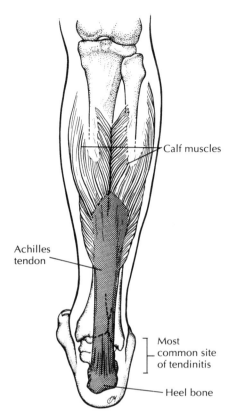

Tendinitis frequently occurs in the Achilles tendon, which connects the calf muscles to the heel bone.

the area of inflammation are also evaluated because unusually short or inflexible muscles are often the cause of tendinitis.

Treatment for tendinitis begins with resting the affected area. Pain relievers and anti-inflammatory drugs are used to ease immediate symptoms, but they will not by themselves cure the condition or keep it from recurring. Injecting cortisone and a local anesthetic into the area surrounding the tendon usually provides substantial relief within 24 to 72 hours.

In rare cases, surgery is necessary to repair damaged tendons. In the past, tendons were replaced with artificial tissues that never achieved the strength and flexibility of natural tissues. More effective techniques and materials have since been developed.

People participating in sports can prevent tendinitis by taking time for warm-up prior to exercise. For example, stretching the leg and calf muscles before and after running may help prevent inflammation of the Achilles tendon.

Wearing supports in shoes during physical activity can correct instability of the foot and lessen pain when tendinitis does occur.

# Testes, undescended

See Undecended testes.

# Tetanus

Tetanus is an infectious disease, commonly associated with improperly cleaned deep wounds, that causes severe muscle contractions.

Tetanus is caused by toxins (poisonous substances) that are produced by *Clostridium tetani* bacteria. These bacteria may be present on the skin at the time of the injury or may enter the body through a wound caused by an object that has been in contact with material, such as soil, in which bacterial spores are present. Puncture wounds and animal bites, because of their depth, are especially vulnerable to tetanus infection since they are difficult to clean and medicate.

Tetanus symptoms are varied, depending on the extent of the infection and the body part that is affected. A common symptom is lockjaw, in which the muscles of the jaw go into severe, continuous contraction, thus rendering the jaw immobile. Other symptoms include bowing or arching of the body (a rare occurrence) because of contraction of lower back muscles, back muscle spasms, and throat spasms, which can cause blockage of the airway. The affected body parts become immobile because of the simultaneous and continuous contraction of opposing muscle groups.

In severe cases, the contractions involve most of the fibers in an affected muscle, similar to what would be required to lift a heavy weight or to marshal all the potential force of a muscle against a great resistance. Such violent and prolonged muscle contractions can be very painful.

Treatment includes muscle relaxant drugs, such as diazepam, to ease the contractions. Antimicrobial drugs, such as penicillin, are used to fight the infection. Tetanus antitoxin is injected intramuscularly (into a muscle) in the hope of lessening the severity of the disease. However, the antitoxin does not counteract the toxin already in the nervous system, nor does it act to relieve symptoms already present.

Immunization with the tetanus vaccine is the best preventive against the disease. Infants begin at two months of age to receive the initial series of tetanus shots combined with diphtheria and whooping cough. Boosters are given at 18 months and five years and then every ten years after that through adulthood. Also, wounds should be attended to immediately, especially puncture wounds and animal bites. It is especially important that the tetanus booster be administered periodically if small skin wounds are a common occurrence in the course of the workday.

# Throat

See Ear, nose, and throat.

# Thrombocytopenia

Thrombocytopenia is a disorder characterized by a decrease in the number of platelets in the blood. Platelets are tiny components of the blood that act to promote clotting when there is an injury or another problem that requires bleeding to be stopped. Normally, about five to ten times the number of platelets needed for clotting circulate in the bloodstream; this amounts to about 200,000 to 500,000 per milliliter. In general, thrombocytopenia is considered to be present when the platelet count is less than 100,000. Abnormal bleeding commonly does not occur, however, until the count is less than 50,000, and serious or unprovoked bleeding usually does not occur with counts above 20,000.

There are basically two mechanisms whereby thrombocytopenia occurs: decreased production of platelets and increased destruction of platelets. In the former, the elements in the bone marrow responsible for the production of platelets may malfunction or be severely diminished. Increased destruction of platelets occurs in essential, or idiopathic (of unknown cause), thrombocytopenia. In this disorder, which is most common in children, antibodies are made against the person's own platelets, thereby causing their destruction. Thrombocytopenia can also be due to the use of some medications. Severe, overwhelming infection can also cause increased destruction of platelets. In pregnancy, platelets from the fetus can sometimes enter the circulation of the mother, causing antibody formation and the consequent destruction of fetal platelets, with abnormal bleeding at birth.

An obvious sign of thrombocytopenia is a rash of reddish to reddish-purple spots. These are due to bleeding within and underneath the skin. Abnormal or easily provoked bleeding is the most dangerous symptom of thrombocytopenia. This bleeding may be minor, such as oozing from the gums while brushing the teeth or bruising caused by merely leaning on or brushing up against something. The bleeding can be much more serious, however, as in spontaneous internal bleeding, which may go unrecognized until the person goes into shock (collapse of the circulatory system).

Laboratory evaluation of the blood is the basis of a diagnosis of thrombocytopenia. Examination of a sample of bone marrow may also be performed.

Treatment depends on the cause. If infection is present, this must be remedied; usually, the platelet count will then return to normal on its own. In essential thrombocytopenia, corticosteroids (cortisone or prednisone) are the initial treatment. In drug-induced thrombocytopenia, the first step is generally to discontinue the drug. This will usually result in improvement; if not, corticosteroids may be helpful. In severe immune thrombocytopenia of the newborn, exchange transfusion (whereby all or most of the blood is exchanged with transfused blood) may be necessary. If the platelet count in any of these conditions is dangerously low (around 20,000 per milliliter), transfusion of platelets may be indicated until the disease process has been brought under control.

Thrombocytopenia may not be preventable in most cases. Nevertheless, the recognition of symptoms, such as rash and easy bleeding, at an early stage of the disorder, may lead to prevention of serious complications.

See also Platelets.

# Thrombophlebitis

Thrombophlebitis is a condition in which both inflammation and blood clots exist in a vein. This can be caused by a number of factors. Commonly, when a person is immobilized, blood stagnates in the veins of the legs; this induces clotting, which in turn prevents blood from returning to the heart. The blood below the clot remains there, causing a buildup of pressure that forces fluid into the tissues, resulting in swelling. Simultaneously, the veins and surrounding area may become quite inflamed and tender. This condition is most often found in the deep veins of the legs, but it can also occur in veins of the pelvis and arms.

Thrombophlebitis itself may not be too serious, but it can lead to a life-threatening condition called pulmonary embolism if a blood clot formed in a deep leg vein breaks loose, travels through the bloodstream, and becomes lodged in a blood vessel in the lung. Pulmonary embolism can lead to chest pain, shortness of breath, coughing up of blood, and even death.

The development of thrombophlebitis is favored by any condition that inhibits the free flow of blood through the veins, such as prolonged bed rest or inactivity, perhaps following illness or surgery; congestive heart failure, which affects the ability of the heart to pump blood throughout the body; and injury or infection that damages a vein. Other factors that may lead to an increased tendency toward thrombophlebitis are pregnancy, the use of birth control pills by susceptible individuals, occupations that require long periods of standing or sitting, obesity, old age, and chronic infections. In some cases, thrombophlebitis may indicate the presence of a blood disorder or a tumor in the pancreas or lung.

Symptoms of deep-vein thrombophlebitis (which often appear only in advanced cases) are swelling, aching, and a feeling of heaviness in the leg or affected area. The skin may appear white and will be painful to the touch. If the veins of the leg are affected, the condition is characterized by increased pain when walking or when the foot is flexed backward or forward.

Thrombophlebitis of a surface vein (known as superficial thrombophlebitis) can be diagnosed by a simple physical examination, which usually reveals a red, warm, tender cordlike vein.

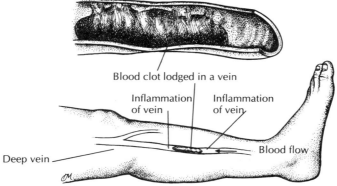

Blood clot lodged in a vein

Inflammation of vein

Inflammation of vein

Deep vein

Blood flow

Thrombophlebitis (inflammation of a vein accompanied by the formation of a blood clot) often occurs in the deep veins of the legs. The condition is suspected if moving the foot forward or backward causes pain.

Diagnostic tests for thrombophlebitis include Doppler imaging (a technique used to detect obstructions by changes in the sounds made by flowing blood), nuclear medicine scans, plethysmography (a test to measure the resistance to blood flow in the veins), and venography. Venography involves the injection of a special dye into the veins so that a clot, if present, will be visualized on an X ray. This is the most sensitive and specific test for thrombophlebitis. Ultrasound imaging is also quite accurate and virtually risk free; however, it does not replace venography.

Treatment of the superficial form of thrombophlebitis begins with bed rest with elevation of the leg. Warm compresses are also helpful, as are anti-inflammatory drugs. Superficial thrombophlebitis rarely, if ever, leads to pulmonary embolism.

Deep-vein thrombophlebitis, because of the potential for pulmonary embolism, is treated much more aggressively. The patient is usually hospitalized and put on bed rest with the leg elevated. Heparin (an anticoagulant, which inhibits the normal clotting mechanism of the blood) is given intravenously, usually for about seven days (up to ten days if pulmonary embolism has occurred). The patient is also usually given the oral anticoagulant warfarin for about six weeks (three to six months if pulmonary embolism has occurred). These drugs do not dissolve an existing clot, but serve to prevent new clots from forming while the old ones are resolving. Newer drugs do dissolve clots but are still used only in special situations.

Prevention of thrombophlebitis is a controversial subject. In hospitalized patients who are immobilized for long periods or who are about to undergo major surgery, doing leg exercises, wearing long support stockings or compression boots (soft plastic bags or sacks that are wrapped around the legs and rapidly inflated and deflated), and increasing activity as soon as feasible may be helpful. Heparin therapy has also been beneficial in preventing deep-vein thrombophlebitis in certain patients. For nonhospitalized patients who are susceptible to this condition, regularly exercising the legs, elevating the legs when lying down, and wearing support hose may be helpful. Heparin or warfarin may be prescribed.

See also Pulmonary embolism.

# Tic

A tic is a spasmodic movement or twitching that is generally a brief, repetitive, purposeless, semivoluntary or involuntary muscle contraction, most commonly seen in the face, shoulders, or arms.

Tics are caused by involuntary muscle contractions. With the exception of the tics that develop as a result of nerve or brain damage and other specific conditions, however, the physiological basis of most tics is largely unknown. They often accompany emotional upset or some hidden psychological problem. Tics in children may be a sign of Gilles de la Tourette's syndrome, a disorder marked by multiple tics and compulsive use of profane language.

A typical "nervous tic" is a twitching of the corner of the eye or the mouth, grimacing, blinking, or making repetitive motions with the arms or shoulders. Tics in children often occur between the ages of five and ten years and may gradually disappear as the child grows older; however, they can persist into adulthood. When nervous tics first arise, they can usually be voluntarily controlled, but persistent tics often become automatic after a period of time.

Many tics are, at the beginning, hard to distinguish from many neurologically based illnesses.

For mild childhood or adult tics, tranquilizers or muscle relaxants may be prescribed. Gilles de la Tourette's syndrome responds to medication. Psychotherapy may help to relieve the emotional stress that precipitates attacks or intensifies the symptoms of some tics.

See also Gilles de la Tourette's syndrome.

# Tonsillitis

Tonsillitis is an inflammation or infection of the tonsils. It occurs most commonly in children from 5 to 15 years old and only rarely in those under the age of two.

The tonsils are two small, almond-shaped lumps of specialized lymph node tissue located in the throat at the back of the mouth. They are barely visible in infants, increase in size during the preschool and early school years, and shrink by adulthood.

The function of the tonsils has not been pinpointed, but scientists believe that they perform at least two vital jobs: they release antibodies (protective agents) into the throat to prevent infection from spreading into the lungs (a useful service to children, who are highly susceptible to ear, nose, and throat infections); and they attract bacterial infection, thereby stimulating the production of antibodies, which accumulate in the body and are then available to prevent future, and potentially much more serious, infections. (Antibodies normally do not develop unless infection is present.) If the tonsils do indeed perform these two functions, then each attack of tonsillitis may help immunize a child against disease; once resistance has been developed, the function of the tonsils is complete.

There are two types of tonsillitis: acute tonsillitis, in which the infection flares up and then disappears in a short time; and chronic tonsillitis, in which the tonsils seem to be permanently inflamed and have abscesses (pus-filled cavities) on them.

Tonsillitis is caused by many different infectious agents, both viral and bacterial. *Streptococcus* bacterium is the most common bacterial cause; acute tonsillitis is usually a "strep" infection. Chronic tonsillitis, however, is more of a mystery; it is not known why chronic tonsillitis occurs in certain people or what causes it.

The symptoms of acute tonsillitis are a sore throat, fever (up to about 101°F), chills, headache, and muscle aches. These symptoms worsen for one to three days and then subside. Nausea, vomiting, stomachache, and swelling of lymph nodes in the neck may also occur and may last for about a week.

The symptoms of chronic tonsillitis include a persistent or recurrent sore

Tonsils

Infected tonsils are reddened and may have gray or yellow patches.

throat, difficulty in swallowing or breathing, and foul breath.

Tonsillitis is diagnosed by examination of the tonsils for redness, swelling, and the presence of gray or yellow infectious material. The doctor will take a sample of this material with a cotton swab in order to identify the particular organism causing the infection.

Bed rest or reduced activity and the use of antibiotics, often penicillin, are recommended to treat tonsillitis if the inflammation is due to bacteria. Gargling with warm salt water can help relieve sore throat.

Surgical removal of the tonsils (called a tonsillectomy) is performed only if the tonsils are abscessed (filled with pus) or so enlarged that they are blocking the air passages. Tonsillectomies are seldom performed today, because research has found that even when tonsils are enlarged, they almost always shrink over time. Furthermore, removing the tonsils does not necessarily prevent recurrent sore throats and colds, as was once believed.

Complications resulting from tonsillitis seldom occur today because of effective, fast-acting antibiotics; rheumatic fever and infections of the sinuses, ears, and kidneys are rare but possible complications.

Since it is not yet known why some people suffer from chronic tonsillitis, preventive measures have not been established. Because episodes of acute tonsillitis may be useful in the development of immunities in the body, prevention of such episodes may not be appropriate. More research is needed in this area.

# Tooth decay

Tooth decay (dental cavities, or caries) is the gradual process of destruction and mineral loss that affects the enamel (outer layer) and dentin (the bony second layer) of a portion of a tooth, causing it to become soft, discolored, and porous.

A combination of factors causes tooth decay. A substance called plaque, made up of sugars, starches, bacteria, and proteins, builds up on dental surfaces, especially near the gums and in other hard-to-clean areas. The plaque prevents the saliva from performing its natural protective function. The bacteria in the plaque feed on the sugars and starches that cling to the teeth and produce acid as a by-product of their metabolism. That acid is probably the agent of destruction of dental tissue.

When the cavity has progressed into the dentin or the surface of an exposed root, the tooth becomes sensitive to touch and rapid temperature changes. Sweet foods can cause pain as dissolved sugar enters the cavity. Bacteria may pass through tiny channels in the dentin and inflame the pulp, which contains blood vessels and nervous tissue, producing toothache.

The cavity reveals itself to the examining dentist as a darkened area or as an area of softness when probed with a sharp instrument. It is also apparent on X rays.

Cavities are treated by drilling out the decayed material and replacing it with a filling. In front teeth, where appearance is important, the filling may be of porcelain or a plastic resin (which is also used to fill pits and tiny cracks in the enamel). In other teeth, the filling is usually silver-colored or an alloy of gold, which is the most durable material. When a tooth is badly damaged, with involvement of the root, the dentist removes all decay, fills the cavity and root canal with dental cement, then grinds and tapers the outer surface and covers it with what is known as a gold crown.

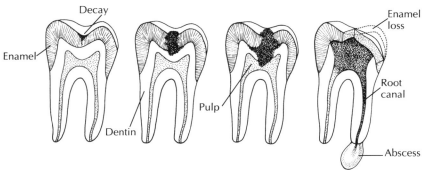

Tooth decay, if untreated, can progress from the surface enamel to the dentin, then to the pulp, and finally through the root canal to form an abscess (pus-filled cavity).

On teeth toward the front, the gold crown is overlaid with porcelain to provide a natural appearance.

To prevent decay, teeth should be cleaned daily with a soft-bristled brush, preferably after each meal, to remove food particles and plaque. Equally important is the use of dental floss to remove debris between the teeth. Avoiding sweet, sticky foods, or at least rinsing or brushing shortly after eating them, may also help prevent decay. A child's teeth will be more resistant to decay if the child drinks water containing the proper amount of fluoride in the first 12 years of life, while the teeth are developing. If the water supply is not fluoridated, a vitamin supplement containing fluoride can be taken daily. Adults and children alike can benefit by using a fluoride-containing toothpaste or mouthwash.

See also Periodontal disease.

# Toxemia of pregnancy

Toxemia of pregnancy is a severe condition that sometimes occurs in the last stage of pregnancy and is characterized by high blood pressure; swelling of the extremities, especially the hands, feet, and ankles; and the presence of protein in the urine. If toxemia is allowed to worsen, convulsions and coma may develop.

The term *toxemia of pregnancy* is actually a misnomer; formerly it was thought that the condition was caused by toxic (poisonous) substances in the blood. The illness is more accurately called preeclampsia before the convulsive stage and eclampsia afterward.

The causes of toxemia of pregnancy are not clearly understood. It tends to be more common among mothers from lower socioeconomic groups. One theory is that dietary deficiencies may be at the root of some cases. Some types of toxemia may be the result of a deficiency of blood flow in the uterus.

Toxemia is divided into three progressively more serious stages, each with its own characteristic symptoms. *Mild preeclampsia* is marked by edema (swelling due to fluid retention), hypertension (high blood pressure), and the presence of protein in the urine. The symptoms of *severe preeclampsia* may include headache, dizziness, fever, drowsiness, tachycardia (abnormally rapid heart rhythm), tinnitus (ringing in the ears), double vision, nausea, vomiting, and scanty or absent urine production. In full-blown *eclampsia*, convulsions may be followed by severe hypotension (low blood pressure) and coma. The condition ultimately leads to death if not treated.

Toxemia cannot be completely cured until the pregnancy is over. Until then, treatment includes stimulation of kidney function, control of high blood pressure and convulsions, and, in severe cases, early delivery of the infant to ensure the survival of the mother.

There is no known preventive for toxemia of pregnancy. The first line of defense is the monitoring of all bodily functions in order to spot symptoms as they begin to appear.

# Toxic shock syndrome

Toxic shock syndrome (TSS) is a rare, sometimes fatal disease that develops very suddenly and progresses rapidly when a bacterial infection spreads through the bloodstream. The disorder was first defined in 1978, when its link to the use of tampons was suspected. Most of the reported cases have occurred in menstruating women under the age of 30 who use tampons. A significant number of these cases have been fatal.

Most researchers believe that TSS occurs when the *Staphylococcus aureus* bacterium enters the bloodstream and produces a toxin (poison) that causes leaks in blood vessel walls, allowing blood to seep into the tissues. This results in a sudden, very dangerous drop in blood pressure; shock; and sometimes death.

In serious cases, low blood pressure and weakening of the cell membranes can leave the victim susceptible to further complications, such as heart and liver damage. Often, the body cannot produce enough antibodies (protective substances) to fight

off the invasion of organisms through the weakened cell membranes, so TSS can easily recur.

Although the use of tampons is considered to be a definite risk factor, tampons do not actually cause the disease but rather promote the growth of bacteria that leads to the disorder. The tampons swell to fill the vagina and thereby inhibit the elimination of blood, creating a breeding ground for infection. Also, if tampons are left in the vagina for long periods of time, the chances for infection are increased. Tampon applicators, moreover, may scratch the walls of the vagina, allowing bacteria to enter.

Since about 25 percent of cases now occur in men and nonmenstruating women, it is clear that the bacteria can enter the body in ways other than through the vagina. In these cases, TSS often occurs when the body has been weakened by major surgery, severe burns, or boils or abscesses. Also, women who have recently given birth are at a higher risk of contracting TSS because the vagina is more susceptible to the invasion of bacteria at this time.

The symptoms of TSS are high fever, vomiting, diarrhea, a rash that looks like sunburn, peeling of skin on the soles of the feet and the palms of the hands, blurred vision, and disorientation.

The occurrence of the high fever, the characteristic rash, low blood pressure, and involvement of several organ systems strongly points to the diagnosis of TSS. Cultures of the blood and mucous membranes will be performed to search for evidence of infection by the *Staphylococcus aureus* bacterium.

Emergency medical treatment should be sought immediately. This will necessitate hospitalization, during which the patient will be given therapy similar to that administered to poisoning victims. Fluids or whole-blood transfusions are given to raise blood pressure, an ice blanket is used to reduce fever, and antibiotics are administered to fight the infection.

The best precaution is probably to discontinue or limit the use of tampons. Tampons can still be worn safely, but they should be changed every three to four hours and alternated with sanitary napkins as often as possible, especially before going to bed.

# Transient ischemic attacks

Transient ischemic attacks (TIAs) are neurologic deficits (such as loss of vision in one eye, inability to speak, paralysis, or weakness of one side of the body) of sudden onset that last for less than 24 hours. Although they are symptomatically similar to minor strokes, they do no discernible lasting damage to brain function.

The major importance of TIAs is their role as a predictor of stroke. When a person describes a "light stroke," it is often a TIA that is meant. If left untreated, TIAs can indeed lead to major strokes, with permanent damage to all affected parts.

TIAs are probably due to a temporary interruption in blood flow to an area of the brain. They can be caused by a narrowing in the carotid arteries (the arteries in the neck that supply the brain with oxygenated blood). This narrowing is usually due to the presence of atherosclerosis (clogging of the arteries). Blood vessel spasms and showers of tiny emboli (clots that travel through the bloodstream) are also possible causes.

The symptoms of TIAs are both varied and frightening to the victim. They can include weakness on one side of the face, numbness in various parts of the body, blindness in one eye, weakness in the arms or legs on one side, difficulty in speaking and understanding speech, and a prickling ("pins and needles") sensation in parts of the body. Vertigo (a sensation of spinning) combined with any of these or other symptoms can also be due to TIAs (this is rare). Fainting spells alone and light-headedness are usually not due to TIAs.

The first step in diagnosis is a complete examination, including a history and physical, neurologic, and eye examinations. Bruits (noises caused by narrowing in an artery) may be heard in a carotid artery. Detailed testing, commonly with angiography (also called arteriography) is performed to pinpoint the problem. In this procedure, a thin catheter is inserted into an artery in the arm or leg and advanced to the site to be studied; a special dye is then injected through the catheter to outline the area so that X rays may be taken. Prior to angiography, an ultrasonic examination of the carotid arteries is usually done to determine if disease (narrowing) is present.

Treatment of TIAs is aimed at preventing more TIAs and, hopefully, stroke. There are two basic methods of treatment: medical, with anticoagulant drugs; and surgical, with the opening and "cleaning out" of the obstructed arteries (endarterectomy). Anticoagulation is usually done with aspirin or heparin and warfarin. Which of these methods—medication or surgery—is more effective in preventing further TIAs or a stroke is dependent on many factors and is a subject of considerable controversy. TIAs can be an indication of more serious problems and must be brought to the attention of a physician immediately.

See also Atherosclerosis and Stroke.

# Traveler's diarrhea

Of all the illnesses likely to afflict travelers to foreign countries, the most common is "traveler's diarrhea." This disorder, an intestinal infection caused by microorganisms to which the traveler is unaccustomed, is characterized by loose, watery stools (bowel movements), often accompanied by nausea and abdominal cramps.

The organism most commonly responsible is probably the *Escherichia coli* (*E. coli*) bacterium. This bacterium is a normal inhabitant of the intestines, but in some areas of the world it has evolved into a strain called enterotoxigenic (poisonous to the intestines) E. coli, or ETEC, which can cause moderate to severe diarrhea. Other organisms that can cause traveler's diarrhea include Campylobacter, Salmonella, and Shigella bacteria; parasitic protozoa (one-celled organisms), such as Entamoeba histolytica (the cause of amoebic dysentery) and Giardia lamblia; and a number of viruses.

The major symptom of the illness is, of course, diarrhea, which can range in intensity from mild (three to four loose, watery stools per day) to severe (10 to 20 bloody stools per day). The severity of traveler's diarrhea is largely dependent on the type of organism that is causing the infection and the health status of the individual. Traveler's diarrhea caused by bacteria usually begins a few days after the beginning of the trip and may last for several days to a few weeks if not properly treated. *Campylobacter* and *Shigella* infections commonly are marked by severe, bloody diarrhea. The diarrhea caused by *Giardia* organisms is usually characterized by abundant stools (rarely blood-tinged) and can be asso-ciated with other symptoms, such as fever, weight loss, and weakness. Traveler's diarrhea caused by protozoa can be mild or very severe, with involvement of other organs, such as the liver.

Knowledge of which foreign countries have been visited recently will help the doctor in making a preliminary diagnosis. Because it is very difficult to differentiate among the various infectious causes of diarrhea, laboratory studies, such as stool cultures and blood tests, are often needed. Parasitic diarrhea is especially difficult to diagnose; occasionally, multiple cultures are necessary, as well as proctosigmoidoscopy (visual examination of the rectum and lower portion of the large intestine with a special instrument).

Prescription antidiarrheal medications are often sought by individuals about to leave on a trip so that they can treat themselves if they suffer some form of traveler's diarrhea. Physicians are justifiably reluctant to prescribe these medications routinely because in many forms of diarrheal illness, such drugs can actually cause complications and prolong the course of the disease. These medications should never be taken except on the advice of a physician.

Mild cases of traveler's diarrhea usually clear up without treatment in a few days. Diarrhea that lasts for more than several days or that is associated with persistent fever or with the presence of blood, pus, or mucus in the stools calls for immediate medical attention.

Much has been written in recent years about prevention of traveler's diarrhea by taking medication before and during the trip. It must be remembered that all medications have potential side effects and that the indiscriminate use of antibiotics and antidiarrheal medications can be dangerous. Except in special circumstances (for example, a person with severe health problems, for whom an episode of severe diarrhea could be catastrophic), routine prophylaxis (preventive treatment) with antibiotics is not recommended.

Because there are no vaccines or universally effective prophylactic drugs to use against traveler's diarrhea, caution should be exercised when eating or drinking in many foreign countries. Avoid unboiled water (and ice made from unboiled water). Be careful of water that you use to brush your teeth, too. Do not assume that bottled water available locally is safe. Lettuce and other fresh vegetables are common culprits. Fruit with intact skin is usually safe if you wash it with safe water and peel it yourself before eating. Beer, wine, and carbonated beverages are usually safe, but it must be remembered that the addition of alcoholic beverages to water does not kill infectious organisms and make such drinks safe. Food obtained from local street vendors should be avoided.

# Trichinosis

Trichinosis is a condition caused by the infestation of the body by *Trichinella spiralis*, a parasitic worm sometimes found in pork.

Trichinosis is most commonly caused by eating pork that has not been cooked for a sufficient length of time or at a sufficiently high temperature to kill the *Trichinella spiralis* worms. The worms are encapsulated in the meat itself. When the meat is eaten, the worms emerge from it and begin their life cycle in the human host. This begins in the small intestine, where the larvae (an immature form of the worms) mature within two days after they emerge from the meat. The adults breed, the males die, and the females produce more larvae, which invade the tissues of the bowel and are then dispersed to muscles throughout the body, where they lodge. The muscles around the eyes, the tongue, and the diaphragm (the muscle separating the chest cavity from the abdomen) and the muscles between the ribs are the most commonly affected.

Quite often, the infested patient is entirely unaware of the presence of trichinosis. When large infestations do occur, however, they are accompanied by symptoms. One to two days after consumption of the contaminated meat, a severe flulike illness consisting of fever, nausea, vomiting, diarrhea, and abdominal pain occurs. Tenderness and swelling around the infested muscles are common occurrences. After a period of about seven days, rash, swelling of the eyelids, and neurologic disorders may develop. Myocarditis (inflammation of the heart muscle) can also occur at this stage. Eventually the larvae in the muscles die and become calcified. Symptoms gradually disappear within a few months.

Since there is no way to get the larvae out of the muscles, treatment is aimed at relief of discomfort. Analgesics, such as aspirin, are administered for pain, and anti-inflammatory steroids (cortisone drugs, such as prednisone) are administered for allergic symptoms, myocarditis, and central nervous system involvement. Thiabendazole (which tends to kill worms such as the *Trichinella*) is often given with good results. It is advisable to keep a close watch for fever, abdominal pain, vomiting, and dermatitis (skin inflammation).

The only preventive measure is to make sure that any meals that contain pork are sufficiently cooked (to an internal temperature of at least 170°F) to kill the larvae.

# Trigeminal neuralgia

Trigeminal neuralgia, or tic douloureux, primarily affects elderly persons (most commonly, those over age 70), although it may also occur in younger persons with multiple sclerosis. The pain arises from the trigeminal nerve, which controls sensation in the face, teeth, mouth, and nasal cavity and movement of the jaw. The pain, usually excruciating, covers one side of the face and can be set off by eating, by washing, or even by being exposed to a gust of air. With time, the stabbing pains occur more and more frequently, until they become constant. The cause is unknown. Although the condition is not life-threatening, it can become very disabling.

Treatment for the various types of neuralgia depends on the location of the damaged nerves, the severity of the pain, and the reason behind the impairment. Therapy may vary from cold or hot packs and aspirin to stronger prescription painkillers. For shingles, ointments may soothe and dry up blisters, and the antiviral drug acyclovir may shorten the course of the illness. A physician may refer a patient to a neurologist. In rare instances, neurosurgery to sever a damaged nerve is necessary to halt pain.

There is virtually no way to prevent neuralgia, except to treat underlying diseases that may precipitate nerve damage and to avoid overexposure to chemicals and drugs.

# Tuberculosis

Tuberculosis is a bacterial infection caused by *Mycobacterium tuberculosis* organisms. Because the body's defense system has difficulty fighting this type of bacterium, it attempts to wall off invading organisms within small nodules, called granulomas or tubercles, which contain both the infecting bacteria and the tissue produced by the body in reaction to them.

Of all persons who are infected by the tuberculosis bacteria, 80 percent will never experience the symptoms of the disease. Usually, the body is able to surround the offending bacteria with granulomas; the tuberculosis bacteria then lie dormant in the body, and active disease does not develop. However, because the body cannot kill the bacteria—only contain them within granulomas—the infection can become active at a later time, often when some other disease has weakened the body's defenses.

Of the 20 percent of infected persons in whom an active case of tuberculosis does develop, only half will become sick within three months of contracting the infection; the other half will suffer from the disease at some time in their lives, perhaps years later. Tuberculosis usually affects the lungs, but it can also involve other parts of the body, such as the spine, the kidneys, the digestive tract, and the lining of the heart.

Tuberculosis is contracted when a person breathes in droplets containing *Mycobacterium tuberculosis* organisms that have been coughed or sneezed into the air by an infected person. Tuberculosis is contagious, especially for persons living in crowded conditions. Also highly susceptible to this disease are those who are undernourished, in poor health, or living in poor urban areas, as well as the very young, the very old, and those in the medical professions. People with AIDS or other conditions affecting the immune system are also at high risk. Anyone who has been in close contact with a tuberculosis patient should be tested for the disease.

Early signs include fever, fatigue, loss of appetite, and weight loss. Later signs include coughing up of blood-tinged sputum, chest pain, and shortness of breath.

The symptoms of tuberculosis are similar to those of many other diseases, and its characteristic symptoms frequently do not appear until the disease is in its advanced stages. For these reasons, this disorder often remains untreated or misdiagnosed for some time before the patient is finally tested for it. Recently the incidence of tuberculosis has been on the rise. Awareness of this by physicians and patients leads to early treatment, fewer complications, and less spreading of the disease. Tuberculosis may be accompanied by an infection due to *Streptococcus bacteria*, which often further complicates diagnosis.

Patients can be tested for tuberculosis with a tuberculin skin test. If the bacteria are present, whether active or inactive, the patch of skin that has been treated with dead tuberculosis bacteria will swell. Chest X rays or sputum analysis may also help to identify the site of infection.

Tuberculosis is treated with a variety of antibacterial drugs simultaneously. Each medication acts on a different portion of the tuberculosis bacterium; only in combination do these drugs have the greatest probability of eliminating the infection. The drugs are usually prescribed for a long period of time, perhaps 9 to 18 months, but usually after two weeks the patient is no longer contagious and can resume normal activities. With this type of treatment, the disease is rarely fatal. Severe side effects, such as liver or hearing damage, can result from certain antituberculosis drugs.

An active case of tuberculosis can be prevented in some high-risk per-

sons by the administration of certain antituberculosis drugs. (High-risk persons include those under the age of 35, especially children, who have been exposed to the disease, as well as those with chronic diseases that have weakened their respiratory systems.) Liver damage from these drugs is more likely to occur in those over the age of 35, so people in this age group are not good subjects to receive these drugs.

Regardless of age or physical condition, anyone who has been in close contact with a person who has an active case of tuberculosis should be tested for the disease.

# U

# Ulcer

An ulcer is an erosion (open sore) on the surface of an organ or tissue. Ulcers most commonly erupt in the esophagus, stomach, and duodenum, in which case they are known as peptic ulcers.

Although the cause of peptic ulcers has not been fully established, scien-

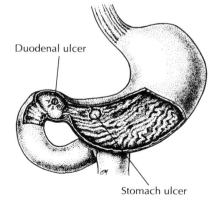

Duodenal ulcer

Stomach ulcer

The most common ulcers are those that affect the stomach or the duodenum (the first segment of the small intestine).

tists believe that the more common duodenal ulcers may result from the presence of excessive amounts of acid produced by the stomach. The stomach may increase acidic secretions after coffee, alcohol, and certain medications are consumed or after cigarettes are smoked. Therefore, these substances are thought to contribute to the development of ulcers. Aspirin and aspirinlike compounds exert a direct damaging effect on the lining of the stomach.

The less common stomach ulcers may be due to an inherent weakness in the wall of the stomach. However, this weakness may result from the same environmental conditions that aggravate duodenal ulcers.

Emotional stress may play a role in ulcer development. However, physicians distinguish between stress as a factor by itself and certain ways of dealing with stress that may increase susceptibility to ulcers.

Heredity plays an important role in contributing to ulcers. Persons who have a family history of ulcers seem to have a greater likelihood of acquiring the condition, as do persons with type O blood. In addition, liver disease, rheumatoid arthritis, and emphysema may increase vulnerability to ulcers.

Ulcers can produce mild symptoms resembling heartburn or severe pain radiating throughout the upper portion of the body. The most common discomfort of ulcers is a burning sensation in the abdomen above the navel that may feel like hunger pangs. Pain comes about 30 to 120 minutes after eating or in the middle of the night when the stomach is empty. At this time, the acidic stomach juices are more apt to irritate the unprotected nerve endings in the exposed ulcer. Usually, pain subsides after eating or drinking something or taking an antacid to neutralize stomach acid.

Some people experience nausea, vomiting, and constipation. Blood in the feces (discoloring them black), blood in the vomit, extreme weakness, fainting, and excessive thirst are all signs of internal bleeding, and may appear in more advanced cases.

While ulcers are not usually lifethreatening, they can cause serious damage if left untreated. Ulcers may erode nearby blood vessels and cause internal seepage of blood or hemorrhage (massive internal bleeding). A perforated ulcer may penetrate an adjoining organ, causing infection. In addition, scar tissue growing around the ulcer may lead to an obstruction or narrowing.

Physicians diagnose peptic ulcers primarily on the basis of an X-ray examination after the patient has swallowed a special chalky substance called barium. The barium makes the digestive tract visible on X-ray film, allowing the doctor a view of any abnormalities.

A second diagnostic technique is called an upper GI endoscopy (also called gastroscopy). The doctor inserts an endoscope (a flexible, lighted, tubelike instrument) through the mouth and down the esophagus to directly view the lining of the esophagus, stomach, and duodenum. An endoscopic examination and a biopsy (removal of a tissue sample for analysis) are necessary to confirm that an apparent ulcer is not actually a cancerous growth.

Treatment of ulcers involves relieving the irritation so that healing is able to progress naturally. Antacids counteract stomach acid and relieve symptoms, but they can cause complications. For example, sodium bicarbonate, a primary antacid ingredient, contains large amounts of sodium, which can aggravate kidney disease or high blood pressure.

For treatment of ulcers, a physician may prescribe other preparations to promote healing. Sucralfate coats the stomach, protecting it against gastric acid. Cimetidine, ranitidine, and other medications known as "H$_2$ blockers" inhibit gastric acid production and secretion. Omeprazole, a newer drug that is not an H$_2$ blocker, strongly inhibits gastric acid secretion and is very effective in healing ulcers and esophagitis resistant to other medication.

Although recent studies have shown that a bland diet is not necessary for ulcer management, such a diet may be recommended until acute symptoms disappear. Thereafter, many doctors suggest avoiding only foods known to cause distress.

The effect of milk on ulcers is also questionable. Its neutralizing action on stomach acid is mild and temporary at best. Nevertheless, people who substitute milk for known irritants, such as alcohol and caffeine, are less likely to irritate their ulcers.

Most ulcers heal within two to six weeks after treatment begins. To prevent recurrence, patients should continue to refrain from use of cigarettes, caffeine, alcohol, and other substances that stimulate stomach acid production or irritate the digestive tract lining.

When drug therapy and diet cannot cure an ulcer, surgical repair may be necessary. Surgery is appropriate for repeated ulcers that recur or are life-threatening, such as perforated ulcers. Sometimes, surgeons remove a portion of the stomach and parts of the vagus nerve (which controls digestive secretions) to reduce stomach acid production. Usually, ulcers do not reappear after surgery.

Recently, endoscopic cautery (burning of tissue through the endoscope), direct injection of medications, and laser surgery have been quite successful in stopping bleeding, reducing the size of tumors, and correcting strictures (narrowing due to scar formation). These procedures and medications have spared many individuals a surgical procedure.

# Ulcerative colitis

Ulcerative colitis is a chronic inflammatory disease of the large intestine characterized by bloody diarrhea and the development of erosions (open sores) on the lining of the colon.

Although there is a familial tendency to develop ulcerative colitis, the cause of the disorder is unknown. Any age group may be affected, but it tends to begin in persons between the ages of 15 and 40.

Among possible contributing factors are infection, immunologic derangement (a breakdown in the body's defense system), lack of protective elements in the bowel wall, nervous or psychological disturbances, and alterations in the connective tissue in the colon.

The first sign of ulcerative colitis is usually a series of attacks of bloody

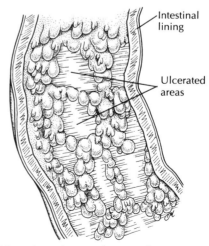

Ulcerative colitis is a chronic inflammatory disease characterized by bloody diarrhea and ulcerated areas in the lining of the colon.

diarrhea. The attacks can vary in intensity and duration and are usually interspersed with periods of normal bowel movements. The onset of the attacks may be severe, with sudden violent diarrhea, high fever, symptoms of abdominal inflammation, and bacterial invasions. Often, an attack will be preceded by mild lower abdominal cramps and the appearance of small amounts of blood or mucus in the feces.

If ulceration is confined to the rectum and the terminal portion of the colon (ulcerative proctitis), the bowel movements may be normal or bloody, with discharges of mucus containing red and white blood cells between stools. If the disorder extends to other portions of the colon, however, stools become looser and more frequent (perhaps as many as 10 to 20 per day), and the patient suffers severe cramps, watery stools, fever, anemia (due to blood loss), and loss of appetite.

If the condition persists in this severe form, hemorrhage (internal bleeding) is the most common complication. In toxic colitis, a serious complication, the colon loses muscular tone and dilates almost completely, resulting in perforations of the organ. The risk of colon cancer and cancer of the bile ducts is also increased in patients with ulcerative colitis. Arthritis, skin and eye disorders, and biliary tract disease are among other problems associated with ulcerative colitis.

Ulcerative colitis is diagnosed with the use of a stool examination and colonoscopy (in which a lighted, flexible, tubelike instrument is inserted through the anus and into the entire colon for a visual examination of the interior). X-ray studies with a barium enema are indicated, except in cases in which risk of perforation makes the barium enema procedure a potential danger for the patient.

Mild cases of ulcerative colitis may sometimes be treated with adequate physical and mental relaxation (since the severity of the disease appears to be stress-related in some patients); a diet low in milk, milk products, nuts, kernels, and seeds; and antidiarrheal medication. More severe cases may respond to the drug sulfasalazine. Salicylate drugs (aspirinlike compounds), either in oral or enema form, and antibiotics have also been helpful. In cases that do not respond to salicylate or sulfasalazine therapy, hydrocortisone (a steroid hormone) may be given by enema, along with oral cortisone preparations. The only cure for ulcerative colitis is total colectomy (removal of the entire colon) sometimes with the rectum left in. Newer surgical techniques have, in many cases, eliminated the need for ileostomy. In ulcerative proctitis, surgery is usually unnecessary, and individuals do not usually progress to full-blown ulcerative colitis.

# Undescended testes

Undescended testes is a condition in which one or both of the testes (male sex glands) do not descend into the scrotum (the sac between the legs that normally contains the testes), but remain in the abdomen, where they developed before birth. This condition is also called cryptorchidism or cryptorchism and is not uncommon.

If the testes do not descend, they often degenerate or atrophy (shrink), and thus do not secrete the male sex hormones that they ordinarily supply. This, in turn, can cause the elimination or suppression of the development during puberty of secondary male sex characteristics such as body hair, heavier musculature, deepening voice, and so forth. Damaged sperm, or insufficient production of them,

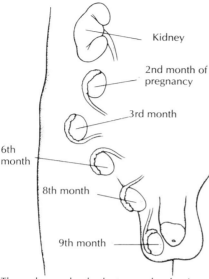

Kidney

2nd month of pregnancy

3rd month

6th month

8th month

9th month

The male sex glands, the testes, develop in the abdomen and gradually descend downward into the scrotum before birth.

can also result from undescended testes, especially if the situation is still present in adolescence or adulthood. If one testis is damaged but the other has descended and is normal, sexual development will be normal.

The causes of this condition are not clearly understood. It is conjectured that a membrane in the abdomen gets in the way of normal testicular positioning. If only one testis is undescended, the problem is most likely mechanical in nature; if both are involved, the underlying cause may well be hormonal.

Treatment for this condition is controversial. In deciding on treatment, three important considerations must be kept in mind: the potential lack of fertility if the testes do not descend, the likelihood that they will descend without intervention, and the risk that the undescended testes will become cancerous. Hormone therapy is sometimes an effective treatment, but in many cases in which it has apparently been successful, some doctors think that the testes would probably have

descended by themselves anyway. Surgery to bring the testes into the scrotum is usually successful if done before the age of five years. The physician can sometimes cause the testes to descend by manipulation of the tissues around them.

A male with an undescended testis is at increased risk for cancer of the testes even if the testis is brought down surgically. All males who have had an undescended testis should be taught to examine their testes for the presence of lumps on a monthly basis throughout adolescence and adulthood.

There is no known means of preventing undescended testes.

# Urethritis

Urethritis is an infection or inflammation of the urethra (the tube that runs through the penis and connects the bladder to the outside of the body). It is the most common condition affecting the male reproductive system and may occur in all men.

Two sexually transmitted diseases, gonorrhea and chlamydia, are the most common causes of urethritis in both men and women. Irritation may also be caused after sexual intercourse by chemicals contained in vaginal spermicides and douches. Once inside the urethra, these bacteria and chemicals will cause the urethra to become irritated and swollen.

The most common symptoms of urethritis are burning during urination and a creamy white or yellow discharge from the penis. Unlike a bladder infection, urethritis does not cause an increase in the frequency of urination.

Urethritis is diagnosed by an examination of the penis to check for discharge. The doctor will then take specimens of the discharge for examination under a microscope and for bacterial culture.

Infections of the urethra are treated with antibiotics. A person who has urethritis should abstain from sexual activity until a full course of antibiotics has been taken and until all tests indicate that the infection is no longer present. Every sexual partner of the infected person needs to be examined and, if necessary, treated.

Urethritis can be prevented by avoiding sexual contact with someone who is infected with either gonorrhea or chlamydia. Using condoms also helps reduce the risk of contracting these infections. If urethritis is caused by chemical irritation from vaginal spermicides or douches, these substances should be avoided or a condom should be used.

# Urinary system

The urinary system includes those organs of the body that produce and eliminate urine (a combination of water and waste products that passes out of the body as fluid). By controlling urine flow, the system maintains proper water balance throughout the body. Individual parts of the urinary system monitor the concentration of salts and other necessary nutrients.

The organs most responsible for the control of the balance of chemicals and water in the blood are the two kidneys. The kidneys are bean-shaped structures located in back of the abdomen. Their chief functions are to filter wastes from the blood and to ensure reabsorption of essential chemicals back into the bloodstream. They also play a major role in blood pressure regulation, and they influence the production of red blood cells. In the kidneys, waste products combine with water and salts to form urine.

Urine passes from each kidney into the bladder through tubes called ureters. The bladder stores the urine prior to elimination from the body. A

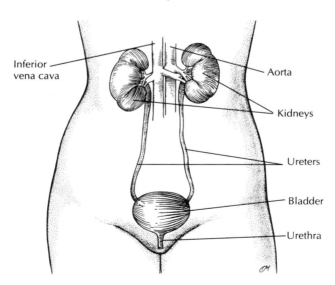

Inferior vena cava

Aorta

Kidneys

Ureters

Bladder

Urethra

The role of the urinary system (the female urinary tract is shown here) is to cleanse the blood. Arterial blood is filtered through the kidneys and returned to the circulation. Waste products, plus excess water, are sent through the ureters to the bladder, to be excreted as urine.

sphincter muscle around the exit from the bladder prevents urine from escaping. When the bladder is about half full, the body feels an urge to empty the organ. At this time, the muscle can be relaxed voluntarily to release the urine.

The urethra is a tube that conveys urine from the bladder to the exterior of the body. The female urethra is about an inch and a half long and is enclosed within the body. The male urethra passes through the penis and is approximately eight inches long. For the male, the urethra serves the dual function of transporting urine and semen (the fluid from the male reproductive organs). Semen is released during sexual intercourse, at which time urine is blocked from leaving the bladder.

Changes in urine and urinary habits that do not seem to have an obvious cause may be symptoms of disease.

Some symptoms that require medical attention are changes in frequency, timing, and control of urination; changes in the quantity and color of urine; and the presence of pain accompanying urination. A doctor should be contacted immediately if any of the following symptoms is noted: extreme pain while urinating, blood in the urine, a noticeable increase or decrease in frequency of urination (a symptom of kidney failure), marked changes in the color of the urine, or cloudiness in the urine accompanied by pain or fever.

Changes in urine or urinary habits may be caused by a variety of disorders involving the kidneys, urinary tract, bladder, and prostate (a gland that surrounds the male urethra).

Increased frequency may be caused by inflammation of the kidneys, bladder, or urethra; diabetes mellitus (a disorder of carbohydrate utilization); or an enlarged prostate gland.

A change in timing of urination, usually in the form of very frequent nighttime awakenings accompanied by the urge to urinate (a condition called nocturia), is often coupled with painful urination, a poor stream, or difficulty in starting urination. These may be symptoms of an enlarged prostate gland or an inflammatory or infectious disease within the urinary tract. They could also be symptoms of tumors or other disorders that result in increased pressure on the bladder.

Difficulty in controlling, starting, and maintaining the flow of urine may also be symptoms of an inflammation of the prostate gland. Inability to hold back urine is a common problem of elderly people, as their control of the sphincter muscle of the bladder weakens. Also affected by this problem are women in the late stages of pregnancy, when the enlarged uterus continuously presses on the bladder.

Changes in the quantity of urine normally produced can also signal disease. Producing an excessive amount of urine (called polyuria) may be a symptom of kidney disease, diabetes, or glandular disorders. Decreased production of urine may indicate the presence of dehydration, internal hemorrhaging, or acute renal failure.

Slight changes in the color and clarity of the urine from day to day are normal, but strikingly obvious color changes and extreme cloudiness may signal infection, tumors, kidney stones, prostate problems, or other abnormalities in the urinary tract.

Pain while urinating, most commonly in the form of a burning sensation felt along the urethra, may be a sign of a lower urinary tract infection. Excruciating pain across the abdomen or the back may signal the presence of kidney stones.

Treatment of urinary problems usually involves treating the underlying cause of the change, which can range all the way from a mild infection to a very serious disease. An accurate diagnosis by a physician is the first step in receiving proper treatment for these disorders.

See also Cystitis and Prostatitis.

# Uterine cancer

This disease is most common in women over the age of 50. Especially susceptible are women who have never given birth, those who are obese or diabetic, and those who suffer from high blood pressure. Women who have taken the female hormone estrogen are probably at higher risk of suffering from uterine cancer than those who have not.

Vaginal bleeding after menopause is the most common symptom of uterine cancer. If a Pap smear shows no abnormalities, a minor surgical procedure known as dilatation and curettage (D&C) may be performed. This involves scraping the interior walls of the uterus in order to examine the tissue for the presence of cancer. If cancer is identified, a hysterectomy (surgical removal of the uterus) is usually performed. (Often, the ovaries are removed as well.) Cancer of the uterus is harder to detect than that of the cervix; it is often discovered when it is too advanced for successful treatment.

See also Cancer.

# Urinary tract infection

See Cystitis.

# Vaginal cancer

Once confined to women over 50 years of age, vaginal cancer has begun to appear in women between the ages of 17 and 20. The mothers of most of these young women took artificial estrogens, particularly diethylstilbestrol (DES), during pregnancy to prevent miscarriage. A woman whose mother took artificial estrogens during pregnancy should have a Pap smear twice a year. Symptoms of vaginal cancer include vaginal pain and bleeding. The disease is usually treated with radiation and surgery.

See also Cancer.

# Vaginitis

Vaginitis is an inflammation of the vagina, usually marked by burning and itching of the external genital organs.

Vaginitis is most commonly caused by an imbalance of the microorganisms normally present in the vagina, resulting when some factor causes one of the strains to reproduce more quickly than the others. Possible causes of overgrowth of microorganisms include the use of birth control pills, which produce changes in the vaginal lining; the use of certain antibiotics, which may kill some types of bacteria but allow others to flourish. Other causes include the presence of a warm, moist environment (such as may be created by wearing tight pants or panty hose, nylon underwear, or a wet bathing suit), which acts as a breeding ground for infection; and,

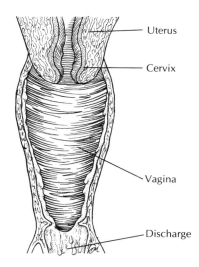

Vaginitis is an infection or often inflammation of the vagina, characterized by a discharge from the vagina. It is commonly caused by a protozoan, a fungus, or a bacterium, each of which is shown here as it would appear under a microscope.

particularly for infection by *Hemophilus vaginalis* or *Trichomonas vaginalis*, the introduction of an infectious microorganism through sexual contact with an infected individual. Vaginitis tends to occur more often in the summer, because excessive heat and moisture are known to promote the disease.

One variety of the disease, called noninfectious vaginitis, is not caused by overproduction of microorganisms, but rather by direct irritation of the vagina by some outside agent, such as the chemical irritation that arises from the excessive use of douches, feminine hygiene sprays, bubble baths, talcum powder, and scented or colored toilet paper.

Pregnant women and those who have diabetes or gonorrhea (a sexually transmitted disease) are at a higher risk of developing vaginitis than other women.

Infection by *Candida albicans* causes severe itching of the external genital organs and pain during intercourse. Because of the thick, white vaginal discharge, which resembles cottage cheese in texture and has a "yeasty" odor, this condition is commonly known as a yeast infection. This is the type of vaginitis most frequently contracted by diabetic and pregnant women.

Infection by *Hemophilus vaginalis* causes a creamy white or grayish, foul-smelling discharge.

The presence of *Trichomonas vaginalis* is indicated by itching and burning, as well as by a greenish-white discharge and foul odor. These symptoms are likely to appear during or immediately following the woman's menstrual period.

Noninfectious vaginitis is characterized only by irritation and dryness, usually with no discharge.

Vaginitis is diagnosed by determining which microorganism is causing the infection. Microscopic examination of a sample, or "smear," of vaginal secretions is used to make the diagnosis.

Treatment will vary according to the type of microorganism. Fungal infections are generally treated with an antifungal cream, which is applied directly to the vagina, or as a vaginal suppository (forms of which are now available without a doctor's prescription).

Bacterial infections are treated with antibiotics, administered either orally or as vaginal suppositories. Because bacterial infections can be transferred between sexual partners, both are usually treated with oral antibiotics.

An oral antibiotic called metronidazole is given to women with protozoan infections and to their partners. Because some studies have linked this drug to cancer and genetic damage in laboratory animals, it should not be taken during the first half of pregnancy.

Noninfectious vaginitis is usually treated simply by avoiding the irritants that may cause it, such as perfumed soaps, chemical sprays, and scented tissues, and by not wearing tight-fitting clothing.

Some types of vaginitis can probably be prevented by using only non-scented, white toilet paper; wearing cotton underwear and loose-fitting pants; avoiding the overuse of douches, feminine hygiene sprays, and scented toiletries; and having any sexual partners use condoms.

# Varicose veins

Varicose veins are swollen, stretched veins in the legs, close to the surface of the skin, caused by pooling of blood. Varicose veins alone are not too serious, but they may lead to a more serious condition, such as a skin ulcer, phlebitis (inflammation of a vein), or thrombosis (blood clot formation).

Blood from the legs must return to the heart uphill, against the force of gravity, so the veins in the legs have one-way valves to prevent blood from flowing back down toward the feet. When pressure on the veins stretches them or when the valves are injured in some way, the valves cannot close properly, and some blood travels back down. This blood accumulates in pools, which, in turn, stretch the veins even more.

Varicose veins are caused by a number of factors that put excess pressure on the veins in the legs: prolonged standing; prolonged sitting, especially with the legs crossed; lack of exercise; confining clothes; obesity (which puts excess pressure on the legs and contributes to the inability of the muscles to push blood upward); heredity (a tendency toward weak vein walls and valves seems to

Blood returning to heart

Valve closed to prevent backflow of blood

Normal

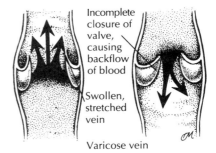

Incomplete closure of valve, causing backflow of blood

Swollen, stretched vein

Varicose vein

The drawing at the top shows the interior of a normal vein, in which the action of a valve prevents blood returning to the heart from flowing backward. In the drawing of a varicose vein, the valve has been weakened and cannot completely close, causing the blood to accumulate.

be inherited); and even height (tall people may be more susceptible because their blood needs to travel farther in its return trip to the heart).

Women are more susceptible to varicose veins than men, largely due to hormonal factors. Pregnancy accentuates this difference because special hormones released at this time tend to relax the walls of the veins. Also, varicose veins often appear during the last few months of pregnancy due to the increased strain from the weight of the growing uterus. These veins may recede, however, after the birth of the baby.

Varicose veins are very noticeable since they form close to the skin. They appear as bulging, bluish, cord-like lines running down the legs. Symptoms that accompany varicose veins are feelings of achiness, heaviness, and fatigue in the legs, especially at the end of the day; itchy, scaly skin covering the affected areas; and, in advanced cases, swollen ankles, pain shooting down the leg, and leg cramps at night.

Diagnosis can most often be made on the basis of physical examination because the affected superficial veins can be readily seen and palpated. If involvement of deeper veins is suspected, Doppler imaging (a technique used to detect obstructions by observing the changes in the sounds brought about by flowing blood) may be performed.

Varicose veins are usually treated by wearing elastic stockings, which act to aid the muscles pushing the blood upward. Very severe cases may require a surgical procedure called vein stripping, in which the afflicted veins are tied off and removed; other healthy veins in the area will take over the job of pushing blood toward the heart. A chemical can also be injected into the veins, closing them off and forcing the blood to find other channels to the heart.

Those with varicose veins may need to lose weight, exercise regularly, and stretch their legs or put their feet up whenever possible. Exercises to improve circulation in the legs may help relieve pressure.

Varicose veins tend to recur even after corrective procedures, particularly if adequate preventive measures are not undertaken.

# Vertigo

See Dizziness and vertigo.

# Vital signs

*Vital signs* is a term used in diagnostic medicine for four easily observed variables—body temperature, pulse rate, respiratory rate, and blood pressure. Although evaluation of the vital signs is not sufficient to arrive at a clear diagnosis of a patient's condition, these four items taken together serve as important indicators of the presence of disease or injury. They

Varicose vein

Because varicose veins are close to the surface, they are very visible.

are usually the first step in a diagnostic evaluation.

Temperature is a useful index of a patient's condition, since a fever (an abnormal rise in body temperature) is usually a significant indicator of disease. Fever is generally a sign of infection, but it can be present whenever there is tissue destruction (from a severe sunburn, for example, or when large amounts of tissue deteriorate due to lack of blood supply).

The pulse rate reflects the heart rate. The heart rate varies with a person's level of physical activity; for example, the heart beats faster during exercise and more slowly during rest. An inappropriate heart rate may indicate disease. A feverish patient will have an increased heart rate, while a weak but rapid pulse is characteristic of severe blood loss or diseases of the heart itself. An irregular pulse rate may also indicate a reaction to stress or to overconsumption of caffeine.

The respiratory rate is the rate of breathing. Patients with fever hyperventilate (have an increased respiratory rate), which lowers body temperature. Hyperventilation is a common response to pain or stress, as well. Any condition that leads to acidosis (the presence of abnormally high acid levels in the body) drives the respiratory rate upward. Diseases of the lungs, which decrease their ability to oxygenate the blood, also increase respiratory rate.

The blood pressure is an indicator of the amount of blood in circulation and the pumping force of the heart. A decrease in circulating blood volume, such as occurs in cases of severe bleeding, lowers blood pressure and deprives the tissues of adequate blood flow. Reflexes then are initiated that compensate, in part, for the reduced blood volume and pressure. For example, the heart rate increases in an attempt to make up for the reduction in blood volume, and the blood vessels supplying the digestive organs narrow, which diverts blood to more vital areas, such as the brain. Sustained elevation of blood pressure constitutes a disorder in its own right—hypertension.

# Vitamins

A vitamin is any of a large group of organic substances often identified as "enzyme components," which are found in many foods in small amounts and are necessary for normal body functioning. Many vitamins help to regulate the rate at which chemical reactions take place in the human body.

Vitamins are not themselves direct sources of energy. As enzyme components, they can act only in the presence of nutrients contained in food. Hence, taking massive doses of supplements in place of normal eating is useless and dangerous.

In general, vitamin megadoses (large doses far beyond daily requirements) are not needed. Many reputable nutritional guides suggest that for persons on restricted-calorie diets (containing less than 1,000 to 1,200 calories daily), a multivitamin preparation may be useful, but higher potency or "therapeutic" formulas are not generally necessary.

The Food and Drug Administration has developed a system of nutrition labeling for foods, the U.S. Recommended Daily Allowances (USRDAs). The USRDAs for selected vitamins for adults and children four years and older are as follows:

| | |
|---|---|
| Vitamin A | 5,000 international units |
| Vitamin $B_1$ | 1.5 milligrams |
| Vitamin $B_2$ | 1.7 milligrams |
| Vitamin $B_6$ | 2 milligrams |
| Vitamin C | 60 milligrams |
| Vitamin D | 400 international units |

Vitamin E      30 international units
Folic acid         0.4 milligrams
Biotin             0.3 milligrams
Niacin             20 milligrams

**Vitamin A** Vitamin A is found in fish-liver oils, liver, butter, egg yolks, cheese, dark-green vegetables, and yellow vegetables and fruits. Deficiency of this vitamin in the diet causes inadequate production of rhodopsin (important in the functioning of the eye), resulting in night blindness. Vitamin A deficiency can also result in disorders of the skin and mucous membranes and decreased resistance to infection. Megadoses of this vitamin in the absence of deficiency may cause serious health problems.

**Vitamin B** The name vitamin B may refer to any member of the vitamin B complex, including thiamin, riboflavin, niacin, niacinamide, the $B_6$ group, biotin, pantothenic acid, folic acid, para-aminobenzoic acid, inositol, cyanocobalamin (vitamin $B_{12}$), and choline.

Vitamin $B_1$, or thiamin, is found in enriched and whole-grain breads and cereals, meat (especially pork and liver), dried beans and peas, and nuts. A deficiency can result in beriberi, a disease characterized by abnormal heart function, swelling, and inflammation of the nerves.

Vitamin $B_2$, or riboflavin, is found in milk, meats (especially liver), eggs, dark-green vegetables, and enriched cereal products. It acts as a catalyst in bodily processes that involve oxidation (use of oxygen). Dietary deficiencies may result in stomatitis (inflammation of the mucous membranes of the mouth), cheilitis (inflammation of the lips), and eye disorders.

Vitamin $B_6$ is a group of substances (pyridoxine, pyridoxal, and pyridoxamine) that are widely distributed in animal and plant tissues. These substances are involved in the metabolism of amino acids (the building blocks of protein) and in the breakdown of glycogen (a stored sugar). Vitamin $B_6$ is found in wheat, bran, yeast, and seeds. A deficiency can result in functional disturbances of the nervous system.

Vitamin $B_{12}$, or cyanocobalamin, affects the formation of red blood cells and is found in all animal products, especially liver and other meats, fish, cheese, and eggs. When vitamin $B_{12}$ is absent from the diet or is not absorbed by the body, anemia (deficiency of red blood cells) may result.

Biotin acts as a coenzyme, or biologic catalyst, in several metabolic reactions. Some of these reactions are important for the manufacture of fatty acids; others are essential for the synthesis of glucose, a primary source of energy. Some biotin is normally produced in the intestinal tract by bacteria that live there. Because of the difficulty of measuring how much biotin these bacteria actually make, nutritionists have been unable to establish how much biotin the body needs each day. However, it has been found that ordinary mixed diets usually provide from 100 to 300 micrograms of biotin a day. This amount, plus the amount produced by intestinal bacteria, is apparently enough. Biotin deficiency is almost unheard of in humans.

Folic acid is found in dark-green vegetables, liver, and legumes. Folic acid functions as a coenzyme, or catalyst, in a number of biological reactions. One of the most important of these is the synthesis of deoxyribonucleic acid (DNA). When plants and animals grow, cells must divide and multiply. To do this, a cell has to synthesize DNA—to double its supply so that each of the two new cells has a full supply of the gene-containing material.

In adults, symptoms of folic acid deficiency—such as anemia, nerve damage, and sore, red, swollen tongue—may not appear for months because the body tends to hold on to its supply of the vitamin. In infants and children, however, symptoms may appear much more quickly. Because they are growing rapidly, infants and children need proportionally more folic acid than do adults; a deficiency slows and stunts growth.

Symptoms of deficiency may also occur rapidly in pregnant women because they need more of the vitamin. Pregnancy increases the need for folic acid because it is a time of rapid growth and manufacture of new cells. Anemia caused by folic acid deficiency is quite prevalent among pregnant women subsisting on restricted diets, such as those of low-income populations in developing countries.

**Vitamin C** Vitamin C, or ascorbic acid, is found in many vegetables and fruits, especially green peppers and most citrus fruits. It is an essential element in the human diet. A deficiency may result in a disease called scurvy, in which the victim suffers anemia, spongy gums, bleeding, and edema (excess fluid retention in the tissues). An overdose of vitamin C (such as may result from taking "megadoses") may cause gout, kidney stones, and decreased fertility.

**Vitamin D** Vitamin D includes any of several related antirickets compounds. These compounds are present in fish-liver oils, liver, butter, cream, egg yolks, and fortified milk; they are also produced in the body on exposure to sunlight. A vitamin D deficiency may cause rickets in children and osteomalacia (softening of the bones) or osteoporosis (decreased bone mass) in adults. As with vitamin A, large doses of this vitamin in the absence of deficiency can be quite toxic, especially in young children.

**Vitamin E** Vitamin E is necessary in human diets for normal muscular and reproductive functioning and development, normal red blood cell functioning, and other biochemical processes. Vitamin E is found in wheat germ oil, vegetable oils, whole-grain products, egg yolks, organ meats (especially liver), and dark-green vegetables.

**Vitamin K** Vitamin K is a group of vitamins found in their natural state in spinach, cabbage, and other leafy green vegetables and in egg yolk and liver. These vitamins play a role in clotting of the blood by increasing the production of prothrombin, the clotting agent in the blood. A deficiency can result in blood coagulation abnormalities. Individuals who are on anticoagulant drugs, such as warfarin, should consult their physician about the appropriate dosage of vitamin K, because too much of the vitamin will lessen the effect of the drug and too little of the vitamin will increase the drug's effect.

See also Minerals.

# W

# Warts

Warts are infectious growths in the outer layers of the skin. Because they are contagious, they can spread from person to person or from one site to another on the same person. Most frequently, warts appear on the hands and fingers and on the soles of the feet. However, they can emerge anywhere on the skin, including the genital and anal areas.

Common warts are caused by exposure to a virus called the human papilloma virus. The virus can remain inactive for up to six months after contact before causing the eruption of abnormal skin masses.

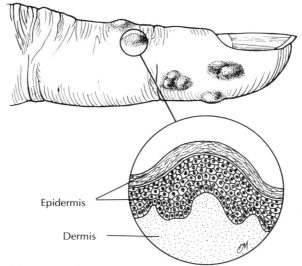

Epidermis

Dermis

Warts (infectious swellings in the outer layer of the skin) are caused by a virus.

The virus is transmitted to another person or another site on the body by direct contact. For example, brushing or combing the hair can spread the virus from a wart on the scalp. Shaving or scratching a given area on the body and then touching another area will also transmit the virus. In addition, moist parts of the body, such as the soles of the feet, provide a breeding ground for growth of the virus.

As people become older, they seem to develop an immunity, or resistance, to the wart virus. For this reason, children tend to acquire warts more frequently than adults, though warts can occur at any age.

Usually, warts appear as firm gray masses that feel tender or itchy. Their size and shape vary depending on the location and severity of the viral infection. Children are most likely to have flat warts, particularly on the face. This variety looks smooth, flat, and yellowish brown.

Plantar warts grow on the soles of the feet, where they can become as large as two inches in diameter. These warts cause considerable pain because the tissue swelling pushes inward with the pressure of each step; the discomfort from plantar warts feels like walking with a pebble in your shoe.

Most warts are not health-threatening. However, they can be so extensive in number as to cause extreme sensitivity or pain.

Studies have shown that two out of every three warts disappear on their own, usually within two years. Consequently, physicians usually recommend leaving warts alone unless they cause discomfort or obstruction.

Doctors sometimes treat one or two warts and find that the patient's other warts also clear up. A possible explanation is that the original treatment stimulates manufacture of antibodies (protective substances) that fight the virus in other warts.

There are over-the-counter preparations to aid removal of warts. Most of these remedies contain a form of acid, which is dangerous if not used according to directions. Although some of these drugs are effective, only a doctor should remove a wart.

Physicians may try a variety of topical preparations to loosen the warts.

A solution containing cantharidin, a substance that causes blistering, may be applied directly to the wart. About one week after application, the doctor should be able to remove the wart with a surgical knife or scissors. Corn plasters containing salicylic acid often soften the wart so that it can be scraped away.

When a wart persists, physicians may advise surgery to remove affected tissue. Electrosurgery dissolves wart tissue with electric current. Cryotherapy freezes the area with dry ice or liquid nitrogen; freezing allows the wart to be lifted off easily.

# Z

# Zygote

When a female sex cell (an ovum or egg) is fertilized by a male sex cell ( a gamete or sperm), the two fuse together to form a single cell called a zygote. This single cell contains genetic information in the form of 46 chromosomes (microscopic chemical strings made up of genes) 23 of which come from each parent.

The zygote is the first stage of the process that begins with the fertilization of the egg and ends with the birth of a fully formed infant. Within a few days after fertilization, the second stage begins, as the zygote starts to divide into a multiple-celled body. About three days later, a spherically shaped structure called a morula is formed, consisting of many cells all joined together.

The word *zygote* applies only to the single cell that is formed by fertilization.

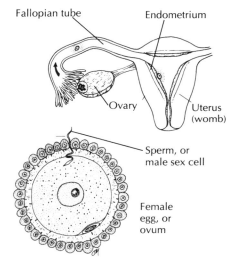

Under normal circumstances, a ripe egg cell, or ovum, is expelled once a month from the ovary to travel up the fallopian tube. If it is fertilized by the male sex cell, or gamete, the two together form a zygote that travels to the endometrium (the lining of the uterus) where it embeds itself and begins to form an embryo, the first stage of human life.

# Emergency
# first aid
# action guide

# Emergency first aid action guide

Successfully handling an emergency requires training, nerve, a calm hand, and the ability to work effectively under pressure. Nobody has an instinctive knowledge of what to do during a medical emergency. If you do not know what to do, you will assuredly do more harm than good. The purpose of this section is to acquaint you with the basic types of emergencies you may someday face and to teach you the accepted procedures for handling those emergencies.

Note that this section is not intended as a substitute for professional medical care. Instead, it is just what it says it is: a guide that will tell you what you can do during an emergency to keep a victim alive until the professionals arrive. For fast reference, it is arranged in alphabetical order—except for the section on unconsciousness and cardiopulmonary resuscitation. This section appears first because the technique is vital to almost every first-aid emergency, and it must be mastered first. Read this section thoroughly, and discuss it with your family and friends. Someday your life or theirs may depend on what you learned as you read this section. The approach is simple and step-by-step. The emphasis is on *how to do what needs to be done.*

Before learning about specific emergency procedures, you should know some facts about emergency situations themselves, regardless of what the particular emergency may be. Imagine that you have just walked into an emergency situation. A victim needs help. What do you do first? And what do you do next? Here are the first steps to follow in such a situation.

**Make certain that the environment poses no threat to you or to the victim.** Take a few seconds to look around for safety hazards. If the emergency is an auto accident, is the victim still in the car? Is there leaking gasoline? Are power lines down? Is the car on fire? Are other cars bearing down on you? Do you have lighting equipment to warn other drivers? If you get into the victim's car to try to get him or her out, will the car then roll off the edge of a cliff? Many would-be rescuers have wound up being rescued themselves (or killed) when they did not assess the situation in terms of hazards.

**Check the victim to see if he or she is breathing.** Sometimes a victim will have a blocked airway (the passage by which air goes through the mouth, down the throat, and into the windpipe is called the airway). This means that he or she cannot breathe even if nothing else is wrong. Look to see if the victim is breathing or not. If not, then immediately check the airway to see if it is blocked by food, broken teeth, tissue, blood, or any other obstruction. If the airway is blocked, remove the obstruction. Use your fingers. In case of food choking, you may want to perform chest compression techniques such as the Heimlich maneuver (see the section on Choking). The main objective is to *clear the airway* so the victim can breathe. If the victim cannot breathe, then death will occur within a matter of a few minutes. And you have only a few seconds to do something about the problem so the victim will not die. If the airway was open, or if you have unblocked it, proceed to the next step.

**Make certain that the victim is now breathing.**

Just because the airway is unblocked, do not assume that the victim will start breathing. Absence of breathing can be caused by factors other than a blocked airway. If the airway is open yet the victim is still not

breathing and is unconscious, it is time to begin cardiopulmonary resuscitation, or CPR (see the section on CPR). If you do not succeed in getting the victim to breathe within a few seconds, it may be too late.

**Check to see if the heart is beating.**

Absence of a heartbeat can be the result of a number of circumstances, ranging from cardiac arrest (sudden halt of heartbeat), to a heart attack, to an interruption in the heart's electrical impulses because of electric shock (as might be caused by an accidental electrocution, for example). The objective is to get the heart beating again as soon as possible.

If the victim is not breathing and has no heartbeat, seconds count. If the airway is blocked, the victim will not be able to breathe. If the victim cannot breathe, it will do no good to restart the heart, because if there is no oxygen in the lungs there will be no way that the blood pumped into the lungs by the heart can be oxygenated.

By the same token, if the airway is clear and the breathing cycle has been restarted by forcing breaths down the victim's throat, without the heartbeat the blood will not go into the lungs to become oxygenated. It is useless to restore breathing without restoring the heartbeat or to restore a heartbeat without restoring breathing. This is why the fundamental technique for victim revival is called *cardiopul-*

*monary* resuscitation: "Cardio" refers to the heart and "pulmonary" refers to the lungs.

In addition to breathing and heartbeat, there are other matters to consider.

## Check for heavy bleeding.

While heavy bleeding will not lead to death immediately, if left unattended, it will surely cause death in a short time. Furthermore, some people are more prone to shock than others, and even a small drop in blood pressure caused by bleeding will put them in shock (see the section on Shock). Once you have made certain that the victim is breathing and has a pulse, attend to any heavy bleeding (see the section on Bleeding). If you cannot completely stop the bleeding, you can at least slow it down so that clotting can begin.

There is one more important objective:

## Do no harm to the victim.

Your task is to save victims, not harm them. If you are not sure about what to do, find someone to take over who does know what to do. If no such person is available, then immediately call medical professionals and try to prevent further injury to the victim until they arrive.

In order to be fully prepared for an emergency, you should first be aware of the services available through the 911 emergency number in your area. Local emergency services that use the easily-remembered 911

system are becoming more widely available. Fire and police assistance can usually be reached this way, as well as paramedics in some locations. In addition to the 911 system, or in places that do not use it, the following numbers should be at your fingertips at all times:

- Police
- Fire department
- Poison control center
- The nearest hospital emergency department
- The nearest ambulance service (especially if the hospital or fire department in your area does not provide ambulance service)
- Your own physician

This information should be posted near every telephone in your home and at your place of work. You should also carry this list in your purse or wallet.

You now have the framework within which you can act decisively and effectively during an emergency. The next step is to learn first-aid techniques for specific problems. The following sections will instruct you about particular emergencies, beginning with cardiopulmonary resuscitation—the most important procedure you can learn.

Cardiopulmonary resuscitation (CPR) is the fundamental victim-revival technique. Without both heartbeat and breathing, no victim can survive. Regardless of the cause of an emergency, if a victim is not breathing and there is no heartbeat, CPR will mean the difference between life and death. You will have only a few seconds to act.

You cannot learn CPR simply by reading about it. CPR involves not only knowing why certain actions are taken and how they should be done; it involves *actually doing* them as well.

For this reason, it is strongly recommended that you attend one of the CPR courses offered by the Red Cross and through the American Heart Association. You will be taught by professionals, and you will receive a certificate that shows you have developed some skill in performing the technique. You might also check the fire department, the ambulance companies, and your local college or university. Most hospitals do not offer such courses.

When you sign up for a CPR course, you should look for the following elements to make certain that you are enrolling in a legitimate program of study and practice:

- How long is the program? (It should last for at least six hours.)
- How much time will you spend actually working with the simulation mannequin? (You should spend at least two hours with the mannequin so that you will "get the feel" of how to apply the various techniques.)
- Does the course teach how to clear a blocked airway? (If it doesn't, then you won't be able to learn the first step to follow if the victim you try to help has a blocked airway.)
- What is the ratio of students to instructors? (Classes with more than six students for each instructor are not recommended.)
- Do you get a certificate or card if you complete the course successfully? (If you do not receive some kind of certificate or card from either the Heart Association or the Red Cross, the course may fall short of their minimum standards—which means that it should not be up to your minimum standards either.)

In the next few pages you will learn what to do when you must revive an unconscious victim. Remember, CPR is a skill that has to be learned; it is the only way to keep victims alive when their breathing or heartbeat has stopped.

# Unconsciousness

### 1. Try to get the victim to respond.

• Prod the victim or pinch their shoulder or another spot on the body near the head.

• Shout in the victim's ear. If you know the victim's name, shout that.

• **Warning:** Do not shake or roll the victim suddenly or vigorously. There may be a back, head, or neck injury that would be aggravated by such a move.

### 2. If there is no response, call for help.

### 3. Gently place the victim on their back.

• **Do not** let the victim's head hit the ground.

• **Do not** let the victim's neck bend or twist.

• **Do not** give the victim anything to eat or drink.

### 4. Open the victim's airway.

• Place one hand on the victim's forehead and press down, causing the head to tilt back.

• Hook the fingers of your other hand under the bony portion of the lower jaw, then lift up and forward.

• Do not press on the soft area under the jaw, as you might obstruct the airway.

Step 4. Press forehead down and lift jaw.

## 5. Check to see if the victim is breathing.

- Lean over the victim's face and listen for breathing sounds.

- Place your cheek close enough to the victim's mouth to feel breathing exhalations.

- Watch the chest to see if it rises and falls with breathing movements.

- **Warning:** Take about 5 seconds for these actions.

Step 5. Listen, feel, and look for breathing.

## 6. If breathing is absent, give 2 slow breaths.

• Pinch the victim's nose between the thumb and forefinger of the hand resting on the victim's forehead.

• Open your mouth widely, take a deep breath, and fill your lungs with air.

• Cover the victim's mouth (which should be slightly open due to chin lift) with your open mouth and make an airtight seal.

• Deliver 2 slow (1½ to 2 seconds each) independent breaths, watching for chest to rise. Remove your mouth, allowing the victim to fully exhale between the 2 breaths.

Step 6. Pinch victim's nose and give breaths.

## 7. Check for a pulse.

- Keep one hand on the victim's forehead and put the fingers of the other hand on the victim's Adam's apple.

- Slide your fingers from the Adam's apple to the side groove.

- Feel with your fingertips for a pulse. Feel for about 10 seconds. Move to the next step quickly.

## 8. If there is a pulse, blow in a breath every 5 seconds.

- Pinch the victim's nose between your thumb and fingers.

- Take a deep breath and fill your lungs with air.

- Cover the victim's mouth. Blow a full breath (1½ to 2 seconds) every 5 seconds.

- Between each breath, take your mouth off the victim's mouth and watch for a natural rise and fall of the victim's chest.

- Repeat this procedure every 5 seconds.

Step 7. Feel for pulse.

• Check the pulse periodically as you keep up the breathing cycle.

9. **Continue giving breaths until the victim can breath alone, unless there is no pulse.**

10. **If there is no pulse, begin external compressions.**

• Place your hands on the center of the victim's chest and feel with your fingers for the notch at the bottom of the breastbone.

• Measure the distance equal to the width of about two fingers from the notch toward the head.

Step 10. Find notch at tip of breastbone.

- Place the heel of your hand on the lower breastbone, above your fingers.

- Place the other hand on top.

Step 10. Place heel of hand on lower breastbone above your fingers.

Step 10. Place other hand on top.

• Straighten your arms and press straight down to compress (push in) the chest 1½ to 2 inches.

• Each compression takes ¾ of a second.

• Make 15 compression movements, then give 2 deep breaths.

## 11. Call for help again.

• Whoever comes should call an ambulance while you continue compressions and breaths.

• If no one responds, continue CPR for about 5 minutes.

## 12. Call the ambulance or rescue squad yourself.

• Tell the person who answers:

Address

Telephone number from which you are calling

That the victim is unconscious

Step 10. Compress chest 1½ to 2 inches.

### 13. Restart CPR.

• Continue CPR until either A) the victim's pulse and breathing return, or B) the ambulance or rescue squad arrives.

### 14. If victim is breathing and there is a pulse, keep the airway open.

• **Do not** pour liquids in the victim's mouth.

• Stay with the victim for about 5 minutes until you see some improvement. Then call the ambulance.

• If someone else is there, have them call the ambulance while you stay with the victim and watch for signs of improvement.

### 15. Check the skin to see if it:

• Looks red
• Feels very hot
• Is dry, even under the arms

### 16. If these skin conditions exist, move the victim to a cooler place.

• See the section on Heatstroke for treatment procedures.

### 17. Periodically check the pulse and breathing.

**Note:** In an unconscious victim, putting anything in the mouth could cause aspiration and/or airway obstruction. Wait for ambulance personnel to give glucose. In a conscious but confused victim, sugar may be given.

# Reasons for your actions:

## Unconsciousness

Your main objective is *to keep the brain alive and undamaged.*
You are trying to prevent:

a. insufficient oxygen to the brain (from absence of a heartbeat and insufficient breathing)

b. very high temperature (over 105° F) that can injure the brain.

All of the steps of CPR are directed toward achieving that objective.

The "pinch, prod, and shout" technique is done to see if the victim is really unconscious. You should never start CPR on someone whose heart is beating or who is breathing, because you may upset the heartbeat or breathing cycle if you administer CPR. In short, you may do more harm than good.

When you roll the victim over onto their back to begin CPR, make sure that there are no injuries that could be worsened by such a movement.

Since the victim cannot survive without oxygen, you must first make sure that the victim can breathe. This means that you must inspect the airway and see if it is blocked. It will do no good to initiate mouth-to-mouth resuscitation techniques if the airway is obstructed.

If the airway is clear, then the victim can breathe. If he or she is not breathing, mouth-to-mouth resuscitation is started. Mouth-to-mouth technique is the most effective method known.

If the airway is clear and breathing has begun, blood still has to be pumped through the lungs so that it can be oxygenated. Oxygenated blood is then taken back to the heart to be pumped to the rest of the body. See if you can detect a heartbeat (feel for a pulse with your fingers). It is absolutely imperative that you know for sure that the heart is not beating before you commence CPR. Feel for a pulse for at least 10 seconds. If you have definitely failed to find any pulse, then begin CPR.

The chest compressions squeeze the heart between the breastbone and spine. This helps the heart to begin pumping again.

Compared to a normal heartbeat, CPR is about 30 percent as effective in getting blood through the heart. And the air that you breathe into the victim's lungs contains only about 16 percent oxygen. Nevertheless, this combination of 16 percent oxygen per volume of air and 30 percent efficiency in heart action is enough to keep a victim alive and enough to prevent the brain from being damaged.

Whatever the causes of unconsciousness, you should stay with the victim until professional help arrives. If you have restarted the victim's breathing and heartbeat, watch them carefully in case they stop again. The causes of unconsciousness discussed here are the most dangerous ones; the ones where a few seconds mean the difference between life and death. Read the 17 steps that should be followed in cases of unconsciousness over and over until you are familiar enough with them to perform the procedures without having to look them up. Take a CPR course.

# Bleeding

In the case of bleeding, minutes count (unless the person has been bleeding for some time, in which case *seconds* count). Further, because some people are more susceptible to shock from loss of blood than are other people, you must never assume that bleeding is unimportant.

1. **Apply pressure to the wound.**

   • Cover the wound with some kind of bandage material:
   A cloth
   A paper napkin
   A piece of torn clothing
   A handkerchief
   A sterile dressing if you have one
   A sanitary napkin

   • If possible, wear rubber gloves to avoid contact with the blood.

   • Place your hand over the bandage and press down firmly.

   • Keep the pressure applied until the bleeding stops or slows.

   • **Do not** remove a bandage. If the bandage becomes soaked, place another one on top of it, and keep the pressure on the wound.

2. **Raise the bleeding part of the body (unless it is broken) so that it is higher than the level of the heart.**

Step 2. Elevate wound above heart.

3. **Do not allow the victim to move the wounded part.**

4. **Do not pour antiseptics on or into the wound.**

5. **If the bleeding does not stop under pressure within 5 minutes, do the following:**

   • Apply pressure to a pressure point between the wound and the heart.

   • **Arm wound**–press your fingers into the groove between the two big muscles on the inside of the arm.

Step 5. Pressure point for arm wound.

• **Leg wound**–press your fingers into the middle of the crease where the thigh joins to the body at the groin.

Step 5. Pressure point for leg wound.

• **Neck wound**–press your fingers into the groove to the side of the Adam's apple on the same side as the wound.

**NOTE:** As soon as the bleeding stops, lift your fingers from the pressure point.

• If the victim is going into shock (pale, cool, clammy skin and rapid pulse) stop the bleeding immediately, even if you have to use a tourniquet. Do not allow a 5-minute period to elapse, as mentioned above.

**6. If the victim has suffered an amputation, or is bleeding and going into shock, do the following:**

• Use material–cloth, bandage, tie, belt, sock–at least 1½ inches wide. Do not use a rope, a piece of string or twine, or a piece of wire.

• Position the tourniquet above and near to, but not on, the wound.

• Tie a small stick to the tourniquet with a single knot.

Step 6. Use a cloth for a tourniquet.

• Twist the stick until the bleeding stops, but no tighter.

Step 6. Tighten the tourniquet with a stick.

• Tie a strip of cloth to one end of the stick and attach the stick to the limb to maintain tightness.

Step 6. Attach stick to limb.

• Note the exact time that you apply the tourniquet.

• Once you put the tourniquet on, do not take it off.

• Use a tourniquet only as a last resort when all other methods of stopping the bleeding have failed.

## 17. Treat for shock.

• Lay victim down.

• Prop up legs (12 inches), but not if you suspect head injury or broken leg.

• Cover victim with blanket or coat.

• Do not move victim.

• Do not give victim anything to eat or drink.

## 18. Call ambulance.

Step 17. Cover victim with a blanket and prop up feet about 12 inches.

# Reasons for your actions:

## Bleeding

Your main objective is to stop the blood loss at once.

The major risk in heavy bleeding is that the victim's circulation will decrease to a point that insufficient oxygen (which is carried in the blood) will reach the brain.

In most cases, you can stop bleeding by applying direct pressure to the wound. You should put on plenty of bandage material and apply pressure on top of the wound.

Wearing rubber gloves, if possible, will help you to avoid contact with blood and decrease your chances of contracting infectious diseases such as HIV or hepatitis.

Do not take off the soaked bandages. This can break up the clots that have already formed to slow the bleeding, thus making the treatment ineffective. Apply clean bandages over the soaked ones.

If the wound is in the arm or leg, raise it above the level of the heart to help the blood in the limb flow back toward the body and slow the bleeding even more. Keep the wounded limb immobile to slow the bleeding even further and prevent the breakage of the blood clots.

An antiseptic is not needed. Some antiseptics can actually damage healthy tissues. You do not need to worry about infection at this point. Your main job now is to stop the bleeding.

Sometimes you will need to shut off the blood supply to an area in order to stop the bleeding. That is what happens when you push on a pressure point. However, this procedure can be dangerous since all the tissues beyond that point also need blood. You might cause permanent damage to a limb or other body area by using pressure points to stop bleeding, but you should do it if necessary to save the victim's life. To minimize the risk of this kind of damage, release the pressure on the point as soon as the bleeding stops. Push on it when the bleeding starts again. This will help stop the bleeding while doing the minimum damage to the rest of the area. If you keep up this off-on pressure, the bleeding will usually stop in a few minutes.

In rare instances, neither direct pressure nor pressure on pressure points will stop the bleeding. Then you may want to use a tourniquet to save the victim from bleeding to death. Tourniquets are very dangerous and should be used only as a last resort. Use a tourniquet only in cases of amputation, where part of the limb has already been lost, or when shock occurs and the bleeding has not been stopped by other measures.

Do not loosen or remove a tourniquet if you put one on. Poisons from the crushed tissue under the tourniquet can return to the body via the bloodstream and cause shock.

If a great deal of blood has been lost, the victim should be treated for shock. In this situation, remember to keep the blood flowing back to the brain. Elevate the victim's legs, if possible, to help the blood flow back to the body (trunk) and brain. The only two exceptions pertain to cases involving a head injury (you want to avoid increasing the pressure and swelling in the victim's brain) and a broken leg.

# Broken bones

Broken bones can be dangerous, not only in terms of the bones themselves, but in terms of the damage that sharp bone edges can do to blood vessels and nerves around the area of the break.

When you treat a victim with broken bones, keep in mind that the sharp end of a broken bone can be as destructive as a knife.

## 1. Check that the airway is clear.

- If the victim is unconscious, do not lift or bend the neck.

- Open the mouth by pulling the jaw down and/or forward.

- Refer to the material on opening the victim's airway in the section on Unconsciousness.

- Clear the mouth and throat of any broken teeth, bones, or other debris.

Step 1. Lift jaw and tongue to check airway.

## 2. Control any heavy bleeding.

• Cover the bleeding area or wound with one of the following:
A sterile bandage
A piece of cloth or clothing
A sanitary napkin or a handkerchief

• Press on bandage until the bleeding stops.

• Do not cause movement or pain if you can help it.

• Refer to the section on Bleeding.

## 3. Examine the victim for shock.

• Look for the following symptoms:
Pale, cool, clammy skin
Rapid pulse (pulse rate over 100 beats per minute)
Victim is restless or drowsy

• If the victim displays symptoms of shock, refer to the section on Shock.

## 4. Examine the injury to see if it is open (a wound at or near the breakpoint) or closed (no break in the skin).

• If the break is *open,* cover the wound with a clean cloth, bandage, sanitary napkin, or handkerchief.

• Do not try to clean the wound.

• Check the pulse and the skin color on the limb on the side of the break farthest away from the heart.

• See if the victim can feel you touch the skin on either side of the break.

## 5. Immobilize the broken bone.

• First: Immobilize the joint above and the joint below the break so that they cannot move.

• Second: Do not try to straighten bent arms or legs at their joints.

• Third: Do not try to move the bone(s) when trying to put on a splint.

• Here is a list of materials from which splints can be made.
Pillows
Boards
Newspapers
A baseball bat
An umbrella
The other leg
A light barbell bar
Blankets
Magazines
Cardboard
A golf club
A broomstick
A hockey stick

• To tie the splint on, here is a list of things that can be used:
A belt
Masking tape
Adhesive tape
A shirt sleeve
A tie
Electrical tape
Duct tape
A pair of pants
A scarf
A curtain sash
A curtain

• Remember not to tie a splint so tightly as to cut off circulation. Loosen the ties if the extremity begins to turn cool and blue.

• In the case of broken fingers, you can splint with the following:
A small stick
A table knife
A tongue depressor
A pencil or pen
A watercolor brush

• In the case of a broken hand, wrist, or forearm, apply the splint as follows:

Run splints up both sides of the forearm, from the wrist to the elbow.

Step 5. Splint forearm from elbow to and including wrist.

Position the arm so the thumb points up, then put it into a sling that wraps around the arm and loops around the neck.

• In the case of an upper arm, collarbone, shoulder, or elbow break in which the elbow is bent, do the following:

Use a sling to immobilize the arm and support its weight.

Loop this sling around the neck.

Tie another sling so that it wraps around the chest, bringing the arm close to the body.

Step 5. For upper arm injury, tie sling to chest.

• In the case of a broken elbow that is straight, do the following:

Use a splint that reaches from the armpit all the way to the wrist. Wrap the arm so that the elbow does not shift from side to side or off the splint.

Step 5. For elbow injury, use splint from armpit to and including wrist.

• In the case of a broken pelvis, do the following:

Keep the victim still, and tie his or her legs together to keep them from moving.

Do not move the victim unless it is absolutely necessary.

Examine the victim and treat for shock if necessary.

• In the case of a broken leg, do the following:

Place some padding between the legs, and tie them together.

Use a single splint between the legs or a splint along the side of each leg.

Wrap the legs so that they do not move.

Step 5. For leg or pelvis injury, tie legs together.

• In the case of a broken and bent knee, do the following:

Keep the knee bent, and use a splint between the upper and lower leg that will keep the knee from moving from a bent position.

Step 5. For knee injury, keep knee bent and splint between upper and lower leg.

• In the case of a broken foot or ankle, do the following:

Remove the victim's shoe or boot carefully. Cut it off if necessary.

Use a pillow or a blanket for the splint. Make sure that it is soft, and that it wraps around the foot or ankle.

Step 5. Use a thick, soft splint for foot injury.

6. **Call an ambulance.**

7. **Make periodic checks of the splinted part.**

   • Watch for the following symptoms:

   An increase in pain

   Decreased feeling on the skin in the area

   Lack of pulse in the affected area

   Paleness or blueness of the skin.

8. **If any of the symptoms described in Step 7 are noted, do the following:**

   • Check to see if the ties holding the splints are too tight.

   • Check to see if an unbroken joint is bent to the extent that the normal circulation is impaired.

   • If either of these problems exists, loosen and/or reset the ties or wraps. Be careful not to disturb the injured area.

# Reasons for your actions:

## Broken bones

Your objectives are to:

a. stop blood loss

b. keep blood flowing to the brain

c. prevent further damage

d. prevent infection

e. reduce pain

Broken bones in themselves are not fatal and need not be serious. However, they can do a great deal of damage with jagged edges (which can cut muscles and veins and can also cause bleeding in the area of the break). The edge of the break can cut nerves and major blood vessels, especially in the case of breaks near joints such as the elbow and knee. Here, the edges can poke through the skin (this is called an open break, rather than a closed break that does not penetrate the skin). Bacteria then enter the area and cause infection. However, in both open and closed breaks, the edges of the bone will grind against one another, causing intense pain.

The break itself is not the major concern. Instead, first concern yourself about the more life-threatening problems: blocked airways, lack of breathing or pulse, and bleeding.

Your first step is to make certain that the airway is open and that the victim is breathing. Your next step is to control any bleeding that is taking place. Do this with the pressure-bandage method. Use a sterile bandage, a piece of cloth, a strip of clothing, a sanitary napkin, and/or a handkerchief.

If the broken bones are large, or if there are several breaks, there may be enough internal bleeding to cause shock. Therefore, you should examine the patient and treat for shock, if necessary, to keep oxygen flowing to the brain. (Review section on Shock, if necessary).

After you have taken care of bleeding and determined that the victim is not in shock, you should next examine the victim to see if any nerves are damaged. If this is the case, the skin area below the break will be numb. Also look to see if any large blood vessels have been cut. In this case, there may be no pulse beneath the break and skin color will be abnormal.

If you can immobilize the broken bone(s), this will prevent further damage, because the jagged edges of the bone will not be moving around and slicing the tissue. This will also reduce pain, since the edges will not grind together. To immobilize the break successfully, you will have to keep both the joint above and the joint below from moving.

Do not try to straighten broken or displaced bones. Moving the bone could cause more slicing of tissue or nerves. Put the splint on the limb in the position you find it (especially in the case of the elbow and knee where nerves and blood vessels are close to the bone).

If the break is open, cover it. Do not try to clean the wound; you might force germs and dirt in more deeply.

Make sure an ambulance is called. The victim will need to have the broken bone(s) set as soon as possible.

# Burns

Burns are frightening and painful injuries, especially in severe cases. The first step is to reassure and try to calm the victim. Move swiftly and decisively.

1. **Determine the severity of the burn.**

   • *First degree burn:* The skin will be red in color and painful (such as occurs due to sunburn).

   • *Second degree burn:* The affected area will be red in color, painful, and there will be blisters.

   • *Third degree burn:* The affected area may be black or white in appearance, though there may be no pain.

2. **Treatment for first degree burns.**

   • Place the burned body part in cold water (**do not** put salt or ice in the water).

   • If you cannot immerse the burned body part, put cold water on it by gently pouring the water or by soaking and squeezing a sponge over the burn.

3. **Treatment for second degree burns.**

   • Place the burned body part in cold water (**do not** put salt or ice in the water).

   • Place cold, wet dressings on the burn. Use only clean cloths (freshly ironed sheets, for example) or, preferably, sterile bandages.

   • Call a doctor or an emergency department.

   • Do not break blisters.

   • Do not put oil, butter, or ointments on the burned area.

   • Do not remove burned or blistered skin.

## 4. Treatment for third degree burns.

• Do not remove burned clothes. Leave them on the skin.

• If the face is burned, keep the victim sitting upright.

• Make sure that the airway is kept open. Tilt the head back if necessary.

• Call an ambulance or rescue squad.

• Keep the burned areas higher than the heart: elevate arms, hands, feet, and legs.

Step 4. Keep the burned area higher than the heart.

# Reasons for your actions:

## Burns

Your main objectives are:

a. for first-degree burns: relieve pain

b. for second-degree burns: prevent infection and relieve pain

c. for third-degree burns: keep oxygen flowing to the brain, prevent infection, and reduce swelling.

Many first-degree burns can be treated at home. The chief goal in such cases is to relieve pain. These burns are not severe and will generally heal rapidly once the pain subsides.

In second-degree burns, the skin is damaged to the point of risking infection. The blisters at the site of the burn are potential areas of infection and should not be broken. As long as such blisters are not broken, there is no danger of infection. However, if they are, often the tissue beneath becomes infected and is severely scarred later on. Do not use butter and ointments since they may carry bacteria and may actually cause infection. The best treatment is to use freshly ironed cloths, which will be nearly sterile and will not be a source of infection. You can then treat the pain with cold water.

If you use salt and ice together in the water, the water temperature could be lowered enough to increase damage to the tissues. It is better to use plain cold water.

Third-degree burns signal extensive damage to the skin and to other tissues, including blood vessels (hence the white or pale skin) and nerves (there will be no pain; though in this case the absence of pain is worse than pain).

Remember that with a third degree burn or burns, your goals are to keep oxygen flowing to the brain, to prevent infection, and to reduce swelling.

If the victim's face is burned, the hairs in his or her nose are singed, the mouth cavity is black or dark, or there is a deep cough, suspect burns to the lungs and airway. This may cause the airway to swell shut, so check frequently to see that the airway is still open. Remember that burned lungs collect fluid, and that leads to shortness of breath. It may be easier to keep victims with burned lungs breathing if they remain sitting up.

Seek medical care for all third-degree burns, for second-degree burns involving the face or genitals, or circumferential burns to the extremities. Any victim who may have inhaled smoke or hot gasses should also be seen immediately in an emergency department because of the significant risk of airway burns and possible airway loss.

Serious burns can cause a tremendous loss of fluid from the bloodstream. Even when there is no apparent bleeding, the victim may be in shock. Treat as for blood loss shock, since the problems are the same: low blood pressure and low blood supply to the brain.

Most burn victims in shock should have nothing to drink, since vomiting may be a problem in severe burn cases.

In some cases, clothing will be burned directly onto the skin. Removing the clothing or fabric could cause more damage by opening up infection-prone tissue. Any clothing or fabric that is actually smoldering or still burning should be removed, however.

Medical attention is especially important if the burned area involves the face, hands, feet, and/or genitals. Swelling of burned arms or legs might increase tissue damage. Thus, swelling should be reduced by elevating affected limbs.

# Chemicals in the eyes

Eye tissues are extremely delicate. A few seconds can mean permanent loss or impairment of sight if the victim is not properly treated. You will have to take charge immediately.

1. **Take over the victim's actions. Do not let victims rub their eyes.**

   • Do not let victims keep their eyes closed.

   • Assure the victim that you are going to help, that you know what you are doing, and that you are going to do it immediately.

2. **Rinse the eye with clean water for 15 minutes. Do not use hot water.**

   • Have the victim lie down near a source of water (a bathtub or a sink).

   • Hold the victim's eyelids open. Do not touch the eyeball.

   • Pour water slowly over the eyeball. Do not pour it directly on the eyeball, but at the inner corner of the eye instead.

   • Let the water flow across the eye from the inner corner and out the outer corner.

   • Keep pouring clean water for 15 minutes by the clock.

Step 2. Rinse eye with clean water for 15 minutes.

3. **Do not use antidotes or other chemicals, such as vinegar, unless a doctor tells you to do so.**

4. **Take victim to emergency room or doctor's office.**

**If you are alone:**

**NOTE:** Someday, you might be the victim, and if you are alone, it will be up to you to save your eyes. Read this section thoroughly, and learn it well enough to be able to help yourself without looking at the guide. Remember: You will not be able to read this if you are the victim.

1. **Get to a source of water. Fill a deep bowl or the sink with water and put your face into it. Blink your eyes open and closed continuously while they are under water.**

Step 1. If you are alone, immerse face in water and blink eyes continuously.

2. **Change the water every 3 to 5 minutes for 15 minutes.**

3. **If only one eye is involved, do the following:**

   • If you have a sink with a faucet that you can get your head under, set the flow at a gentle stream and put your head under the faucet. Position your head so that the water flows from the inner corner of your eye at the nose over the eyeball and runs down your cheek. If you cannot put your head under the faucet, use the bowl or sink but keep the unaffected eye tightly clenched shut to make sure that none of the chemical gets into the unaffected eye.

4. **Do not use antidotes or other chemicals, such as vinegar, unless a physician orders you to do so.**

5. **Have someone take you to an emergency room or a doctor's office as soon as you have rinsed the affected eye(s) for 15 minutes.**

# Reasons for your actions:

## Chemicals in the eyes

Your main objective is to remove the chemical as quickly as possible.

Some chemicals are extremely harmful to eyes and can cause permanent scars and damage to the eyeball of the victim. This can lead to partial or total blindness if the chemicals are not removed at once.

Time is important. Do not waste time. Start rinsing the eyes immediately, before the damage is done. Remember that you must rinse the eyeball itself and not just the outside of the eyelids.

It helps to have the victim lie down near a source of water, such as a bathtub or a sink. The victim may be in so much pain that he or she resists opening the eyes, but you must force the eye open. If necessary, hold the eyelids open yourself. Be careful not to touch the eyeball if you can avoid it.

The water should not be poured directly on the eyeball but at the inner corner of the eye instead. Let the water flow from inner to outer corner for more complete cleansing. In order to get all the chemicals out, continue to rinse for a full 15 minutes.

When you are through rinsing, even if the victim says that his or her eyes feel fine, make certain they are checked by a doctor. Sometimes scarring of the eyes can take place and the doctor will need to examine the eyes and treat the victim accordingly.

If you are victim yourself, place your eye under a running faucet or immerse your upper face in water from a sink, pan, or deep bowl. If none of these options is available, cup your hand, fill it with water, and immerse the affected eye in it. Blink the eyes continuously while they are under the water. When you have rinsed the eye(s) thoroughly for 15 minutes, be certain you have someone take you to a doctor or hospital to have your eyes checked.

# Choking

When a person is choking, a few seconds can mean the difference between life and death. You must act quickly.

1. **Ask the victim if it is possible to speak.**

2. **If the victim can speak, wheeze, or moan, the following applies:**

   • Stay with the victim and tell them to try to expel or cough out whatever is stuck in the throat.

   • **Do not** slap the person's back.

3. **If the victim cannot make any sounds, reach around the person's waist with your arms, and do the following:**

   • Find the spot halfway between the navel and the breastbone.

   • Place thumb side of other fist in that spot.

Step 3. Find spot between navel and breastbone.

• Grasp your fist with your other hand, and press your fist in and upward in a short, snappy movement (this is called the Heimlich Maneuver).

• Repeat the movement 4 times for a total of 5 thrusts.

• Perform a second series of 5 thrusts until the obstruction is cleared or the patient becomes unconscious.

Step 3. Press fist in and upward.

**NOTE:** If the victim is pregnant or very fat, do the following:

• Stand behind the victim, reach around under their armpits, and position your hands in the middle of the breastbone (not at the bottom tip). If the victim is a woman, be careful not to injure her breasts.

• Place the thumb of your left fist against the middle of the breastbone and grasp your fist with your right hand.

• Squeeze the victim's chest 5 times with short, snappy squeezes. Make sure that you squeeze with sufficient force to compress the chest.

• Continue until obstruction is cleared or patient becomes unconscious.

Step 3. If victim is pregnant, give chest squeezes.

### 4. If the victim becomes unconscious, do the following:

- Lower the victim to the floor on their back.

- Do not let the victim's head hit the floor.

- Call for help—911 or the equivalent—and activate Emergency Medical Services (EMS).

### 5. Open the airway. Remove any visible foreign body and give a forced breath.

- Check the victim's airway (refer to material on opening the victim's airway in the section on Unconsciousness).

- Look in the patient's mouth and perform a finger sweep to remove any foreign material. Try to remove the object causing the choking by turning the victim's head to one side, opening the victim's mouth, and pulling the jaw down. Then lift the tongue out of the way and sweep deeply into the back of

Step 5. Perform finger sweep to remove foreign material.

the mouth with a hooked finger.

• Push back on the victim's forehead and pinch the nose between your thumb and fingers.

• Take a deep breath, cover the victim's mouth with yours, and forcefully blow air in.

• Check to see if the chest is rising.

Step 5. Pinch victim's nose and give breaths.

### 6. If the air goes into the victim's lungs and the chest rises, do the following:

• Give the victim another forced breath every 5 seconds.

• Take your mouth away from the victim's mouth between breaths.

### 7. If no air goes into the victim's lungs during Step 5, do the following:

• Place the heel of one hand halfway between the bottom of the breastbone and the navel. Place other hand on top.

• Push inward and upward toward the upper parts of the abdomen with 5 quick thrusts.

Step 7. Find position for abdominal thrust midway between breastbone and navel.

**NOTE:** If the victim is pregnant or very fat, do the following:

• Place the heel of one hand (with the other hand on top of it) on a spot in the middle of the breastbone (not at the bottom tip).

• Push straight down quickly and forcefully 5 times. Use enough force to compress the chest 1½ to 2 inches. Start with the arms almost straight.

Step 7. Give pregnant woman chest thrusts.

## 8. Try to remove the object that is causing the choking.

• Turn the victim's head to one side.

• Open the victim's mouth and pull the jaw down so that you can get your hand into the victim's mouth.

• Lift the tongue out of the way and sweep deeply into the back of the mouth with a hooked finger.

## 9. Try to give another breath.

## 10. Repeat the following:

• 5 abdominal thrusts (or 5 chest thrusts if the victim is pregnant or very fat).

• Try to remove the object.

• Try to give a breath.

## 11. Final advice

• Do not leave the victim until breathing has begun.

• Do not begin heart compressions.

• Do not give any other first aid.

Step 8. Sweep deeply into the back of the mouth with a hooked finger.

# Reasons for your actions:

## Choking

Your main objectives are to

a. decide if the blockage causing the choking is complete or partial;

b. watch to see that a partial blockage does not become complete;

c. get air into the victim somehow if the blockage is complete.

In the step-by-step emergency procedure above, you are reminded in Step 1 to ascertain whether or not the victim can talk. Remember that so long as speech is possible or the victim can make any noises at all—even if words are not distinct—it is a sign that air is moving from the lungs. As long as the person is able to talk or make noises, try to encourage the coughing up of whatever object or bit of food is causing the blockage.

If the blockage is complete, the victim will be unable to make any sound at all. You must then try to "blow" out the chunk of food or the object by forcing air out of the lungs –an action very similar to the way a pea shooter works. This is accomplished by the 5 upward abdominal thrusts directed toward the spot just between the navel and the breastbone.

The reason for this procedure is simple: When the abdomen is squeezed it will push up the diaphragm, the muscle between the abdomen and chest, and thus will force the air out of the chest.

The procedure differs somewhat for a pregnant woman or a very fat person. The abdominal thrust could be dangerous to a pregnant woman and might be impossible to use with an obese person, so you vary the technique and use a chest thrust. The results are the same, but you do not run the risk of injuring the patient.

You must try to get air into an unconscious victim quickly—or death will occur. And you must try to give a breath following the procedure outlined above in Step 5. You always run a slight risk of forcing the chunk of food or other object down farther, but you might also manage to open up one lung so the victim can breathe.

If no air goes into the victim even by using this procedure, repeat the 5 abdominal thrusts, then try once again to provide a breath. Keep repeating this sequence until the airway becomes clear enough for the victim to breathe without assistance.

Even if the victim's heart stops, there is no value to any other kind of first aid until you clear the airway and the person can get some breaths.

**Remember: The first step in any emergency is always to open the airway and allow the victim to breathe.** Do not move on to another emergency procedure until that is done and the person is breathing again.

# Convulsions

Some people are so startled by a person having convulsions that they are practically useless when it comes to giving first aid. What is required of someone giving first aid is calmness, decisiveness, and quick action.

1. **If the victim is still standing, gently ease them to the floor or ground.**

2. **Hold onto the victim firmly, but gently.**

- **Do not** allow the victim's head to strike the floor or ground.

- **Do not** allow the victim to hurt himself or herself.

3. **Do not try to open the victim's mouth (it will probably be clenched shut).**

- **Do not** put your fingers into the victim's mouth.

- **Do not** insert any object into the victim's mouth.

4. **Place the victim on their side.**

Step 4. Place victim on their side.

5. **Stay with the victim until the seizure is over, and do the following:**

- Make sure that the airway is open.

- Roll the victim over onto his or her back.

- Refer to material on opening the victim's airway in the section on Unconsciousness.

- Check for easy, regular breathing.

7. **Call an ambulance and tell them the following:**

- What has happened and where you and the victim are located.

- A telephone number where you can be reached.

8. **Do not let the victim stand, walk, drive, or engage in any activity after the convulsion has ended.**

9. **Do not give the victim anything to drink or eat.**

10. **If the victim is a child with a high temperature, do the following:**

   • Remove the child's clothes and place cold, wet towels on their body until the fever comes down.

   • Give a child's dose of acetaminophen (Tylenol) if the child is awake.

   • Call for an ambulance.

# Reasons for your actions:

## Convulsions

Your main objective is to protect the victim.

Two ideas should be understood at the beginning: Persons experiencing a seizure or convulsion should not be feared, nor should they be treated with force. What is needed is to protect them from hurting themselves during the seizure.

A convulsion is actually a massive electrical stimulation to the brain. It will cause all the muscles to become stiff, causing the victim to twitch and temporarily stop breathing. There is nothing you can do to stop this process.

But you can protect victims by keeping them from falling on sharp objects, from knocking their heads on the floor, or striking furniture with their arms and legs. Move any heavy or sharp objects or furniture. If the victim must be held or restrained, do so gently.

Do not try to pry the mouth open or insert any object into the mouth. The tongue will heal in time if it is bitten.

After the seizure is over, the victim may be groggy and disoriented. Protect the victim from having vomitus inhaled into airways and lungs by placing him or her on side. Also avoid giving food or drink that might cause vomiting and thus endanger the open airway.

Stay with the victim until the seizure is completely over. Call an ambulance and return to the victim, because another seizure may occur.

Remember that in small children, a high fever can actually cause convulsions even if the child is not epileptic. In a case such as this, you can prevent a seizure from occurring by using first aid to lower body temperature (see instructions in Heatstroke section).

# Drowning

Drowning can result from a variety of mishaps. And if the victim is still in the water, you must be careful to avoid making matters worse by becoming a victim yourself.

**1. Do not become a victim.**

- Throw the victim a life preserver, a float, a rope, or an inner tube.

- Reach out to the victim with a pole.

- Row out to the victim in a boat.

- Swim out only as last resort.

- Watch out for rocks, reefs, submerged trees, snakes, or sharks.

**2. If the victim is still in the water, but is not breathing, do the following:**

- Turn the victim's face up out of the water.

Step 2. Turn the victim faceup.

- Keep the victim's neck straight.

- Pinch the victim's nose between your thumb and fingers.

- Take a deep breath.

- Cover the victim's mouth with your own, and blow 1 quick, deep puff of air into their mouth every 5 seconds.

Step 2. Give the victim a breath while in the water.

3. **Move the victim to the edge of the water and then out of the water.**

4. **If a neck injury is suspected, do the following:**

   - Keep the neck from twisting or bending.

   - Continue breaths of air if necessary.

• Get help and place a board (surfboard, wood) under the victim.

• Raise the board until the victim's body is supported.

• Carry the victim on the board to a safe place.

## 5. Check the victim's pulse.

• Place your other hand on the victim's neck.

• Slide the fingers from the Adam's apple to the side groove in the neck.

• Feel for a pulse.

Step 4. Using a board, carry a victim with a neck injury to shore.

• Continue to give breaths of air.

• Do not bend the victim's neck or let head roll from side to side.

• Continue feeling for a pulse for about 10 seconds.

## 6. If you feel a pulse, give 1 breath of air every 5 seconds.

• Pinch the victim's nose between your thumb and fingers.

• Take a deep breath and hold it.

• Cover the victim's mouth with your own and blow forcefully into the victim's mouth.

• Take your mouth off of the victim's mouth between each puff of air.

• Watch the chest to see if it is rising and falling.

• Repeat the puffs of air every 5 seconds.

7. **If there is no pulse, refer to the section on Unconsciousness.**

8. **If the victim vomits, do the following:**

• Turn the victim's head to the side quickly.

Step 8. If victim vomits, turn head.

• If you suspect a neck injury, keep the neck straight and turn the whole body to the side.

Step 8. If victim with neck injury vomits, turn entire body to the side.

• Clean out the victim's mouth.

• Continue to give breaths of air.

9. **When the victim recovers, cover them with a blanket, towels, or a jacket.**

10. **Call an ambulance or rescue squad.**

• Tell them your location.

• Tell them that CPR is in progress.

• Tell them that you suspect a neck injury.

# Reasons for your actions:

## Drowning

Your main objectives are to:

a. keep oxygen flowing to the brain

b. prevent damage to the spinal cord

c. maintain normal body temperature in the victim.

When you are rescuing or planning the rescue of a drowning person, first remember that it is risky to reach them by swimming to them. Drowning victims are often panicky and frightened: They can be very difficult to control. This could result in serious danger to you as well as the victim. So try other measures before swimming to them. Swim or dive in your attempt to rescue the victim only as a last resort.

The major problems in drowning cases are suffocation and low body temperature. Sometimes, however, a victim whose head hits bottom can suffer a neck injury. Therefore, remember that your major objectives are to keep oxygen flowing to the brain, to prevent damage to the spinal cord if the neck is injured, and to maintain normal body temperature.

As soon as you have reached the victim, try to correct any breathing problems. If you are a particularly strong swimmer, you may be able to start some artificial respiration before you reach the shore. Certainly you can do so if the victim is rescued in a boat. But do not become overtired and risk your own life.

If CPR is needed, begin it regardless of how long the victim has been underwater. If the victim is still in the water but not breathing, follow the procedure in Step 2 using artificial breaths to start them breathing again.

There is always danger of a neck injury and consequent risk of spinal injury in drowning cases. If there is a neck injury, you will need help in getting the victim out of the water without further injury. During the rescue effort, try to keep the neck straight and immobile by supporting it with your hand or a flat surface (surfboard, piece of wood, life preserver).

Be alert for the possibility of vomiting. You can save the victim's life with CPR only to lose them if vomit flows into their lungs, reducing the chances for survival. Watch and make sure that any vomit does not go down the airway.

If the victim needs CPR but you suspect neck injury, be certain to administer CPR without bending the neck.

Remember that a drowning victim has suffered exposure and is in danger of severely lowered body temperature. Cover them with a blanket, towel, jacket, beach gear, or tent cover in order to raise body temperature. Make certain that an ambulance or rescue squad is called as soon as possible.

# Heart attack

Most sudden deaths from heart attacks occur in the first 2 hours after the pain starts. Fast action is essential.

**NOTE:** If the victim is conscious, go directly to Step 11.

1. **If the victim is unconscious, lay the victim on their back on the floor, the ground, or a bed.**

2. **Call for help.**

   • If someone responds to your call, tell them to call an ambulance or rescue squad.

   • If no one comes to help, call an ambulance or rescue squad yourself.

3. **When the ambulance or rescue squad is called, they should be told the following:**

   • The telephone number from which the call is made.

   • The address at the victim's location.

   • That CPR is being given.

4. **Return to the victim immediately.**

5. **Check that the airway is open.**

Step 5. Press forehead down and lift jaw.

## 6. Check that the victim is breathing.

• Look at the chest to see if it is rising or falling.

• Lean over the victim's face and listen for breathing sounds.

• Place your cheek next to the victim's mouth or nose and try to feel breaths of air.

• Continue these steps for 5 seconds.

Step 6. Listen, look, and feel for breathing.

## 7. If the victim is not breathing, start CPR.

• Pinch the victim's nose between your thumb and fingers.

• Take a deep breath and hold it.

• Cover the victim's mouth with your mouth.

• Gradually blow 2 deep breaths into the victim's mouth.

• Take your mouth away from the victim's mouth after each breath.

Step 7. Pinch victim's nose and give breaths.

## 8. Check the victim's pulse.

• Place your fingers on the victim's Adam's apple, then slide them to one side into the neck groove.

• Feel gently for a pulse.

• Keep feeling for a pulse for 10 seconds.

Step 8. Feel for pulse.

## 9. If you feel a pulse, provide breaths.

• Give a forced breath every 5 seconds.

• Check the victim's pulse periodically.

## 10. If you do not feel a pulse, begin compressions.

- Find notch at tip of the breastbone.

- Measure the distance equal to the width of about two fingers from the notch toward the head.

- Place your other hand on top and straighten your arms.

- Place the heel of your hand on this spot on the lower half of the breastbone.

Step 10. Find notch at tip of breastbone.

Step 10. Place heel of hand on lower breastbone above your fingers.

• Press straight
downward to compress
chest inward about 1½ to
2 inches.

• Each compression of
the chest should last
about ¾ of a second.

Step 10. Compress chest 1½ to 2 inches.

• After 15 compressions,
give 2 slow deep breaths.
Then repeat the compres-
sions. Continue until you
get a heartbeat.

11. **If the victim is conscious, call an ambulance or rescue squad and tell them the following:**

   • The number of the telephone from which you are calling.

   • The address at your location.

   • That the victim has possibly had a heart attack.

   • That the victim is conscious.

12. **Help the victim to get into a comfortable position, but do not insist that the victim must lie down.**

13. **If the victim has nitroglycerin tablets, they can be taken as prescribed.**

14. **Stay with the victim until the ambulance or rescue squad arrives, and do the following:**

   • Be alert for a sudden lapse into unconsciousness or a sudden cessation of heartbeat and/or breathing.

   • If the symptoms indicate that it is needed, be prepared to administer CPR instantly.

15. **Do not take the victim to the hospital yourself unless there is no ambulance or rescue squad available.**

16. **Do not allow the victim to refuse to go to the hospital.**

# Reasons for your actions:

## Heart Attack

Your main objectives are to:

a. recognize a heart attack immediately

b. bring medical care to the victim at once

c. be prepared to treat sudden heart stoppage

d. keep oxygen flowing to the brain, if the heart stops.

At any minute during the first 2 hours after a heart attack, the victim's heart could suddenly stop. CPR (including artificial breathing and external compressions) must be started immediately if the victim is to survive. Early defibrillation is the best predictor of survival. Therefore, it is important to call for help promptly.

The first symptom of a heart attack is usually chest pain, described as a feeling of "heavy pressure" or a sense of burning over the breastbone that is like indigestion. The pain may extend to the jaw and arms (usually the left arm and left side of the body).

Other signs include shortness of breath, sweating, pale or bluish skin, nausea, and apprehension.

If the victim is already a heart patient and has nitroglycerin pills for heart pain (another term for chest pain is angina pectoris) they may be taken as prescribed. But if the pain does not subside once the pills are taken, heart attack should be suspected rather than simple angina pains.

If you suspect a heart attack, do not drive the victim to the hospital or clinic. If you are the victim, do not attempt to drive yourself. The reason is that no one will be able to give CPR, nor will there be sufficient room to perform CPR, while in a vehicle, and CPR is the only way to save the victim's life. Thus, it is important to call an ambulance, which will be equipped, staffed, and otherwise prepared to deal with heart stoppage if it occurs. Therefore, your first priority is to call the ambulance yourself or have some trustworthy person call it.

Do not waste time "waiting to see what happens." The greatest risk period is the first 2 hours, and during this time the patient should be in the hospital or at least in an ambulance where lifesaving equipment and professionals are at hand. While you are waiting for the ambulance, however, be sure to stay with the victim and watch for sudden heart stoppage so that you can start CPR and continue it until the ambulance arrives.

Ask the victim what position feels most comfortable and put him or her in that position. If the heart is weak, the patient's shortness of breath will often be worse lying down.

If the victim suddenly becomes unconscious, go through the CPR procedure step by step. Once you have started the procedure, do not interrupt CPR for more than five seconds.

You should call an ambulance before starting CPR in order to get an ambulance with a defibrillator to the victim as soon as possible.

# Heatstroke

Heatstroke can result in brain damage if the victim does not receive competent care. Seconds count.

### 1. Decide if it is heatstroke.

• Observe the victim and see if these conditions exist:

The skin is red instead of pale.

The skin is hot to the touch instead of cool.

The skin is dry instead of wet or clammy.

Step 1. Red, hot, and dry is heatstroke.

Step 1. Pale, cool, and wet skin is *not* heatstroke.

The victim's temperature is 105°F or above as measured by a thermometer.

The environment is warm (or hot) and humid.

• If these conditions exist, then the victim is probably suffering from heatstroke.

2. **Do not give the victim anything to eat or drink.**

3. **Move the victim into a cooler environment.**

   • An air conditioned home or building.

   • An air conditioned automobile or bus.

   • A shady place with a breeze.

4. **Remove almost all of the victim's clothing.**

5. **Cover the victim's body with wet, cold cloths.**

   • Use towels, washcloths, tablecloths, or even clothlike paper towels.

   • Change the cloths as soon as they begin to get warm, and replace them with cool ones, or keep wetting the cloths.

6. **Fan the victim.**

**7. If possible, immerse the victim in cold water.**

A bathtub

A creek or stream

A pond or cool inlet of a lake

A calm section of beach water if you are near the ocean

**NOTE:** Do not use ice. Keep the victim's head above water.

**8. Recheck the victim's temperature periodically.**

• Take the victim's temperature with a thermometer.

• Feel the victim's skin if you have no thermometer.

**9. Call an ambulance as soon as you safely can.**

• Do not stop treatment to call the ambulance.

• Do not leave the victim alone until the body temperature reaches a safe level.

**10. Final note: From time to time, check the victim's pulse and breathing.**

# Reasons for your actions:

## Heatstroke

Your main objective is to quickly lower the body temperature.

Heatstroke is a critical condition and is very common in the summertime, especially in very hot or very humid climates. Occasionally, the part of the brain that controls the body's temperature fails for various reasons and heatstroke can occur. In drier climates the risk is reduced; it is much higher in hot, very humid environments, especially when the person has been working or exercising vigorously.

In heatstroke, the skin does not sweat and thus does not cool the body by evaporation of sweat, so the body temperature climbs. Blood vessels in the skin will swell to give off heat, and the person's skin will look red. The body's temperature will continue to rise, while sweating still does not occur. The condition is serious because permanent brain damage can result if the body temperature remains high for too long a time.

Remember that your main goal is to reduce body temperature as quickly as possible. The best way to do this is to put the victim in a cold shower or tub of water. If this is not possible, cold, wet towels or cloths will do. The most important fact to remember is that fast action is essential.

# Poison swallowed

The first rule is always to keep poisons out of the reach of children or others who do not understand the danger. This applies to many cleaning preparations and medications. Above all, stay calm: fewer than 20 percent of all suspected poisonings actually require hospital treatment.

1. **Look immediately for the poison's container or look for signs of the poison itself (powder or liquid on the floor).**

2. **Call the nearest Poison Control Center, hospital, or emergency room, and tell them the following:**

   • Who you are and where you are located.

   • A telephone number where you can be reached.

   • The name of the poison and the ingredients as they are described on the label of the container.

   • The amount of poison you think was swallowed.

   • The size of the victim, especially if it is a child.

3. **Follow the instructions given.**

4. **Do not give antidotes. Do not induce vomiting unless you are directed to do so by the Poison Control Center, hospital, or emergency room.**

5. **Do not give any (salt) solutions.**

6. **Take the poison container to the hospital or emergency room along with the patient.**

# Reasons for your actions:

## Poison swallowed

Your main objectives are to

a. find out exactly what poison was swallowed

b. call for help.

Since there are so many Poison Control Centers and emergency departments throughout the country, you do not need to take any emergency measure without guidance. If you can find out exactly what poison was swallowed, you are well on your way toward resolving the problem.

The important thing is to call a Poison Control Center (PCC) at once with the information you have obtained. Then do exactly what you are told to do.

Although inducing vomiting is the right measure in many cases, it is not necessarily right in all cases. For example, when someone swallows corrosives, such as acid or lye, or petroleum products, such as lighter fluid, vomiting could cause more harm than good. In addition, some solutions that induce vomiting—salt, for instance— can be hazardous.

Remember that diluting the poison by giving lots of milk or water may also make things worse, since such action increases the speed at which the poison is absorbed throughout the system.

This is a case where the cardinal rule of first aid applies in every instance: *Do no harm.* The main task is to identify the poison accurately and quickly and then call the PCC. Do exactly what the Poison Control Center tells you to do.

# Shock

Quick attention is necessary when a victim goes into shock. No visible wounds are necessary for a person to go into shock.

1. **Examine the victim for shock symptoms.**

   • Pale skin.

   • Cool, clammy, and sweating skin.

   • Restlessness, drowsiness, or mental confusion.

   • Thirst.

   • Rapid pulse (over 100 beats per minute).

   • Rapid and weak breathing.

   • Dilated (enlarged) pupils.

2. **If any or all of these symptoms are present, the victim should lie down immediately and not be allowed to walk, sit, or stand.**

3. **Prop up the victim's legs (to a height of about 12 inches) unless you suspect a head injury or a broken leg.**

Step 3. Cover victim with a blanket and prop up feet about 12 inches.

## 4. Stop any bleeding.

• Cover the wound with one of the following:

Step 4. Pressure point for arm wound.

A sterile dressing or bandage

A clean cloth

Some piece of clothing

A sanitary napkin

• Place the covering over the wound, then place your hands on the bandage and press firmly against the wound.

• If possible, use plastic gloves to protect yourself from contact with the victim's blood.

• If the bleeding does not slow or stop immediately, apply pressure to the appropriate pressure point:

**Arm wound**–place your fingers in the groove between the two large muscles on the inside of the upper arm.

**Leg wound**–place fingers in the crease where the thigh joins to the torso at the groin.

**Neck wound**–place the fingers in the groove at the side of the Adam's apple on the side of the neck that is bleeding.

• When the bleeding stops, ease up on the pressure point.

If the bleeding starts again, reapply pressure.

• If you are dealing with an amputation victim and the bleeding does not stop in 2 to 3 minutes, use a tourniquet. Refer to the section on Bleeding for directions.

5. **Call an ambulance.**

6. **Keep the victim warm by covering them with a blanket or clothing.**

7. **Do not move the victim unless it is necessary to ensure survival.**

8. **Do not give the victim anything to eat or drink. In particular, do not offer any beverage containing alcohol.**

Step 4. Pressure point for leg wound.

# Reasons for your actions:

## Shock

Your main objective is to keep as much blood flowing as possible in order to supply oxygen to the brain.

Where there has been a great deal of bleeding or loss of fluid due to burns, the blood pressure decreases. The result is shock. In cases of shock, the following happens:

- The brain is "starved" for blood and oxygen.
- The victim is thirsty because of the loss of fluid in the body.
- The victim becomes drowsy, restless, and confused at the same time.
- The victim will breathe rapidly or gasp for breath in an effort to draw in more oxygen.
- The victim develops a rapid pulse because the heart beats faster to maintain the blood pressure.
- The blood vessels in the skin narrow to divert blood from the skin to the brain, and the victim's skin becomes pale and cool to the touch.

The best treatment, of course, is to provide fluids into the veins and to administer oxygen and blood transfusions. These steps raise the oxygen level and blood pressure, which is exactly what a physician, paramedic, or hospital staff member does for a person in shock. However, until a victim receives such medical help, you must try to stop further blood loss, if possible, and try to divert blood from the legs and extremities toward the brain. To do this, lay the patient down. Raise the legs about 12 inches to send blood toward the brain—unless you suspect a head injury. In the case of a head injury, avoid increasing pressure and swelling in the brain by keeping the victim lying flat. And if the victim has a broken leg, moving the broken limb will only increase the damage and bleeding. In this case, it is also best to simply keep the victim lying flat.

You can control external bleeding by using the usual techniques: direct pressure, then pressure points, then a tourniquet as a last resort. Stop the bleeding as quickly as you can. Go directly to a tourniquet if the blood flow is heavy. The victim who is in shock is already near death and cannot afford to lose any more blood.

The shock victim is also losing body heat and should be covered with blankets or warm clothing to protect against loss of body heat.

Since shock victims will often go directly into surgery once they are in the hospital, it is advisable to give them nothing to eat or drink. Alcohol, which could be dangerous in this situation, is to be particularly avoided.

# Spinal Injury

Spinal injuries can result in permanent paralysis of a portion or all of the body. Consequently, you should proceed with extreme caution any time that you treat a victim who has, or is suspected of having, a spinal injury. The basic rule is "Always assume spinal injury in accident cases." If you follow this rule you will avoid possible additional injury to the victim.

**1. The following situations may indicate that a spinal injury has occurred:**

- An accident victim is unconscious.

- The victim is unconscious and has bruises or cuts on his or her head.

- The circumstances of the accident indicate that a fall from a height occurred, that the head was struck, or that the neck or back was flexed or extended.

- The accident victim is awake, but is not moving.

- The accident victim complains of pain in neck or back.

**NOTE:** In each of these cases, spinal injury may be present. Always treat victims who show these symptoms as if they have spinal injuries until you know for sure that they do not.

**2. Check the victim's airway to see if it is clear of obstruction.**

- Do not bend the neck or lift the neck as you would if the victim were not a spinal injury case.

- Look at the chest to see if it is rising and falling.

- Lean over the victim and listen for breathing sounds.

- Place your cheek near the victim's mouth and see if you can feel breaths of air.

• If the victim has difficulty breathing, do the following:

Pull the mouth open by grasping the jaw.

Lift the tongue out of the way. If the jaw will not hinge downward, try to pull it forward without shifting the position of the neck.

**Warning:** Do not move the neck unless you absolutely cannot open the mouth otherwise.

3. **Do not move the victim unless the victim's life is in danger.**

• Move the victim only under the following or similar circumstances:

There is a fire.

There is danger of an explosion.

There is danger of drowning.

There is danger of a cave-in.

There is no way to protect the victim from approaching traffic.

There is no pulse.

4. **If you must move the victim, do the following:**

• Keep the neck and back straight.

• Support the neck and back.

• Do not let the head fall and the neck twist.

• Do not let the back twist or arch from side to side.

Step 2. Pull the mouth open by grasping the jaw to check airway.

**5. If the victim is conscious, instruct the victim to remain still and not move the back or neck.**

**6. If the victim is lying down, do the following:**

• Support the spine so that it will not move.

• **Do not** place a pillow under the victim's head.

• Place rolled-up blankets, clothes, rocks, or pieces of wood at each side of the head so that it will not roll from side to side.

• If the neck is bent at an odd angle, do not try to straighten it. Prop the head on either side to keep the neck in the position in which you found it.

• Call an ambulance.

**7. If the victim is in a sitting position, do the following:**

• Get behind the victim.

• Place your hands at the sides of the victim's head to support the head so it will not move.

• Support the head until someone comes who can call an ambulance.

**NOTE:** In all cases of spinal injury, whether of the neck or the upper, middle, or lower back, the key step is to prevent movement.

Step 6. Place rolled-up blankets or clothes on either side of head to immobilize the head.

# Reasons for your actions:

## Spinal injury

Your main objective is to prevent damage to the spinal cord by preventing movement of the broken or shifted vertebrae (the bones that make up the spine).

Sometimes, as the result of an accident, one or more of the bones in the victim's spine will shift or be broken. While this condition is painful, it seldom causes any permanent damage—unless the broken or shifted vertebrae damage the spinal cord, which is encircled by the vertebral bones. Thus, your main objective in administering first aid is to prevent damage to the spinal cord.

This is an important "prime directive" for any person practicing first-aid or emergency procedures. All too often, well-meaning people try to "help" a victim of an accident by pulling or dragging the individual away from the scene of an auto or other kind of accident. Remember, if the victim's spinal cord is damaged by any twisting or bending movements, that person could become paralyzed. Therefore, do not move anyone you suspect of having a spinal injury unless it is absolutely necessary to avoid traffic, fire, water, or a similar threat.

If the victim is unconscious when you arrive on the scene, assume that he or she has a spinal injury and act accordingly. If there is an injury to the head or neck, a spinal injury can be considered likely.

If the victim is awake and conscious, ask if there is any pain in the neck or back. If the victim appears dazed or uncertain, treat for spinal injuries and tell the person to remain as is.

The first step, as always, is to make sure the airway is open. If it is necessary to open the airway, do so without bending the neck. Instead, keep the neck still and lift the victim's jaw or pull forward from the angles of the jaw. You can even give forced breaths using this technique.

If faced with the choice between risking the death of the victim by not moving them, on the one hand, or risking further injury by moving them, on the other, then you must try to save the victim's life. Check Step 4 regarding ways to minimize damage if you must move a patient. Similarly, if the patient is not breathing and there is no airway open, do what is necessary to give breaths—but again, minimize the risk of paralysis as much as possible.

If CPR is needed (in cases where there is no pulse) you may have to move the victim to a solid surface in order to perform CPR. If the victim is in a car that is burning, about to explode, or sinking in water, and the victim must be moved, do so. Try to minimize risk by keeping the neck and shoulders immobilized as much as possible, however. Refer to Steps 4 and 6 for additional pointers.

To prevent accidental damage to the spinal cord while waiting for the ambulance, keep the neck stable by holding the head of a sitting victim or immobilizing the head, neck, and spine of a victim who is lying down. This will keep the spinal bones in line so that the spinal cord does not kink. Maintain this support until the ambulance crew or paramedics have attached the necessary splints and tell you that it is all right to release the victim from your grasp.

# Home first-aid kit

The following items should be in every home first-aid kit.

Syrup of ipecac. You should have enough for 1 ounce for each member of the family. You should get syrup of ipecac, not the fluid extract.

A roll of 1-inch adhesive tape

A roll of 2-inch duct tape (for splints)

The following supply of sterile bandages:
    A dozen 4-inch by 4-inch
    A dozen 3-inch by 3-inch
    A dozen 2-inch by 2-inch

Sterile vaseline gauze

Two 4-inch elastic bandages

Two 2½-inch elastic bandages

A bottle of hydrogen peroxide

Scissors

Tweezers

One insect sting kit (if a member of the family has insect sting allergies)

Acetaminophen (Tylenol) with a child-proof cap

Two thermometers (one rectal, one oral)

Cotton-tipped swabs

One triangle bandage

Antibacterial ointment

One roll of 1-inch-wide gauze bandage

One roll of 4-inch-wide gauze bandage

Assorted adhesive bandages

Antihistamines for allergic reactions

Corticosteroid cream for bites, stings, and minor rashes

# Emergency telephone numbers

Poison Control Center _____

Paramedics _____

Doctor _____

Doctor _____

Doctor _____

Hospital emergency dept. _____

Fire department _____

Police department _____

Ambulance _____

Work phone numbers _____

Local pharmacy _____

24-hour pharmacy _____

Dentist _____

Neighbor _____

Relative _____

**Your address and phone number (for baby-sitters and visitors)**

_____

_____

# Family medical history

Detailed family medical records are helpful in diagnosing and treating potential health problems, especially those that tend to recur in some families. To help your doctor become fully informed about your family's medical history, note any serious diseases in your family. The list below should be consulted when filling out the form. In addition to listing diseases that have occurred in the family, be prepared to discuss with your doctor your personal habits and lifestyle (diet, exercise, smoking, and so forth), any medications you take on a regular basis, and your past health history (hospitalizations, operations, illnesses).

Is there any history in your family of:

| | |
|---|---|
| Allergies | Hypertension |
| Arthritis | Mental disorders |
| Cancer | Mental retardation |
| Cystic fibrosis | Muscular dystrophy |
| Diabetes | Sickle cell anemia |
| Epilepsy | Stroke |
| Hearing defects | Tay-Sachs disease |
| Heart defects | Visual defects |
| Hemophilia | Other recurring |
| Huntington's chorea | family diseases |

| Name | Birth date | Blood type and Rh | Allergy and disease history |
|---|---|---|---|
| Mother | | | |
| Her mother | | | |
| Her father | | | |
| Father | | | |
| His mother | | | |
| His father | | | |
| Child | | | |
| Child | | | |
| Child | | | |

SCHEDULE OF PHYSICAL EXAMS

# The practice of preventive medicine involves having certain tests

| Age | 20 to 29 | | 30 to 39 | | 40 to 49 |
|---|---|---|---|---|---|
| **Sex** | **Male** | **Female** | **Male** | **Female** | **Male** |
| General Physical Exam | Every 3 years | Every 3 years | Every 3 years | Every 3 years | Yearly |
| Pelvic Exam | | Yearly | | Yearly | |
| Pap Test | | Yearly | | Yearly | |
| Rectal Exam | | | | | Yearly |
| Stools for Occult Blood | | | | | |
| Self-Testicular Exam or Self-Breast Exam | Monthly | Monthly | Monthly | Monthly | Monthly |
| Mammography | | | | Baseline test between 35-40 | |
| Cholesterol | Every 5 years if under 200* | Every 5 years if under 200* | Every 5 years depending on level | Every 5 years depending on level | 1-3 years depending on level |
| EKG Electrocardiogram of heart | | | | | Baseline test between 40-45 |

These guidelines apply only to people who are symptom-free. Your general physical exam should include:
• Health counseling on diet, exercise, dental care, smoking, alcohol/drug abuse, seat belt use, and exposure to sun.
• A cancer check-up including mouth, skin, thyroid, lymph nodes, breasts, testes, and prostate.
• A blood count, urinalysis, and blood pressure check. Further tests may be ordered by your physician based on your age, sex, personal/family health history, and other risk factors.
Source: Northwestern Memorial Hospital, Chicago (for immunization schedule see section on immunization).

# completed as recommended by primary care physicians.

| 40 to 49 | 50 to 59 | | 60 to 69 | |
| Female | Male | Female | Male | Female |
| --- | --- | --- | --- | --- |
| Yearly | Yearly | Yearly | Yearly | Yearly |
| Yearly | | Yearly | | Yearly |
| Yearly | | Yearly | | Yearly |
| Yearly | Yearly | Yearly | Yearly | Yearly |
| | Yearly | Yearly | Yearly | Yearly |
| Monthly | Monthly | Monthly | Monthly | Monthly |
| Every 1-2 years | | Yearly | | Yearly |
| 1-3 years depending on level | Yearly | Yearly | Yearly | Yearly |
| Baseline test between 40-45 | Yearly (as needed) | Yearly (as needed) | Yearly (as needed) | Yearly (as needed) |

**\*If cholesterol is over 200, follow physician's directions**

# Index

# B

# C

# G

# H

# I

# J